THE CARDIAC CARE UNIT

Survival Guide

EDITOR

Eyal Herzog, MD

Director, Cardiac Care Unit
St. Luke's-Roosevelt Hospital Center
Associate Professor of Clinical Medicine
Columbia University College of Physicians and Surgeons
New York, New York

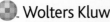 Wolters Kluwer | Lippincott Williams & Wilkins
Health

Philadelphia · Baltimore · New York · London
Buenos Aires · Hong Kong · Sydney · Tokyo

Acquisitions Editor: Frances DeStefano
Product Manager: Leanne Vandetty
Production Manager: Alicia Jackson
Senior Manufacturing Manager: Benjamin Rivera
Marketing Manager: Kimberly Schonberger
Creative Director: Doug Smock
Production Service: S4Carlisle

© 2012 by LIPPINCOTT WILLIAMS & WILKINS, a WOLTERS KLUWER business
Two Commerce Square
2001 Market Street
Philadelphia, PA 19103 USA
LWW.com

Printed in the United States of America

Library of Congress Cataloging-in-Publication Data

The CCU survival guide / editor, Eyal Herzog.
    p. ; cm.
  Includes bibliographical references and index.
  ISBN-13: 978-1-4511-1047-0 (alk. paper)
  ISBN-10: 1-4511-1047-2 (alk. paper)
  I. Herzog, Eyal.
  [DNLM: 1. Acute Coronary Syndrome—therapy. 2. Coronary Care Units. 3. Heart Diseases—therapy. WG 300]

  616.1'2—dc23

2011036403

Care has been taken to confirm the accuracy of the information presented and to describe generally accepted practices. However, the authors, editors, and publisher are not responsible for errors or omissions or for any consequences from application of the information in this book and make no warranty, expressed or implied, with respect to the currency, completeness, or accuracy of the contents of the publication. Application of the information in a particular situation remains the professional responsibility of the practitioner.

The authors, editors, and publisher have exerted every effort to ensure that drug selection and dosage set forth in this text are in accordance with current recommendations and practice at the time of publication. However, in view of ongoing research, changes in government regulations, and the constant flow of information relating to drug therapy and drug reactions, the reader is urged to check the package insert for each drug for any change in indications and dosage and for added warnings and precautions. This is particularly important when the recommended agent is a new or infrequently employed drug.

Some drugs and medical devices presented in the publication have Food and Drug Administration (FDA) clearance for limited use in restricted research settings. It is the responsibility of the health care provider to ascertain the FDA status of each drug or device planned for use in their clinical practice.

To purchase additional copies of this book, call our customer service department at (800) 638-3030 or fax orders to (301) 223-2320. International customers should call (301) 223-2300.

Visit Lippincott Williams & Wilkins on the Internet: at LWW.com. Lippincott Williams & Wilkins customer service representatives are available from 8:30 a.m. to 6 p.m., EST.

10 9 8 7 6 5 4

Dedication

To my patients who have taught me so much over the years.

Contents

Patient and Family Information Contents

Contributing Authors

Jeanine B. Albu, MD
Associate Clinical Professor of Medicine
Department of Medicine
College of Physicians & Surgeons
Columbia University
Senior Attending
Department of Medicine
St. Luke's-Roosevelt Hospital Center
New York, New York

Edgar Argulian, MD, MPH
Division of Cardiology
St. Luke's-Roosevelt Hospital Center
Columbia University College of Physicians & Surgeons
New York, New York

Emad F. Aziz, DO, MB, CHB
Assistant Professor of Clinical Medicine
Columbia University
Director of ACAP Research Program
St. Luke's-Roosevelt Hospital Center
New York, New York

Eric M. Bader MD
Fellow
Department of Cardiology
Columbia University College of Physicians and Surgeons
St. Luke's and Roosevelt Hospitals
New York, New York

Sandhya K. Balaram, MD, PhD, FACS
Assistant Professor of Clinical Surgery
Columbia University College of Physicians and Surgeons
Chief, Division of Cardiothoracic Surgery
St. Luke's-Roosevelt Hospital Center
New York, New York

Anip Bansal, MD
Assistant Attending
Department of Nephrology
St. Luke's-Roosevelt Hospital Center
New York, New York

Louis Brusco, Jr., MD, FCCM
Assistant Professor of Clinical Anesthesiology
Department of Anesthesiology
Columbia University College of Physicians & Surgeons
Vice Chair
Department of Anesthesiology
St. Luke's-Roosevelt Hospital Center
New York, New York

Matthew A. Cavender, MD
Fellow
Department of Cardiovascular Medicine
Cleveland Clinic
Cleveland, Ohio

Farooq A. Chaudhry, MD
Associate Professor of Clinical Medicine
Department of Medicine
Columbia University
Director of Echocardiography
Associate Chief of Cardiology
Department of Medicine
St. Luke's-Roosevelt Hospital
New York, New York

Neel P. Chokshi, MD, MBA
Cardiovascular Fellow
Division of Cardiology
Columbia University
St. Luke's-Roosevelt Hospital Center
New York, New York

Amy Chorzempa, MS, RN, ANP-BC
Nurse Practitioner
Department of Interventional Cardiology
St. Luke's-Roosevelt Hospital Center
New York, New York

David L. Coven, MD, PhD
Assistant Professor of Medicine
Columbia University College of Physicians and Surgeons
Attending Physician
Division of Cardiology
St. Luke's-Roosevelt Hospital Center
New York, New York

Mithilesh K. Das, MD
Associate Professor of Clinical Medicine
Indiana University School of Medicine
Krannert Institute of Cardiology
Chief, Cardiac Arrhythmia Service, Roudebush VA
    Medical Center
Indianapolis, Indiana

Gregory B. Dodell, MD
Fellow
Department of Endocrinology, Diabetes, and Nutrition
St. Luke's-Roosevelt Hospital Center
New York, New York

Barry A. Franklin, PhD
Professor, Internal Medicine
Oakland University
William Beaumont School of Medicine
Rochester, Michigan
Director, Preventative Cardiology and
    Cardiac Rehabilitation
William Beaumont Hospital
Royal Oak, Michigan

Tiberio M. Frisoli, MD
Medical Resident
Department of Internal Medicine
Columbia College of Physicians & Surgeons
St. Luke's-Roosevelt Hospital
New York, New York

Horiana B. Grosu, MD
Fellow
Department of Pulmonary and Critical Care
St. Luke's-Roosevelt Hospital Center
New York, New York

Dan G. Halpern, MD
Department of Medicine
Columbia University College of Physicians and Surgeons
Cardiovascular Fellow
Department of Medicine
St. Luke's-Roosevelt Hospital
New York, New York

Seongwook Han, MD, PhD
Krannert Institute of Cardiology
Indiana University
Methodist Hospital
Indianapolis, Indiana

Eyal Herzog, MD
Director, Cardiac Care Unit
St. Luke's-Roosevelt Hospital Center
Associate Professor of Clinical Medicine
Columbia University College of Physicians and Surgeons
New York, New York

Mun K. Hong, MD
Associate Professor of Clinical Medicine
Department of Medicine
Columbia University College of Physicians
    and Surgeons
Director, Cardiac Cath Lab and Interventional Cardiology
Department of Medicine
St. Luke's-Roosevelt Hospital Center
New York, New York

Gregory Janis, MD
Attending Physician
Department of Cardiology
St. Luke's-Roosevelt Hospital Center
New York, New York

Fahad Javed, MD
Attending Physician
Department of Internal Medicine
Columbia University
St. Luke's-Roosevelt Hospital Center
New York, New York

Michael A. Jolly, MD
Interventional Cardiology Fellow
Department of Cardiovascular Disease
Cleveland Clinic
Cleveland, Ohio

James P. Jones, MD
Assistant Professor of Clinical Medicine
Department of Medicine
Columbia University
Attending Physician
Department of Medicine
St. Luke's-Roosevelt Hospital
New York, New York

Ulrich P. Jorde, MD
Associate Professor of Medicine
Department of Medicine – Cardiology
New York-Presbyterian Hospital
Columbia University Medical Center
New York, New York

Rajeev Joshi, MD
Fellow
Department of Cardiology – Electrophysiology
Columbia University
St. Luke's-Roosevelt Hospital
New York, New York

Sandeep Joshi, MD
Cardiology Fellow
Department of Medicine
St. Luke's-Roosevelt Hospital Center
New York, New York

Eitan Moshe Klein, MD
Department of Medicine
St. Luke's-Roosevelt Hospital Center Columbus Cardiology
    Associates
New York, New York

Itzhak Kronzon, MD
Director of Cardiac Imaging
Department of Cardiovascular Medicine
Lenox Hill Hospital
New York, New York

Marrick L. Kukin, MD
Director, Heart Failure Program
Department of Cardiology/Medicine
St. Luke's Roosevelt Hospital
Professor of Clinical Medicine
Department of Medicine
Columbia University College of Physicians & Surgeons
New York, New York

Prabhat Kumar, MD

A. Michael Lincoff, MD
Professor of Medicine
Cleveland Clinic Lerner College of Medicine of Case Western
    Reserve University
Vice Chairman
Department of Cardiovascular Medicine
Cleveland Clinic
Cleveland, Ohio

Harikrishna Makani, MD
Post Doctoral Clinical Fellow
St. Luke's Roosevelt Hospital
Columbia University College of Physicians
    and Surgeons
New York, New York

Anuj Mediratta, MD
Clinical Instructor
Department of Medicine
Northwestern University Feinberg School of Medicine
Chicago, Illinois

Venu Menon, MD
Director, Coronary Care Unit
Department of Cardiovascular Medicine
Cleveland Clinic
Cleveland, Ohio

Franz H. Messerli, MD, FACC, FACP
Professor of Clinical Medicine
Columbia University College of Physicians
    and Surgeons
Division of Cardiology
St. Luke's-Roosevelt Hospital
New York, New York

Ruth Minkin, MD
Assistant Professor of Clinical Medicine
College of Physicians and Surgeons
Columbia University
Assistant Director of the MICU
St. Luke's Site
Director, Pulmonary Hypertension Program
Attending Physician
St. Luke's-Roosevelt Hospital Center
New York, New York

Merle Myerson, MD, EdD, FACC
Assistant Professor
Department of Medicine and Epidemiology
Columbia University College of Physicians
    and Surgeons
Attending Cardiologist and Director
Cardiovascular Disease Prevention Program
St. Luke's-Roosevelt Hospital
New York, New York

Kishore Nallu, MD

Mary M. O'Sullivan, MD
Associate Clinical Professor
Department of Medicine
Columbia University
Senior Attending
Department of Medicine
St. Luke's-Roosevelt Hospital
New York, New York

Aastha Pal, MD
Post Doctoral Residency Fellow
Department of Medicine
St. Luke's-Roosevelt Hospital Center
New York, New York

Angela M. Palazzo, MD
Assistant Professor of Clinical Medicine
Department of Medicine
Columbia University
Associate Division Chief
Division of Cardiology
St. Luke's-Roosevelt Hospital Center
New York, New York

Vishal P. Patel, DO
Fellow
Pulmonary, Critical Care, & Sleep Medicine
St. Luke's-Roosevelt Hospital Center
New York, New York

Gila Perk, MD
Associate Director
Echocardiography Laboratory
Lenox Hill Hospital
New York, New York

Xavier Pi-Sunyer, MD, MPH
Professor
Department of Medicine
Columbia University
Chief, Endocrinology, Diabetes, and Nutrition
Department of Medicine
St. Luke's-Roosevelt Hospital
New York, New York

Bruce Polsky, MD
John H. Keating, Sr. Professor of Clinical Medicine
Department of Medicine
Columbia University College of Physicians and Surgeons
Chairman
Department of Medicine
St. Luke's-Roosevelt Hospital Center
New York, New York

Balaji Pratap, MD
Resident
Department of Internal Medicine
St. Luke's-Roosevelt Hospital Center
New York, New York

Vera H. Rigolin, MD
Associate Professor of Medicine
Department of Medicine/Cardiology
Northwestern University Feinberg School of Medicine
Cardiologist
Northwestern Memorial Hospital
Medical Director
Echocardiography Laboratory
Northwestern Memorial Hospital
Chicago, Illinois

David S. Roffman, PharmD
Professor
Department of Pharmacy Practice and Science
University of Maryland School of Pharmacy
Therapeutic Consultant
Division of Cardiology
University of Maryland Medical System
Baltimore, Maryland

Ronald E. Ross, MBBS
General Surgery Chief Resident
Department of Surgery
Columbia University College of Physicians and Surgeons
St. Luke's-Roosevelt Hospital Center
New York, New York

Alan Rozanski, MD
Professor of Medicine
Columbia University College of Physicians and Surgeons
Director, Cardiology Fellowship Program
Division of Cardiology
St. Luke's-Roosevelt Hospital
New York, New York

Gagangeet Sandhu, MD
Nephrology Fellow
Deparment of Nephrology
St. Luke's-Roosevelt Hospital Center
Columbia University College of Physicians and Surgeons
New York, New York

Muhamed Saric, MD, PhD
Associate Professor
Leon H. Charney Division of Cardiology
Director, Echocardiography Lab
New York University Langone Medical Center
New York, New York

Janet M. Shapiro, MD
Associate Clinical Professor of Medicine
Department of Medicine
Columbia University
Director, Medical Intensive Care Unit
Department of Medicine
St. Luke's and Roosevelt Hospital Center
New York, New York

Mark Sherrid, MD
Professor
Department of Medicine
St. Luke's-Roosevelt Hospital Center
New York, New York

Daniel B. Sims, MD
Assistant Professor of Medicine
Division of Cardiology
Emory University School of Medicine
Center for Heart Failure Therapy and Transplantation
Division of Cardiology
Emory University Hospital
Atlanta, Georgia

Jagmeet P. Singh, MD, PhD
Associate Professor of Medicine
Harvard Medical School
Cardiac Arrhythmia Service
Cardiology Division
Massachusetts General Hospital
Boston, Massachusetts

Vikas Soma, MD
Post Doctoral Clinical Fellow
Department of Medicine
St. Luke's-Roosevelt Hospital Center
New York, New York

Jacqueline E. Tamis-Holland, MD
Assistant Professor of Clinical Medicine
Columbia University College of Physicians and Surgeons
Interventional Cardiologist
Site Director, Roosevelt Hospital Cardiac
    Catheterization Laboratory
Department of Medicine – Cardiology
St. Luke's-Roosevelt Hospital
New York, New York

Seth Uretsky, MD
Assistant Professor of Clinical Medicine
Department of Medicine
Columbia University College of Physicians & Surgeons
Director, Cardiac CT & MRI
Department of Medicine
St. Luke's-Roosevelt Hospital Center
New York, New York

Tracy Zivin-Tutela, MD
Assistant Professor
Department of Medicine
St. Luke's-Roosevelt Hospital
Department of Medicine
Division of Infectious Diseases
St. Luke's-Roosevelt Hospital Center
New York, New York

Preface

Heart disease is the leading cause of death in the world. Advances in the treatment of heart disease are considered among the greatest achievements of modern medicine. For physicians, nurses, and all health care providers who care for patients with heart disease, the most exciting place in the hospital is the cardiac care unit (CCU).

The Cardiac Care Unit Survival Guide is truly a survival book that discusses the most important information needed to "survive" the CCU. It is practically two books combined into one. Each chapter has two parts: Part A for physicians and other health care providers, and Part B for patients and their families.

Part A of each chapter is aimed towards physicians (interns, residents, fellows, and attendings), medical students, nurses, physician assistants, and other health care providers who rotate or practice in the CCU. It is organized in a way that the reader will not need to review any additional text book regarding the topics discussed and will be able to understand the simplified pathophysiology of the disease, the diagnostic modalities, the initial critical care management in the CCU and the follow-up care in a step down unit, and the plan for discharge. Algorithms and pathways for management are provided in most chapters for easy implementation in any health care system.

Part B of each chapter for patients and their families covers the same topics discussed in the first part but is directed to the patients and their families. The language and the medical terminology are simpler and geared towards the general public.

Specifically the second part of each chapter is written for:

- patients and their families who survived acute heart disease

- the general public and patients and their families to *prevent* heart disease

- doctors, nurses, and medical students who need to explain the cardiac diagnosis and treatment to patients and their families in simple terms

- health care executives who need to establish a systematic standard of care to reduce cost and to improve effectiveness.

It is my hope that this book will serve as a teaching tool to save the lives of patients with heart disease.

Eyal Herzog

Acknowledgments

I would like to acknowledge the extraordinary work of LaToya Selby from my office at St. Luke's Hospital in New York, who is always my right hand in helping my trainees and patients in the hospital and is also the editing coordinator for this book.

Thank You,
Eyal Herzog

SECTION I

Acute Coronary Syndrome

Eyal Herzog
Fahad Javed
Emad F. Aziz
Mun K. Hong

CHAPTER

1

Pathway for the Management of Acute Coronary Syndrome

The practice of medicine is changing at unprecedented speed. Today's reasonable assumption is outdated by tomorrow's evidence. A deluge of data faces us as we deal with acute coronary syndrome (ACS). ACS subsumes a spectrum of clinical entities, ranging from unstable angina (UA) to ST-elevation myocardial infarction (STEMI; often referred to as "Q-wave myocardial infarction"). The management of ACS is deservedly scrutinized, as it accounts for 2 million hospitalizations and a remarkable 30% of all deaths in the Unites States each year. Clinical guidelines on the management of ACS, which are based on clinical trials, have been updated and published.[1,2]

This chapter will outline the current modalities available for the prompt diagnosis and optimal management of ACS patients. In this chapter, we describe a novel pathway for the management of ACS at our institution.[3,4]

The pathway has been designated with the acronym of *P*riority risk, *A*dvanced risk, *I*ntermediate risk, and *N*egative/low risk (*PAIN*) that reflects patient's most immediate risk stratification upon admission (Figure 1.1). This risk stratification reflects patient's 30 days risks for death and MI following the initial ACS event.

The pathway is color-coded with "PAIN" acronym (P—red, A—yellow, I—yellow, and N—green) that guides patient

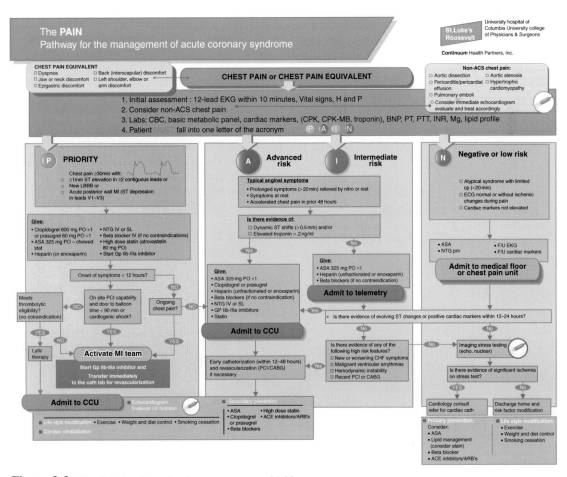

Figure 1.1. The PAIN pathway for the management of ACS.

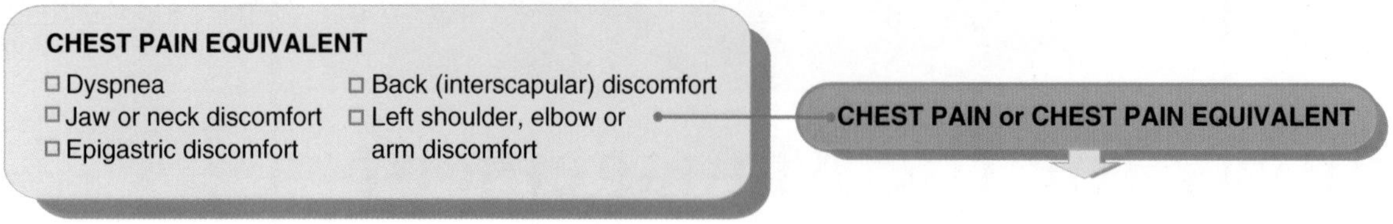

CHEST PAIN EQUIVALENT

☐ Dyspnea   ☐ Back (interscapular) discomfort
☐ Jaw or neck discomfort   ☐ Left shoulder, elbow or
☐ Epigastric discomfort   arm discomfort

CHEST PAIN or CHEST PAIN EQUIVALENT

Figure 1.2. Chest pain and chest pain equivalent symptoms.

management according to patient's risk stratification. These colors—similar to the road traffic light code—have been chosen as an easy reference for the provider about the sequential risk level of patients with ACS.[5]

INITIAL ASSESSMENT OF PATIENTS WITH CHEST PAIN OR CHEST PAIN EQUIVALENT

Patients who present to emergency departments with chest pain or chest pain equivalent will be enrolled into this pathway.

Figure 1.2 shows the chest pain equivalent symptoms. The initial assessment is seen in Figure 1.3. All patients should have an electrocardiogram (ECG or EKG, abbreviated from the German *Elektrokardiogramm*) performed within 10 minutes as well as detailed history and physical exam.

Non-ACS chest pain should be excluded urgently. Causes include aortic dissection, pericarditis and pericardial effusion, pulmonary emboli, aortic stenosis, and hypertrophic cardiomyopathy. If any of these emergency conditions is suspected, we recommend obtaining immediate echocardiogram or CT and to treat accordingly.

Our recommended initial laboratory tests include CBC, basic metabolic panel, cardiac markers (to include CPK, CPK-MB, and Troponin), BNP, PT, PTT, INR, magnesium, and a lipid profile.

INITIAL MANAGEMENT OF PRIORITY PATIENTS

"PRIORITY" patients are those with symptoms of chest pain or chest pain equivalent lasting longer than 30 minutes with one of the following EKG criteria for acute MI:

1. ≥1 mm ST elevation in two contiguous leads, or
2. New left bundle branch block (LBBB), or
3. Acute posterior wall MI (ST segment depression in leads V1–V3).

The initial treatment of these patients includes placing an intravenous line, providing oxygen, treating patients with oral aspirin (chewable 325 mg stat), clopidogrel (600 mg loading dose) or prasugrel (60 mg loading dose), *intravenous β-blocker* (if no contraindication), heparin (unfractionated or enoxaparin), nitroglycerin, oral high-dose statin, and to consider using intravenous glycoprotein IIb to IIIa inhibitors if it will not delay the transfer of the patient to the cardiac catheterization laboratory (Figure 1.4).

The key question for further management of these patients is the duration of the patients' symptoms. For patients whose symptoms exceed 12 hours, presence of persistent or residual chest pain determines the next strategy. If there is no evidence of continued symptoms, these patients will be treated as if they had been risk stratified with the advanced risk group.

For patients whose symptoms are <12 hours or with ongoing chest pain, further management is based on the availability of on-site angioplasty (percutaneous coronary intervention or PCI) capability with expected door to balloon time of <90 minutes or the presence of cardiogenic shock. Patients with expected door to balloon time of <90 minutes should be transferred immediately to the cardiac catheterization lab for revascularization. The MI team is activated for this group of patients (Figure 1.5).

In our institution, a single call made by the emergency department physician to the page operator activates the MI team, which includes the following health care providers:

1. The interventional cardiologist on-call (who is considered the "team leader").
2. The director of the CCU.
3. The cardiology fellow on-call.
4. The interventional cardiology fellow on-call.

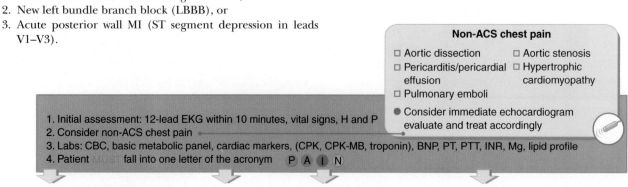

Non-ACS chest pain

☐ Aortic dissection   ☐ Aortic stenosis
☐ Pericarditis/pericardial   ☐ Hypertrophic
    effusion   cardiomyopathy
☐ Pulmonary emboli

● Consider immediate echocardiogram evaluate and treat accordingly

1. Initial assessment: 12-lead EKG within 10 minutes, vital signs, H and P
2. Consider non-ACS chest pain
3. Labs: CBC, basic metabolic panel, cardiac markers, (CPK, CPK-MB, troponin), BNP, PT, PTT, INR, Mg, lipid profile
4. Patient MUST fall into one letter of the acronym   P A I N

Figure 1.3. Initial assessment of patients with chest pain.

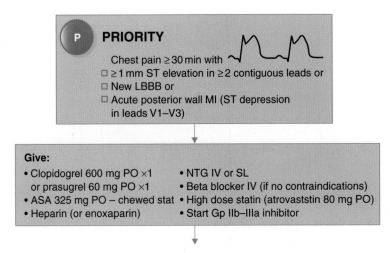

Figure 1.4. The initial management of PRIORITY patients (patient with ST-elevation MI).

5. The cath lab nurse on-call.
6. The cath lab technologist on-call.
7. The CCU nursing manager on-call.
8. The senior internal medicine resident on-call.

Activating this group has been extremely successful in our institution and has markedly reduced our door to balloon time. These strategies have been recently shown to decrease door to balloon time in the range of 8 to 19 minutes.[6]

For hospitals with no PCI capability or in situations when door to balloon time is expected to exceed 90 minutes, we recommend thrombolytic therapy if there are no contraindications.

CCU MANAGEMENT AND SECONDARY PREVENTION FOR PATIENTS WITH PRIORITY MI

Patients with "PRIORITY" MI should be admitted to the CCU (Figure 1.6). All patients should have an echocardiogram to evaluate left ventricle systolic and diastolic function and to exclude valvular abnormality and pericardial involvement. We recommend a minimum CCU stay of 24 hours to exclude arrhythmia complication or mechanical complication. For patients with no evidence of mechanical complications or

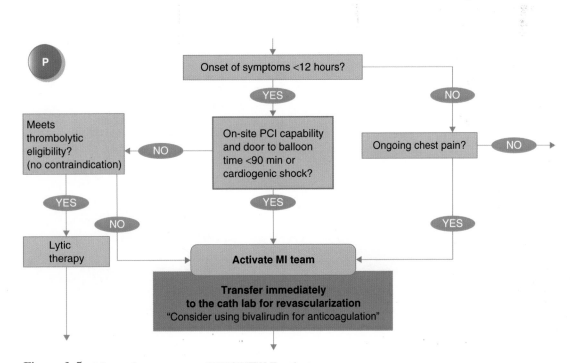

Figure 1.5. Advanced management of PRIORITY MI patients.

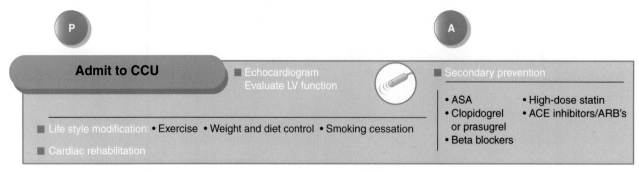

Figure 1.6. CCU management and secondary prevention for patients with PRIORITY MI.

significant arrhythmia, secondary prevention drugs should be started, including aspirin, clopidogrel or prasugrel, high-dose statin, β-blocker, and ACE inhibitor or angiotensin receptor blocker (ARB).

Most patients can be discharged within 48 hours with recommendations for life style modification including exercise, weight and diet control, smoking cessation, and cardiac rehabilitation. Secondary prevention drugs should be continued on discharge.

MANAGEMENT OF ADVANCED RISK ACS

Typical anginal symptoms must be present in patients, who will enroll in the advanced or the intermediate risk groups.

These symptoms include the following:

1. prolonged chest pain (>20 minutes) relieved by nitroglycerine or rest;
2. chest pain at rest; or
3. accelerated chest pain within 48 hours.

In order to qualify for the advanced risk group, patients must have either dynamic ST changes on the EKG (>0.5 mm) and/or elevated troponin (>0.2 ng per /ml) (Figure 1.7).

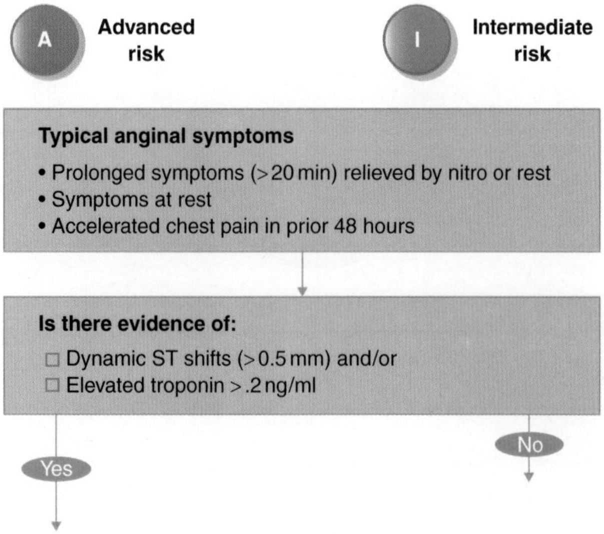

We recommend that patients be admitted to the CCU and be treated with aspirin, clopidogrel or prasugrel, heparin, glycoprotein IIb–IIIa inhibitor, β-blocker, statin, and nitroglycerin if there are no contraindications (Figure 1.8).

These patients should have early cardiac catheterization within 12 to 48 hours and revascularization by PCI or coronary artery bypass surgery (CABG) if necessary. All patients should have an echocardiogram to evaluate LV function. Recommendation for secondary prevention medication, life style modification, and cardiac rehabilitation should be provided similar to the patients with PRIORITY risk group (Figure 1.6).

MANAGEMENT OF INTERMEDIATE RISK GROUP

Both intermediate risk group and advanced risk patients present to the hospital with typical anginal symptoms. Compared with the advanced risk patients, the immediate risk patients *do not* have evidence of dynamic ST changes on the EKG or

Advanced risk / **Intermediate risk**

Typical anginal symptoms

• Prolonged symptoms (>20 min) relieved by nitro or rest
• Symptoms at rest
• Accelerated chest pain in prior 48 hours

Is there evidence of:

☐ Dynamic ST shifts (>0.5 mm) and/or
☐ Elevated troponin > .2 ng/ml

Yes   No

Figure 1.7. Risk stratification as advanced risk ACS.

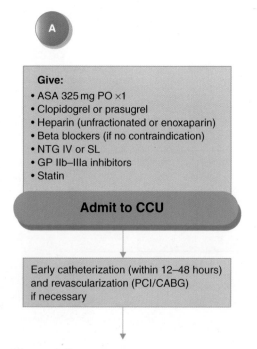

Give:

• ASA 325 mg PO ×1
• Clopidogrel or prasugrel
• Heparin (unfractionated or enoxaparin)
• Beta blockers (if no contraindication)
• NTG IV or SL
• GP IIb–IIIa inhibitors
• Statin

Admit to CCU

Early catheterization (within 12–48 hours) and revascularization (PCI/CABG) if necessary

Figure 1.8. Management of patients with advanced risk ACS.

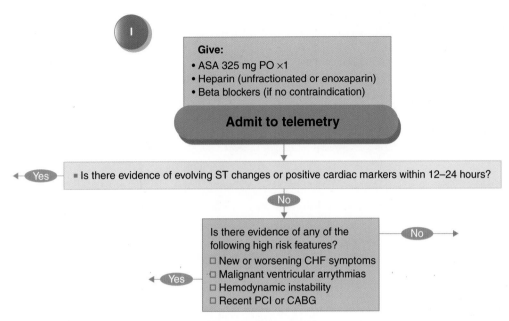

Figure 1.9. Management of patients with intermediate risk ACS.

evidence of positive cardiac markers. These patients should be admitted to the telemetry floor and be given aspirin, heparin, and β-blocker if no contraindication (Figure 1.9). We recommend a minimum telemetry stay of 12 to 24 hours. If during this period of time there is evidence of dynamic ST changes on the EKG or evidence for positive cardiac markers, the patients should be treated as if they had been stratified to the advanced group.

The intermediate risk group patients are assessed again for the following high risk features:

1. New or worsening heart failure symptoms;
2. Malignant ventricular arrhythmias;
3. Hemodynamic instability; or
4. Recent PCI or CABG.

If there is an evidence of any of these high risk features, we recommend transferring the patient for cardiac catheterization within 12 to 48 hours and for revascularization by PCI or CABG if necessary. Patients with no evidence of high-risk features should be referred for cardiac imaging stress testing (stress echocardiography or stress nuclear test).

MANAGEMENT OF NEGATIVE- OR LOW-RISK GROUP PATIENTS:

These groups of patients have atypical symptoms and do not have significant ischemic EKG changes during pain and do not have elevated cardiac markers.

These patients should be treated only with aspirin and given sublingual nitroglycerin if needed. If a decision was made to admit them to the hospital, they should be admitted to a chest pain unit or to a regular medical floor. They should be followed up for 12 to 24 hours with repeated EKG and cardiac markers (Figure 1.10). If there is evidence of evolving ST changes on the EKG or evidence of positive cardiac markers, the patients

should be treated aggressively as with the advanced risk group patients.

If there are no significant EKG changes and all cardiac markers are negative, we recommend cardiac imaging stress testing by stress echocardiography or stress nuclear test (Figure 1.11).

Evidence of significant ischemia on any of these stress imaging modalities will be followed by a referral for cardiac catheterization. If there is no evidence of significant ischemia on stress testing, the patients can be discharged home with a recommendation for risk factor modification to include primary prevention medication and life style modification (Figure 1.12).

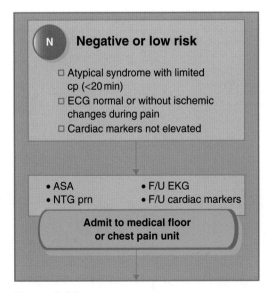

Figure 1.10. Initial management of patients with negative or low-risk ACS.

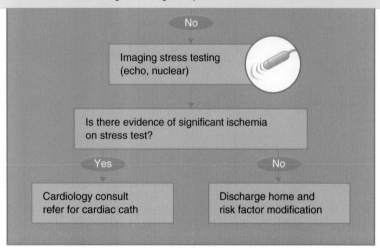

Figure 1.11. Risk stratification of low-risk patients by using cardiac imaging stress testing.

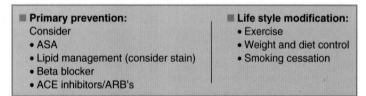

Figure 1.12. Primary prevention for low-risk patients.

REFERENCES

1. Anderson JL, Adams CD, Antman EM, et al. ACC/AHA 2007 guidelines for the management of patients with unstable angina/non-ST-elevation myocardial infarction: a report of the American College of Cardiology/American Heart Association Task Force on Practice Guidelines (Writing Committee to Revise the 2002 Guidelines for the Management of Patients with Unstable Angina/Non-ST-Elevation Myocardial Infarction) developed in collaboration with the American College of Emergency Physicians, the Society for Cardiovascular Angiography and Interventions, and the Society of Thoracic Surgeons endorsed by the American Association of Cardiovascular and Pulmonary Rehabilitation and the Society for Academic Emergency Medicine. *J Am Coll Cardiol.* 2007;50(7):e1–e157.
2. Kushner FG, Hand M, Smith SC Jr, et al. 2009 focused updates: ACC/AHA guidelines for the management of patients with ST-elevation myocardial infarction (updating the 2004 Guideline and 2007 Focused Update) and ACC/AHA/SCAI guidelines on percutaneous coronary intervention (updating the 2005 Guideline and 2007 Focused Update): a report of the American College of Cardiology Foundation/American Heart Association Task Force on Practice Guidelines. *Circulation.* 2009;120(22):2271–2306.
3. Herzog E, Saint-Jacques H, Rozanski A. The PAIN pathway as a tool to bridge the gap between evidence and management of acute coronary syndrome. *Crit Pathw Cardiol.* 2004;3:20–24.
4. Herzog E, Aziz EF, Hong MK. A novel pathway for the management of acute coronary syndrome. In: Herzog E, Chaudhry F. *Echocardiography in Acute Coronary Syndrome: Diagnosis, Treatment and Prevention.* London: Springer; 2009:9–19.
5. Saint-Jacques H, Burroughs VJ, Watowska J, et al. Acute coronary syndrome critical pathway: chest PAIN Caremap—a qualitative research study-provider-level intervention. *Crit Pathw Cardiol.* 2005;4:145–156.
6. Bradley EH, Herrin J, Yondfei Wang YF, et al. Strategies for reducing the door-to-balloon time in acute myocardial infarction. *N Engl J Med.* 2006;355:2308–2320.

PATIENT AND FAMILY INFORMATION FOR:

Management of Acute Coronary Syndrome

MANAGEMENT OF ACUTE CORONARY SYNDROME (ACS)

ACS is the world's number one killer disease accounting for nearly half of all deaths worldwide. About a third of heart attack victims do not even reach a doctor: it kills suddenly and unexpectedly. There are many complexities and variations in the presentation of ACS. Seconds and minutes count once a person presents with ACS. High-level training and expertise are needed to quickly evaluate this condition and to ensure appropriate management. Immediate diagnosis and effective management very often mean the difference between life and death.

VARIOUS FORMS OF ACS

The term ACS is an umbrella term to identify patients who have evidence of heart tissue necrosis or are believed to be at high risk for it, in the immediate future. The concept of ACS provides a simplified diagnosis to approach a patient with chest pain or its equivalent symptoms and helps to rationalize therapeutic interventions on basis of clinical evidence. ACS encompasses a spectrum of coronary artery diseases, including Unstable Angina (UA), STEMI, and non-STEMI (often referred to as "non-Q-wave myocardial infarction"). These types are named according to the different appearances of the EKG, a common diagnostic test used to determine the electric activity of the heart providing valuable pertinent information concerning heart's function.

ALARMING SYMPTOMS/WARNING SIGNS OF A HEART ATTACK OR ACS

The red flag of decreased blood flow to the heart is chest pain or "angina" as it is called in medical literature, experienced either as constricting pressure-like pain over the chest or tightness around the chest, and sometimes radiating to the left arm and the left angle of the jaw. *You may simply say that when heart muscle does not receive enough blood and therefore oxygen, it reacts by complaining or causing pain.* This may be coupled with diaphoresis (sudden, heavy sweating), nausea (feel like throwing up), and vomiting, as well as shortness of breath (a sensation of hunger for air that cannot be satisfied) sometimes referred to as chest pain equivalent. In many cases, the sensation is "atypical," with pain experienced in different ways or even

being completely absent (which is more likely in female patients and those with diabetes). Some patients may report palpitations, anxiety or a sense of impending doom, and a feeling of being acutely ill. Some unusual heart attack symptoms may present as abdominal pain, heartburn-type pain, clammy skin, lightheadedness, dizziness or fainting, unusual or unexplained fatigue, and feeling of being apprehensive.

BEST THING TO DO IF YOU THINK THAT YOU ARE HAVING ACS

Get medical help right away if you have the above mentioned signs and symptoms and think that you are having a heart attack. Whenever possible, get emergency medical assistance rather than driving yourself to the hospital. You could be having a heart attack.

INITIAL ASSESSMENT OF PATIENTS WITH CHEST PAIN OR CHEST PAIN EQUIVALENTS

Over the previous couple of decades, clinical guidelines on the management of ACS, which are based on clinical trials, have been continuously updated. Based on these clinical data and practical outcomes from various clinical trials, we have developed a novel pathway for the management of ACS patients to ensure optimal and prompt management in our institute (Figure 1.1). This pathway allows physicians to identify the ACS by a comprehensive strategy based on your history, physical examination, imaging techniques, and laboratory work up. An EKG is obtained immediately and laboratory testing is performed. Initial laboratory testing includes basic tests of kidney, liver, and thyroid function, as well as CBCs and chemical markers of heart muscle damage called cardiac biomarkers (Figure 1.3). This initial assessment helps to differentiate ACS chest pains from the other causes of chest pain (Figure 1.3).

EKG

An EKG is a graphic produced by an electrocardiograph, which records the electrical activity of heart. Its name is made of different parts: *electro*, because it is related to electrical activity; *cardio*, Greek for heart; *gram*, a Greek root meaning "to write." In the United States, the abbreviation "EKG" is often preferred over "ECG." This is the first "emergent" test that is done by a medical personnel on any patient who presents with the complaint of chest pain or is considered at risk of having ACS. The technician will apply the electrodes/leads to your chest, arms, and legs. During the test, be as still as possible, and breathe normally. Any unnecessary movement can give a false reading. The EKG is supposed to be done within 10 minutes of your presentation into a health care facility to identify your cardiac function. The EKG machine is able to show if you are having a heart attack in a real time, and it is able to show if you have had a heart attack in the past. It can differentiate between a new and an old heart attack. The machine can also pinpoint irregularities in the heart rhythm. An EKG provides a graph of the heartbeat. Portions of the graph are labeled as P, Q, R, S, and T. A heart attack or ACS may result in changes in these particular segments on the radiograph. Common ones are ST-segment (portion of radiograph between S and T portion) elevations or depressions, T wave inversions or flattening, and LBBB. A LBBB may occur as a primary abnormality of the heart's electrical system, but often occurs in the setting a heart attack. Patients who have ST-segment elevation may ultimately develop a Q-wave myocardial infarction (heart attack). (The Q-wave describes another part of an ECG graph.) Patients who have ischemic discomfort without an ST-segment elevation are having either UA, or a non-ST-segment elevation MI that may lead to a non-Q-wave MI.

HISTORY:

An important component of the diagnosis of the ACS is the patient's previous medical history. Physicians will ask you about any prior episode of chest pain, shortness of breath, fainting or other signs, which are described earlier. In addition, physicians will be inquiring if you have any other medical disease including but not limited to high blood pressure (hypertension), high blood glucose levels (diabetes mellitus), high blood cholesterol levels (dyslipidemias or hypercholesterolemia), thyroid problems, kidney problems (renal insufficiency or renal failure), peripheral arterial disease (atherosclerosis causing narrowing of the arteries of extremities, particularly the feet and legs) because these can predispose patients to ACS. Physician will also ask you about your social habits including your smoking status, intake of alcohol, life style to ascertain how frequently you participate in exercise, eating habits, or use of any illegal drugs especially cocaine as these all contribute to ACS. You will need to provide a list of medications that you are taking, especially those that may have been recently started. Finally, a family history is very important. Is there a history of immediate family members (parent and siblings) or close relatives who have had heart attack at an early age?

PHYSICAL EXAM:

The physical examination is highly variable among different ACS patients. Physicians start with the vital signs that consist of your blood pressure, heart rate, respiratory rate, temperature, and oxygenation levels of your blood, which all can be affected during ACS episodes. Sometimes if ACS results in abnormal function of heart, certain abnormal sounds called bruits or murmurs can be heard when the physician listens to your heart sounds with the help of stethoscope. In addition to these, general appearance of patients sometimes indicates the severity of the condition, which range from nervousness, fright to cold, or pale skin.

THE "PAIN" PATHWAY FOR THE MANAGEMENT OF ACS PATIENTS

Prompt, efficient treatment greatly improves one's chance of surviving a heart attack. In 2004, considering the fact that key to successful treatment in ACS is early treatment, we used published guidelines to define the strategy and resolved differences in the literature by consensus of local experts in the form of a clinical pathway to reduce variations in ACS patient care and improve outcomes. The pathway is based on the hypothesis that following a simplified and unified algorithmic approach for the management of patients with ACS by the physicians can enhance prompt initiation of optimized goal-directed therapy based on established guidelines in a hospital setting. This can be helpful as there will be no time wasted to figure out what to do first and what next once a patient with ACS is diagnosed.

After initial assessment, patients are placed in one of the following four categories according to the severity of the risk they are at as per our clinical pathway that is designed with the acronym PAIN: (1) **P**riority risk (2) **A**dvanced risk (3) **I**ntermediate risk, or (4) **N**egative risk/ Low risk (as shown in Figure 1.1). These four categories reflect patient's most immediate risk stratification on admission based on astute observation and skillful application. We have made the pathway color-coded with "PAIN" acronym (P—red, A—yellow, I—yellow, and N—green) to guide patient management according to patient's risk stratification. These colors—similar to the road traffic light code—have been chosen as an easy reference for the providers and patients about the sequential risk level of patients with ACS.

INITIAL MANAGEMENT OF PRIORITY PATIENTS (PATIENTS WITH ST ELEVATION MI)

According to our pathway, we place patients immediately into "priority risk" category, who show warning signs of chest pain or chest pain equivalent exceeding 30 minutes, and they also have one of the following changes on the EKG (Figure 1.4):

(a) ≥1 mm ST-segment elevation in two adjacent leads of EKG demonstrating that an artery supplying certain portion of the heart is blocked; or

(b) New LBBB denoting blockage of the coronary artery supplying portion of heart conduction system; or

(c) ST-segment depression in leads V1 to V3 of EKG, which demonstrates that back wall of the heart has blocked/ impaired blood supply.

As soon as it is ascertained that the patient belongs to the priority risk group, initial treatment is started, which consists of providing oxygen to maintain good supply of oxygen to the body usually by means of nasal prongs or the face mask and an intravenous access is established as certain medications may need to be given directly into the veins. Pharmacologic medications that are given immediately to each patient in this group include aspirin given orally (dose of 325 mg), clopidogrel (initial dose of 600 mg to build up blood levels of this drug initially) or prasugrel (dose of 60 mg), nitroglycerine under the tongue commonly to reduce/alleviate the chest pain, ß-blocker directly into the veins (provided patient does not have any contraindication like history of asthma, slow heart rate, or active heart pump failure), heparin (a blood thinner that reduces the ability of the blood to clot), and high dose of oral statins (usually a drug named atorvastatin at dose of 80 mg) to lower blood cholesterol. Aspirin, clopidogrel, or prasugrel by inhibiting the sticking of platelets (blood cells involved in the clotting, which lead to blood clots and subsequently heart attacks) are the most effective treatment modalities in ACS which along with heparin, a blood thinner, certainly provide a shield against vicious circle of blood clot formation/propagation during initial phases of ACS and minimize the damage to heart tissue.

After the initial stabilization of the patient with ACS in priority risk group, the next and the most vital question to be addressed is the duration of patient's symptoms (Figure 1.5). For patients whose symptoms started more than 12 hours ago, management depends on they still are having persistent or residual chest pain. If they no longer have ongoing chest pain, they are treated like the patients who are risk stratified as advanced risk groups, and their treatment plan details will be discussed in the next section.

Those patients who started having chest pain or chest pain equivalents more than 12 hours ago but still are having chest pain or discomfort and those patients who are brought earlier to the health care facility site and their duration of symptoms is <12 hours, further treatment plan depends on the availability of on-site advanced heart intervention termed angioplasty (medically mostly referred as percutaneous coronary intervention or PCI). It is also important to make sure that the door to balloon time (a terminology used to demonstrate how fast a patient with ST-segment elevation MI can be taken to PCI facility in the hospital once the patient enters the hospital door) is <90 minutes. The presence of heart pump failure resulting in inability of the heart to pump blood to different parts of the body called cardiogenic shock) also requires emergent intervention. If the door to balloon time is <90 minutes (which is the national goal), another antiplatelet medication named glycoprotein IIb/IIIa inhibitor can be given directly into the veins of these patients, and they are transferred immediately to the cardiac catheterization laboratory (the place where PCI is done) for prompt intervention. The procedure is called PCI or angioplasty—dilation of occluded coronary vessels by a long, hollow tube (catheter) passed through a large artery in your groin or arm, sometimes requiring placement of scaffoldings (called stents) to maintain the flow of blood in these vessels after initial dilation and prevent renarrowing.

For hospitals with no PCI capability or in situations where door to balloon time is expected to exceed 90 minutes,

thrombolytic therapy (certain medications with the goal of dissolving/break up clogged clots) can be considered, provided there are no contraindications (like history of bleeding in the brain, extremely elevated blood pressures, or active bleeding). Our hospital is well-equipped with the cardiac catheterization laboratory and door to balloon time is also <90 minutes. Whenever we receive a patient designated as priority risk, a team called MI team is activated in our hospital, and every effort is made to transfer the patient to the cardiac catheterization laboratory as early as possible to open up the blocked coronary artery.

CCU MANAGEMENT AND SECONDARY PREVENTION OF PATIENTS WITH PRIORITY RISK HEART ATTACK

Patients belonging to priority risk group are admitted to the CCU for intense, continuous, and highly skilled monitoring for a minimum of 24 hours to make sure that patients do not suffer from any complication that might occur after a heart attack (Figure 1.6). These complications include heart pump failure, rhythm abnormalities, recurrence of chest pain, or extension of the heart attack as discussed later in the book.

In the CCU, patients are evaluated to determine whether they need further treatment. Each patient gets a test called "echocardiogram—an ultrasound of the heart." This test makes it possible to "look" directly into your heart without penetrating your skin. It tells us about the function of your heart, heart valves, and the anatomy of your heart (A detailed description of echocardiography is provided in Chapter 5). Once we make sure that you do not have any complication of heart attack, for example, any arrhythmia (abnormal rhythm of your heart) or any structural abnormality (like valvular malfunction), we start drugs to prevent any further damage to your heart, medically called secondary prevention. These drugs include aspirin, clopidogrel or prasugrel, high-dose statin, ß-blocker and ACE inhibitor, or ARBs (details about these drugs are discussed in Chapter 7). Most patients can be discharged within 48 to 72 hours with recommendations for life style modification including exercise, weight and diet control, smoking cessation, and heart rehabilitation (heart/cardiac rehabilitation helps people who have had a heart attack or heart operation to lead active, productive lives—mentally, physically, and socially).

MANAGEMENT OF ADVANCED RISK ACS PATIENTS

There are patients who have chest pain or chest pain equivalent symptoms of >20 minutes but their pain is resolved after receiving nitroglycerin or by rest. These patients do not have abnormal EKG changes as we have explained in the priority risk section. These patients are further divided into either advanced risk or intermediate risk groups (Figure 1.7).

Our pathway emphasizes the need for frequent reevaluation of advanced risk patients mainly by repeat EKGs and blood tests. We look to see if the EKG shows any new ST-segment change (>0.5 mm) and/or the laboratory work up shows any increase in the markers of heart tissue damage/death in the blood called cardiac biomarkers (of which troponin is the most important one). Consider these markers as chemical clues to your heart's health—they leak into the blood from damaged heart cells after a heart attack.

Patients who have ST-segment change of >0.5 mm and/or have levels of troponin in blood of ≥0.2 ng per/dl are classified as advanced risk patients and are admitted directly into the CCU for close monitoring and treatment (Figure 1.8). These patients are treated with aspirin, clopidogrel or prasugrel, heparin, glyoprotein IIb/IIIa inhibitor, ß-blocker, statin, and nitroglycerin.

If you belong to this group, after getting the medication you will undergo an echocardiogram (ultrasound of heart) to determine the current status of your heart's pumping ability. We recommend that these patients get an early cardiac catheterization within 12 to 48 hours and revascularization by PCI or CABG if necessary. Recommendations for secondary prevention medication, life style modification, and cardiac rehabilitation should be provided similar to the patients with PRIORITY risk group.

MANAGEMENT OF INTERMEDIATE RISK GROUP

As mentioned in previous section, both the advanced risk group and the intermediate risk patients present to the hospital with same symptoms. Compared with the advanced risk patients, the intermediate risk patients *do not* have any new ST-segment changes on the EKG or any elevation of biomarkers of cardiac tissue damage/death in blood (no troponin spillage into blood >0.2 ng per ml).

If you belong to this group, then you will be admitted to a telemetry unit (telemetry units are used to monitor your heart rhythm activity around-the-clock, which is displayed on monitors usually watched by a health care personnel continuously). You will receive aspirin, heparin, and ß-blocker if no contraindication. We recommend that you should undergo minimum telemetry stay of 12 to 24 hours as to ascertain that you are not at any urgent risk of any heart attack (Figure 1.9). If during this period of time, we observe any new ST-segment changes on the EKG or increase in the level of cardiac markers in blood, you will be transferred to the CCU and will be treated further as advanced risk patient.

The intermediate risk group patients are further assessed during their stay for the following conditions (Figure 1.9):

1. New or worsening heart failure symptoms (mostly shortness of breath, enlarged neck veins, cough, and unable to lie flat on bed).
2. Malignant ventricular arrhythmias (life threatening abnormal rhythm of the heart).
3. Hemodynamic instability (abnormal blood pressure, pulse rate, respiratory rate, and oxygen level in blood).
4. Any history of recent PCI or CABG.

If you have any of these high-risk features, we recommend performing cardiac catheterization within 12 to 48 hours and for revascularization by PCI or CABG if necessary. If you do not have any of above mentioned high-risk features, you will be referred for cardiac imaging stress testing (stress echocardiography or stress nuclear test), details of which are discussed in Chapters 5 and 6. You will be managed thereafter as per the results of these tests (Figure 1.11).

MANAGEMENT OF NEGATIVE OR LOW-RISK GROUP PATIENTS

This is the group of patients who have atypical symptoms and do not have significant EKG changes even during an episode of chest pain. These patients also do not have any indication of heart tissue damage by means of increased cardiac biomarkers in the blood. This group is therefore marked by green color in the pathway denoting that no "immediate" risk of heart attack is present in these patients (Figure 1.10).

If you belong to this group, then you will be treated only with aspirin on presentation. If you are found to have chest pain, you will be given nitroglycerin under the tongue if needed. If a decision is made to admit you to the hospital based on the severity of your symptoms or functional impairment, you will be admitted to a chest pain unit or to a regular medical floor (Figure 1.10). You will be closely followed up for 12 to 24 hours with repeated EKGs and cardiac markers testing periodically (usually we check them every 6 to 8 hours for a total of three times if all stay negative). If there is an evidence of evolving ST-segment changes on the EKG or an evidence of positive cardiac biomarkers, your management plan will be changed and you would be treated aggressively as with the advanced risk group patients.

If there are no significant EKG changes and all cardiac markers are negative, we recommend cardiac imaging stress testing by stress echocardiography or stress nuclear test after discussion with your physician.

Evidence of significant ischemia on any of these stress imaging modalities means that you likely have a disease of the coronary arteries will be followed by a referral for cardiac catheterization to see how much and where the narrowing or blockages. If there is no evidence of significant ischemia on stress testing, you will be discharged home with a recommendation for risk factor modification to include primary prevention medication (medications given to prevent disease), and life style modification (Figure 1.12). Common tools for primary prevention are low-dose aspirin daily, maintaining lower levels of cholesterol as per recommendations of your doctors, strict control of high BP if present with drugs like ß-blockers and ACE/ARBs, and regular exercise. Risk factor modification includes abstaining from health hazard behaviors like smoking, drinking alcohol or illicit drugs, and includes weight reduction and exercise.

Vikas Soma
Kishore Nallu
Eyal Herzog
Mun K. Hong

CHAPTER

2

ST-Segment Elevation Myocardial Infarction

ST-segment elevation myocardial infarction (STEMI; often referred to as Q-wave myocardial infarction [MI]) accounts for approximately 30% new cases of MI every year in the United States.[1] STEMI represents the most urgent group of patients for immediate therapy and thus, represents the priority group of the *P*riority risk, *A*dvanced risk, *I*ntermediate risk, and *N*egative/low risk (PAIN) pathway.[2] Prompt recognition is the key step in the management of these patients because reperfusion therapy is most beneficial when performed early in presentation. Early reperfusion is the key to maximizing the preservation of ischemic myocardium at risk, and minimizing the acute and late morbidity and mortality associated with STEMI.[3,4]

PATHOPHYSIOLOGY

The likely mechanism of STEMI is the plaque rupture of a previously non-flow-limiting lesion or less likely, endothelial erosion.[5] These events result in the sudden development of a flow-limiting stenosis with eventual thrombus formation and cessation of blood flow. The inciting factors are unknown, although hypersympathetic state, including early morning hours and associated with strenuous physical or mental stress, has been hypothesized to increase the likelihood of plaque rupture.

INITIAL ASSESSMENT

The American College of Cardiology/American Heart Association (ACC/AHA) guidelines on STEMI[6] suggest that all patients presenting to the emergency department (ED) with a history of chest pain or symptoms suggestive of STEMI should undergo the following:

1. Triaged and managed through a predetermined, guideline-based, institution-specific chest pain protocol such as the PAIN pathway.[2] The protocol should address, in order of importance, those findings that permit rapid triage and initial diagnosis and management, and should include the following top six differential diagnostic possibilities:

   a. Acute coronary syndrome (ACS)
   b. Acute aortic dissection
   c. Acute pulmonary embolism
   d. Tension pneumothorax

   e. Acute perforation of peptic ulcer or esophageal tear or rupture
   f. Acute pericarditis.

In addition, the 2009 ACC/AHA STEMI guidelines focused update[7] recommended that each community develop a STEMI system of care that includes the following:

   a. Ongoing multidisciplinary team collaboration (including emergency medical services, nonpercutaneous coronary intervention [non-PCI] capable hospitals/STEMI referral centers, and PCI capable hospitals/STEMI receiving centers) to evaluate outcomes and measures of performance.
   b. A process for prehospital identification and activation
   c. Transfer protocols for patients who arrive at STEMI referral centers and are candidates for primary PCI.
   d. Destination protocols for STEMI receiving centers.

2. The 12-lead ECG is the most critical data for establishing the diagnosis of STEMI, as initial biomarkers can be negative. A 12-lead electrocardiogram (ECG) should be performed and interpreted by an experienced physician within 10 minutes of ED arrival.

   a. If the initial ECG is nondiagnostic, but there is a high clinical suspicion of STEMI, then an ECG should be repeated every 5 to 10 minutes to assess for evolving ST-elevation.
   b. In patients with suspected inferior STEMI, a right-sided ECG should be obtained to assess for right ventricular (RV) infarction, which manifests as ST-elevation in leads V_{3R} and V_{4R}.
   c. In patients with suspected posterior wall or high lateral wall infarction, leads V_7, V_8, and V_9 should be obtained by extending the lateral chest leads to the back.

3. If STEMI is present, the decision to establish reperfusion either by primary PCI, the preferred revascularization option,[8] or fibrinolytic therapy should be made within 20 minutes of ED arrival. The goal is to achieve a door-to-needle time for fibrinolytics within 30 minutes or perform primary PCI within 90 minutes of first medical contact by persons skilled in the procedure.[6] These goals should not be understood as the ideal times for reperfusion but as the longest times that should be considered acceptable for effective reperfusion therapy.

4. During this time, a focused history and physical examination should be performed with the following objectives:

   a. Risk stratify patients using scoring systems such as the thrombolysis in myocardial infarction (TIMI) risk score[9] or Grace score.[10] As opposed to patients with unstable angina or NSTEMI, in whom risk stratification identifies a high-risk subset of patients who derive the greatest potential benefit from an early invasive approach, all patients with STEMI (presenting <12 hours of symptoms onset) benefit from early reperfusion. Risk stratification in STEMI patients helps to identify those with higher morbidity and mortality. These high-risk features include patients with advanced age, cardiogenic shock or heart failure, large anterior wall MI, and those who develop electrical (e.g., ventricular arrhythmias) or mechanical complications from the STEMI.[11,12] Patients who do not either receive any reperfusion therapy or achieve successful reperfusion after primary PCI or fibrinolytic therapy also have a higher risk of in-hospital mortality.

   b. Perform a quick but thorough review of exclusion criteria for fibrinolytic treatment whether STEMI is confirmed and whether the patient is in a nonprimary PCI center with long (>60 minute) transfer time for primary PCI.

MANAGEMENT STRATEGIES

INITIAL APPROACH

Immediately after the diagnosis of STEMI, the patients should receive oxygen and adjunct pharmacology based on predetermined, guideline-based, institution-specific protocol, including but not limited to aspirin, clopidogrel/prasugrel, statin, and possibly glycoprotein IIb/IIIa (GP IIb/IIIa) inhibitor. All patients should be placed on a cardiac monitor with a defibrillator on standby.

MODE OF REPERFUSION

The current ACC/AHA guidelines for the treatment of STEMI recommend that a reperfusion strategy, based on either pharmacological management with a fibrinolytic agent or mechanical management with primary PCI, should be implemented as soon as possible after arrival in the ED (class I-A recommendation).[7] Factors affecting the choice of reperfusion therapy include time between onset of chest pain and presentation, patient characteristics at presentation (high vs. low risk), and access to a skilled facility capable of primary PCI.

Time from symptom onset. The most important determining factor is the time from symptom onset, which directly correlates with the clinical outcome in patients with STEMI regardless of the reperfusion method. If the symptom duration is <3 hours, and the door-to-balloon minus door-to-needle time is <1 hour, primary PCI is preferred. However, if the estimated time from first medical contact to balloon inflation is >90 minutes (or door-to-balloon minus door-to-needle time is >1 hour), fibrinolytic therapy is preferred.[7] PCI is the favored strategy when there is a delay between symptom onset and presentation (>3 hours) and when PCI can be performed in a timely manner with a door-to-balloon time goal of 90 minutes.

High-risk patients. Primary PCI has been shown to have better clinical outcomes in high-risk patients, including those elderly who develop shock within 36 hours of MI, patients with severe heart failure and/or pulmonary edema (Killip class III or IV), and symptom onset within 12 hours. If the clinical scenario describes a STEMI with high-risk features, transfer for primary PCI is favored even if the time from first medical contact to balloon inflation modestly exceeds 90 minutes.

Access to skilled facility capable of primary PCI. The biggest obstacle to the use of primary PCI for all STEMI patients is the lack of a skilled facility capable of primary PCI. For those patients presenting to facilities without this capability, rapid transfer to a PCI center can produce better outcomes than fibrinolysis, as long as the door-to-balloon time, including inter hospital transport time, is <90 minutes. If, however, rapid transfer is not possible, fibrinolytic therapy should be administered. If patient presents very early after symptom onset (<1 hour), and there are no contraindications to fibrinolytic therapy, the therapy should be administered as it may abort the infarction.[13] In patients with high-risk features, rapid transfer to a PCI center is preferred as long as the door-to-balloon time is <90 minutes. Patients who do receive fibrinolytic therapy, especially those with high-risk features (e.g., elderly, anterior MI location), should be electively transferred to a PCI center in the event that rescue PCI is needed.[14] Table 2.1 summarizes the criteria for selecting a reperfusion therapy.

PRIMARY PCI

The current STEMI guidelines[6] indicate that the benefit of PCI over fibrinolytic reperfusion pertains to primary PCI performed in a skilled facility. A skilled facility is defined as a laboratory that performs approximately 400 PCI procedures annually, and at least 36 of them are primary PCI. The PCI should be performed by experienced interventionalists, defined as operators who perform >75 PCI procedures annually, and at least 11 of them are primary PCI.

The suggested relationship between PCI-capable centers and improved outcomes is illustrated by findings from a retrospective analysis of 1997 Medicare claims data demonstrating that the need for coronary artery bypass graft (CABG) surgery after PCI occurred more frequently (2.25% vs. 1.55%; $P<.001$) when the procedure was performed by inexperienced staff (>60 vs. <30 cases per year) and that the risk of 30-day mortality was higher (4.29% vs. 3.15%; $P<.001$) for patients treated at low-volume PCI centers (<80 vs. >160 Medicare cases per year).[15]

BENEFITS OF PRIMARY PCI OVER FIBRINOLYTICS

RESTORATION OF TIMI 3 FLOW

Several studies have shown that primary PCI results in substantially better rates of normal flow in the culprit artery compared with treatment with fibrinolytic agents (TIMI grade 3: 74% to 93%[16,17] vs. 60% to 63%[18–20]). Fibrinolysis fails to restore blood flow completely in 30% to 40% of patients with STEMI, and analyses of randomized clinical trials comparing primary PCI and fibrinolysis have shown improved clinical outcomes with primary PCI.[8,21]

TABLE 2.1	Criteria for selecting reperfusion therapy

If presentation is <3 hours and there is no delay to an invasive strategy, there is no preference to either strategy; however

AN INVASIVE STRATEGY IS GENERALLY PREFERRED IF:	**FIBRINOLYSIS IS GENERALLY PREFERRED IF:**
1. Late presentation (>3 hours since symptom onset)	Early presentation (<3 hours from symptom onset) and delay to invasive strategy
2. Skilled PCI lab available with surgical backup (11): • Operator experience: >75 PCI cases/year • Team experience >36 primary PCI cases/year	Invasive strategy is not an option: • Cath lab is occupied/not available • Vascular access difficulties • No access to skilled PCI lab
3. Medical contact to balloon or door to balloon time <90 minutes	Delay to invasive strategy: • Prolonged transport • Door to balloon time > 90 minutes
4. <1 hour delay vs. time to fibrinolytic therapy with a fibrin-specific agent	• >1 hour delay vs. immediate fibrinolytic therapy with a fibrin-specific agent
5. High risk STEMI: • Cardiogenic shock • Killip class III or IV	
6. Contradications to fibrinolysis, including increased risk of bleeding and intracranial hemorrhage	
7. Diagnosis of STEMI is in doubt	

ADVERSE EVENTS

Meta-analysis of 23 randomized trials has shown that primary PCI was superior to fibrinolytic therapy in reducing mortality (7% vs. 9%, $P = .0002$), nonfatal reinfarction (3% vs. 7%, $P < .0001$), stroke (1.0% vs. 2.0%, $P = .0004$), and the combined endpoint of death, nonfatal reinfarction, and stroke (8% vs. 14%, $P < .0001$).[8]

REOCCLUSION

Fibrinolytic therapy, albeit widely available, is limited by early and late reocclusions of the infarct-related artery. The incidence of reocclusion after successful fibrinolysis increases over time as shown in a series of studies.[22–24] It is up to 25% to 30% within months of STEMI.[25,26] Reocclusion of a previously patent artery is a cause of increased in-hospital mortality and is detrimental to the long-term recovery of left ventricular function.[27] However, coronary stenting virtually eliminates vascular recoil, and multiple studies have shown low reocclusion rates between 0% and 6% on follow-up angiography ranging from 6.2 days to 7.7 months after angioplasty with stent placement for STEMI.[28–32]

ANATOMIC RISK STRATIFICATION

A subset of patients may have severe three-vessel or left main disease or anatomic features unfavorable for PCI and may be candidates for urgent or emergency CABG. These patients may be missed if a fibrinolytic strategy is used. Another subset of patients will have spontaneously reperfused coronary arteries or may have acute pericarditis or other nonthrombotic causes of ST-segment elevation, such as epicardial or microvascular spasm or Tako-tsubo cardiomyopathy (TCM).[33] These patients can be treated medically and conservatively, avoiding the risks of fibrinolytic therapy. In addition, identification of high-risk patients by cardiac catheterization, such as those with concomitant valvular disease, may facilitate additional strategies that will improve outcome, whereas low-risk patients may be eligible for early hospital discharge.

HIGH-RISK PATIENTS

Primary PCI in patients with anterior STEMI reduces mortality compared with fibrinolytic therapy although there is no difference in patients with non anterior STEMI.[34,35] Patients with cardiogenic shock treated with coronary revascularization experienced an absolute 9% reduction in a 30-day mortality compared with those managed with medical stabilization.[36] In Second National Registry of Myocardial Infarctions (NRMI-II)[12] acute MI patients with congestive heart failure (CHF) had a 33% relative risk reduction in mortality with primary PCI compared with a 9% relative risk reduction with fibrinolytic therapy.

STRATEGIES TO MINIMIZE THE DOOR-TO-BALLOON TIME

There are many strategies to reduce the door-to-balloon time, and a report by Bradley et al.[37] suggests practical ways to achieve this important goal. In their survey of hospitals and review of 28 different strategies, 6 of them were found to significantly reduce the door-to-balloon time. They included the following, and we already have majority of them in place at our institution:

1. ED physicians activate the catheterization laboratory or the MI team (reducing 8.2 minutes).
2. A single call to a central page operator activates the catheterization laboratory or the MI team (13.8-minute reduction).
3. ED physicians activate the catheterization laboratory or the MI team while the patient is being transported by the ambulance to the hospital (saving 15.4 minutes).

4. The on-call staff is expected to arrive in the catheterization laboratory within 20 minutes after being paged (reducing 19.3 vs. >30 minutes).
5. The on-call interventionalist stays in the hospital for these emergencies (14.6-minute reduction).
6. A collaborative feedback is provided between the ED and the catheterization laboratory (8.6-minute reduction).

Most of these strategies can be implemented without undue stress on the system, except for the attending interventionalist taking the call in the hospital. These reductions in precious minutes are especially important when many patients still present late after the onset of their symptoms.

TRANSFER FOR PRIMARY PCI

Data from a meta-analysis of five trials evaluating safety and feasibility of emergent transfer for PCI showed that despite the inherent delay involved in transfer, primary PCI was associated with a significant reduction in nonfatal reinfarction, total stroke, and the combined endpoint of death, nonfatal reinfarction, and stroke compared with on-site fibrinolysis.[8] This was true even in high-risk patients. However, most of these transfer studies were performed in Europe where the distances are shorter, the time required for transfer is shorter, and the use of dedicated emergency vehicles resulted in efficient transfer. Thus, it is unknown whether these results could be replicated elsewhere.

PREHOSPITAL FIBRINOLYTICS AND PRIMARY PCI IN FACILITIES WITHOUT CARDIAC SURGERY

An observational cohort study in patients with STEMI showed lower mortality rates in patients treated with primary PCI compared to both in-hospital fibrinolysis and prehospital fibrinolysis.[38] The randomized comparison of primary angioplasty and prehospital fibrinolysis in acute myocardial infarction (CAPTIM) trial (stopped prematurely because of poor recruitment) showed no significant difference in the rate of death, nonfatal MI, and stroke between patients treated with primary PCI and those treated with prehospital fibrinolytic therapy.[39]

The cardiovascular patient outcomes research team (C-PORT) trial evaluated whether treatment of acute MI with primary PCI is superior to thrombolytic therapy at hospitals without on-site cardiac surgery. At 6-month follow-up, the composite endpoint of death, reinfarction, and stroke was significantly lower in the primary PCI group (12.4% vs. 19.9%, $P = .03$).[40] The ACC/AHA guidelines for the management of patients with STEMI considers the performance of primary PCI in a community hospital without on-site cardiac surgery as a class IIb indication, provided the hospital meets the skilled PCI facility requirements and the procedures performed by an experienced interventionalist. Nonetheless, a protocol for rapid transfer to a hospital with cardiac surgery should be in place in case of procedural complications or other surgical emergencies, such as concomitant mechanical complications.

FIBRINOLYTIC THERAPY

As stated earlier, the time from onset of symptoms to fibrinolytic therapy is an important predictor of MI size and patient outcome.[41] The efficacy of fibrinolytic agents in lysing thrombus diminishes with the passage of time.[42] Fibrinolytic therapy administered within the first 2 hours (especially the first hour) can occasionally abort MI and dramatically reduce mortality.[43,44] The National Heart Attack Alert Working Group recommends that EDs strive to achieve a 30-minute door-to-needle time to minimize treatment delays.[45] Prehospital fibrinolysis by skilled emergency medical service (EMS) personnel reduces treatment delays by up to 1 hour and reduces mortality by 17%.[46]

CONTRAINDICATIONS TO FIBRINOLYTIC THERAPY IN STEMI

ABSOLUTE CONTRAINDICATIONS

1. Any prior intracranial hemorrhage.
2. Known structural cerebral vascular lesion (arteriovenous malformations, aneurysms, etc.).
3. Known malignant intracranial neoplasms (primary or metastatic).
4. Ischemic stroke within 3 months except acute ischemic stroke within 3 hours.
5. Suspected aortic dissection.
6. Active bleeding or bleeding diathesis (excluding menses).
7. Significant closed-head or facial trauma within 3 months.

RELATIVE CONTRAINDICATIONS

1. History of chronic, severe, and poorly controlled hypertension.
2. Severe uncontrolled hypertension on presentation (systolic blood pressure [SBP] >180 mm Hg or diastolic blood pressure [DBP] >110 mm Hg).
3. History of prior ischemic stroke >3 months, dementia, or known intracranial pathology not covered under absolute contraindications.
4. Traumatic or prolonged (>10 minutes) cardiopulmonary resuscitation (CPR).
5. Major surgery within the last 3 weeks.
6. Recent internal bleeding (within 2 to 4 weeks).
7. Noncompressible vascular punctures.
8. Pregnancy.
9. Active peptic ulcer.
10. Current use of anticoagulation: the higher the international normalized ratio (INR), the higher the risk of bleeding.
11. For streptokinase/anistreplase: prior exposure (more than 5 days ago) or prior allergic reaction to these agents.

CONCLUSION ON REPERFUSION STRATEGY

Given the logistical issues, it is not possible to state definitively that a particular reperfusion approach is indicated for all patients, in all clinical settings, and at all times of day. The most important recommendation is that a reperfusion therapy should be selected immediately for all patients with suspected STEMI. The appropriate and timely use of any reperfusion therapy is likely more important than the type of therapy, as time is muscle and the latter determines the long-term outcome.

ROLE OF PCI AFTER FIBRINOLYTIC THERAPY

PCI after fibrinoytic therapy can be considered in various clinical settings such as the following:

Facilitated PCI. Performed following administration of reduced-dose fibrinolytic therapy, GP IIb/IIIa inhibitors, or a combination of both.
Rescue PCI. Performed emergently following failed fibrinolysis.
Immediate PCI. Performed within 24 hours following presumed successful fibrinolysis.
Delayed PCI. Performed within days following presumed successful fibrinolysis.

FACILITATED PCI

A meta-analysis of trials comparing primary PCI with facilitated PCI showed that STEMI patients who received facilitated PCI had initial higher TIMI 3 flow in infarct-related artery, but the final TIMI 3 flow rates were the same.[47] Furthermore, facilitated PCI was associated with significantly increased rates of nonfatal reinfarction, urgent target vessel revascularization, stroke, and death when compared with primary PCI.

In the facilitated intervention with enhanced reperfusion speed to stop events (FINESSE) trial,[48] STEMI patients who presented within 6 hours of symptom onset were randomized to primary PCI with adjunctive abciximab, upfront abciximab administered prior to catheterization laboratory arrival, or the combination of half-dose reteplase and abciximab administered prior to catheterization laboratory arrival. After a 90-day follow up, there was no difference in the primary outcome (all-cause mortality, rehospitalization, ventricular function more than 48 hours after randomization, cardiogenic shock, and congestive heart failure) among the three strategies. However, bleeding increased significantly in patients who were randomized to facilitated PCI, especially those who received half-dose reteplase and abciximab. Thus, the randomized trial data available to date do not support a strategy of facilitated PCI.

RESCUE PCI

Reperfusion after fibrinolytic therapy is considered to have failed if at 90 minutes after initiation of fibrinolytic therapy, there is <50% ST-segment resolution in the lead that showed the greatest degree of ST elevation at presentation.[49] The ACC/AHA STEMI guidelines recommend rescue PCI in the following cases: fibrinolytic-treated STEMI patients meeting high-risk criteria (i.e., cardiogenic shock [<75 years of age, class I; 75 years of age or older, class IIa]; hemodynamic or electrical instability; persistent ischemic symptoms) and for certain moderate- and high-risk patients who did not strictly meet the above criteria (class IIb).[7] These recommendations were based on results of the rescue angioplasty versus conservative treatment of repeat thrombolysis (REACT) trial,[50] which showed that event-free survival was significantly higher in patients treated with rescue PCI compared to conservative therapy or repeat fibrinolysis (84.6% vs. 70.1% vs. 68.7%, respectively). A recent meta-analysis[51] of eight trials (including REACT trial) showed that when compared with conservative therapy, rescue PCI was associated with a trend toward reduction in all-cause mortality, a significant reduction in the risk for heart failure and reinfarction when compared with conservative therapy. The expected benefits of rescue PCI are greater with earlier PCI after the onset of ischemic symptoms.

IMMEDIATE PCI

Several trials have evaluated the outcomes of immediate PCI and have shown significantly better clinical outcomes with immediate PCI and no significant increase of bleeding in high-risk patients.

The trial of routine angioplasty and stenting after fibrinolysis to enhance reperfusion in acute myocardial infarction (TRANSFER-AMI)[52] tested the immediate PCI concept in high-risk STEMI patients. Patients with high-risk STEMI who were treated with fibrinolytics were randomized to a pharmacoinvasive strategy (immediate transfer for PCI within 6 hours of fibrinolytic therapy) or to a standard treatment after fibrinolytic therapy, which included rescue PCI as required. The 30-day composite of death, reinfarction, recurrent ischemia, new or worsening heart failure, and cardiogenic shock were significantly lower in the immediate PCI group compared to standard therapy group (11.0% vs 17.2%, *P* = .004). These results lend further support to the routine, early transfer of high-risk, fibrinolytic treated patients to a PCI center for early PCI supported by contemporary antiplatelet and antithrombotic therapy.

DELAYED PCI AND THE OPEN ARTERY HYPOTHESIS

Should stable, high-risk STEMI patients with persistent, complete occlusion of the infarct-related artery presenting outside the currently accepted period for myocardial salvage of 12 hours receive only optimal medical therapy, or should they, in addition, undergo PCI of the infarct-related artery? The answer to this question is still unclear. The open artery hypothesis asserts that the restoration of antegrade flow in the infarct-related artery days, weeks, or even several months after MI would improve long-term outcome and survival even if left ventricular function did not improve. Two pivotal trials led to this assertion: the Western Washington trial[53] in which fibrinolytic therapy, using streptokinase, improved survival without improving left ventricular function, and the Second International Study of Infarct Survival (ISIS-2 trial), in which streptokinase improved mortality even in patients receiving it between 13 and 24 hours after the onset of STEMI.[54] The open artery hypothesis is also strongly supported by several nonrandomized, retrospective studies.[55–57] However, the recently published results of the multicenter, randomized open artery trial (OAT) did not corroborate the open artery hypothesis within the first 30 days after the MI.[58] The OAT trial, which randomized 2,166 patients with total occlusion of the infarct-related artery within 3 to 28 days after STEMI and mean left ventricular ejection fraction (LVEF) below 50% to optimal medical therapy alone or optimal medical therapy with PCI, showed no reduction in major cardiovascular events (death, reinfarction, or heart failure) during a mean follow-up of up to 4 years. There was a statistically nonsignificant trend toward excess reinfarction in the PCI cohort. TOSCA-2, a substudy of 381 patients in OAT, failed to demonstrate any significant improvement in LVEF in patients with PCI than in those receiving medical therapy (48.3% to 52.5% and 48.0% to 51.2%, respectively).[59] At 1 year, there was no significant difference between the PCI and medical therapy groups with regard to the increases seen in LVEF (48.3% to 52.5% and 48.0% to 51.2%, respectively). In patients presenting late after STEMI, rigorous selection criteria that include demonstrating a large area of myocardium at risk and ascertainment of myocardial viability using noninvasive tests may be necessary before PCI of the infarct-related artery is undertaken.

Although the 2009 ACC/AHA STEMI guidelines[7] focused update does not recommend the use of terms such as facilitated, rescue, immediate or delayed PCI in discussing reperfusion strategies, a good understanding of these strategies is, however, needed.

DRUG-ELUTING STENTS VERSUS BARE-METAL STENTS

The use of drug-eluting stents (DES) in STEMI has been controversial. Many randomized controlled trials comparing primary angioplasty to primary PCI with bare-metal stents (BMS) have shown a clear benefit with stent placement in rates of restenosis, reocclusion, and target vessel revascularization, although no significant difference in mortality was seen.[60–62]

The recent randomized harmonizing outcomes with revascularization and stents in acute myocardial infarction (HORIZONS-AMI) trial compared DES with BMS in 3,006 STEMI patients undergoing primary PCI. At 1-year follow-up there was no difference in the composite endpoint of death, reinfarction, stroke, or stent thrombosis. The rates of target vessel and target lesion revascularization were significantly lower in the DES group compared to BMS group (5.8% vs. 8.7% and 4.5% vs. 7.5%, respectively).[63] Patient selection, just as with elective PCI, is crucial to minimize the risk of late stent thrombosis with DES.

THROMBUS ASPIRATION

The 2009 ACC/AHA STEMI guidelines focused update has added manual thrombus aspirations as a class IIa indication. This recommendation is based on data from Thrombus Aspiration During Percutaneous Coronary Intervention in Acute Myocardial Infarction Study (TAPAS) and Thrombectomy with Export Catheter in Infarct-related Artery During Primary Percutaneous Coronary Intervention. (EXPIRA) trials.[64,65] In the TAPAS trial, 1,071 patients were randomized to manual thrombus aspiration before PCI or PCI with balloon angioplasty followed by stenting. Thrombus aspiration before PCI group had significantly higher rates of complete resolution of ST-segment elevation and at 1-year follow-up had significantly lower rates of cardiac death and nonfatal reinfarction. In the EXPIRA trial, TIMI myocardial blush grade of 2 or more and 90-minute ST-segment resolution >70% occurred more frequently in the thrombus aspiration group. Furthermore, only the thrombus aspiration group showed significant reduction in infarct size measured by contrast-enhanced magnetic resonance imaging. These trials compared routine use of thrombus aspiration to no thrombus aspiration; therefore, the benefit of selective thrombus aspiration in patients with large thrombus burden remains unclear.

ADJUNCT MEDICAL THERAPY

ANTIPLATELET AGENTS

As mentioned earlier, plaque rupture leads to flow-limiting stenosis and eventual thrombus formation and cessation of blood flow.[5] Persistent cessation of blood flow leads to acute MI. The adhesion, activation, and aggregation of platelets at the ruptured plaque play an important role in the thrombus formation. Additional platelet recruitment occurs through the release of thromboxane A2 (TXA2) and ADP, and activation of GP IIb/IIIa receptors[66] leading to further propagation of the thrombus. A thrombus rich in platelets is much more resistant to fibrinolytic therapy and promotes reocclusion even after successful fibrinolysis.[67] Increased platelet activation is also seen after primary PCI in patients with acute STEMI,[68] thus increasing thrombotic reocclusion. Antiplatelet agents thus play a vital role in patients with STEMI.

Types of antiplatelet agents and their mechanism of action are as follows:

- *Aspirin*: Blocks the enzyme cyclooxygenase, which is the mediator of initial step in the synthesis of TXA 2 and arachidonic acid.[69]
- *Thienopyridines*: This class includes clopidogel, ticlopidine and prasugrel. These medications block the binding of ADP to the P2Y12 receptors in the platelets and prevent activation of the GP IIb/IIIa receptor complex and subsequent aggregation of platelets.[70]
- *GP IIb/IIIa receptor inhibitors*: As the name suggests, they inhibit the GP IIb/IIIa receptors and thus prevent platelet aggregation by blocking the binding of the GP IIb/IIIa receptor to fibrinogen, thereby inhibiting fibrinogen–platelet bridging.[71]

ASPIRIN

Aspirin use in patients with STEMI is associated with both short- and long-term benefit. When started within 24 hours of STEMI, at 5 weeks, aspirin use was associated with a 23% reduction in vascular mortality and when used with streptokinase was associated with a 42% reduction.[72] A meta-analysis of 15 trials showed aspirin use to decrease vascular events by 30% at 30-day and by 25% at 2-year follow-up.[73]

DOSING AND DURATION

For STEMI patients' post-PCI, the current ACC/AHA STEMI guidelines recommend a dose of 162 to 325 mg of aspirin for at least 1 month in patients who received a BMS, for 3 months in those who received a sirolimus-eluting stent, and for 6 months for those who received a paclitaxel-eluting stent. Following this minimum period, a dose of 75 to 162 mg is recommended indefinitely.[49]

THIENOPYRIDINES

These include clopidogrel, ticlopidine, and prasugrel. Thienopyridines have an additive benefit when used with aspirin.

Clopidogrel. In two randomized trials (COMMIT/CCS-2 and CLARITY-TIMI 28) of patients treated with fibrinolytic therapy and heparin, there was benefit from early administration of clopidogrel in addition to aspirin.[74,75] In patients who have received fibrinolytic therapy, the current ACC/AHA guidelines recommend a loading dose of 300 to 600 mg, with continuation of clopidogrel at 75 mg per day for at least 14 days. In patients undergoing primary PCI for STEMI, indirect evidence from subset analysis of patients enrolled in CLARITY-TIMI 28 and other randomized trials in patients with non-ST elevation MI shows additive benefit of clopidogrel when used with aspirin.[76–78] In the HORIZONS AMI trial, a 600-mg loading dose, compared to 300-mg loading dose was a significant independent predictor of lower rates of major adverse cardiac events with no increase in the rate of major bleeding at the higher dose.[79]

Ticlopidine. Owing to its association with higher hematologic complications, such as neutropenia[80] and thrombotic thrombocytopenic purpura, the use of ticlopidine is almost nonexistent. Clopidogrel is preferred over ticlopidine due to its better side-effect profile.

Prasugrel. In the TRITON-TIMI 38 trial, 13,608 patients with moderate to high-risk ACS including 3,534 patients with STEMI were randomized to prasugrel versus clopidogrel.[81] At 15-month follow-up the primary endpoint of cardiovascular death, nonfatal MI, or nonfatal stroke was significantly lower with prasugrel compared to clopidogrel (10% vs. 12.4%). The rate of stent thrombosis was also significantly lower in the prasugrel group (1.6% vs. 2.8%). In a subset analysis, prasugrel was found to be especially beneficial in patients with diabetes.[82] In patients at high risk for bleeding (age ≥ 75 years, weight ≤ 60 kg, or those with prior stroke or transient ischemic attack), prasugrel was associated with significantly higher bleeding and hence should be avoided.

In patients undergoing primary PCI, the current ACC/AHA guidelines recommend a loading dose of 600 mg of clopidogrel or 60 mg of prasugrel to be given as early as possible before or at the time of PCI. In patients receiving a stent (BMS or DES) during PCI for ACS, a daily dose of 75 mg of clopidogrel or 10 mg of prasugrel should be given for at least 12 months.[7]

TICAGRELOR AND CANGRELOR

Ticagrelor is a cyclopentyltriazolopyrimidine, which has a more rapid onset of action than clopidogrel and binds reversibly rather than irreversibly with the P2Y12 platelet receptor.[83] In the PLATO trial with 18,624 patients (38% with STEMI) ticagrelor had significantly better outcomes than clopidogrel.[84] Cangrelor is an intravenous non-thienopyridine P2Y12 receptor blocker that has not been shown to be superior to clopidogrel in patients with ACS undergoing PCI.[85]

GLYCOPROTEIN IIB/IIIA INHIBITORS

The currently available agents in this class include abciximab, tirofiban, and eptifibatide. Although no major studies with head-to-head comparison are available, based on the data from smaller trials, all are considered equally efficacious.[86,87] In the setting of primary PCI for STEMI, abciximab has been studied the most. In patients with STEMI undergoing primary PCI, the current guidelines recommend the used of GP IIb/IIIa inhibitors in selected cases, such as patients with a large thrombus burden or in patients with inadequate thienopyridine loading. GP IIb/IIIa inhibitors should be used as adjunct therapy with dual-antiplatelet therapy and anticoagulation with unfractionated heparin or bivalirudin.[7]

CLOPIDOGREL RESISTANCE

Clopidogrel resistance is defined as incomplete blockade of the platelet membrane P2Y12 receptor, as measured by various laboratory tests specific to clopidogrel's mechanism of platelet inhibition, in patients on clopidogrel therapy. The mechanism of clopidogrel resistance is multifactorial, including variations in the absorption or metabolism of clopidogrel, or in the combination of clopidogrel with its specific platelet receptor.[88] The clinical outcomes in patients with clopidogrel resistance have been worse compared to patients with no resistance.[89] A higher loading dose (600 mg) and a higher maintenance dose (150 mg daily) have shown to increase P2Y12 receptor blockade in several studies. However, preliminary data from the gauging responsiveness with a verifyNow assay impact on thrombosis and safety (GRAVITAS) trial, the largest randomized trial to date in patients with clopidogrel resistance, comparing a higher loading (600 mg) and maintenance dose (150 mg daily) of clopidogrel to regular maintenance dose (75 mg), showed increased P2Y12 receptor blockade with a higher dose, but there was no additional clinical benefit.[90] The correct approach to improve clinical benefits in patients with clopidogrel resistance is unclear, but alternative medications such as prasugrel and ticagrelor might be of benefit and further studies are needed.

ANTICOAGULATION

Several anticoagulants are currently available for adjunct therapy in patients with STEMI. These include the following:

Unfractionated heparin (UFH)
Low-molecular-weight heparin (enoxaparin)
Direct-thrombin inhibitors (bivalirudin)
Synthetic heparin pentasaccharide (fondaparinux)

The choice of anticoagulant is dependant of the patients' risk of bleeding and treatment strategy.

For primary PCI. According to the current ACC/AHA guidelines, in patients with STEMI undergoing primary PCI, UFH with planned GP IIb/IIIa inhibitors or bivalirudin with provisional GP IIb/IIIa inhibitors is recommended. In patients with higher risk of bleeding bivalirudin is a reasonable choice. In patients who have received enoxaparin, if the last subcutaneous dose was administered at least 8 to 12 hours earlier, an additional IV dose of 0.3 mg per kg of enoxaparin is recommended. If the last subcutaneous dose was administered within the prior 8 hours, no additional enoxaparin is recommended.[7] The anticoagulation should be stopped at the end of the intervention, except in complicated cases and if there is ongoing ischemia.

For fibrinolytic therapy. In patients with STEMI undergoing reperfusion with fibrinolytics therapy, enoxaparin or fondaparinux are recommended. UFH is a reasonable alternative especially in patients undergoing PCI after fibrinolytic therapy.[7] Anti-coagulation therapy should be continued until hospital discharge.

No reperfusion therapy. In patients with STEMI who do not undergo reperfusion therapy, anticoagulation with enoxaparin or fondaparinux is recommended over UFH and should be continued until hospital discharge.[7]

β-BLOCKERS

Oral β-blockers are recommended within the first 24 hours in all patients with STEMI, who do have any contraindications. Patients with contraindications should be reevaluated after

24 hours for β-blocker therapy. IV β-blockers are a reasonable alternative in patients who are hypertensive at the time of presentation. IV β-blockers are contraindicated in patients with signs of heart failure or evidence of a low output state or with increased risk for cardiogenic shock or other relative contraindications to β blockade.[7]

NITRATES

IV nitrates can be used in patients with persistent chest pain or hypertension. Nitrated should be avoided in patients with severe aortic stenosis, right ventricular infarction, and with concomitant use of phosphodiesterase inhibitors.

SECONDARY PREVENTION

For secondary prevention after an acute MI, the following are recommended[49]:

1. *Blood pressure (BP) control.* It is recommended to initiate lifestyle modifications and/or medical therapy after an acute MI to achieve a goal of <140/90 mm Hg or <130/80 mm Hg if patient has diabetes or chronic kidney disease.
2. *Lipid management.* It is recommended to initiate dietary and lifestyle modifications for lipid management immediately after an acute MI. In patients with an LDL-C of 100 mg per dl or more, LDL-C lowering drug therapy should be initiated to achieve a goal of <100 mg per dl. Further reduction of LDL-C to <70 mg per dl is also considered reasonable.
3. *Diabetes.* Glucose control in coordination with a primary care physician or an endocrinologist is recommended with a target HA1c of <7%.
4. *Physical activity and weight reduction.* Medically supervised cardiac rehabilitation is recommended for patients after a recent MI and/or heart failure. A goal of 30 to 60 minutes of moderate aerobic activity every day or at least 5 days a week is recommended. An initial weight reduction goal of 10% from baseline should be targeted and further weight loss encouraged to achieve a BMI between 18.5 and 24.9 kg per m^2 and waist circumference of <40 inches in men and <35 inches in women.
5. *Smoking and alcohol.* Complete smoking cessation and avoidance of environmental tobacco smoke is highly recommended. Regular counseling to quit smoking should be given to all tobacco users and family members who smoke, and a plan for quitting should be developed to assist the patients.
6. *Medications.* β-blockers, as stated earlier should be started within 24 hours of an STEMI and continued indefinitely. Angiotensin converting enzyme (ACE) inhibitors should be started and continued indefinitely after STEMI in patients with LVEF <40%, hypertension, diabetes, chronic renal insufficiency or those who do not undergo revascularization. In patients intolerant to ACE inhibitors, angiotensin receptor blockers (ARB) can be used.

FUTURE DIRECTIONS

There is still much public education necessary to improve the symptom onset to presentation time for medical evaluation. This is especially true in those patients, for whom English is not the first language. In addition, therapies aimed at preventing microcirculatory disturbance are needed to further improve the reperfusion therapy. Finally, novel therapies to "regenerate" infarcted myocardium, such as stem cell or bone marrow precursor therapy in the infarcted area, may further improve the long-term outcome.

REFERENCES

1. Lloyd-Jones D, Adams RJ, Brown TM, et al.; for the American Heart Association Statistics Committee and Stroke Statistics. Heart disease and stroke statistics—2010 update: a report from the American Heart Association Statistics Committee and Stroke Statistics Subcommittee. *Circulation.* 2010;121(7):e46–e215.
2. Herzog E, Saint-Jacques H, Rozanski A. The PAIN pathway as a tool to bridge the gap between evidence and management of acute coronary syndrome. *Crit Pathw Cardiol J Evid Based Med.* 2004;3(1):20–24.
3. Berger PB, Ellis SG, Holmes DR Jr, et al. Relationship between delay in performing direct coronary angioplasty and early clinical outcome in patients with acute myocardial infarction: results from the Global Use of Strategies to Open Occluded Arteries in Acute Coronary Syndromes (GUSTO-IIb) trial. *Circulation.* 1999;100:14–20.
4. Cannon CP, Gibson CM, Lambrew CT, et al. Relationship of symptom-onset-to-balloon time and door-to-balloon time with mortality in patients undergoing angioplasty for acute myocardial infarction. *JAMA.* 2000;283:2941–2947.
5. Shin J, Edelberg JE, Hong MK. Vulnerable atherosclerotic plaque: clinical implications. *Curr Vasc Pharmacol.* 2003;1:183–204.
6. Antman EM, Anbe DT, Armstrong PW, et al. ACC/AHA guidelines for the management of patients with ST-elevation myocardial infarction: a report of the American College of Cardiology/American Heart Association Task Force on Practice Guidelines (Committee to Revise the 1999 Guidelines for the Management of Patients with Acute Myocardial Infarction). *Circulation.* 2004;110:282–292.
7. Kushner FG, Hand M, Smith SC Jr, et al. 2009 focused updates: ACC/AHA guidelines for the management of patients with ST-elevation myocardial infarction (updating the 2004 guideline and 2007 focused update) and ACC/AHA/SCAI guidelines on percutaneous coronary intervention (updating the 2005 guideline and 2007 focused update): a report of the American College of Cardiology Foundation/American Heart Association Task Force on Practice Guidelines. *Circulation.* 2009;120:2271.
8. Keeley EC, Boura JA, Grines CL. Primary angioplasty versus intravenous thrombolytic therapy for acute myocardial infarction: a quantitative review of 23 randomized trials. *Lancet.* 2003;361:13–20.
9. Antman EM, Cohen M, Bernink PJ, et al. The TIMI risk score for unstable angina/non-ST elevation MI: a method for prognostication and therapeutic decision making. *JAMA.* 2000;284(7):835–842.
10. Granger CB, Goldberg RJ, Dabbous O, et al. Predictors of hospital mortality in the global registry of acute coronary events. *Arch Intern Med.* 2003;163(19):2345–2353.
11. Marrrow DA, Antman EM, Parsons L, et al. Application of the TIMI risk score for ST-elevation MI in the National Registry of Myocardial Infarction 3. *JAMA.* 2001;286:1356.
12. Wu AH, Parsons L, Every NR, et al. Hospital outcomes in patients presenting with congestive heart failure complicating acute myocardial infarction: a report from the Second National Registry of Myocardial Infarction (NRMI-2). *J Am Coll Cardiol.* 2002;40:1389–1394.
13. Taher T, Fu Y, Wagner GS, et al. Aborted myocardial infarction in patients with ST-segment elevation: insights from the Assessment of the Safety and Efficacy of a New Thrombolytic Regimen-3 Trial Electrocardiographic Substudy. *J Am Coll Cardiol.* 2004;44:38–43.
14. Keeley EC, Grines CL. Should patients with acute myocardial infarction be transferred to a tertiary center for primary angioplasty or receive it at qualified hospitals in the community? The case for emergency transfer for primary percutaneous coronary intervention. *Circulation.* 2005;112:3520–3532; discussion 33.
15. McGrath PD, Wennberg DE, Dickens JD Jr, et al. Relation between operator and hospital volume and outcomes following percutaneous coronary interventions in the era of the coronary stent. *JAMA.* 2000;284:3139–3144.
16. A clinical trial comparing primary coronary angioplasty with tissue plasminogen activator for acute myocardial infarction. The Global Use of Strategies to Open Occluded Coronary Arteries in Acute Coronary Syndromes (GUSTO IIb) Angioplasty Substudy Investigators. *N Engl J Med.* 1997;336:1621–1628.
17. Grines CL, Cox DA, Stone GW, et al. Coronary angioplasty with or without stent implantation for acute myocardial infarction. Stent Primary Angioplasty in Myocardial Infarction Study Group. *N Engl J Med.* 1999;341:1949–1956.
18. The effects of tissue plasminogen activator streptokinase or both on coronary artery patency ventricular function and survival after acute myocardial infarction. The GUSTO Angiographic Investigators. *N Engl J Med.* 1993;329:1615–1622.
19. Bode C, Smalling RW, Berg G, et al. Randomized comparison of coronary thrombolysis achieved with double bolus reteplase (recombinant plasminogen activator) and front loaded accelerated alteplase (recombinant tissue plasminogen activator) in patients with acute myocardial infarction. The RAPID II Investigators. *Circulation.* 1996;94:891–898.
20. Cannon CP, Gibson CM, McCabe CH, et al. TNK tissue plasminogen activator compared with front loaded alteplase in acute myocardial infarction results of the TIMI 10B trial thrombolysis in myocardial infarction (TIMI) 10B investigators. *Circulation.* 1998;98:2805–2814.
21. Weaver WD, Simes RJ, Betriu A, et al. Comparison of primary coronary angioplasty and intravenous thrombolytic therapy for acute myocardial infarction a quantitative review. *JAMA.* 1997;278:2093–2098.
22. Neuhaus KL, Von Essen R, Tebbe U, et al. Improved thrombolysis in acute myocardial infarction with front loaded administration of alteplase results of the rt-PA-APSAC patency study (TAPS). *J Am Coll Cardiol.* 1992;19:885–891.

23. White HD, French JK, Hamer AW, et al. Frequent reocclusion of patent infarct related arteries between 4 weeks and 1 year effects of antiplatelet therapy. *J Am Coll Cardiol.* 1995;2:218–223.
24. Wilson SH, Bell MR, Rihal CS, et al. Infarct artery reocclusion after primary angioplasty stent placement and thrombolytic therapy for acute myocardial infarction. *Am Heart J.* 2001;141:704–710.
25. Meijer A, Verheugt FW, Werter CJ, et al. Aspirin versus coumadin in the prevention of reocclusion and recurrent ischemia after successful thrombolysis a prospective placebo controlled angiographic study. Results of the APRICOT Study. *Circulation.* 1993;87: 1524–1530.
26. Takens BH, Brugemann J, Van der Meer J, et al. Reocclusion three months after successful thrombolytic treatment of acute myocardial infarction with activated plasminogen streptokinase activating complex. *Am J Cardiol.* 1990;5:1422–1424.
27. Nijland F, Kamp O, Verheugt FW, et al. Long term implications of reocclusion on left ventricular size and function after successful thrombolysis for first anterior myocardial infarction. *Circulation.* 1997;95:111–117.
28. Antoniucci D, Santoro GM, Bolognese L, et al. A clinical trial comparing primary stenting of the infarct related artery with optimal primary angioplasty for acute myocardial infarction: results from the Florence Randomized Elective Stenting in Acute Coronary Occlusions (FRESCO) trial. *J Am Coll Cardiol.* 1998;31:1234–1239.
29. Antoniucci D, Valenti R, Buonamici P, et al. Direct angioplasty and stenting of the infarct-related artery in acute myocardial infarction. *Am J Cardiol.* 1996;78:568–571.
30. Kastrati A, Pache J, Dirschinger J, et al. Primary intracoronary stenting in acute myocardial infarction: long-term clinical and angiographic follow-up and risk factor analysis. *Am Heart J.* 2000;139:208–216.
31. Rodriguez A, Bernardi V, Fernandez M, et al. In-hospital and late results of coronary stents versus conventional balloon angioplasty in acute myocardial infarction (GRAMI trial). Gianturco-Roubin in Acute Myocardial Infarction. *Am J Cardiol.* 1998;81:1286–1291.
32. Suryapranata H, Vanít HAW, Hoorntje JC, et al. Randomized comparison of coronary stenting with balloon angioplasty in selected patients with acute myocardial infarction. *Circulation.* 1998;97:2502–2505.
33. Kurisu S, Sato H, Kawagoe T, et al. Tako-tsubo-like left ventricular dysfunction with ST-segment elevation: a novel cardiac syndrome mimicking acute myocardial infarction. *Am Heart J.* 2002;143:448–455.
34. Stone GW, Grines CL, Browne KF, et al. Influence of acute myocardial infarction location on in-hospital and late outcome after primary percutaneous transluminal coronary angioplasty versus tissue plasminogen activator therapy. *Am J Cardiol.* 1996;78:19–25.
35. Henriques JP, Zijlstra F, vanít Hof AW, et al. Primary percutaneous coronary intervention versus thrombolytic treatment: long term follow up according to infarct location. *Heart.* 2006;92:75–79.
36. Hochman JS, Sleeper LA, Webb JG, et al. Early revascularization in acute myocardial infarction complicated by cardiogenic shock. SHOCK Investigators. SHould we emergently revascularize Occluded Coronaries for cardiogenic shocK. *N Engl J Med.* 1999;341:625–634.
37. Bradley EH, Herrin J, Wang Y, et al. Strategies for reducing the door-to-balloon time in acute myocardial infarction. *N Engl J Med.* 2006;355:2308–2320.
38. Stenestrand U, Lindback J, Wallentin L. Long-term outcome of primary percutaneous coronary intervention vs prehospital and in-hospital thrombolysis for patients with ST-elevation myocardial infarction. *JAMA.* 2006;296:1749–1756.
39. Bonnefoy E, Lapostolle F, Leizorovicz A, et al. Primary angioplasty versus prehospital fibrinolysis in acute myocardial infarction: a randomized study. *Lancet.* 2002;360:825–829.
40. Aversano T, Aversano LT, Passamani E, et al. Thrombolytic therapy vs primary percutaneous coronary intervention for myocardial infarction in patients presenting to hospitals without on-site cardiac surgery: a randomized controlled trial. *JAMA.* 2002;287:1943–1951.
41. Boersma E, Maas AC, Deckers JW, et al. Early thrombolytic treatment in acute myocardial infarction: reappraisal of the golden hour. *Lancet.* 1996;348:771–775.
42. Zeymer U, Tebbe U, Essen R, et al. Influence of time to treatment on early infarct related artery patency after different thrombolytic regimens. ALKK-Study Group. *Am Heart J.* 1999;137:34–38.
43. Appleby P, Baigent C, Collins R, et al. Indications for fibrinolytic therapy in suspected acute myocardial infarction: collaborative overview of early mortality and major morbidity results from all randomized trials of more than 1000 patients. Fibrinolytic Therapy Trialists' (FTT) Collaborative Group. *Lancet.* 1994;343:311–322.
44. Weaver WD, Cerqueira M, Halistrom AP, et al. Prehospital-initiated vs hospital initiated thrombolytic therapy. The Myocardial Infarction Triage and Intervention Trial. *JAMA.* 1993;270:1211–1216.
45. Emergency department: rapid identification and treatment of patients with acute myocardial infarction. National Heart Attack Alert Program Coordinating Committee, 60 Minutes to Treatment Working Group. *Ann Emerg Med.* 1994;23:311–329.
46. Morrison U, Verbeek PR, McDonald AC, et al. Mortality and prehospital thrombolysis for acute myocardial infarction: a meta-analysis. *JAMA.* 2000;283:2686–2692.
47. Keeley EC, Boura JA, Grines CL. Comparison of primary and facilitated percutaneous coronary interventions for ST-elevation myocardial infarction: quantitative review of randomized trials. *Lancet.* 2006;367:579–588.
48. Ellis SG, Tendera M, de Belder MA, et al. Facilitated PCI in patients with ST-elevation myocardial infarction. *N Engl J Med.* 2008;358:2205–2217.
49. Antman EM, Hand M, Armstrong PW, et al. 2007 focused update of the ACC/AHA 2004 guidelines for the management of patients with ST-elevation myocardial infarction: a report of the American College of Cardiology/American Heart Association Task Force on Practice Guidelines: 2007 Writing Group to Review New Evidence and Update the ACC/AHA 2004 Guidelines for the Management of Patients with ST-Elevation Myocardial Infarction. *J Am Coll Cardiol.* 2008;51:210–247.
50. Gershlick AH, Stephens-Lloyd A, Hughes S, et al. Rescue angioplasty after failed thrombolytic therapy for acute myocardial infarction. *N Engl J Med.* 2005;353:2758–2768.
51. Wijeysundera HC, Vijayaraghavan R, Nallamothu BK, et al. Rescue angioplasty or repeat fibrinolysis after failed fibrinolytic therapy for ST-segment myocardial infarction: a meta-analysis of randomized trials. *J Am Coll Cardiol.* 2007;49:422–430.
52. Cantor WJ, Fitchett D, Borgundvaag B, et al. Routine early angioplasty after fibrinolysis for acute myocardial infarction. *N Engl J Med.* 2009;360:2705–2718.
53. Kennedy JW, Ritchie JL, Davis KB, et al. Western Washington randomized trial of intracoronary streptokinase in acute myocardial infarction. *N Engl J Med.* 1983;309:1477–1482.
54. ISIS 2 (Second International Study of Infarct Survival) Collaborative Group. Randomised trial of intravenous streptokinase oral aspirin both or neither among 17,187 cases of suspected acute myocardial infarction ISIS 2. *Lancet.* 1988;2:349–360.
55. Cigarroa RG, Lange RA, Hillis LD. Prognosis after acute myocardial infarction in patients with and without residual anterograde coronary blood flow. *Am J Cardiol.* 1989;64:155–160.
56. Lange RA, Cigarroa RG, Hillis LD. Influence of residual antegrade coronary blood flow on survival after myocardial infarction in patients with multivessel coronary artery disease. *Coron Artery Dis.* 1990;1:59–63.
57. Lamas GA, Flaker GC, Mitchell G, et al. Effect of infarct artery patency on prognosis after acute myocardial infarction. *Circulation.* 1995;92:1101–1109.
58. Hochman JS, Lamas GA, Buller CE, et al.; for the Occluded Artery Trial Investigators. Coronary intervention for persistent occlusion after myocardial infarction. *N Engl J Med.* 2006;355:2395–2407.
59. Dzavik V, Buller CE, Lamas GA, et al. Randomized trial of percutaneous coronary intervention for subacute infarct-related coronary artery occlusion to achieve long-term patency and improve ventricular function: the Total Occlusion Study of Canada (TOSCA)-2 trial. *Circulation.* 2006;114:2449–2457.
60. Pasceri V, Patti G, Speciale G, et al. Meta-analysis of clinical trials on use of drug-eluting stents for treatment of acute myocardial infarction. *Am Heart J.* 2007;153:749–754.
61. Kastrati A, Dibra A, Spaulding C, et al. Meta-analysis of randomized trials on drug-eluting stents vs. bare-metal stents in patients with acute myocardial infarction. *Eur Heart J.* 2007;28: 2706–2713.
62. De Luca G, Stone GW, Suryapranata H, et al. Efficacy and safety of drug-eluting stents in ST-segment elevation myocardial infarction: a meta-analysis of randomized trials. *Int J Cardiol.* 2009;133:213–222.
63. Mehran R, Brodie B, Cox DA, et al. The harmonizing outcomes with revascularization and stents in acute myocardial infarction (HORIZONS-AMI) trial: study design and rationale. *Am Heart J.* 2008;156:44–56.
64. Svilaas T, Vlaar PJ, van der Horst I, et al. Thrombus aspiration during primary percutaneous coronary intervention. *N Engl J Med.* 2008;358:557–567.
65. Sardella G, Mancone M, Bucciarelli-Ducci C, et al. Thrombus aspiration during primary percutaneous coronary intervention improves myocardial reperfusion and reduces infarct size: the EXPIRA (thrombectomy with export catheter in infarct-related artery during primary percutaneous coronary intervention) prospective, randomized trial. *J Am Coll Cardiol.* 2009;53:309–315.
66. Furie B, Furie BC. Mechanisms of thrombus formation. *N Engl J Med.* 2008;359:938.
67. Jang IK, Gold HK, Ziskind AA, et al. Differential sensitivity of erythrocyte-rich and platelet-rich arterial thrombi to lysis with recombinant tissue-type plasminogen activator. A possible explanation for resistance to coronary thrombolysis. *Circulation.* 1989;79(4):920–928.
68. Gawaz M, Neumann FJ, Ott I, et al. Platelet function in acute myocardial infarction treated with direct angioplasty. *Circulation.* 1996;93(2):229–237.
69. Patrono C. Aspirin as an antiplatelet drug. *N Engl J Med.* 1994;330:1287.
70. Foster CJ, Prosser DM, Agans JM, et al. Molecular identification and characterization of the platelet ADP receptor targeted by thienopyridine antithrombotic drugs. *J Clin Invest.* 2001;107(12):1591–1598.
71. White HD. Non-ST-elevation acute coronary syndromes: unstable angina and non-ST elevation myocardial infarction. In: Topol EJ, ed. *Textbook of Cardiovascular Medicine.* 2nd ed. Philadelphia, PA: Lippincott, Williams & Wilkins; 2002:chap 17:351–384.6.
72. Randomised trial of intravenous streptokinase, oral aspirin, both, or neither among 17,187 cases of suspected acute myocardial infarction: ISIS-2. *Lancet.* 1988;2(8607):349–360.
73. Collaborative meta-analysis of randomised trials of antiplatelet therapy for prevention of death, myocardial infarction, and stroke in high risk patients. *BMJ.* 2002;324(7329):71–86.
74. COMMIT collaborative group. Addition of clopidogrel to aspirin in 45 852 patients with acute myocardial infarction: randomised, placebo-controlled trial. *Lancet.* 2005;366:1607–1621.
75. Sabatine MS, Cannon CP, Gibson CM, et al. Addition of clopidogrel to aspirin and fibrinolytic therapy for myocardial infarction with ST-segment elevation. *N Engl J Med.* 2005;352(12):1179–1189. Epub 2005 Mar 9.
76. Sabatine MS, Cannon CP, Gibson CM, et al. Effect of clopidogrel pretreatment before percutaneous coronary intervention in patients with ST-elevation myocardial infarction treated with fibrinolytics: the PCI-CLARITY study. *JAMA.* 2005;294(10):1224–1232. Epub 2005 Sep 4.
77. Mehta SR, Yusuf S, Peters RJ, et al. Effects of pretreatment with clopidogrel and aspirin followed by long-term therapy in patients undergoing percutaneous coronary intervention: the PCI-CURE study. *Lancet.* 2001;358(9281):527–533.
78. Steinhubl SR, Berger PB, Brennan DM, et al. Optimal timing for the initiation of pretreatment with 300 mg clopidogrel before percutaneous coronary intervention. *J Am Coll Cardiol.* 2006;47(5):939–943. Epub 2006 Feb 9.
79. Stone GW, Witzenbichler B, Guagliumi G, et al. Bivalirudin during primary PCI in acute myocardial infarction. *N Engl J Med.* 2008;358(21):2218–2230.
80. Haushofer A, Halbmayer WM, Prachar H. Neutropenia with ticlopidine plus aspirin. *Lancet.* 1997;349:474.
81. Morrow DA, Wiviott SD, White HD, et al. Effect of the novel thienopyridine prasugrel compared with clopidogrel on spontaneous and procedural myocardial infarction in the Trial to Assess Improvement in Therapeutic Outcomes by Optimizing Platelet inhibition with Prasugrel-Thrombolysis in Myocardial Infarction 38: an application of the classification system from the universal definition of myocardial infarction. *Circulation.* 2009;119(21):2758–2764. Epub 2009 May 18.

82. Wiviott SD, Braunwald E, Angiolillo DJ, et al. Greater clinical benefit of more intensive oral antiplatelet therapy with prasugrel in patients with diabetes mellitus in the trial to assess improvement in therapeutic outcomes by optimizing platelet inhibition with prasugrel-thrombolysis in myocardial infarction 38. *Circulation*. 2008;118(16):1626–1636. Epub 2008 Aug 31.

83. Schomig A. Ticagrelor—is there need for a new player in the antiplatelet-therapy field? *N Engl J Med*. 2009;361:1108.

84. Wallentin L, Becker RC, Budaj A, et al. Ticagrelor versus clopidogrel in patients with acute coronary syndromes. *N Engl J Med*. 2009;361(11):1045–1057. Epub 2009 Aug 30.

85. Bhatt DL, Lincoff AM, Gibson CM, et al. Intravenous platelet blockade with cangrelor during PCI. *N Engl J Med*. 2009;361(24):2330–2341.

86. Raveendran G, Ting HH, Best PJ, et al. Eptifibatide vs abciximab as adjunctive therapy during primary percutaneous coronary intervention for acute myocardial infarction. *Mayo Clin Proc*. 2007;82(2):196–202.

87. Valgimigli M, Campo G, Percoco G, et al. Comparison of angioplasty with infusion of tirofiban or abciximab and with implantation of sirolimus-eluting or uncoated stents for acute myocardial infarction: the MULTISTRATEGY randomized trial. *JAMA*. 2008;299(15):1788–1799. Epub 2008 Mar 30.

88. Gurbel PA, Mahla E, Antonino MJ, et al. Response variability and the role of platelet function testing. *J Invasive Cardiol*. 2009;21:172.

89. Sibbing D, Morath T, Braun S, et al. Clopidogrel response status assessed with multiplate point-of-care analysis and the incidence and timing of stent thrombosis over six months following coronary stenting. *Thromb Haemost*. 2010;103(1):151–159.

90. Price M. Late breaking clinical trial at the American Heart Association Scientific Sessions; November 16, 2010; Chicago, IL.

PATIENT AND FAMILY INFORMATION FOR:

ST-Segment Elevation Myocardial Infarction

Heart attack or ST Elevation Myocardial Infarction (STEMI) is an emergency situation for patients. It occurs when one or more of the arteries supplying blood to the heart muscle become completely closed. Heart attacks are one of the most common diagnoses in hospitals and in the United States, it is a leading cause of death. Heart attacks are considered an emergency because the heart muscle dies permanently without blood flow after 30 minutes; therefore, it is important for the patients experiencing these symptoms to call 911 immediately.

CAUSES

Patients at risk for heart attack usually have mild blockages, caused by plaque accumulation in the wall of the blood vessel, which normally do not cause any symptoms or decrease blood flow to the heart muscle. These plaques develop over many years and as they increase in size, they become more unstable. With an inciting event, such as a physical exertion that increases the heart rate and force of contraction of the heart muscle, the plaque can rupture. As the blood continues to flow through that damaged vessel and around the plaque, blood components called platelets begin to form a clot and cause complete cessation of blood flow to the heart muscle. The cause of a heart attack is multifactorial, but it occurs most often in the presence of "risk factors" although a minority of patients, especially younger patients, can experience heart attacks without risk factors. The risk factors that have been identified to cause coronary artery disease and STEMI include a family history of heart attack or heart disease, diabetes or blood sugar elevation, high blood pressure, high cholesterol levels, cigarette smoking or tobacco use, and male gender.

FAMILY HISTORY

A patient's risk of having a heart attack is greatly increased by a family history of premature coronary artery disease defined as male relatives with a heart attack/disease before age 45 and female relatives with heart condition before age 55. This hereditary condition is also associated with high cholesterol levels. Family history is one of the nonmodifiable risk factors, although the associated high cholesterol levels can be treated with proper diet (low fat, low cholesterol) and medications when necessary.

DIABETES MELLITUS

Both childhood onset (type I) and adult onset (type II) diabetes are strong risk factors for STEMI for several reasons.

Diabetes adversely affects the balance of lipids in the body and accelerates the progression of the atherosclerotic plaques. It also causes the platelets to form blood clots more readily.

HYPERTENSION (HIGH BLOOD PRESSURE)

There is a direct correlation between high BP and STEMI. Medications prescribed to lower blood pressure have reduced the risk of STEMI.

HYPERLIPIDEMIA (HIGH CHOLESTEROL)

The lipid profile, a common laboratory test, includes measurement of LDL (bad cholesterol), HDL (good cholesterol), triglyceride levels, and total cholesterol. The risk for STEMI increases when HDL levels are low (<40 mg per dl), and LDL, total cholesterol, and triglyceride levels are elevated.

TOBACCO

Some of the toxins associated with cigarette smoking damage blood vessel walls. This leads to increased thrombus (clot) formation by platelets. Some studies have shown that these platelet thrombi accumulate more in vessels that have turbulent blood flow secondary to stenosis.

MALE GENDER

The overall incidence of STEMI is higher among men than women. However, as age increases, the disparity of STEMI incidence between males and females narrows.

Heart attacks are more common in older patients; however, approximately 50% of heart attacks occur in patients under 65 years. In younger patients, drugs such as cocaine or severe exertion such as heavy weight lifting in young men can also cause heart attacks.

INITIAL ASSESSMENT

The way that a heart attack presents can be variable, but most commonly patients experience profound chest tightness or heaviness, often associated with shortness of breath, dizziness, cold sweats, and anxiety. The chest pain is typically located in the center of the chest and often described as radiating to the left shoulder, arm, or jaw.

The symptoms usually begin during a period of vigorous physical exertion or mental and emotional stress and do not resolve during a period of rest following the exertion. When an individual presents with this type of history to the Emergency Department (ED), medical personnel use a chest pain protocol, which systematically permits rapid triage, initial diagnosis, and management.

The mainstay of diagnosis of a STEMI is the EKG. An EKG with electrodes attached to the outside of the chest wall measures the electrical conduction through the heart. It is essential to perform and interpret this test by an experienced physician within 10 minutes of ED arrival. The first visible change on the EKG is elevation of the "ST segment." This elevation distinguishes heart attack from other heart conditions. If the initial EKG does not indicate STEMI but a physician has a high suspicion, then an EKG is ordered every 5 to 10 minutes to assess an evolving ST-elevation. Other important tests for the diagnosis include laboratory markers of myocardial (heart) cell injury, including troponin and creatine kinase. These proteins and enzymes are normally contained inside the heart cells; however, when the cells die during a heart attack, these markers are released into the blood stream and can be measured.

If a STEMI is present on EKG, there are two options available to reopen a blocked vessel, both aimed at restoring blood flow to the dying heart muscle. Both of these treatments can be performed only in the hospital setting. The first treatment is the administration of a powerful blood clot dissolver called fibrinolytic therapy. The second treatment is a procedure called angioplasty, in which a balloon and/or stents are used by a cardiologist to open up the occluded artery. Recent research has shown that angioplasty and stent placement are the better option for effective therapy, and the ambulance crew in most cases can transport the patient to the nearest angioplasty hospital rather than smaller hospitals that cannot offer this procedure. The goals of an effective therapy are to administer fibrinolytic therapy within 30 minutes or to perform angioplasty within 90 minutes after presentation.

TREATMENT

The four most important elements in improving prognosis of STEMI are (1) prompt recognition of symptoms and seeking medical attention; (2) rapid deployment in emergency medical services; (3) transporting the patient to a facility with skilled physicians and nurses trained in taking care of patients with heart attack; and (4) employing an appropriate treatment, which efficiently relieves the blockage in the artery. The major delay in management of a STEMI is not so much in the medical facility or in transportation but in the patient's ability to recognize the symptoms and call for help. Once the diagnosis of a STEMI is established, supportive therapies are initiated that include oxygen, blood vessel dilator called nitrates, pain medicine such as morphine, and potent antiplatelet therapies. All patients should be placed on a cardiac monitor with a defibrillator on standby. Deciding between the two modes of reperfusion strategies depends on several factors. These factors include time between onset of chest pain and presentation, patient characteristics at presentation, and the availability of a skilled facility capable of angioplasty. Time is the most important factor in determining the therapy to be employed. Fibrinolytic therapy is preferred when there is an early presentation, generally <1 hour. The reason is that the efficacy of fibrinolytic agents in dissolving clots diminishes with the passage of time. Angioplasty is the preferred method when there is a delay between symptom onset and presentation to emergency room. Angioplasty has been shown to have better clinical outcomes in high-risk patients such as elderly or patients with heart failure. Finally, the biggest obstacle to the use of primary angioplasty for STEMI patient is the lack of a skilled facility capable of primary angioplasty. For those patients with STEMI who present to the facility without angioplasty capability, it is still recommended that they be transferred to another center with this capability as long as the patient undergoes the procedure within 90 minutes. On most occasions when an angioplasty is performed, a stent is placed in the vessel to prevent reocclusion. The two types of stents are BMS and DES. However, when angioplasty centers are not available or if the procedure is difficult to perform owing to the anatomy, fibrinolytic therapy is preferred. Fibrinolytic therapy is not recommended in certain situations, such as in patients with prior bleed in the brain, known brain aneurysms, or active bleeding anywhere in the body.

PREVENTION

There are two types of heart attack prevention. Primary prevention is aimed at minimizing the risk for the first heart attack. The goal of secondary prevention is to minimize the risk of a second heart attack. Primary prevention requires treatment of any risk factor and lifestyle modification, such as smoking cessation, avoidance of drug abuse, moderate exercise, and a healthy diet. Studies have shown that these measures can reduce the risk of a first heart attack, especially in those with high cholesterol levels. In addition, medications prescribed to lower cholesterol levels can also reduce the risk of a heart attack. Secondary prevention requires more effort on the part of the patient with a history of a previous heart attack. Not only do they need to adhere to the measures for primary prevention, but they must also be compliant with medications prescribed following the first heart attack. These medications usually include aspirin, a type of blood thinner, either clopidogrel or prasugrel, cholesterol lowering medications, statins, and other medications to improve the heart function. Furthermore, close follow-up with a cardiologist is very important to prevent complications from the heart attack and lower the risk of recurrence. The good news is that the death rate from heart attack continues to decrease. This trend can continue only if the patients and physicians work as a team, with each party contributing to the prevention of the heart attacks. Another important factor is the education of the population at risk and the certification of the public on CPR to save those suffering from heart attack and sudden death.

Non-ST Elevation Myocardial Infarction and Unstable Angina

EPIDEMIOLOGY

Unstable angina (UA) and non-ST-segment elevation myocardial infarction (NSTEMI) are part of the clinical spectrum known as acute coronary syndromes (ACS). They are often grouped together as one entity owing to their similar presenting characteristics and pathophysiology and are collectively referred to as the non-ST-segment elevation ACS (NSTE-ACS). NSTE-ACS is a highly prevalent and serious manifestation of coronary heart disease. There are approximately 1.36 million hospitalizations in the United States alone (765,000 males and 600,000 females) for all ACS (including ST-elevation MI [STEMI] and NSTE-ACS).[1] The estimated proportion of all ACS patients who present with NSTE-ACS varies with different registries; in the second Euro-Heart Survey, 53% of all cases of ACS were NSTE-ACS, whereas 68% of ACS cases reported by the AHA Get with the Guidelines Project, and 62% of cases reported in the study of the Global Registry of Acute Coronary Events (GRACE) were NSTE-ACS.[2]

PATHOPHYSIOLOGY

NSTE-ACS often occurs when there is an imbalance of myocardial oxygen supply and demand resulting in myocardial ischemia. By definition, UA is angina that has changed in quality. This includes new onset angina, angina that occurs with little or no activity, or prolonged episodes of angina. When myocardial ischemia is very prolonged, myocardial necrosis ensues. This is referred to as NSTEMI. Most cases of UA and NSTEMI are the result of severe atherosclerotic plaque causing impingement of the arterial lumen and partially impairing myocardial blood flow. Typically, atherosclerotic plaques comprise cellular debris, cholesterol, and a fibrous cap. In some cases, platelets accumulate on the surface of a ruptured plaque resulting in transient clot formation with occlusion of the lumen or distal micro-emboli and myocardial necrosis. NSTE-ACS can sometimes be seen in situations where there is less severe epicardial coronary artery obstruction. This includes (1) smooth muscle cell spasm with transient arterial occlusion (vasospastic angina); (2) moderate or severe obstruction accompanied by a severe imbalance in myocardial blood supply and demand (as a result of severe anemia, severe hypotension, or hypertensive crisis); (3) inflammation of the blood vessel walls resulting in thickening of the walls and luminal narrowing (vasculitis); or (4) conditions resulting in paradoxical coronary emboli such as atrial fibrillation, atrial myxoma, left ventricular (LV) clot, or vegetations of the heart valves.

DIAGNOSIS

HISTORY AND PHYSICAL EXAM

It is important that physicians maintain a high index of suspicion for all suspected cases of NSTE-ACS, so that rapid diagnosis can be made, allowing for early institution of medical therapies. Obtaining a detailed clinical history should be the first step in making the diagnosis. Myocardial ischemia typically produces symptoms that are commonly described as chest "squeezing," "heaviness," or "pressure," although it is not uncommon for patients to complain of a "stabbing," "sharp," "aching" or "burning" chest pain. Symptoms may radiate to the jaw, left arm/shoulder, or the back, and may be accompanied by shortness of breath, nausea, or diaphoresis. A history of progressive pain that is aggravated by physical activity or relieved with rest and culminates in symptoms with minimal activity or resting pain is very suggestive of UA, although many patients may present for the first time with rest symptoms. Not all patients have these classic symptoms, and NSTE-ACS should still be considered in patients who present only with shortness of breath, epigastric pain, or back pain. Up to 20% of patients with ACS do not have chest pain on hospital presentation. Older patients, female patients, and patients with diabetes mellitus are more likely to have no chest pain.[3] The remainder of the clinical history should be focused on related cardiac risk factors, and prior cardiac conditions including prior MI, percutaneous coronary interventions or coronary artery bypass (CABG) surgery as this will help to define a patients' cardiac risk. (See "Risk Stratification.")

The physical exam does not usually help in the diagnosis of NSTE-ACS as most patients have an unremarkable exam. However, the abnormalities including tachycardia, hypotension, heart murmurs, respiratory crackles, or poor distal pulses may indicate that the patient is at higher risk and therefore warrant therapies that are more aggressive.

ELECTROCARDIOGRAM

The ACC/AHA guidelines for the management of patients with UA/NSTEMI state that a 12-lead ECG should be performed as soon as possible after arrival in the emergency room (ER) and ideally within 10 minutes of presentation for all patients with suspected ACS.[4] This will allow for the immediate differentiation of patients with NSTE-ACS from those who have STEMI, as initial therapies will vary depending on the presenting type of ACS. ECG changes that are considered suspicious for NSTE-ACS include ST segment depressions of ≥0.5 to 1 mm or T-wave inversions of ≥2 mm in two or more contiguous leads. It is not uncommon however for a patient to have a normal ECG.

CARDIAC BIOMARKERS

The cardiac biomarkers are intracellular macromolecules that are released into the blood stream when myocardial necrosis and cell death occurs. The cardiac biomarkers, most commonly used today, include the cardiac troponins and creatinine phosphokinase (CPK-MB). There are three components of the troponin gene, Troponin T, Troponin I, and Troponin C. Troponin C can be found in both cardiac and skeletal muscles, whereas Troponin T or I are derived from "heart specific genes" and hence are collectively referred to as the cardiac troponins. The cardiac troponin assays are extremely sensitive and specific and are the test of choice when assessing for myocardial necrosis. Cardiac troponin elevations directly correlate with the degree of myocardial injury. There is an independent increased risk for death among the troponin positive patients when compared with those patients with negative troponins. Furthermore, there is an incremental relationship between the risk of death and the cardiac troponin level.[5] CPK-MB is a cytosolic carrier protein for high-energy phosphates. It is less sensitive and less specific for myocardial necrosis than the cardiac troponins; low levels of CPK-MB are sometimes found in the blood of healthy athletes or in association with skeletal muscle damage. CPK-MB should be used in cases when troponin assays are not available.

The cardiac biomarkers can be detected in the blood at anytime between 2 and 12 hours following myocardial necrosis. The cardiac troponin levels generally return to baseline at 4 to 14 days after the index event, whereas the CPK-MB levels will normalize much earlier (within 2 to 3 days).[6] Therefore, the CPK-MB is useful when evaluating patients with suspected reinfarction. Cardiac biomarkers should be obtained in all patients with suspected ACS. This allows the physician to classify patients further into UA and NSTEMI and provides the physician with an important tool used for risk stratification. It is recommended that a patient have an initial blood test on presentation and that this blood test be repeated 6 to 9 hours after admission and then again 12 to 24 hours.

RISK STRATIFICATION

There are two main questions one should ask when examining a patient with suspected ACS: (1) Are the symptoms the patient complains of indicative of cardiac ischemia? (2) If this is an ischemic event, what is the likelihood that this patient will suffer an adverse outcome from this event? The initial assessment will help to answer the former question and provide the clinician with a potential working diagnosis including noncardiac chest pain, and rule out ACS, UA, or NSTEMI. Assuming a working diagnosis of NSTE-ACS based on the initial assessment, the next step is to perform a detailed and accurate risk

assessment. Risk stratification provides the clinician with important information about a patient's prognosis and guides the use of subsequent medical and invasive therapies. For example, high-risk patients are usually treated with IV glycoprotein IIb/IIIa (GP IIb/IIIa) receptor antagonists and early catheterization. (See "Medical Treatment–Antiplatelet Therapy and Initial Conservative versus Initial Invasive Approach.")

The information used to estimate a patient's risk is derived from the patient's clinical history, physical exam, ECG findings, and cardiac biomarkers. In general, a patient can be stratified into three categories: low, intermediate, or high-risk groups. Low-risk patients include younger patients with a normal ECG who do not have any prolonged or recurrent symptoms, have no physical signs of CHF or shock, and have normal cardiac biomarkers. High-risk patients generally have evidence of extensive ischemia or infarction, with pathologic ST and T wave changes on ECG, or moderately to severely elevated cardiac biomarkers, or congestive heart failure/shock. Patients at intermediate risk are those who fall in between these categories.

Cardiac risk scores are simple tools that allow the clinician to estimate qualitatively a patient's risk based on the interplay of multiple clinical variables. There are various risk scores that have been derived and shown to correlate with clinical outcomes.[7-10] The Thrombolysis In Myocardial Infarction (TIMI) risk score[7] is the most commonly used tool for risk assessment and has been shown to have superior prognostic accuracy to that obtained using a physician's "in-formal" assessment.[11] This is a simple 7-point system that provides an estimate of a patient's risk of death, recurrent MI, or severe refractory ischemia requiring urgent revascularization at 2 weeks. The variables that are used in the score include (1) age >65 years, (2) prior known coronary stenosis of >50%, (3) the presence of at least three coronary artery disease risk factors, (4) elevated cardiac enzymes, (5) ST-segment deviation on ECG, (6) recurrent angina prior to presentation, and (7) aspirin use within the last week. One point is allocated for each of the seven variables used in the score, resulting in a total possible score of 7. Event rates increase significantly with increasing risk score (Figure 3.1). As an example, a 60-year-old otherwise healthy

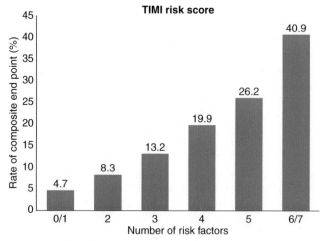

Figure 3.1. TIMI risk score rates of all-cause mortality, myocardial infarction, and severe recurrent ischemia prompting urgent revascularization through 14 days after non-ST elevation myocardial infarction or unstable angina.

male patient who has no previous medical history and is not taking any medications presents with onset of chest pain lasting for 20 minutes, without recurrence. His ECG and cardiac troponins are all normal. His TIMI risk score is zero, and he has a low likelihood for a cardiac event. However, a 78-year-old male with prior CABG surgery on aspirin presents with recurrent resting chest pain, ST-segment depression on ECG, and elevated cardiac troponins. He has a score of 6. Among patients like him, 40% will suffer a cardiac event in the ensuing 2 weeks.

The GRACE risk score[8] was designed to assess the likelihood of in-hospital death among patients with ACS including STEMI, NSTEMI, or UA using variables from an unselected population of patients enrolled in an international clinical registry. Although the TIMI risk score assigns an equal value to each risk, the GRACE risk score assigns values to each variable depending on the strength of the risk. In addition, because the GRACE score was derived from an unselected population of patients, it incorporates a larger range of clinical variables than the TIMI risk score including congestive heart failure, chronic kidney disease, and resuscitated cardiac arrest. In this score eight factors were identified as important predictors of risk (http://www.outcomes-umassmed.org/grace/). The GRACE risk score has been shown to have superior ability to differentiate risk groups and subsequent outcomes when compared with other risk scores.[12,13]

MEDICAL TREATMENT

The goal of medical therapy is to stabilize the patient, by relieving chest pain/symptoms (anti-ischemic agents) and protecting the patient from subsequent events including recurrent ischemia, MI, or death (antiplatelet/anticoagulants and statins).

ANTI-ISCHEMIC AGENTS

Oxygen. Oxygen use may cause comfort and provide relief from breathlessness that patients with myocardial ischemia sometimes feel. It should be used routinely in patients with NSTE-ACS who present with hypoxemia or respiratory distress.[4] Oxygen should be administered with caution to patients with concomitant chronic obstructive pulmonary disease (COPD).

Nitroglycerin. Nitroglycerin causes nitric-oxide-mediated vasorelaxation, with effects on both the coronary and peripheral vascular beds. By dilating the venous circulation, it results in a reduction in preload, which decreases wall stretch, and results in a decrease in myocardial oxygen demand and improvement in ischemic symptoms. Nitroglycerin causes a more modest reduction in afterload, further reducing myocardial oxygen demand. Nitroglycerin has direct effects on the epicardial coronary arteries, with dilatation of normal or diseased vessels. Because of the effects on the venous and arterial circulation, nitroglycerin is used to treat concomitant hypertension or congestive heart failure too. There is no role for the routine initiation of nitroglycerin in the absence of ischemic symptoms, congestive heart failure, or hypertension.[14]

Nitroglycerin should be administered sublingually for relief of ischemic chest pain at a dose of 0.4 mg every 5 minutes. The patient's blood pressure should be monitored carefully between each dose. After initial treatment with three sublingual tablets, consideration should be given to the initiation of IV nitroglycerin if chest pain persists. IV nitroglycerin should be administered at a starting dose of 10 μg per minute and increased by 10 to 20 μg per minute every 3 to 5 minutes as needed to control symptoms while maintaining adequate blood pressure. Once stabilized, a transition to oral long-acting formulations or trans-dermal dosing of nitroglycerin may be considered when clinically indicated for the treatment of intermittent chest pain, or in cases where optimization of medical therapy is planned.

Nitroglycerin should not be used in patients with hypotension or in patients with suspected right ventricular (RV) infarction/ischemia or volume depletion as the negative effect on preload may exacerbate hypotension. In addition, because phosphodiesterase inhibitors cause smooth muscle cell relaxation, they may potentiate the vasodilating effects of nitroglycerin. Therefore, nitroglycerin should also be avoided in patients who have recently taken an oral phosphodiesterase inhibitor.

Morphine. There is invariably some degree of discomfort as well as anxiety and apprehension in most of the patients presenting with NSTE-ACS. This often leads to an increase in sympathetic tone that can exacerbate the supply demand imbalance already seen in the ischemic myocardium. Morphine sulfate is the preferred agent for the relief of pain and anxiety related to ischemic chest discomfort. It can be administered intravenously at starting doses of 1 to 2 mg and repeated as needed to achieve the desired effect of pain relief. Morphine causes veno-dilation with a resultant decrease in preload and therefore is of special benefit in those patients with accompanying acute pulmonary edema or congestive heart failure. Morphine can lower blood pressure, and on occasion cause bradycardia (through increased vagal tone) or respiratory depression. Therefore, a patient's vital status should be carefully monitored for signs or symptoms of hypotension, bradycardia, or respiratory depression. Naloxone can be administered intravenously in doses of 0.1 to 0.2 mg every 15 minutes when indicated to reverse the narcotic effects of morphine. Of note, in a large observational registry of 443 hospitals in the United States enrolling 53,039 patients with NSTE-ACS,[15] the use of IV morphine sulfate was associated with a higher adjusted likelihood of death (propensity adjusted OR: 1.41, 95% CI 1.26, 1.56). Although not randomized, this information raises some concern regarding the use of morphine in patients with ACS.

β-Adrenergic blocking agents. β-Adrenergic blocking agents work by competitively blocking the effects of catecholamines on the β-receptors of cell membranes. Blockade of the B-1 receptors on cardiac myocytes produces slowing of the heart rate and decreased myocardial contractility. This results in decreased myocardial oxygen demand, which favorably shifts the supply demand imbalance toward decreased demand. β-Blockers are therefore indicated for the initial treatment of patients with presumed ACS. Oral β-adrenergic blocking agents should be initiated within the first 24 hours of presentation in the absence of a contraindication to use including hypotension, bradycardia (or high-grade atrioventricular block), congestive heart failure, or severe symptomatic reactive airway disease.

The utility of early intravenous β-blockers has been challenged recently by results of the ClOpidogrel and Metoprolol in Myocardial Infarction Trial (COMMIT) study. In this large randomized trial[16] 45,852 patients with acute MI (93% STEMI and 7% NSTEMI) were randomized to treatment with 15 mg of intravenous metoprolol given over 15 minutes followed by a dose of 200 mg of extended release oral metoprolol daily or placebo. The use of early intravenous β-blockers had a neutral effect on the combined endpoint of mortality, recurrent infarction, or cardiac arrest. There was a lower incidence of recurrent infarction in the treated group (2.0% vs. 2.5% $P = .0002$) that was balanced by a significantly higher rate of cardiogenic shock in this same group (5.0% vs. 3.9% $P < .00001$). Therefore, intravenous β-blockers should be reserved for those patients with refractory hypertension who do not appear to be at increased risk for developing cardiogenic shock.

There are various β-blocker regimens available to physicians for use, with only slight differences in their physical properties. The decision to use one β-blocking agent over another will be largely based on individual patient characteristics and physician/hospital preference: For example, when instituting a β-blocking agent, one may wish to use a short-acting regimen while titrating the initial dose. In addition, if a patient has a history of reactive airway disease, one might choose a predominantly β-1 selective β-blocker (metoprolol and atenolol) to minimize the β-2 effects of these agents that might potentiate bronchoconstriction. Finally, if a patient has a history of congestive heart failure or LV dysfunction one might consider the use of carvedilol or long-acting metoprolol as they have been proven beneficial for use in patients with compensated heart failure.[17–19]

Calcium channel blockers. Calcium channel blockers prevent the influx of calcium across the smooth muscle cell membrane thereby causing relaxation of the smooth muscle cells. There are two general classes of calcium channel blockers, the dihydropyridine calcium antagonists (nifedipine, felodipine, and amlodipine) and the non-dihydropyridine calcium antagonists (verapamil and cardizem). The dihydropyridine calcium antagonists predominantly exert their effects through relaxation of the peripheral vascular smooth muscle cells, whereas the non-dihydropyridines predominantly work by reducing myocardial contractility and AV nodal conduction. Both classes of agents have some effects on coronary vasodilatation. Small randomized controlled studies performed in the 1980s demonstrated that calcium channel blockers decrease ischemic symptoms and improve outcome in patients with UA or NSTEMI.[20,21] However, the short-acting dihydropyridine calcium channel blockers can cause a reflex tachycardia, thereby worsening ischemia. In the absence of concomitant β-blocker use the dihydropyridines have been shown to have a negative impact on outcome.[22] However, both verapamil and diltiazem have the potential to worsen congestive heart failure in patients with significant LV dysfunction. Therefore, calcium channel blockers are generally not considered first line therapy for the treatment of NSTE-ACS. However, if a patient has significant reactive airway disease preventing the administration of a β-blocker, a non-dihydropyridine may be considered as an alternative anti-ischemic agent, provided the patient does not have significant LV dysfunction or symptoms of congestive heart failure.

ANTIPLATELET THERAPY

Aspirin. Aspirin inhibits the synthesis of thromboxane A2, resulting in irreversible inhibition of the COX-1-mediated platelet aggregation for the life of a platelet. In a study of patients with UA, the use of aspirin resulted in a 51% reduction in risk of cardiac death or nonfatal infarction at a mean follow-up of 18 months.[23] As such, aspirin has since become part of the standard therapies used for all patients presenting to the hospital with NSTE-ACS. Aspirin should be given as an initial dose of 325 mg, followed by maintenance doses of 75 to 162 mg daily. If a patient undergoes percutaneous coronary intervention with stent placement, then doses of 162 to 325 mg may be considered post procedure. Aspirin allergy is rare and anyone reporting an allergy to aspirin should be further questioned as to the validity of this statement. In patients with true hypersensitivity to aspirin (hives or angioedema) alternative agents including clopidogrel may be substituted. Alternately, aspirin desensitization may be performed.

P2Y12 receptor blockers. The P2Y12 receptor antagonists include the thienopyridines (clopidogrel, prasugrel, and ticlopidine) that cause platelet inhibition by actively binding to the P2Y12 receptors of platelets resulting in irreversible inhibition of ADP-mediated platelet aggregation and activation for the life of the platelet, and ticagrelor that reversibly binds to the P2Y12 receptor on the surface of platelets. These agents differ slightly in their pharmacokinetics, and side effects; therefore, careful consideration should be given to a patient's clinical characteristics when choosing one agent over another. Ticlopidine was the first agent available for use and has been shown to be of benefit in the secondary prevention of stroke or MI. However, ticlopidine has the potential for serious hematologic side effects including neutropenia, thrombotic thrombocytopenia purpura, and bone marrow aplasia. Given the availability of several other alternative agents, ticlopidine is seldom used in modern practice. The remainder of this section will focus on a review of the more commonly used agents.

Dual antiplatelet therapy with clopidogrel plus aspirin is now standard practice for the treatment of patients presenting to the hospital with NSTE-ACS; this was largely based on the results of the Clopidogrel to Prevent Recurrent Events (CURE) trial.[24] In this study, 12,562 patients with NST-ACS were randomized to 300 mg oral load of clopidogrel followed by 75 mg daily in addition to aspirin or aspirin alone. Patients were followed up for 3 to 12 months. The primary outcome, which was a composite of death from cardiovascular causes, nonfatal MI, or stroke was significantly lower in the clopidogrel group compared to the placebo group (relative risk with clopidogrel as compared with placebo, 0.80; 95% CI, 0.72 to 0.90; $P < .001$). In this study, the group of patients assigned to clopidogrel had a significantly higher rate of major bleeding when compared with those in the placebo group although life-threatening bleeding or hemorrhagic stroke was similar in the two groups. Increased bleeding was notable among the patients undergoing urgent CABG surgery. Therefore, although there is a clear benefit to the routine use of dual antiplatelet therapy for patients with NSTE-ACS, one must exercise caution in patients who are at high bleeding risk, or among those patients in whom urgent cardiac surgery is planned. If cardiac surgery is planned, the ACC/AHA guidelines recommend withholding clopidogrel for 5 days prior to elective surgery if possible.[4]

Unlike aspirin, there is a delayed onset of optimal platelet inhibition following clopidogrel dosing; this varies with each person and with different doses, and can be as late as 12 to 24 hours. Studies have suggested shorter time to optimal platelet inhibition with a larger loading dose,[25] although the optimal loading dose of clopidogrel is not well established. In a recent clinical study examining this question,[26] patients with ACS were randomly assigned to one of two treatment strategies including a loading dose of 600 mg of clopidogrel followed by 150 mg daily for 1 week and then 75 mg daily thereafter, or a loading dose of

300 mg followed by 75 mg daily. In this trial there was no difference in cardiovascular death, MI, or stroke at 30 days for either of the two treatment strategies. However, an analysis examining outcome only among those patients who underwent percutaneous coronary intervention demonstrated a 32% reduction in the incidence of stent thrombosis in the double dose clopidogrel group (Hazard ratio 0.68, 95% CI 0.55 to 0.85, $P = .001$). Major bleeding was significantly higher in the double dose clopidogrel group. Given this information, consideration may be given to a 600 mg loading dose and 150 mg daily initial dose of Clopidogrel for the first week for patients with ACS who undergo percutaneous coronary intervention; there appears to be little added benefit to double dose therapy of clopidogrel among NSTE-ACS who are medically treated or who require surgical intervention.

Clopidogrel is a pro-drug requiring conversion to an active metabolite by the hepatic cytochrome P450 isoenzymes to exhibit antiplatelet effects. It has been shown that certain genetic subtypes have a loss of function of the allele of the *CYP2C19* gene (encoding for one of the hepatic isoenzymes responsible for the metabolism of clopidogrel) resulting in reduced conversion of clopidogrel to its active metabolite. Many studies have suggested that patients with genetic variants of this gene have a reduced pharmacodynamic response to clopidogrel and a higher rate of cardiovascular events when compared with those patients with normal genetic subtypes.[27–30] CYP2C19 is also inhibited by certain medications including the proton pump inhibitors. The co-administration of proton pump inhibitors attenuates the degree of platelet inhibition that occurs with clopidogrel.[31] It is important to realize that there are inconsistencies in these clinical studies. Other studies have not demonstrated an adverse association with clinical outcome related to either an acquired or inherited deficiency in the CYP2C19 isoenzyme.[32,33] The discrepancy in these reports may be related to differences in the populations examined or the number of patients included in the analyses. A large meta-analysis exploring the impact of deficiencies in the CYP2C19 enzyme on cardiovascular events among clopidogrel-treated patients reported higher rates of cardiovascular events and a higher mortality for those patients with loss of function CYP2C19 genetic variants (odds ratio: 1.79, 95% CI 1.10 to 2.91, $P = .019$) or who were taking proton pump inhibitors (odds ratio: 1.18, 95% CI 1.07 to 1.30, $P < .001$).[30]

Taken together this information suggests that caution must be entertained when administering clopidogrel to patients who are poor metabolizers (owing to either genetic polymorphisms or acquired defects in the CYP2C19 enzyme). Although not clearly proven to be of benefit, laboratory assessment of platelet inhibition while on therapy may be helpful in these patients. These tests are generally referred to as a "platelet-reactivity test." The response to clopidogrel is measured by looking at the PRU (P2Y12 reactivity unit) or the percent platelet inhibition.[34,35] In general, a patient with appropriate response to clopidogrel should have a PRU of <240 and >40% platelet inhibition. If a patient exhibits persistently high platelet reactivity despite standard dosing of clopidogrel, consideration should be given to the administration of higher doses of clopidogrel or the use of an alternative P2Y12 receptor blocker.

PRASUGREL. Prasugrel, another thienopyridine, also acts by irreversibly inhibiting the P2Y12 receptor on platelets. Prasugrel appears to be a "stronger" antiplatelet agent than clopidogrel. In a head-to-head comparison study, prasugrel demonstrated higher platelet inhibition and less interindividual variability in

platelet inhibition than clopidogrel.[36] Prasugrel has not been shown to have any clinically relevant interactions with drugs that alter the cytochrome P450 system.

The TRial to assess Improvement in Therapeutic Outcomes by optimizing platelet inhibition with prasugrel-Thrombolysis In Myocardial Infarction 38 (TRITON-TIMI 38)[37] randomized 13,608 patients with moderate- to high-risk ACS to treatment with clopidogrel or prasugrel for a median of 14 months. The primary endpoint, a composite of cardiovascular death, nonfatal MI, or nonfatal stroke was significantly lower in the prasugrel group compared with the clopidogrel group (9.9% vs. 12.1%, hazard ratio, 0.81; 95% CI, 0.73 to 0.90; $P < .001$). This study reported a significantly higher rate of non-CABG-related major bleeding in the prasugrel arm (2.4% vs. 1.8%, hazard ratio, 1.32; 95% CI, 1.03 to 1.68; $P = .03$). Despite this finding, there appeared to be a net benefit from prasugrel (incorporating ischemic and bleeding endpoints) when compared with clopidogrel. However, patients who reported a history of a prior TIA or CVA, demonstrated more bleeding with Prasugrel, and a net negative benefit from treatment was noted in this subgroup. Patients >75 years of age, or weighing <60 kg also demonstrated more bleeding, but there was a net neutral benefit from Prasugrel in these subgroups. Therefore, based on these findings, Prasugrel is not recommended in those patients who report a prior transient ischemic attack (TIA) or cerebrovascular accident (CVA), and caution is advised when using prasugrel in patients who are over the age of 75, or in patients weighing <60 kg. Prasugrel is given as a loading dose of 60 mg, followed by a daily dose of 10 mg. A reduced dose of prasugrel of 5 mg daily should be given to patients who are >75 years of age or weighing <60 kg.

TICAGRELOR. Ticagrelor is a reversible oral P2Y12 antagonist. Unlike the thienopyridines, ticagrelor does not require hepatic conversion to an active metabolite, thus exhibiting the potential for a more rapid onset of action and less interindividual variability. Clinical studies[38] have shown a higher degree of and more predictable intrinsic platelet aggregation following loading and initial dosing of this agent when compared with clopidogrel. The PLATelet inhibition and patient Outcomes (PLATO) trial[39] was a head-to-head comparison of the use of ticagrelor plus aspirin versus clopidogrel plus aspirin in 18,624 patients with ACS. In this study, Ticagrelor reduced the rate of cardiovascular events (CV death, MI, or stroke) from 11.7% to 9.8% compared with clopidogrel (hazard ratio, 0.84, 95% CI, 0.77 to 0.92; $P < .001$). There was no increased risk of major bleeding. This benefit was seen irrespective of the presence or absence of CYP2C19 and ABCB1 genetic polymorphisms.[27] Ticagrelor is given as a loading dose of 180 mg followed by 90 mg twice daily dosing.

Glycoprotein IIB/IIIA receptor inhibitors. Glycoprotein IIB/IIIA receptor inhibitors (GPI) act by inhibiting the glycoprotein receptor on the surface of platelets, thereby preventing fibrinogen binding and platelet aggregation. Several agents that inhibit the glycoprotein receptor are currently in use today including abciximab, eptifibatide, and tirofiban. There is a wide variation in the pharmacokinetic properties of the various GPI resulting in varying clinical responses.

ABCIXIMAB. Abciximab is the Fab fragment of a murine antibody with a strong affinity for the glycoprotein receptor on the surface of the platelets resulting in prolonged antiplatelet effects that can persist for up to a week following discontinuation of therapy. Although abciximab has a long affiniation half-life (strong affinity to the glycoprotein receptor), it has a short plasma half-life. Therefore, if a patient develops serious bleeding following abciximab use, this may be offset by transfusion of platelets. Abciximab is typically administered only in patients undergoing percutaneous coronary intervention. Clinical studies have not demonstrated added benefit to the initial use of abciximab for all patients presenting with NSTE-ACS.[40] Therefore, the ACC/AHA guidelines do not recommend the upstream use of this agent.[4]

EPTIFIBATIDE AND TIROFIBAN. Eptifibatide, a cyclic heptapeptide, and tirofiban, a synthetic nonpeptide competitively inhibit the glycoprotein receptor on the surface of platelets. Both agents have a short biologic half-life with return to platelet activity within 3 to 4 hours of discontinuation of the drug. The PRISM (Platelet Receptor Inhibition in ischaemic Syndrome Management) and PURSUIT (Platelet glycoprotein IIb/IIIa in Unstable angina: Receptor Suppression Using Integrilin Therapy) studies demonstrated benefit to the use of tirofiban and eptifibatide, respectively, among patients with ACS, with a reduction in the composite endpoint of death, MI or refractory ischemia at 30 days for tirofiban (18.5% vs. 22.3%, $P = .03$) and of death or MI at 30 days for eptifibatide (14.2% vs. 15.7%, $P = .04$).[41,42] These agents have been associated with a tendency toward increased bleeding and thrombocytopenia, although the rates of major bleeding are not significantly increased. In view of this information, these agents are recommended by the ACC/AHA for high-risk patients who are intended for an invasive strategy.[4] Low-risk patients who are likely to receive a conservative approach to therapy are less likely to derive benefit from this therapy.

ANTICOAGULANT THERAPY

Anticoagulant therapy results in inhibition of various components of the coagulation cascade, thereby preventing thrombus formation. The ACC/AHA guidelines recommend the use of anticoagulant therapy for treatment of NSTE-ACS as a class I indication, in conjunction with aspirin and ADP receptor blockers.[4] There are various anticoagulants available for use, and the decision to use one over another will vary depending on the clinical circumstances. When deciding on which agent to use, consideration should be given to the patient's risk for bleeding, the presence of concomitant renal disease (which may affect clearance of some agents), the intended approach to management (conservative or invasive), the cost of the agent, and local practices.

Unfractionated heparin. Unfractionated heparin (UFH) is a glycosaminoglycan with varying molecular weights that acts by accelerating the action of antithrombin III, an enzyme that inactivates factors IIa (thrombin) and Xa. Earlier studies have shown a benefit to the adjunctive use of UFH for treatment of patients with ACS.[43] Owing to the heterogeneous molecular properties, UFH can bind with plasma proteins, endothelial cells, and blood cells resulting in less predictable therapeutic responses at any given dose. Therefore, the response to heparin measured by the aPTT (activated partial thromboplastin time) should be monitored on a regular basis. UFH is usually given as a loading dose of 60 units per kg (to a maximum of 4,000 units) followed by a weight-adjusted infusion of 12 units/kg/hour (to

a maximum of 1,000 units per hour). Advantages of UFH include the low cost for use of this agent and the ability of this agent to be cleared from the body within hours of discontinuation of the infusion. In emergency circumstances, UFH can be reversed using protamine. UFH has been associated with a rare condition known as heparin-induced thrombocytopenia, and platelet count should be monitored during use.

Low-molecular-weight heparin. Low-molecular-weight heparins (LMWH) are derived by cleaving the large UFH molecule to form smaller molecules. Although they act by inhibiting both Xa and IIa factors, they appear to have more of an anti-Xa:anti-IIa effect. These molecules have a reduced binding affinity for plasma proteins and therefore have more predictable dose–response relationships. Enoxaparin is generally the preferred LMWH for the treatment of NSTE-ACS. Clinical studies have demonstrated a superior efficacy of enoxaparin when compared with UFH with no significant difference in major bleeding episodes.[44] In a meta-analysis of two clinical trials of patients with NSTE-ACS examining treatment effects from these two agents, enoxaparin resulted in a 20% relative reduction in nonfatal MI or death at 43 days when compared with UFH (odds ratio for death/MI: 0.80, 95% CI 0.71 to 0.91, $P < .0005$).[44] Enoxaparin is given in a dose of 1 mg per kg subcutaneous twice daily. The dose should be reduced to 1 mg per kg daily for those patients with a creatinine clearance <30 ml per minute. Advantages of enoxaparin include the convenient twice daily dosing without the need to monitor laboratory response to anticoagulation.

Fondaparinux. Fondaparinux is a synthetic factor Xa inhibitor, shown to have similar efficacy to enoxaparin for the treatment of NSTE-ACS with less major bleeding.[45] The OASIS-5 (Fifth Organization to Assess Strategies in Ischemic Syndromes) trial[45] compared outcomes among 20,078 patients who were randomized to treatment with fondaparinux or enoxaparin in a noninferiority trial. The composite of the primary outcome (death, MI, and refractory ischemia) and major bleeding at 9 days favored fondaparinux (7.3% vs. 9.0%, hazard ratio, 0.81; $P < .001$). Fondaparinux has been associated with catheter-related thrombosis among patients referred for percutaneous coronary intervention. Therefore, it is generally used when treating patients with an intended conservative strategy. If percutaneous intervention is planned, an alternative method of anti-coagulation should be substituted for fondaparinux. This anticoagulant is given in doses of 2.5 mg subcutaneous daily.

Bivalirudin. Bivalirudin is a direct thrombin inhibitor that binds reversibly to thrombin resulting in the inhibition of clot-bound thrombin. Clinical studies have demonstrated that the use of bivalirudin in patients with ACS results in similar efficacy when compared with UFH and GPI but less bleeding.[46] The Acute Catheterization and Urgent Intervention Triage StrategY (ACUITY) trial[46] randomized 13,819 patients with moderate- and high-risk NSTE-ACS to UFH or enoxaparin plus a GPI, bivalirudin plus a GPI, or bivalirudin alone. Treatment with bivalirudin monotherapy as compared with UFH (or enoxaparin) plus GPI was associated with significantly reduced bleeding complications, similar rates of cardiovascular events, and lower net adverse events (ischemic plus bleeding events) (10.1% vs. 11.7% $P = .02$). Bivalirudin is usually given to patients with NSTE-ACS at the time of PCI, or alternatively, it can be used on initial presentation (as an "upstream" agent) in those patients with a planned invasive strategy.[4] When used in conjunction with PCI, it is given as a loading dose of 0.75 mg per kg followed by an infusion of 1.75 mg/kg/hour.

HMG COENZYME A REDUCTASE INHIBITORS

The HMG coenzyme A reductase inhibitors, commonly referred to as the "statins," exert their effects by lowering LDL and TG levels and raising HDL levels. Studies have demonstrated improved LDL levels and lower rates of cardiovascular events including death or MI for those patients with atherosclerotic heart disease who are treated with HMG coenzyme A reductase inhibitors therapy.[47] However, the extent to which HMG coenzyme A reductase inhibitors improve cardiovascular outcomes appears to be out of proportion to their LDL lowering ability. It has been postulated that HMG coenzyme A reductase inhibitors may also contribute to stabilization of the atherosclerotic plaque, inhibition of thrombogenicity, and improvement in endothelial function.[48] Data suggest a benefit to the early initiation of HMG coenzyme A reductase inhibitor therapy at high doses following ACS, when compared with delayed routine therapy.[49] Therefore, among patients with NSTE-ACS, HMG coenzyme A reductase inhibitors should be initiated in high doses during hospitalization unless there is a contraindication. There are various HMG coenzyme A reductase inhibitors available for use in the market today, and the decision to initiate a particular agent while in hospital is generally based on hospital availability and physician/patient preference.

INITIAL CONSERVATIVE VERSUS INITIAL INVASIVE APPROACH

There are two general approaches to treating patients with ACS after initial stabilization. These include an initial conservative approach in which the patients are treated with aggressive medical therapy or an early invasive approach in which diagnostic coronary angiography is performed within the first 24 to 48 hours of admission. In the conservative approach the patients are treated with maximal medical therapy including antiplatelet, anticoagulant, and anti-ischemic agents and then referred for noninvasive stress testing (stress echo or stress nuclear studies) to assess the burden of ischemia. Coronary angiography is reserved for patients with a complicated hospital course including recurrent ischemic pain despite maximal medical therapy, congestive heart failure or LV dysfunction, ventricular arrhythmias, or inducible ischemia on noninvasive studies (dynamic ECG changes or a significant abnormality on imaging studies). The initial conservative approach is usually preferred for stable patients with low-risk features. The advantage of a conservative approach is that it allows for selection of those patients who have significant ischemia (either spontaneous or induced) to undergo coronary angiography while avoiding the risk of an invasive procedure on a large number of otherwise stable patients who can be medically managed. In the early invasive approach, an intended cardiac catheterization is usually performed early in the hospital course to determine coronary artery anatomy and guide decisions regarding the need for revascularization. The early invasive approach allows the physician to assess coronary anatomy directly in a timely manner so that revascularization can be performed in patients with significant disease.

Multiple studies have compared the outcomes of patients treated with each approach in an effort to determine the ideal strategy to manage patients with NSTE-ACS. The more contemporary studies, such as FRagmin and fast revascularization during InStability in Coronary artery disease (FRISC II), treat angina with aggrastat and determine cost of therapy with an invasive or conservative strategy-thrombolysis in myocardial infarction 18 (TACTICS-TIMI 18), and randomized intervention trial of UA-3(RITA-3) trials performed after the introduction of percutaneous stents, and aggressive antiplatelet therapies have supported an early invasive approach to care with lower rates of the composite endpoint of death, recurrent MI, and refractory ischemia in the invasive groups.[50–52] This benefit was particularly notable among patients with elevated cardiac troponins or a high TIMI risk score. However, the Invasive Versus Conservative Treatment in Unstable Coronary Syndromes (ICTUS) study[53] study failed to demonstrate a benefit to an early invasive approach and reported a higher risk of recurrent infarction in the patients assigned to an initial invasive strategy. In a meta-analysis of all trials[54] examining this issue, an early invasive strategy was associated with a 25% relative reduction in mortality at a mean follow-up of 2 years (4.9% vs. 6.5%, RR: 0.75, 95% CI 0.63 to 0.90, $P = .001$), and nonfatal MI (7.6% vs. 9.1%, RR: 0.83, 95% CI 0.72 to 0.96, $P = .012$). Based on this information, the ACC/AHA recommends an early invasive strategy for high-risk patients; Patients without high-risk features may be treated with either approach.[4]

Although it s now accepted that high-risk patients should be referred for an early invasive approach, the next question relates to the timing of this procedure. Some studies have suggested that an earlier time to intervention may be of more benefit.[55,56] The Intracoronary Stenting with Antithrombotic Regimen- COOLing Off (ISAR COOL) trial[55] was designed to determine whether pretreatment with antiplatelet therapy for several days improved the outcome. In this study, early cardiac catheterization (performed within 6 hours) resulted in a lower rate of death and MI at 30 days when compared with delayed catheterization (performed after 3 to 5 days) (5.9% vs. 11.6%, $P = .04$). In the timing of intervention in acute coronary syndromes (TIMACS) study,[56] 3,031 patients with NSTE-ACS were randomly assigned to early intervention within 24 hours of admission or delayed intervention ≥36 hours. There was no significant difference in the primary outcomes between the early or late catheterization groups. However, in a prespecified subgroup analysis examining benefit of early intervention in a high-risk cohort defined using the GRACE risk score, outcome including death, MI, and stroke at 6 months was significantly better for those patients randomized to the early invasive arm (HR: 0.65, 95% CI 0.48 to 0.88). Based on this and other information, the ACC-AHA 2009 focused update[1] suggests that high-risk patients with NSTE-ACS undergo early catheterization within 12 to 24 hours of presentation.

DISCHARGE PLANNING

It is essential to institute patient education and appropriate counseling regarding the patient's medical condition and the importance of lifestyle modification and compliance with medications at the time of discharge planning for all patients and families of patients with NSTE-ACS. Counseling should be done in a language that is easily understood by the patient. By enabling the patient to participate in the discharge planning, the patient may get a sense of control over his/her clinical condition, which in turn may foster better compliance. A brief discussion of the patient's medical condition should be reviewed at the time of discharge as well as a summary of the role of the individual medications, the potential for developing side effects from medications, the likely duration of each therapy, and the importance of regular follow-up. A heart healthy diet, rich in fruits and vegetables and low in saturated fats, cholesterol, and trans-fats should be advised. When indicated weight loss and avoidance of items high in carbohydrates should be discussed. Patients should be advised to stop smoking; if necessary, medical interventions or formal counseling should be employed. Patients should be advised of the importance of regular physical activity. An individualized exercise "prescription" should be given to all patients. Consideration should be given to the patient's cardiac conditions and other medical conditions that may interfere with the ability to exercise including severe degenerative joint disease, motor weakness from prior cerebrovascular accidents, atherosclerotic peripheral vascular disease, or limiting lung conditions. In an otherwise healthy patient, it is reasonable to advise a regimen of moderate physical activity for 30 to 60 minutes each day, most days of the week. This exercise prescription should be discussed with the patient at the first office visit, providing they are clinically stable. A referral for cardiac rehabilitation can be considered for those patients who would benefit from a more structured program. Patients should be instructed on what to do should symptoms recur. In the case of symptom development a patient should be advised to take a sublingual nitroglycerin tablet and stop any physical activity. If symptoms do not resolve after 5 minutes the patient should be instructed to call 911. A second nitroglycerin tablet may be taken while they are awaiting the ambulance arrival.

The selection of a medical regimen for a patient will be based on the patient's concomitant medical conditions (including diabetes, hypertension, and congestive heart failure), and the hospital management that was employed (including revascularization or optimization of medical therapy). In most cases, the patients are discharged on a medical regimen that is similar to the one they had received prior to discharge. These include but may not necessarily be limited to dual antiplatelet agents and HMG coenzyme A reductase inhibitors. β-Blockers should be prescribed for patients with documented infarction or LV dysfunction, and angiotensin converting enzyme (ACE) inhibitors should be given to patients with LV dysfunction or congestive heart failure.

PROGNOSIS

With the introduction of aggressive medical therapies and catheter-based interventions, the prognosis for patients with NSTE-ACS has become quite favorable. Clinical trials have reported mortality rates as low as 3.1% and recurrent MI rates of 3.8% at 30 days.[56] Epidemiologic studies examining nonselected patients presenting with NSTE-ACS have demonstrated similar outcomes, with in-hospital mortality averaging 4% and recurrent infarction rates of 3%.[57] Mortality is affected by aggressiveness of therapy, with lower rates among patients treated with guideline recommended care.[58] Therefore, it is imperative that all physicians treating patients with NSTE-ACS understand the importance of administering guideline recommended care, so that patients have an optimal chance for a successful outcome.

REFERENCES

1. Kushner FG, Hand M, Smith SS, et al. 2009 focused update: ACC/AHA guidelines for the management of ST elevation myocardial infarction (Updating the 2004 guideline and 2007 focused update) and ACC/AHA/SCAI guidelines on percutaneous coronary intervention (updated the 2005 guidelines and 2007 focused update). A report of the American College of Cardiology Foundation/American Heart Association Task Force of Practice Guidelines. *J Am Coll Cardiol.* 2009;54:2205–2241.
2. Lloyd-Jones D, Adams RJ, Brown TM, et al. Heart and stroke statistics 2010 update. A report from the American Heart Association. *Circulation.* 2010;121:e1–e170.
3. Brieger D, Eagle KA, Goodman SG, et al. Acute coronary syndromes without chest pain, an under-diagnosed and under-treated high-risk group: insights from the Global Registry of Acute Coronary Events. *Chest.* 2004;126:461–469.
4. 2011 ACCF/AHA Focused Update of the Guidelines for the Management of Patients With Unstable Angina/Non–ST-Elevation Myocardial Infarction (Updating the 2007 Guideline) : A Report of the American College of Cardiology Foundation/American Heart Association Task Force on Practice Guidelines. *Circulation* 2011;123:2022–2060.
5. Antman EM, Tanasijevic MJ, Thompson B, et al. Cardiac-specific troponin I levels to predict the risk of mortality in patients with acute coronary syndromes. *N Engl J Med.* 1996;335:1342–1349.
6. Shapiro BP, Jaffe AS. Cardiac biomarkers. In: Murphy JG, Lloyd MA, eds. *Mayo Clinic Cardiology: Concise Textbook.* 3rd ed. Rochester, MN: Mayo Clinic Scientific Press; 2007:773–780.
7. Antmen EM, Cohen M, Bernink PJLM, et al. The TIMI risk score of unstable angina/non-ST elevation MI: a method for prognostication and therapeutic decision making. *JAMA.* 2000;284:835–842.
8. Granger CB, Goldberg RJ, Dabbous O, et al. Predictors of hospital mortality in the Global Registry of Cardiac Events. *Arch Intern Med.* 2003;163:2345–2353.
9. Boersma E, Pieper KS, Steyerberg EW, et al. Predictors of outcome with acute coronary syndromes in patients without persistent ST-segment elevation: results from an international trial of 9461 patients. *Circulation.* 2000;101:2557–2561.
10. Jacobs DR, Kroenke C, Crow R, et al. PREDICT: a simple risk score for clinical severity and long term prognosis after hospitalization for acute myocardial infarction or unstable angina: the Minnesota Heart Survey. *Circulation.* 1999;100:599–607.
11. Fernández-Bergés D, Bertomeu-Gonzalez V, Sánchez PL, et al. Clinical scores and patient risk stratification in non-ST elevation acute coronary syndrome. *Int J Cardiol.* 2011;146:219–224.
12. De Araújo Goncalves P, Ferreira J, Aguiar C, et al. TIMI, PURSUIT, and GRACE risk scores: sustained prognostic value and interaction with revascularization in NSTE-ACS. *Eur Heart J.* 2005;26:865–872.
13. Yan AT, Yan RT, Tan M, et al. Risk scores for risk stratification in acute coronary syndromes: useful but simpler is not necessarily better. *Eur Heart J.* 2007;28:1072–1078.
14. ISIS-4 (Fourth International Study of Infarct Survival) Collaborative Group. ISIS-4: a randomised factorial trial assessing early oral captopril, oral mononitrate, and intravenous magnesium sulphate in 58,050 patients with suspected acute myocardial infarction. *Lancet.* 1995;345:669–685.
15. Meine TJ, Roe MT, Chen AY, et al. Association of intravenous morphine use and outcomes in acute coronary syndromes: results from the CRUSADE Quality Improvement Initiative. *Am Heart J.* 2005;149:1043–1049.
16. COMMIT (ClOpidogrel and Metoprolol in Myocardial Infarction Trial) collaborative group. Early intravenous then oral metoprolol in 45 852 patients with acute myocardial infarction: randomised placebo-controlled trial. *Lancet.* 2005;366:1622–1632.
17. MERIT-HF Study Group. Effect of metoprolol CR/XL in chronic heart failure: metoprolol CR/XL randomised intervention trial in-congestive heart failure (MERIT-HF). *Lancet.* 1999;353:2001–2007.
18. Packer M, Bristow MR, Cohn JN, et al. The effect of carvedilol on morbidity and mortality in patients with chronic heart failure. *N Engl J Med.* 1996;334:1349–1355.
19. Fonarow GC, Lukas MA, Robertson M, et al. Effects of carvedilol early after myocardial infarction: analysis of the first 30 days in Carvedilol Post-Infarct Survival Control in Left Ventricular Dysfunction (CAPRICORN). *Am Heart J.* 2007;154:637–644.
20. Gibson RS, Boden WE, Theroux P, et al. Diltiazem and reinfarction in patients with non-Q-wave myocardial infarction. *N Engl J Med.* 1986;315:423–429.
21. The Danish Study Group on Verapamil in Myocardial Infarction. The effect of verapamil on mortality and major events after myocardial infarction, The Danish Verapamil Infarction Trial (DAVIT) II. *Am J Cardiol.* 1990;66:779–785.
22. Lubsen J, Tijssen JG. Efficacy of nifedipine and metoprolol in the early treatment of unstable angina in the coronary care unit: findings from the Holland Interuniversity Nifedipine/metoprolol Trial (HINT). *Am J Cardiol.* 1987;60:18A–25A.
23. Cairns JA, Gent M, Singer J, et al. Aspirin, sulfinpyrazone, or both in unstable angina—results of a Canadian Multicenter Trial. *N Engl J Med.* 1985;313:1369–1375.
24. The Clopidogrel in Unstable Angina to Prevent Recurrent Events Trial Investigators. Effects of clopidogrel in addition to aspirin in patients with acute coronary syndromes without ST-segment elevation. *N Engl J Med.* 2001;345:494–502.
25. von Beckerath N, Taubert D, Pogatsa-Murray G, et al. Absorption, metabolization, and antiplatelet effects of 300-, 600-, and 900-mg loading doses of clopidogrel: results of the ISAR-CHOICE (Intracoronary Stenting and Antithrombotic Regimen: Choose between 3 High Oral Doses for Immediate Clopidogrel Effect) trial. *Circulation.* 2005;112:2946–2950.
26. The CURRENT-OASIS 7 Investigators. Dose comparisons of clopidogrel and aspirin in acute coronary syndromes. *N Engl J Med.* 2010;363:930–942.
27. Wallentin L, James S, Storey RJ, et al. Effect of CYP2C19 and ABCB1 single nucleotide polymorphisms on outcomes of treatment with ticagrelor versus clopidogrel for acute coronary syndromes: a genetic substudy of the PLATO trial. *Lancet.* 2010;376:1320–1328.
28. Mega JL, Close SL, Wiviott SD, et al. Cytochrome p-450 polymorphisms and response to clopidogrel. *N Engl J Med.* 2009;360:354–362.

29. Simon T, Verstuyft C, Mary-Krause M, et al. Genetic determinants of response to clopidogrel and cardiovascular events. *N Engl J Med.* 2009;360:363–375.

30. Hulot JS, Collet JP, Silvain J, et al. Cardiovascular risk in clopidogrel-treated patients according to cytochrome P450 2C19*2 loss-of-function allele or proton pump inhibitor coadministration: a systematic meta-analysis. *J Am Coll Cardiol.* 2010;56:134–143.

31. Gilard M, Arnaud B, Cornily JC, et al. Influence of omeprazole on the antiplatelet action of clopidogrel associated with aspirin: the randomized, double-blind OCLA (Omeprazole CLopidogrel Aspirin) study. *J Am Coll Cardiol.* 2008;51:256–260.

32. Pare G, Mehta SR, Yusuf F, et al. Effects of CYP2C19 genetic subtype on outcomes of clopidogrel treatment. *N Engl J Med.* 2010;363:1704–1714.

33. Dunn SP, Macaulay TE, Brennan DM, et al. Baseline proton pump inhibitor use is associated with increased cardiovascular events with and without the use of clopidogrel in the CREDO trial. [abstract]. *Circulation.* 2009;118:S815.

34. Patti G, Nusca A, Mangiacapra F, et al. Point-of-care measurement of clopidogrel responsiveness predicts clinical outcome in patients undergoing percutaneous coronary intervention results of the ARMYDA-PRO (Antiplatelet therapy for Reduction of MYocardial Damage during Angioplasty–Platelet Reactivity Predicts Outcome) study. *J Am Coll Cardiol.* 2008;52:1128–1133.

35. Breet NJ, Van Werkum JW, Bouman HJ, et al. Comparison of platelet function tests in predicting clinical outcome in patients undergoing coronary stent implantation. *JAMA.* 2010;303:754–762.

36. Brandt JT, Payne CD, Wiviott SD, et al. A comparison of prasugrel and clopidogrel loading doses on platelet function: magnitude of platelet inhibition is related to active metabolite formation. *Am Heart J.* 2007;153:66.e9–66e.16.

37. Wiviott SD, Braunwald E, McCabe CH, et al. Prasugrel versus clopidogrel in patients with acute coronary syndromes. *N Engl J Med.* 2007;357:2001–2015.

38. Storey RF, Husted S, Harrington RA, et al. Inhibition of platelet aggregation by AZD6140, a reversible oral P2Y12 receptor antagonist, compared with clopidogrel in patients with acute coronary syndromes. *J Am Coll Cardiol.* 2007;50:1852–1856.

39. Wallentin L, Becker RC, Budaj A, et al. Ticagrelor versus clopidogrel in patients with acute coronary syndromes. *N Engl J Med.* 2009;361:1045–1057.

40. GUSTO IV-ACS Investigators. Effect of glycoprotein IIb/IIIa receptor blocker abciximab on outcome in patients with acute coronary syndromes without early coronary revascularization: the GUSTO IV-ACS randomized trial. *Lancet.* 2001;357:1915–1924.

41. The PRISM Study Investigators. A comparison of aspirin plus tirofiban with aspirin plus heparin for unstable angina. *N Engl J Med.* 1998;338:1498–1505.

42. The PURSUIT Trial Investigators. Inhibition of platelet glycoprotein IIb/IIIa with eptifibatide in patients with acute coronary syndromes. *N Engl J Med.* 1998;339:436–443.

43. Théroux P, Ouimet H, McCans J, et al. Aspirin, heparin, or both to treat acute unstable angina. *N Engl J Med.* 1988;319:1105–1111.

44. Antman EM, Cohen M, Radley D, et al. Assessment of the treatment effect of enoxaparin for unstable angina/non–Q-wave myocardial infarction TIMI 11B–ESSENCE Meta-Analysis. *Circulation.* 1999;100:1602–1608.

45. Yusef S, Mehta SR, Chrolavicius S, et al. Comparison of fondaparinux and enoxaparin in acute coronary syndromes. *N Engl J Med.* 2006;354:1464–1476.

46. Stone GW, McLaurin BT, Cox DA, et al. Bivalirudin for patients with acute coronary syndromes. *N Engl J Med.* 2006;355:2203–2216.

47. Scandinavian Simvastatin Survival Study Group. Randomized trial of cholesterol lowering in 4444 patients with coronary heart disease: the Scandinavian Survival Study (4S). *Lancet.* 1994;344:1383–1389.

48. Davignon J. Beneficial cardiovascular pleiotropic effects of statins. *Circulation.* 2004;109(23)(suppl 1):III39–III43.

49. Hulten E, Jackson JL, Douglas K, et al. The effect of early, intensive statin therapy on acute coronary syndrome: a meta-analysis of randomized controlled trials. *Arch Intern Med.* 2006;166:1814–1821.

50. FRagmin and Fast Revascularization during Instability in Coronary Artery Disease Investigators. Invasive compared with non-invasive treatment in unstable coronary artery disease: FRISC II prospective randomized multicenter study. *Lancet.* 1999;354(9180):708–715.

51. Cannon CP, Weintraub WS, Demopoulos LA, et al. Comparison of early invasive and conservative strategies in patients with unstable coronary syndromes treated with the glycoprotein IIb/IIIa inhibitor tirofiban. *N Engl J Med.* 2001;344(25):1879–1887.

52. Fox K, Poole-Wilson PA, Henderson RA, et al. Interventional versus conservative treatment for patients with unstable angina or non-ST-elevation myocardial infarction: the British Heart Foundation RITA 3 randomised trial. *Lancet.* 2002;360:743–751.

53. De Winter RJ, Windhausen F, Cornel JH; the Invasive versus Conservative Treatment in Unstable Coronary Syndromes (ICTUS) Investigators. Early invasive versus selectively invasive management for acute coronary syndromes. *N Engl J Med.* 2005;353(11):1095–1104.

54. Bavry AA, Kumbhani DJ, Rassi AN, et al. Benefit of early invasive therapy in acute coronary syndromes: a meta-analysis of contemporary randomized clinical trials. *J Am Coll Cardiol.* 2006;48(7):1319–1325.

55. Neumann FJ, Kastrati A, Pogatsa-Murray G, et al. Evaluation of prolonged antithrombotic pretreatment ("cooling-off" strategy) before intervention in patients with unstable coronary syndromes: a randomized controlled trial. *JAMA.* 2003;290:1593–1599.

56. Mehta SR, Granger CB, Boden WE, et al. Early versus delayed invasive intervention in acute coronary syndromes. *N Engl J Med.* 2009;360:2165–2175.

57. Ryan JW, Peterson ED, Chen AY, et al. Optimal timing of intervention in non-ST-segment elevation acute coronary syndromes: insights from the CRUSADE (Can Rapid risk stratification of Unstable angina patients Suppress ADverse outcomes with Early implementation of the ACC/AHA guidelines) Registry. *Circulation.* 2005;112:3049–3057.

58. Ticoci P, Peterson ED, Roe MT, et al. Patterns of guideline adherence and care delivery for patients with unstable angina and non-ST segment elevation myocardial infarction (from the CRUSADE Quality Improvement Initiative). *Am J Cardiol.* 2006;98:S30–S35.

PATIENT AND FAMILY INFORMATION FOR:

Non-ST Elevation Myocardial Infarction and Unstable Angina

WHAT IS CORONARY ARTERY DISEASE AND WHAT IS A HEART ATTACK?

The coronary arteries are the blood vessels that supply blood and nutrients to the heart muscle. The arteries are like long, hollow, flexible tubes or pipes. The inside of a normal healthy artery is smooth and allows the blood cells to pass easily. Over time these arteries can develop blockages. These blockages are referred to as plaques and comprise fat and cellular materials. "Atherosclerotic heart disease" and "coronary artery disease" are terms commonly used to describe the condition in which blockages develop in the arteries of the heart because of plaque build-up. Conditions that increase the chance of developing plaques in the arteries of the body include high blood pressure (hypertension), high cholesterol (hypercholesterolemia), diabetes, cigarette smoking, family history of coronary heart disease, and older age.

When blockages in the arteries of the heart get very large, they interfere with the flow of blood to the heart muscle. The heart muscle is then "starved" of nutrients and oxygen. Doctors refer to this condition as ischemia. When this happens, patients often develop symptoms: typically chest pain or chest discomfort. However, not all patients experience chest pain; some complain of jaw, arm, back, or abdominal pain, or they have shortness of breath, sweats, or nausea. "Angina" is the medical term used to describe the discomfort or symptoms that occur as a result of a heart muscle that is "starved for blood." If the blockage is severe, the angina may last for long periods or may occur with little movement. This is referred to as unstable angina (UA). Other times tiny bits of the heart muscle die owing to the lack of blood flow to that area of the heart, and this causes a heart attack. Myocardial infarction is the medical term used to describe a heart attack. A heart attack that usually occurs because of very tight blockages in the arteries of the heart is called a non ST-elevation myocardial infarction (NSTEMI). Sometimes the plaque ruptures or breaks open, and a blood clot forms around the cracked plaque to "repair" the injury to the artery. This clot often completely blocks blood flow and causes a larger heart attack. This type of heart attack is called an ST-elevation myocardial infarction (STEMI). (For more information on this type of heart attack, see Chapter 2.) Collectively, these different conditions (UA, NSTEMI and STEMI) are referred to as acute coronary syndrome (ACS).

HOW IS A HEART ATTACK DIAGNOSED?

A heart attack is diagnosed on the basis of patients' symptoms and from information obtained from an ECG (or EKG) and blood tests.

ELECTROCARDIOGRAM (ECG OR EKG)

An EKG is a simple test where electrodes are placed on the skin and connected to a machine to capture the heart's rhythm and the electrical force of the heart muscle from different angles. An EKG allows the physicians to distinguish a heart attack caused by a blood clot that completely blocks an artery (STEMI) from a heart attack or unstable symptoms resulting from critical blockages in the artery of the heart (NSTEMI or unstable angina). It may also help to locate the area of the heart muscle that is affected.

BLOOD TESTS

When a heart attack occurs, tiny bits of the heart muscle are permanently damaged. When this happens the muscle cells burst and release enzymes into the blood stream (cardiac troponins and creatinine kinase-Mb or CK-Mb). These enzymes can be detected by simple blood tests and will indicate whether a patient suffered a heart attack. They also help to estimate the amount of damage caused by the heart attack. Because it can take up to 8 hours for the enzymes to be detected in the blood, often they are not elevated on the initial blood tests that are performed on admission to the hospital. Therefore, blood tests are usually repeated every 8 to 12 hours on the first day of admission and may be repeated on the second or third day after admission to monitor the levels of the enzymes in the blood.

WHAT OTHER TESTS ARE USED TO EVALUATE A HEART ATTACK?

ECHOCARDIOGRAM

An echocardiogram is a test that uses sound waves to take a picture of the heart. It allows the doctor to see the heart muscle (the walls of the heart) and the heart valves (the doorways that allow blood to flow from one chamber of the heart to another). An echocardiogram will give information about the thickness and strength of the heart muscle and helps a doctor see whether the heart valves are opening and closing properly. This permits a more precise estimate of the amount of heart damage that has occurred as a result of blockages in the arteries and whether a patient has other heart conditions. An echocardiogram can be performed as a routine test to determine whether the heart is functioning normally, or it can be performed during a heart attack to see which wall(s) of the heart are affected. A health care provider may also perform an echocardiogram weeks after a heart attack to determine whether the heart has recovered from the heart attack, or whether there has been any permanent damage to the heart. (For more information on echocardiograms see Chapter 5.)

STRESS TEST

Depending on the type of chest pain, the changes noted on EKG, and the blood work results, a doctor may order a "stress test." A stress test shows if there is any area of the heart that does not get enough blood supply either at rest or with exercise. There are different types of stress tests, but all essentially perform the same function. The results of the stress test often guide a doctor's decision to continue with medications or recommend additional tests such as a cardiac catheterization. (For more information on stress testing see Chapters 5 and 6).

CARDIAC CATHETERIZATION (CORONARY ANGIOGRAM)

A cardiac catheterization, also called a coronary angiogram, is an invasive procedure that looks at the arteries of the heart. With this procedure, a small tube (called a "sheath") is placed in the artery of the leg or arm. Longer hollow tubes (that are typically the size of a long piece of spaghetti) are then placed through this sheath up to the heart. Dye is injected through these tubes while X-ray images are taken. This procedure allows the doctor to look for blockages in all the large arteries of the heart, look at the pumping function of the heart, and check some of the valves of the heart. Based on the results of all of these images, the doctor can decide the best treatment for the coronary artery disease. If there are dangerous blockages in the arteries, they may be opened by a procedure called angioplasty using equipment that is inserted through the same tube in the leg that was used to perform the coronary angiogram. Sometimes a "stent" is placed in the artery to assure the artery remains open. At other times surgery is needed to fix the problem. Occasionally, the doctor may only recommend medications. (For more information on these treatment choices see "How Is a Heart Attack Treated?")

HOW IS A HEART ATTACK TREATED?

Heart attacks and unstable symptoms resulting from limited blood flow to the heart muscle are treated with medications to relieve a patient's symptoms, and stabilize the heart. Often additional procedures are required to help open up the blockages of the heart to restore blood flow to the heart muscle.

MEDICATIONS

The primary role of medications used to treat a heart attack is to help prevent additional blood clots from forming and to reduce the physical stress on the heart. (For more information on medications see Chapter 7.)

Antiplatelet medications prevent clotting by interfering with the platelets (the cells in the blood that act like glue to "clump" the components of the blood clot together). Aspirin, clopidogrel, and prasugrel are the most common antiplatelet agents used in hospitals. Sometimes a patient is administered an antiplatelet medication through an IV line. These medications are called glycoprotein IIB/IIIA receptor antagonists.

Antithrombotic medications help to thin the blood and decrease blood clots from forming by interfering with the enzymes in the blood that cause the blood to clot. These agents can be given intravenously or by injection. Some intravenous or injectable medications include unfractionated heparin, lovenox, fondaparinux, and bivalirudin.

Medications are also given to decrease the amount of work the heart has to do. They may also help to alleviate chest pain. Over time these medications may strengthen the heart and limit the damage from the heart attack. These medications are part of a class of medications called ß-blockers and ACE inhibitors. Nitroglycerin and morphine are also sometimes used to help relieve chest pain and relax the heart.

Statins are medications that lower cholesterol and prevent additional plaque build-up in the arteries. Over time they may prevent future heart attacks. Although statins are designed for long-term use after a patient is discharged from the hospital, they are often started in the hospital.

ANGIOPLASTY AND STENTS

An angioplasty refers to a procedure in which a balloon is inflated in the artery of the heart to help to "clear the artery" of blockages. This is done using equipment that is passed through a sheath in the leg or arm in much the same way as a coronary angiogram. (For more information on coronary angiograms see "What Other Tests Are Used to Evaluate a Heart Attack?") A doctor decides on the equipment to be used and how to treat the blockages based on many factors, including the location of the blockages, the size of the arteries, and the number of arteries that are affected. Once the blockage is opened with a balloon or another piece of equipment, the doctor will decide if a stent is needed as well. A stent is a small metal tube that is placed in the artery and helps to "prop" open the artery. Some stents have a layer of medications covering their surface. These are referred to as drug eluting stents. These stents are less likely to narrow over time; however, they require a patient to take more intense medications for longer periods. The nonmedicated stents are referred to as bare-metal stents. Sometimes patients require multiple stents in the same artery. Other times more than one artery is treated with the angioplasty or stent procedure. (For more information on angioplasty and stents see Chapter 4.)

OPEN-HEART SURGERY

In some cases, the best way to treat the blocked arteries is with open-heart surgery or CABG surgery. In open-heart surgery, a patient is given general anesthesia and a breathing tube is inserted to help the patient breathe. A surgeon then opens the chest and takes arteries from the chest wall, or veins from the legs, and plugs them into the heart arteries and "bypasses" the blockages. Obviously, this is a much more invasive procedure than an angioplasty and generally requires a longer recovery time. However, when multiple arteries are blocked, or if the location of the blockage is in a critical part of the artery, then bypass surgery is preferred. A decision to proceed with surgery is usually based on the number and location of the blockages in the arteries as well as the strength of the heart muscle. A persons' age and other medical conditions may also influence a doctor's decision to advise angioplasty or surgery. (For more information on cardiac surgery see Chapter 8.)

RECOVERING FROM A HEART ATTACK

The health care team will review all aspects of a patient's heart condition at the time of discharge from the hospital. Recovery from a heart attack includes both medications and lifestyle changes to help the heart heal and prevent the development of further heart problems.

MEDICATIONS

The medications that are prescribed following a heart attack are often similar to the medications that are used to treat the heart attack while in the hospital. They help prevent future blood clots from forming and help to strengthen the heart over time. (For more information on medications see "How Is a Heart Attack Treated?") It is essential to take medications as prescribed every day. Most medications are covered by insurance companies, or require only a small co-pay. Some patients may not be able to afford the medications that are prescribed. In these situations, hospitals, health centers, and pharmaceutical companies may be able to assist a patient in obtaining financial assistance to cover the cost of these medications.

HEART HEALTHY DIET

Vegetables, fruits, whole grains, and fish are a great start to a healthy heart. Red meat, fried foods, and food high in salt, saturated fats, trans-fats, and cholesterol should be avoided. The American Heart Association advises that a patient with coronary heart disease maintain a low fat (<30% of total calories from fat with <7% coming from saturate fats) low cholesterol (<200 mg of cholesterol a day), and low salt (<2 g of sodium) diet. It is a good idea for patients to monitor how much fat, cholesterol, and salt they eat and to limit "less healthy" foods. Food labels provide information about the amount of fat, cholesterol, and salt contained in processed foods. The amount of salt and cholesterol ingested in any given day can be estimated by totaling the number of milligrams of cholesterol or salt on each food label or portion of food that one eats. Estimating the amount of fat eaten is a little trickier. The total number of calories that comes from fat should be divided by the total number of calories consumed that day (most food labels show both the total number of calories and the number of calories from fat for that item). This number should be <0.30 (30%). Sometimes a patient may be referred for nutritional counseling. This may be especially helpful in patients who are obese, have diabetes or have trouble understanding what they should and should not eat. The nutritionist may be able to help make sense of food labels and plan a heart healthy diet.

EXERCISE

After a heart attack the doctor will advise an exercise program that is suitable to a patient's overall medical condition. Most often, this will consist of a gradual increase in physical activity over the first 4 weeks following the heart attack. By week 4, most patients will be encouraged to begin a regular exercise program that includes some type of aerobic exercise for at least 45 to 60 minutes on all or most days of the week. The exercise should result in an increase in the heart rate and the rate of breathing but should not leave a patient "exhausted." In some cases a patient may be referred for a structured and formal exercise program (cardiac rehabilitation). The patient should choose an exercise regimen that is convenient with his/her lifestyle and will be the easiest to maintain over time. It is important to understand that aerobic activity refers to any kind of physical movement that increases the heart rate and decreases the resistance of the heart. Although typically one depicts aerobic exercise as "jogging" or an "aerobics" class, there are many other forms of aerobic exercise such as moderate or brisk walking, swimming, tennis, basketball, dancing, gardening, golf, and many other interesting activities. Some other changes a patient can do to make a difference include walking to work instead of driving or taking the bus or train, taking the stairs instead of the elevator, or doing gardening or housework.

QUIT SMOKING

There are absolutely no benefits to smoking. A smoker who continues to smoke following a heart attack is twice as likely to suffer another heart attack. It is essential that a patient quit smoking and avoid second-hand smoke. Some patients are able to stop "cold turkey." Others may require prescription medications or formal counseling at a smoking cessation clinic. All patients should discuss the choice to quit with their health care provider and find an approach that is "right" for them.

MEDICAL FOLLOW-UP

It is essential that a patient follows up with a cardiologist on a regular basis. This will allow the doctor to assess a patient's response to medications and adjust the doses as needed to minimize side effects and optimize the benefit of the medications. Doctors may choose to perform a follow-up echocardiogram and stress test to assess a patient's progress. It is of utmost importance that all patients have a strong relationship with their doctor and feel comfortable with all members of the health care team so that they can openly discuss any or all concerns or questions and feel in control of their heart health.

CHAPTER

4

Angela M. Palazzo
Neel P. Chokshi
David L. Coven

Cardiac Catheterization and Percutaneous Intervention

CORONARY ANGIOGRAPHY

CORONARY ANATOMY

Ample arterial circulation is required for effective myocardial function during both systole and diastole. This supply/demand coupling is accomplished through regional matching of the arterial supply to a particular portion of the myocardium.[1]

Arterial circulation of the heart consists of two parts: (1) large epicardial coronary arteries that serve as conduit vessels, and (2) medium-sized and small intramyocardial coronary arterioles that serve as resistance vessels regulating the amount of coronary flow according to myocardial metabolic needs. Perturbation in any portion of this arterial tree will lead to regional myocardial dysfunction. Acute coronary syndrome (ACS) is the clinical manifestation of a diminished coronary arterial blood supply in conduit or resistance coronary vessels with atherosclerosis being the most common cause.

In most humans, the entire epicardial circulation originates from the two initial branches of the aorta: the left coronary artery (LCA) and the right coronary artery (RCA). They originate from the left and the right sinus of Valsalva, respectively. The initial portion of the LCA is referred to as the left main coronary artery (LMCA); it branches into the left anterior descending artery (LAD) and the left circumflex artery (LCx).

In a few individuals, there may be anomalies in the origin of the coronary arteries pertaining to the number and location of coronary ostia within the aortic root as well as anomalies in the initial course of the vessels. The LAD supplies the largest portion of the left ventricle; the size of the LAD territory tends to be relatively constant among individuals and encompasses about 50% of the left ventricle. The LAD initially runs in the anterior interventricular groove parallel to the long axis of the heart then turns over the left ventricular apex and terminates, in most individuals, in the apical region of the posterior interventricular groove. The LAD gives off septal branches that penetrate into the anterior two-thirds of the interventricular septum, and diagonal branches which supply large areas of the anterior wall of the left ventricle (Figure 4.1A).

The other half of the left ventricle is supplied by both the RCA and the LCx in proportions that vary between individuals. In about 70% of humans, the RCA subtends a larger section of the left ventricle than the LCx (the so-called right-dominant circulation). In about 20% of individuals, the contribution of the two arteries is equal (co-dominant or balanced circulation). In the remaining 10%, the LCx is larger than the RCA (left-dominant circulation). The dominance type does not affect the initial course of either the RCA or the LCx; it arises from the pattern of terminal branching in the two vessels.

In all individuals, the initial course of the RCA is within the right atrioventricular groove and thus perpendicular to the long axis of the heart. During this initial course, the RCA gives off acute marginal (AM) branches that run roughly parallel to the long axis of the right ventricle to supply the acute margin of the right ventricle. The RCA is the principal source of arterial blood supply to the right ventricle; when there is right ventricular dysfunction during ACS, it is invariably caused by abnormalities in the RCA tree (Figure 4.1B).

In a roughly mirror-image pattern, the LCx initially runs in the left atrioventricular groove perpendicular to the long axis of the heart and gives off obtuse marginal (OM) branches. They run parallel to the long axis of the heart and supply the obtuse margin of the heart made up by the lateral wall of the left ventricle (Figure 4.1C).

The inferoposterior aspects of the interventricular septum and the left ventricle are supplied by the posterior descending artery (PDA) and one or more posterolateral branches (PLBs). The PDA usually runs along the proximal two-thirds of the posterior interventricular groove, and its course is parallel to the LAD in the anterior interventricular groove. Along its interventricular course, the PDA gives off septal branches to the inferior aspect of the interventricular septum and meets the LAD in the apical portion of the posterior interventricular septum. PLBs are arterial branches that run along the long axis of the left ventricle and roughly parallel to the course of the PDA and the OMs. PLBs supply the inferior and posterior walls of the left ventricle.

It is the origin of the PDA that determines whether the coronary circulation is right dominant, left dominant, or balanced (co-dominant). In the right-dominant circulation, the PDA is a branch of the RCA; in the left-dominant circulation the PDA is a terminal branch of the LCx; in balanced (co-dominant) circulation both the RCA and the LCx supply the PDA.

PREPROCEDURAL MATTERS

Patient consent. Prior to the procedure, the physician performing the angiography should obtain informed consent from the patient. The discussion should include the indication, the general nature of the procedure, and the associated risks. The specific risks include but are not limited to the following:

- Bleeding
- Infection

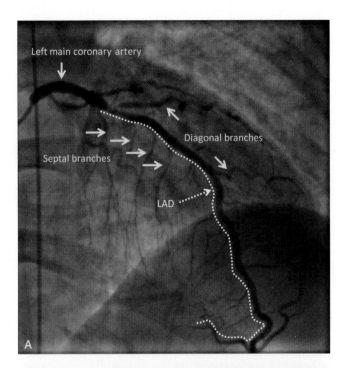

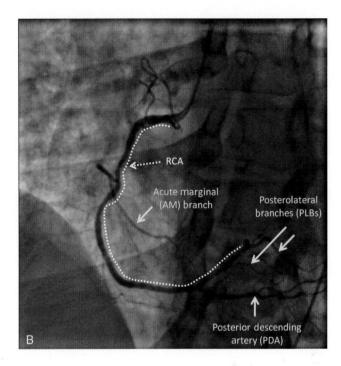

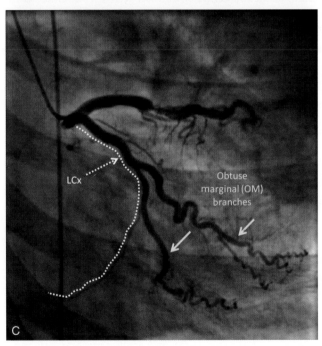

Figure 4.1. Coronary anatomy as visualized by coronary angiography. **A:** Left anterior descending artery (LAD) and its major branches visualized in a cranially and a slightly rightward angulated view (right anterior oblique [RAO] −9°; cranial +36°). **B:** Dominant right coronary artery (RCA) and its major branches visualized in a slightly cranially angulated view (left anterior oblique [LAO] (LAO +28°; cranial +3°). **C:** Nondominant left circumflex (LCx) artery and its major branches visualized in a caudally and a slightly rightward angulated view RAO −6°; caudal −21°).

- Allergic reaction to the contrast
- Contrast induced nephropathy
- Stroke
- Myocardial infarction
- Death

Medications. The patient's active medication list should be reviewed prior to angiography. Individuals on metformin should have this medication held for at least 48 hours post-procedure for the theoretical risk of contrast nephropathy and subsequent lactic acidosis because of the medication. If preexisting renal insufficiency is present, metformin should not be given 48 hours before the procedure as well.

Allergies. Patients should be asked specifically regarding allergies to contrast. If a patient endorses a reaction to this agent, the risks of contrast administration should be weighed prior to proceeding. In instances of a mild reaction, patients can generally proceed after premedication with diphenhydramine without further problems.

Laboratory testing. When possible, all patients should have a recent laboratory evaluation including assessment of renal function, baseline hemoglobin level, and coagulation studies. Although this may not be feasible in the emergent setting, labs should be at least drawn prior to the procedure and monitored afterwards. In patients with renal disease, the risks of contrast nephropathy should be considered prior to proceeding and intravenous fluids should be given *N*-acetylcysteine should be considered if not contraindicated.

Electrocardiogram. The electrocardiogram (ECG) should be reviewed for abnormalities that may be suggestive of an anatomical site of myocardial injury. This may be useful in establishing the culprit coronary vessel and guiding intervention.

Anesthesia. Local anesthesia is generally used at the site of arterial puncture to minimize pain. Conscious sedation can also be administered to reduce anxiety and relieve pain. A variety of short-acting agents can be used.

Arterial access. To perform coronary angiography, the coronary ostia must be directly cannulated with a catheter at the aortic root. This catheter is inserted into the arterial vasculature peripherally and guided up to the root of the aorta under fluoroscopy. To obtain access, an arterial sheath (Figure 4.2) is placed using a modified Seldinger technique at one of three possible peripheral sites. The femoral artery is the most common site of peripheral access for coronary angiography. The sheath is placed in the common femoral artery proximal to the bifurcation into the superficial femoral and profunda femoris arteries and distal to the superficial epigastric artery. Relative to anatomical landmarks, the puncture is made over the palpable pulse just inferior to the inguinal ligament at the level of the midpoint of the femoral head. The large lumen size of this vessel segment minimizes the risk of acute occlusion during the procedure, and the vessel's superficial course allows direct compression for closure of the puncture site. As an alternative to the femoral artery in the leg, cardiac catheterization can be performed either from the brachial artery or from the radial artery in the arm. Both approaches allow for almost immediate ambulation of the patient.

Brachial artery cannulization can accommodate larger diameter catheters but the risk of bleeding is higher than with a radial approach and occlusion of the brachial artery compromises the dual circulation to the hand.

Radial artery access has the lowest bleeding risk of any site. Prior to the performance of a radial catheterization, an Allen's test must be performed to insure that dual circulation to the hand is intact in the event of a radial occlusion. A micropuncture needle is used for cannulation. Vasospasm of the radial artery sometimes occurs and pretreatment through the sheath with nitroglycerin and verapamil can often mitigate this.

For either approach, the sheath is removed immediately following the study and manual compression is applied.

Diagnostic catheterization. With the arterial sheath in place, a guide wire and catheter are inserted into the sheath and advanced from the peripheral artery to the level of the aortic root under fluoroscopy. The wire is then withdrawn, and the catheter is manipulated by the angiographer to visualize the desired coronary artery or the left ventricle. Typically, left ventriculography is performed using a pigtail catheter (Figure 4.3A). Cannulation and visualization of the right and left coronaries are done with their respective catheters (Figure 4.3B, C).

LEFT VENTRICULOGRAPHY. Once at the level of the aortic root, the pigtail catheter is advanced across aortic valve and positioned in the center of the left ventricle. Contrast is injected into the ventricle while recording the radiographic images in a right anterior oblique (RAO) view. This provides a two-dimensional image of the anterior, inferior, and apical walls of the left ventricle (Figure 4.4A, B). Images may also be obtained in the left anterior oblique (LAO) view for visualization of the posterior wall and the interventricular septum. This image modality is useful in assessing wall motion abnormalities and ejection fraction as well as mitral regurgitation as contrast can be directly visualized leaking across the mitral valve. In patients with kidney disease, the left ventriculogram may not be performed to minimize exposure to nephrotoxic contrast.

LEFT HEART PRESSURES. With the pigtail catheter in the left ventricle, intracavitary pressures tracings can be directly measured including the left ventricular end diastolic pressure (LVEDP) which is often useful in the clinical assessment of patients with ACS. Patients can also be evaluated for aortic stenosis by assessing the transvalvular pressure gradient as the catheter is pulled back across the aortic valve.

CORONARY ARTERIES. Assessment of the coronary arteries is performed by cannulating the artery, injecting contrast under fluoroscopy, and assessing the opacification of the artery to identify narrowing and irregularities in contrast flow. The degree of stenosis is quantified based on the lumen width ahead of and following the site of narrowing. The degree of stenosis can also be assessed by grading the quality of contrast flow distal to the site of narrowing.

CORONARY ARTERY BYPASS GRAFTS. In patients with previous coronary bypass surgery, grafts are cannulated and visualized with a variety of specialty catheters. It is helpful to know the patient's bypass graft anatomy prior to the procedure as this can guide the angiographer in searching for saphenous grafts and internal mammary grafts.

Closure of puncture site. Following cardiac catheterization, all sheaths and catheters are removed and hemostasis is achieved

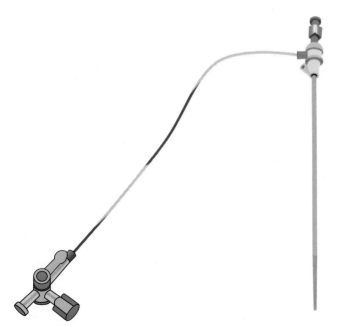

Figure 4.2. An arterial sheath, shown here, is placed in the peripheral artery. This serves as the point of access to perform the cardiac catheterization.

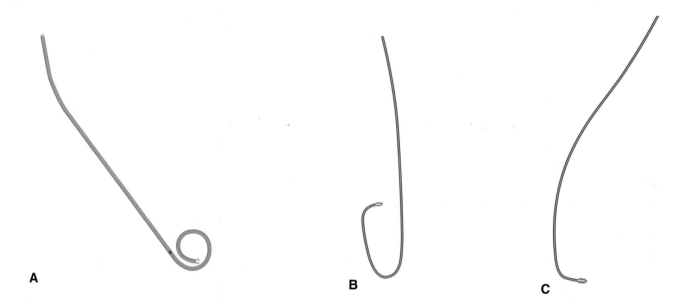

Figure 4.3. Coronary artery catheters used in angiography. A: A pigtail catheter is placed across the aortic valve to assess left ventricular function and hemodynamics. **B:** A Judkins left catheter, shown here, is used to cannulate the left coronary artery. **C:** A Judkins right catheter, shown here, is used to cannulate the right coronary artery.

in a variety of ways. Direct manual pressure can be applied to the arterial site for a minimum of 10 minutes to control the bleeding. Sheath size and anticoagulation status may greatly increase the time necessary to obtain adequate hemostasis. Various compression devices are marketed and are usually used as an adjunct to manual compression when anticoagulation requires longer compression period. Although of different designs, they all exert external pressure over the arteriotomy site. It is important to note that all external compression devices require a high level of vigilance to assure that the device is properly placed and bleeding is successfully controlled.

A number of devices to close the arteriotomy site directly are currently on the market. These include, but are not limited to, the Angio-seal vascular closure device (St. Jude Medical) that has a bioabsorbable intravascular layer and a collagen extra-vascular plug that act together to seal the puncture site. After 60 to 90 days, these components dissolve, and the access site can be used again. A possible complication unique to this device is embolization of the intravascular component. The Mynx vascular closure device (AccessClosure) is a sealant that is introduced into the tissue tract above the arteriotomy site. When exposed to blood this sealant swells to achieve hemostasis. The third example of arteriotomy closure devices is the Perclose device (Abbott Laboratories) that deploys needles percutaneously to suture the arteriotomy site. A possible complication of this device is inadvertent complete ligation of the artery.

Although the time to ambulation is improved using these closure devices, there is scant evidence to suggest that complications rates are reduced. Patient comfort has been cited as an advantage to their usage.

COMPLICATIONS

The risk of complication from cardiac catheterization is low but increases with the acuity of the patient and the baseline medical condition. The risk of death, MI, or major cerebral–vascular event in stable patients who undergo an elective catheterization is approximately 0.1%. The risk of vascular access problems that require further therapy is approximately 0.5% but increases with the presence of peripheral vascular disease. These risks include local bleeding, retroperitoneal bleeding, pseudoaneurysm formation, development of arterio-venous fistulas, dissection, and embolization. Other risks include cardiac arrhythmias or heart block, infection at the puncture site, and renal insufficiency/renal failure, particularly in patients with preexisting renal insufficiency and diabetes. Coronary or aortic dissections are rare complications of diagnostic angiography. Cardiac perforation during right heart catheterization is rare. Hypersensitivity reactions can occur and range from mild to severe, including anaphylaxis. The highest predictor of allergic reaction is a prior history of contrast reactions. The presence of a shellfish allergy is no longer thought to be an indicator of increased risk other than as an indication that the patient may have an atopic predilection. If a history of prior significant reaction to contrast is obtained, pretreatment with steroids and antihistamines should be considered.

POSTPROCEDURE MONITORING

Post procedure, bed rest is necessary and ranges from 2 hours, when vascular closure devices are used, to 4 to 6 hours after manual compression. This varies with the size of the sheaths used and the patient's anticoagulation status. In patients with a femoral access site, the affected leg should be kept straight for the prespecified time to minimize risk of hemorrhage at the puncture site. Vital signs are closely monitored because a change in blood pressure or pulse may be an early indicator of bleeding. Patients with preexisting renal insufficiency should have electrolytes and renal function drawn the next day and in 3 to 5 days if there has been an increase from baseline values."

In addition to the above precautions, those who undergo an intervention are typically monitored for longer periods because of the higher risk of complications such as acute stent thrombosis and procedure-related MI. In these patients, post-procedure

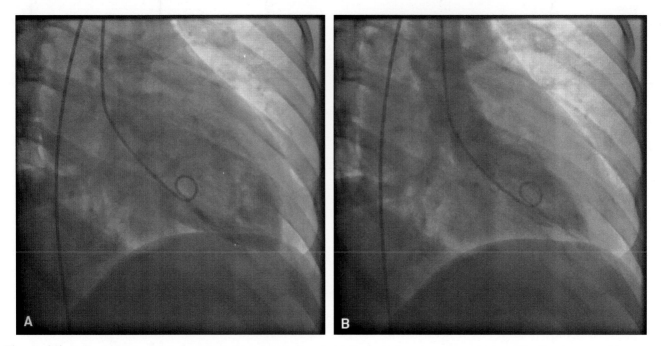

Figure 4.4. Left ventriculogram performed during catheterization. A: A left ventriculogram performed using a pigtail catheter provides assessment of wall motion and left ventricular ejection fraction. The fluoroscopic image here shows the ventricle during diastole as contrast is injected via the catheter. **B:** The left ventriculogram during systole as contrast is injected via the pigtail catheter.

monitoring may include a stay in a telemetry unit. Length of stay will be influenced by the patient's initial clinical presentation.

CORONARY INTERVENTION

Percutaneous transluminal coronary angioplasty (PTCA), first performed in 1977 by Andreas Gruentzig, transformed the practice and treatment of coronary artery disease. Revascularization using balloon angioplasty, in combination with stents, is the contemporary procedure of choice for patients presenting with ST-elevation myocardial infarction (STEMI) and other acute coronary syndromes. It is an effective therapy in many patients with stable angina and persistent symptoms despite medical therapy. A variety of equipment and medications have evolved in the field of interventional cardiology making it a complex, well-studied, and technically diverse area of nonsurgical therapy for coronary artery disease. This therapy can be utilized for patients with simple discrete lesions as well as those with more complex anatomy and left ventricular dysfunction.

DECISION TO INTERVENE

The decision to intervene on a patient is based both on the clinical presentation and on the findings of the diagnostic portion of coronary angiography. According to the American College of Cardiology/American Heart Association (ACC/AHA) guidelines, the class I indications for percutaneous coronary interventions (PCI) are as follows:

- Acute ST-elevation (i.e., transmural) MI (level of evidence A).
- Class II to IV angina or anginal equivalent (e.g., arrhythmia, dyspnea), unstable angina or non-ST-elevation acute coronary syndrome (level of evidence B).
- Asymptomatic or mildly symptomatic patients (class I angina) with noninvasive imaging showing moderate to severe

ischemia or a moderate to large area of viable myocardium (level of evidence B).
- Evidence of recurrent ischemia or infarction after thrombolysis (level of evidence B).

Other indications for PCI that are considered as classes II and III are beyond the scope of this discussion but are clearly defined in recent guidelines.[2,3]

After identifying a coronary lesion on diagnostic angiography, the decision to intervene is based primarily on whether the lesion is suspected to be responsible for a significant reduction in perfusion to the myocardium resulting in ischemia. In general, a lesion appearing to obstruct >70% of the vessel lumen on coronary angiography, as visually estimated by the angiographer, is considered likely to be flow limiting and a functionally significant stenosis. When the degree of the stenosis is in question, or if the lesion does not correlate to the patient's ACS presentation, additional tools within the catheterization lab may be utilized to determine whether the stenosis is responsible for the patient's ischemia.

TECHNIQUE

The basic technique of the most common PCIs involves four basic elements:

1. Guiding catheters
2. Coronary guide wires
3. Balloon dilation catheters
4. Coronary stents

The success of angioplasty is dependent on anatomic factors, such as vessel tortuosity, the degree of calcification, and the location of the stenosis. As distal lesions are potentially more difficult to advance equipment across, it is crucial to select the most appropriate guiding catheters and wires prior to attempting the intervention.

Guiding catheters. The guiding catheter serves three major functions: a conduit to deliver equipment, support for advancing equipment, and pressure monitoring. The guiding catheter resembles the catheters used for diagnostic coronary angiography, but the inner lumen has a larger diameter to accommodate a variety of equipment as well as to allow adequate contrast to be delivered during the procedure. Similar to diagnostic catheters, guiding catheters have preshaped tips and different luminal sizes to seat the left and right coronary arteries. In cases where simultaneous balloon or stent inflation may be necessary as in bifurcation lesions, or when larger devices are required, the selection of the appropriate lumen size of the guide catheter becomes very important. The luminal size of a catheter in millimeters is the French size divided by three; the most common size is 6F, which is approximately 2 mm in diameter. This information can be used to estimate vessel size during angiography when the opacified guiding catheter and the opacified vessel are visualized. Additional characteristics of guiding catheters compared with diagnostic catheters include a thinner wall, which may predispose to more "kinking" or twisting of the catheter during manipulation, and a more flexible tip to reduce trauma to the coronary ostium, and a stiffer shaft to provide support. Finally, guiding catheters provide the ability to monitor aortic pressure during PCI. Manipulations of the catheter in the vessel may cause changes in the pressure wave form suggesting that it is pressed against a plaque causing wave-form dampening, or "ventricularization" characterized by a pressure wave resembling a ventricular wave form seen with significant stenoses in the ostium of a vessel.

Coronary guide wires. After placement of the guiding catheter and administration of anticoagulant for the intervention, the guide wire is advanced across the stenosis where it serves as a platform for balloons, stents, and other devices that need to be advanced and removed during the intervention. Guide wire selection is determined and influenced by anatomic factors of both the vessel and the lesion. Guide wires are very small-caliber "steerable" wires that are generally constructed with an inner core wire and an outer core spring tip. The distance between these determines the stiffness of the wire and contributes to the ability to maneuver the wire in the vessel. Softer wires are less traumatic and easier to advance in tortuous vessels. Stiffer wires provide more support and greater ability to torque the wire. Guide wires may also have different coatings such as a hydrophilic tip that can more easily negotiate highly tortuous vessels or a radio-opaque coating on the distal portion allowing visualization in the vessel to monitor placement in the distal vessel.

Balloon dilation. Once the guide wire has been advanced to the distal vessel, balloon dilation catheters are selected. These are two general types including a monorail or rapid-exchange catheter or an over-the-wire configuration. Monorail balloons were developed to help the single operator by using a short "rail" but may require more manipulations of the balloon, guide wire, and guide catheter as they offer less support. Over-the-wire balloons allow improved delivery to tortuous, calcified vessels and better support to advance across highly stenotic lesions. Over-the-wire systems typically require two operators as the long guide wire extends the entire length of the balloon catheter before it exits the end. Careful planning can avoid the need to exchange a short guide wire for a longer one if an over-the-wire balloon is needed. Balloon dilation prior to stent implantation is

performed for a variety of reasons including to evaluate the characteristics of the stenosis (i.e., fibrotic or calcific), the length of the area to be stented, and the diameter of the stent to be used. Successful predilation of the stenosis occurs when both the pressure and the duration of inflation inside the balloon causes the stenotic lesion to yield completely along its entire length. With increasing balloon diameters and higher pressures, inflation can result in an increased risk of vessel injury. On the contrary, lower inflation pressures may not cause sufficient yielding of the stenosis, complicating adequate stent placement. Inflation of the balloon is accomplished using an accessory device called an indeflator that measures and controls the amount of pressure generated by balloon inflation. Balloons and stent packages come with compliance charts that guide the operator regarding the amount of pressure necessary to achieve a certain diameter of balloon size. This is called the nominal pressure.

In addition to length and diameter, the compliance of a balloon must be considered. Compliant balloons can increase their size by >20% when pressure is increased above nominal pressure, whereas noncompliant balloons change very little. Therefore, noncompliant balloons are better suited for calcified or fibrotic lesions where more tensile strength is needed to expand the lesion. There are many ways to approach balloon inflation including size, inflation time, and pressures but the overall concept is to eliminate the "waist" or area of stenosis. Lower-pressure inflations tend to have fewer complications including vessel dissections, but this may be at the cost of inferior angiographic results. A successful balloon result as a stand-alone procedure is defined as a residual stenosis of ≤50%.

Prior to the advent of stents, plain old balloon angioplasty (POBA) could result in a number of untoward effects. The most dramatic and serious was abrupt closure of the vessel. Abrupt closure was a major cause of MI, emergency coronary artery bypass grafting (CABG), and death prior to the advent of stents.

A barrier to long-term success of stand-alone angioplasty is re-stenosis. This is an exaggerated healing response by smooth muscle cells at the site of the angioplasty leading to neo-intimal hyperplasia and subsequent impingement on the lumen of the vessel that may ultimately lead to ischemia and the reoccurrence of angina.

CORONARY STENTS (FIGURE 4.5). Re-stenosis occurs in about 30% to 40% of lesions with stand-alone balloon angioplasty.[4–6] The FDA approval of bare-metal intracoronary stents in 1994 significantly reduced the rates of re-stenosis from 15% to 25% conferring more durable results. More importantly, stents drastically reduced the need for urgent coronary artery bypass surgery and reduced other procedural complications of balloon angioplasty. A variety of stents are currently available. These differ mainly in their metallic composition, architectural design, and balloon catheter delivery system. These characteristics can affect deliverability, fluoroscopic visualization, and to a lesser degree re-stenosis rates.

The approval of drug-eluting stents (DES) in 2004 had a major impact on re-stenosis rates. These metal stents have a polymer coating with a drug impregnated on its surface that elutes over time reducing neo-intima hyperplasia in a wide variety of lesions and patient types. DES have significantly reduced the rate of re-stenosis and the need for repeat lesion revascularization as compared to POBA and bare-metal stents (BMS).

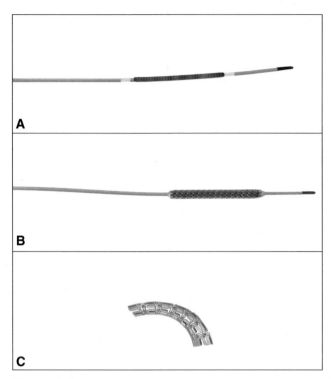

Figure 4.5. Stents are positioned at the site of the coronary lesion and then deployed with the assistance of a balloon. An unexpanded stent on a balloon (**A**); the expanded stent on a balloon (**B**); the expanded stent off the balloon (**C**).

Although intracoronary stents reduce rates of re-stenosis, one significant complication remains. Clotting and occlusion of the vessel within the lumen of the stent known as subacute thrombosis is a rare (~1.0%) complication of DES with a mortality of up to 45% and nonfatal infarction in 30% to 40% cases.[7] The use of dual antiplatelet agents has reduced the occurrence of this complication, but late stent thrombosis can occur >1 year after placement of the stent with cessation of therapy. The pathophysiology of this event is uncertain, but the lack of endothelialization of the stent is thought to play an important role. Endothelialization occurs within a few weeks after BMS implantation but is delayed with DES. Therefore, the type of stent selected is a major consideration for patients because a DES will require a longer duration of dual antiplatelet therapy relative to BMS. The appropriate duration of dual antiplatelet therapy with aspirin and a thienopyridine is still under intense study.

ANCILLARY DEVICES

There is an array of additional equipment that can be used to both identify the characteristics of the lesion and evaluate its functional significance when the angiographic degree of stenosis is in question. In addition to this, modification of the lesion to optimize stent deployment is possible as well as removal of thrombus during acute coronary syndromes.

LESION ASSESSMENT

Intravascular ultrasound. Coronary angiography displays only luminal narrowing and, in essence, is only capable of "luminology." This has distinct drawbacks in the evaluation of not only the length of atherosclerotic disease but also the degree of

stenosis. Intravascular ultrasound (IVUS) has a resolution of 100 to 150 μm allowing for the identification of the luminal border as well as the interface between the media and adventitia. Based on differences in echogenicity, IVUS can also provide important information about the distribution of calcium as well the true extent of atherosclerotic disease in the vessel. The most common uses of IVUS include the assessment of LMCA stenosis and intermediate lesions. It is also a useful tool after stent deployment, to evaluate apposition of the stent to the vessel wall. Post-PCI use of IVUS has become increasingly important since re-stenosis rates and in-stent thrombosis rates are influenced by proper stent deployment.

Optical coherence tomography. Optical coherence tomography (OCT) is based on fiberoptics and uses imaging catheters that emit near infrared light. The higher frequency and bandwidths of the light beam results in a 10-fold increase in image resolution compared with IVUS. OCT is better able to identify the composition of coronary plaques (lipid-rich, fibrous, calcific), the presence of thrombus, prolapse of tissue through stents, and vessel dissection. The technique is limited in that OCT cannot image through red blood cells and requires a brief infusion of contrast into the vessel. The clinical utility of this technique is currently being investigated.

Fractional flow reserve. Fractional flow reserve (FFR) is a technique to assess the physiologic significance of an angiographically indeterminate stenosis. FFR measurement has a strong correlation with noninvasive stress testing for evaluation of hemodynamically significant lesions. Before FFR measurement adenosine is infused to induce maximal hyperemia in the coronary vessels. Following this, the pressure distal to the stenosis is compared with aortic pressure. A measurement below 0.75 to 0.80 is consistent with a hemodynamically significant lesion. The use of FFR has been associated with significant reductions in the risk of death, myocardial infarction and repeat revascularization extending beyond 2 years.[8] FFR can also be used to evaluate left main disease, determine optimal stenting, and confirm the severity of in-stent restenosis.

LESION MODIFICATION—ROTATIONAL ATHERECTOMY

Rotational atherectomy is performed to modify a lesion through ablation of calcific or fibrotic plaque. This may allow successful delivery and deployment of balloon catheters and stents in otherwise technically challenging lesions. The device has a diamond-studded burr at its tip, which rotates at approximately 160,000 rpm causing abrasion and ablation of calcific or fibrotic plaque, leaving normal tissue unaffected. Rotational atherectomy causes microparticles to be released into the distal capillary bed that occasionally may lead to no-reflow resulting in impaired distal coronary flow and possible infarction. In spite of this, rotational atherectomy is successful in 92% to 97% of cases with a low incidence of major complications. Currently, the use of rotational atherectomy is largely confined to fibrotic or heavily calcified lesions.

THROMBECTOMY

Because of the nature of atherosclerotic disease and plaque rupture, the development of thrombus during acute coronary syndromes is an important predictor of short- and long-term prognosis as well as procedural success. Mechanical removal of totally occlusive or partially occlusive thrombus is an important part of many interventional procedures. The use of thrombectomy has been shown to reduce future major adverse cardiovascular events, improve ST-segment resolution during STEMI, and reduce infarct size. Pharmacologic therapy may also be employed to reduce thrombus burden and prevent thrombotic events.

ASPIRATION

During aspiration thrombectomy, a long catheter is advanced to the site of the thrombus and negative pressure is applied through a syringe with a locking plunger controlled with a three-way stopcock. Thrombus is "sucked" out of the vessel and blood flow is improved. This is usually followed by PTCA/stent placement.

RHEOLYTIC DEVICES

The angiojet thrombectomy system (Possis) involves the use of a catheter system, driver, and pump that delivers saline under high pressure into the vessel at the site of thrombus. The saline jet not only causes disruption of the thrombus but also creates a powerful vacuum within the artery. The thrombus is removed from the catheter through the pump.

DISTAL PROTECTION DEVICES

Devices to help protect the distal vasculature are used in obstructive stenoses of heavily diseased saphenous vein grafts after CABG. Distal protection devices are placed in the graft beyond the lesion to trap atherosclerotic debris so that it can be withdrawn eliminating embolization into the native circulation.

FILTERWIRE

The FilterWire EZ (Boston Scientific) is a device with fixed wire and a distal filter, shaped like a basket. The basket is collapsible and can be opened and closed by means of a protective sheath. It can expand to accommodate vessel diameters from 2.25 to 5.5 mm. After stenting, a retrieval sheath is placed over the basket containing the atherosclerotic debris and the system is removed.

GUARDWIRE

The GuardWire (Medtronic) is a temporary occlusion and aspiration device that uses a balloon attached to a wire and an inflation adaptor to inflate the balloon. During occlusion, the lesion is stented followed by the rapid aspiration of the contents of the vessel. The atherosclerotic debris is removed, the balloon is deflated, and flow is restored through the vein graft. Unlike the FilterWire, this device may cause ischemia and thus may be associated with more hemodynamic compromise particularly when the graft subtends large areas of native myocardial circulation.

REFERENCES

1. Saric M. Echocardiography in acute coronary syndrome: anatomy, essential views, and imaging plains. In: Herzog E, Chaudhry F, eds. *Echocardiography in Acute Coronary Sydrome.* London: Springer-Verlag; 2009:17–35.
2. Smith SC Jr, Feldman TE, Hirshfeld JW Jr, et al.; Writing Committee Members. A report of the American College of Cardiology/American Heart Association Task Force on Practice Guidelines (American College of Cardiology/American Heart Association/Society for Cardiovascular Angiography and Interventions Writing Committee to Update the 2001 Guidelines for Percutaneous Coronary Intervention). *Circulation.* 2006;113(1):156–175.
3. Kushner FG, Hand M, Smith SC Jr, et al. 2009 focused updates: ACC/AHA guidelines for the management of patients with ST-elevation myocardial infarction (updating the 2004 guideline and 2007 focused update) and ACC/AHA/SCAI guidelines on percutaneous coronary intervention (updating the 2005 guideline and 2007 focused update) a report of the American College of Cardiology Foundation/American Heart Association Task Force on Practice Guidelines. *J Am Coll Cardiol.* 2009;54(23):2205–2241.
4. Garg S, Serruys PW. Coronary stents: current status. *J Am Coll Cardiol.* 2010;56(10) (suppl):S1–S42.
5. Garg S, Serruys PW. Coronary stents: looking forward. *J Am Coll Cardiol.* 2010;56(10) (suppl):S43–S78.
6. Serruys PW, Kutryk MJ, Ong AT. Coronary-artery stents. *N Engl J Med.* 2006;354(5):483–495.
7. Holmes DR Jr, Kereiakes DJ, Garg S, et al. Stent thrombosis. *J Am Coll Cardiol.* 2010;56(17):1357–1365.
8. Fractional Flow Reserve versus Angiography for Guiding Percutaneous Coronary Intervention Pim A.L. Tonino, M.D., Bernard De Bruyne, M.D., Ph.D., Nico H.J. Pijls, M.D., Ph.D., Uwe Siebert, M.D., M.P.H., Sc.D., Fumiaki Ikeno, M.D., Marcel van `t Veer, M.Sc., Volker Klauss, M.D., Ph.D., Ganesh Manoharan, M.D., Thomas Engstrøm, M.D., Ph.D., Keith G. Oldroyd, M.D., Peter N. Ver Lee, M.D., Philip A. MacCarthy, M.D., Ph.D., and William F. Fearon, M.D. for the FAME Study Investigators N Engl J Med 2009; 360:213-224HYPERLINK "http://www.nejm.org/toc/nejm/360/3/" January 15, 2009.

PATIENT AND FAMILY INFORMATION FOR:

Cardiac Catheterization and Percutaneous Intervention

Cardiac catheterization is a procedure in which a small catheter is inserted into the heart to measure pressures in the right- and left-sided chambers of the heart and to obtain X-ray pictures of the coronary arteries and the left ventricle, which is the major pumping chamber of the heart. This technique is useful in the evaluation of a variety of cardiac diseases:

1. The evaluation of the coronary arteries, the blood vessels that nourish the heart walls. The identification and severity of coronary artery disease or blockages in the arteries is diagnosed by injecting the coronary arteries with a contrast material that is seen under X-ray.
2. Valvular heart disease can be assessed by pressure measurements in the heart chambers and injection of contrast into the ventricles or the aorta.
3. The pumping function of the heart can also be evaluated with similar injections into the left ventricle.
4. Certain congenital forms of heart disease can be evaluated with cardiac catheterization by pressure measurements and oxygen analysis in the chambers of the heart.

Cardiac catheterization is done through a blood vessel either in the leg or in the arm or wrist. It is performed in a cardiac catheterization laboratory that is a specialized X-ray room. Prior to the test, the doctors will obtain an ECG and blood tests. The patient will most likely be asked not to eat for several hours before the test but most medications can be taken with a sip of water. If the patient takes blood thinners other than aspirin, plavix, prasugrel or other antiplatelet drugs the doctor may discontinue these or modify the doses before the test. If the patient is a diabetic, his/her daily medication may be held or reduced prior to the catheterization.

When the patient arrives in the catheterization laboratory an intravenous line will be started in the arm by the nurse so that medication, including sedation, can be given to the patient during the test. He/she will most likely be awake during the test but the sedation will relax him/her and relieve anxiety. ECG monitoring electrodes will be placed on the chest so that continuous recordings of the heartbeat can be monitored by a technician during the test. To reduce the risk of infection, hair will be shaved from the groin area if the doctor chooses to use the femoral artery in the leg for the insertion of the catheter. The groin area or arm area will be cleaned with an antiseptic solution.

For catheterization done by the femoral artery in the leg, the doctor will palpate the area where the maximum pulse is felt and then inject a small amount of numbing medicine into the area before inserting the thin plastic sheath or tube into the artery. If pressures are to be obtained in the right-sided chambers of the heart a similar sheath is placed in the femoral vein in the leg. The catheters, which are placed in the heart under X-ray guidance, are introduced into the blood vessels through these sheaths to minimize trauma to the blood vessels and discomfort.

A similar technique is used if the procedure is done through the artery in the arm or wrist.

In a "left heart catheterization" the catheters are guided under X-ray up the aorta, the main artery leading to the heart. From the aorta, these catheters can access the coronary arteries and the left ventricle or main pumping chamber of the heart.

In a "right heart catheterization" the catheter is introduced into the major vein of the body, the vena cava, and inserted into the right-sided chambers of the heart usually to obtain pressure measurements. A combined "right and left heart catheterization" is often done to help evaluate diseases of the heart valves and muscle.

Coronary angiography is the process of injecting contrast or "dye" into the coronary arteries to diagnose blockages or "stenosis" of the blood vessels of the heart. Digital X-ray images are obtained during the injection of contrast in the arteries, and these will be analyzed by the doctors to diagnose obstructions and plan treatment.

A diagnostic cardiac catheterization and angiogram takes about 30 to 45 minutes.

Following the procedure, if no further intervention such as balloon angioplasty or stent placement is to be done the same day, the small plastic sheath will be removed from the leg or arm. Pressure will be applied manually for several minutes (10 to 20 minutes) to stop the bleeding from the artery. Alternatively, a small collagen seal or other "closure" device can be placed in the artery to seal the hole in the vessel. The use of a seal allows the patient to ambulate earlier. The staff will provide special instructions for post-procedure care if this is done. The patient will be required to stay in bed on his/her back for 2 to 4 hours after the procedure.

CORONARY ARTERY INTERVENTIONS

After the coronary angiogram, the doctor will review the pictures and decide whether the patient is a candidate for a coronary intervention. If there are blockages in the coronary arteries and the patient has chest pain or other equivalent symptoms or, if the stress test is positive, the patient may be offered a PCI. There are many different treatments for patients with coronary artery disease including medication, coronary bypass surgery, or PCI. The choice of treatment depends on the number of arteries involved and the complexity of the stenoses, the heart function, symptoms and whether the patient has diabetes. The goal of these therapies is to improve quality of life and symptoms and, in some patients, to prolong life.

Patients who are having a heart attack affecting the full thickness of the heart muscle almost always have a coronary artery that is acutely and completely blocked by blood clot known as thrombus. This is referred to as an STEMI and requires prompt treatment to open the artery and rapidly restore blood flow to the heart muscle to reduce permanent damage. If the patient is taken to a hospital equipped with a cardiac catheterization laboratory, he/she will most likely be sent directly to the lab to have a cardiac catheterization and immediate PCI. If done within a short period, this procedure has been shown to reduce mortality or death and minimize damage to the heart. If the hospital does not have a catheterization lab, the patient may be transferred immediately to one that does, or given powerful medications to dissolve the clot.

Some patients who present to the hospital have what is referred to as a non-STEMI or unstable angina. Often the symptoms of this are relieved with medication and the EKG (Electrocardiogram) has more subtle changes. This is sometimes diagnosed with blood tests that are done after admission and frequently predict a narrowed but not completely blocked artery. These patients may benefit from a more elective cardiac catheterization and possible PCI or, depending on the circumstances, further noninvasive testing to determine the future risk of cardiac events.

TECHNIQUES OF PERCUTANEOUS CORONARY INTERVENTION FOR CORONARY ARTERY DISEASE

The different types of coronary interventions will be reviewed in detail. They are all done through similar catheters and sheaths as the diagnostic catheterization and angiography. An intervention may be done ad hoc, at the time of the diagnostic test or scheduled electively after the pictures are reviewed. The timing may depend on the complexity of the narrowing or other active medical issues as well as at the patient's request.

CORONARY ANGIOPLASTY

This procedure is often referred to as percutaneous coronary angioplasty (PTCA). A thin steerable wire called a guide wire is inserted into the diseased artery and advanced across the narrowing under X-ray. Once this wire is in position, a flexible tube with a balloon at the tip is inserted over the wire and across the narrowing or "lesion" and inflated. This compresses the plaque or narrowing in the artery and, when the balloon is deflated, allows the blood to flow through the dilated artery. The balloons come in various lengths and diameters and more

than one may be used to achieve an acceptable result. When the artery is dilated to an acceptable diameter, the balloon and the guide wire are removed. Balloon angioplasty may be used alone or prior to the insertion of a stent.

One of the advantages of balloon angioplasty is the wide variety of sizes of balloons available. Even very small arteries can be successfully treated with balloons. A disadvantage of balloon dilatation as a "stand-alone" procedure is a high rate of re-stenosis caused by excessive scar tissue formation at the site of the dilatation. This may necessitate a repeat procedure.

CORONARY STENT IMPLANTATION

The advent of coronary stents addressed one of the prime long-term problems seen with balloon angioplasty, re-stenosis. The tendency to form scar tissue at the site of balloon dilatation has been as high as 50% or greater in some instances. Stents are metal support devices that stay in place in the artery forever. Most often, these are made of stainless steel, and their rigid structure not only keeps the artery from collapsing on itself (recoil), but as the initial improvement in diameter is greater after insertion of the stent, they can prevent critical renarrowing of the artery from scar tissue formation. Stents can be either "drug eluting" or "non-drug eluting." A DES has substances applied to the surface that prevent cell growth and thus excessive scar formation within the stent. This reduces the rate of re-stenosis or renarrowing even further, often dramatically reducing the need for repeat procedures.

A stent is, in essence, a foreign substance in the body and when the metallic surface of the stent is exposed to blood and platelets, a blood clot or thrombus can form, effectively blocking the blood flow and causing a heart attack. Therefore, patients are given two medications, aspirin plus another antiplatelet drug such as plavix or prasugrel which together greatly reduce the risk of this happening. If the patient is treated with a stent, he/she must be committed to taking this "dual antiplatelet therapy" for as long as the physician prescribes them to prevent this subacute thrombosis or clot formation.

Because "coated" or DES prevent cell growth within the stent, they are recognized as "foreign" to the body for a longer period and are more susceptible to clot formation for longer periods than noncoated stents. In this case, the patient will be asked to continue taking dual platelet therapy for a year or longer as opposed to a few months. If the patient has elective surgery planned, a history of bleeding, or is unwilling or unable to take the antiplatelet therapy for a prolonged period, it is essential to let the doctor know so an appropriate choice of stent can be made.

ROTATIONAL ATHERECTOMY

Sometimes the coronary arteries can be so severely calcified that the insertion of a balloon or a stent is impossible owing to the rigid narrowing. The rotoblator is a rapidly rotating burr with a head embedded with diamond chips mounted on a catheter. When this device is inserted into a calcified section of artery, it pulverizes the calcified plaque.

It can be used as a stand-alone device or followed by coronary stenting.

THROMBECTOMY

During a heart attack, a blood clot or thrombus forms in the artery blocking the flow of blood. This blood clot can be removed using a catheter that actually aspirates the clot into the catheter to remove it from the artery by mechanical suction. Other devices can be used to disrupt the clot before removal by generating high-pressure saline jets that create a suction effect that draws the clot into the catheter and macerates it.

INTRAVASCULAR ULTRASOUND

Because the pictures taken during coronary angiography are two-dimensional images, it is sometimes hard to estimate the extent of narrowing in an artery or the amount of calcium or clot present. Ultrasound, which utilizes a miniature transducer at the end of a catheter can be used to visualize the inside of the artery. It can help to determine the extent of narrowing of the artery, the composition of the plaque, the pattern of calcification, and the presence of clot. After the initial X-ray pictures are taken the doctor may insert this device into the artery to further characterize the narrowing to help plan the therapeutic procedure.

NONCORONARY INTERVENTIONS

CLOSURE OF DEFECTS IN THE HEART STRUCTURE

Occasionally patients will present with small holes between the upper chambers of the heart. These atrial septal defects can be often successfully closed through catheter-based techniques thus avoiding open heart surgery. If the patient has this condition, the doctor will explain the benefits and alternatives to this type of treatment.

FUTURE DIRECTIONS IN CARDIAC INTERVENTIONS

The treatment of valvular heart disease is an active area of research. Catheter-based procedures may be performed for some cases of narrowing of the mitral valve and occasionally for the aortic valve. Transcatheter techniques for replacement or repair of diseased valves are currently being performed in many research centers and will likely become commonplace in the future.

Eyal Herzog
Dan Halpern
Farooq A. Chaudhry

CHAPTER 5

Echocardiography in Acute Coronary Syndrome

The last few decades have witnessed remarkable progress in the understanding of the pathophysiology of acute coronary syndrome (ACS). This, in turn, has led to advances in various imaging techniques for diagnosis and therapeutic options. Developments in the field of echocardiography have paralleled the progress made in ACS. The initial use of echocardiography was to detect pericardial effusions and cardiac tumors. However, the current applications of various forms of echocardiography include an extended list of pathologic and therapeutic indications. Advances in echocardiographic techniques and instrumentation have rivaled those in management of ACS.[1] This chapter focuses on the role of echocardiography in ACS.

ASSESSMENT OF REGIONAL SYSTOLIC FUNCTION IN ACUTE CORONARY SYNDROME

Occlusion of an epicardial coronary artery at the time of ACS may lead to a loss of contractile function in the myocardial segments subtended by that vessel. The magnitude and duration of wall motion abnormalities depend on the severity, extent, and duration of the coronary occlusion.

In unstable angina (UA), left and right ventricular wall motion maybe normal unless transthoracic echocardiography happens to be performed during an episode of chest pain.

Non-ST-elevation myocardial infarction (NSTEMI) usually results from an occlusion of a coronary branch vessel often in an elderly patient with preexisting collateral coronary circulation. Typically the loss of contractile function is restricted to the subendocardial layer that is most vulnerable to ischemia. However, on standard echocardiography, the contractility loss may be observed in the entire thickness of the affected myocardial segment. This overestimation of contractile loss is attributed to tethering (an apparent passive loss of contractility in normal segments owing to contractile loss in an adjacent area).

ST-elevation myocardial infarction (STEMI) often results from an acute occlusion of a major coronary vessel and tends to occur in a younger age group compared with NSTEMI. If the total session of coronary flow lasts for >3 to 6 hours, myocardial necrosis will occur and the myocardium in the affected segments will be replaced with a fibrous tissue over the ensuing weeks.[2]

The magnitude of regional contractile loss in ACS is usually assessed semi-quantitatively. It is usually interpreted clinically as follows[2]:

1. Interpretation of wall motion abnormalities:
   Normal — Contractility preserved
   Hypokinesis — Partial loss of contractility
   Akinesis — Complete loss of contractility
   Dyskinesis — Paradoxical movement of the affected segment away from the center of the ventricle during systole
   Aneurysmal — Outward movement of the affected segment during both systole and diastole
2. Extent and location of affected segments
3. Suspected coronary artery distribution (left anterior descending artery vs. right coronary artery vs. left circumflex artery).

ASSESSMENT OF GLOBAL SYSTOLIC FUNCTION IN ACUTE CORONARY SYNDROME

Global ventricular systolic function in ACS is assessed through either wall motion scoring and global ventricular ejection fraction.

WALL MOTION SCORING

Wall motion scoring analysis assigns a numeric value to the degree of contractile dysfunction in each segment. Most common scoring criteria are seen in Table 5.1.

Once all segments are assigned individual scores, total score is calculated as a sum of individual scores. A wall motion score index (WMSI) in then calculated as a ratio between the total score over the number of evaluated segments. The WMSI is a dimensionless index.

For a fully visualized normal ventricle the total score is 17 (all segments have normal contractility). Because all 17 segments are evaluated, the WMSI of a normal heart is $17/17 = 1$. For abnormal ventricles, the higher the WMSI, the more significant is the abnormal wall motion.

TABLE 5.1	Left Ventricular Wall Motion Scoring
	Score
Normal	1
Hypokinesis	2
Akinesis	3
Dyskinesis	4
Aneurysmal	5
Wall motion score index =	$\dfrac{\text{Sum of individual segment scores}}{\text{Number of evaluated segments}}$

ASSESSMENT OF VENTRICULAR EJECTION FRACTION

Numerous studies have consistently shown left ventricular ejection fraction (LVEF) as one of the most powerful predictors of future mortality and morbidity in patients with heart disease.[3] LVEF is the single most powerful predictor of mortality and the risk for developing life-threatening ventricular arrhythmias after myocardial infarction.[4] Furthermore, once the ACS resolves, the residual LVEF is important for treatment options as LVEF cutoff values are built into recommendations for both medical and electrical device therapies. Even with treatment and clinical stabilization of heart failure, there is an inverse, almost linear, relationship between LVEF and survival in the patient whose LVEF is <45% (Figure 5.1).[5]

By definition, LVEF is the percentage of the end-diastolic volume that is ejected with each systole as the stroke volume. Thus, to calculate the LVEF one needs to estimate the end-systolic and end-diastolic volume of the left ventricle.

For two-dimensional echocardiography, biplane Simpson's rule is routinely used for estimation of LVEF.[6,7] Most modern ultrasound systems provide a semiautomated software package for the Simpson's rule analysis. Operators are usually required to trace only the left ventricular endocardial border at end-diastolic and end-systolic in the apical four-chamber and two-chamber views; the software package then automatically calculates the left ventricular end-diastolic volume, end-systolic volume, and LVEF (Figure 5.2).

With the advent of real-time three-dimensional (RT3D) transthoracic techniques, left ventricular volumes and LVEF can now be calculated with greater accuracy than is possible with the biplane Simpson's rule (Figure 5.3). RT3D-derived left ventricular volume data are now comparable to those obtained by cardiac magnetic resonance imaging, the prior gold standard for such calculations.[7]

Thus, whenever available, left ventricular volumes and LVEF in ACS should be calculated from an RT3D system. The biplane Simpson's rule should be the next best method for such calculations when only a two-dimensional ultrasound system is available.

THE ISCHEMIC CASCADE

The ischemic cascade refers to a sequence of events that occurs in the myocardium after the onset of ischemia.[8] Myocardial

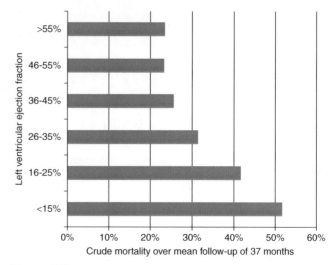

Figure 5.1. Relationship between left ventricular ejection fraction and survival. Note the negative almost linear relationship between survival and left ejection fractions <45%. (Based on numeric data from Curtis JP, Sokol SI, Wang Y, et al. The association of left ventricular ejection fraction, mortality, and cause of death in stable outpatients with heart failure. *J Am Coll Cardiol.* 2003;42(4):736–742.)

perfusion is determined by coronary blood flow and myocardial oxygen consumption. Any imbalance in this supply and demand relationship results in myocardial ischemia.[9] The mechanical, electrographic, and clinical events that follow the development of ischemia were formally described in 1985 by Hauser et al.,[10] and were later termed the "ischemic cascade."[11] Classically, the observable changes occur sequentially (Figure 5.4) starting with perfusion abnormalities leading to abnormalities in wall function, then ischemic electrocardiogram (EKG) changes, and finally angina.[12] Echocardiography has the ability to detect these pathophysiologic changes in the myocardium at the most initial stages and therefore is more sensitive than history, physical examination, and EKG for identification of myocardial ischemia.[13]

Echocardiography for the diagnosis of suspected acute ischemia is most helpful in subjects with a high clinical suspicion but nondiagnostic ECG as it allows real-time assessment of myocardial function. In addition, through stress modalities, it offers assessment and risk stratification in patients who present to the emergency department (ED) with chest pain.

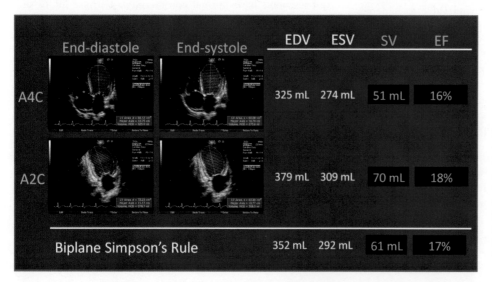

Figure 5.2. Calculation of left ventricular ejection fraction (LVEF) by biplane Simpson's rule. The operator of an ultrasound system is required to trace the endocardial border of an end-diastolic and an end-systolic frame in the apical four-chamber (A4C) and two-chamber (A2C) views. The system then calculates the end-diastolic volume (EDV), end-systolic volume (ESV), stroke volume (SV), and LVEF.

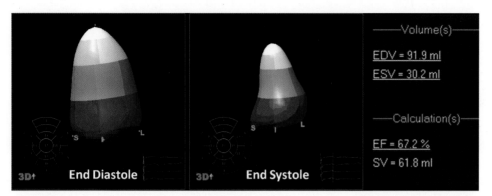

Figure 5.3. Calculation of left ventricular volumes and ejection fraction (EF) by three-dimensional echocardiography. A 3D ultrasound system calculates the end-diastolic volume (EDV), end-systolic volume (ESV), stroke volume (SV), and left ventricular ejection fraction (LVEF) automatically from a 3D data set after an operator manually enters key reference points of the left ventricle.

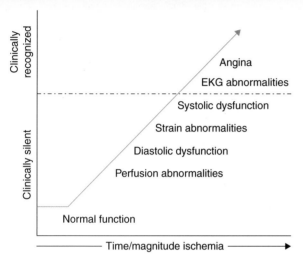

Figure 5.4. The ischemic cascade. Myocardial dysfunction occurs in a predictable sequence that is detectable prior to clinical symptoms.

STRESS ECHOCARDIOGRAPHY

There are different types of stress echocardiography that can be used in the evaluation of patients with coronary artery disease (CAD).[14] For patients who are able to exercise, treadmill and supine bicycle stress echocardiograms are preferred techniques. For patients unable to exercise, pharmacologic stress testing using dobutamine, dipyridamole, or adenosine is an alternative method to provoke ischemia.

Table 5.2 outlines the methods to induce stress. The basic principle of stress echocardiography is the identification of new wall motion abnormalities that occur in the presence of provocable ischemia. This involves the comparison of baseline echocardiographic images obtained under resting conditions with those obtained immediately postexercise in the case of treadmill or peak exercise in the case of bicycle protocol. Parasternal long and short axis as well as apical two-, three-, and four-chamber views are acquired at baseline and post-stress testing. The left ventricle is divided into 17 segments as per the recommendation of the American Society

TABLE 5.2	Methods to Induce Stress
Exercise	*Pharmacological*
Treadmill	Dobutamine
Supine bicycle	Dipyridamole
Isometric	Adenosine

of Echocardiography. All images are digitized in a continuous loop format utilizing a quad-screen format to facilitate the detection of new segmental wall motion abnormalities. The best postexercise image is selected and compared with the baseline image by side-by-side comparison in the quad-screen image format.

In the United States, the most commonly used method for provoking ischemia in patients able to exercise is treadmill testing. The sensitivity of exercise testing is strongly dependent on attaining adequate heart rate and cardiovascular workload. The use of treadmill or bicycle methods of exercise require the patient to achieve a target heart rate of 85% of the age predicted maximum heart rate or attain a workload of at least six metabolic equivalents (METS) to achieve satisfactory sensitivity. In patients who can achieve these workloads, exercise testing is the method of choice to provoke myocardial ischemia.

The most common treadmill protocol used is the Bruce protocol, although other protocols such as the modified Bruce can be used depending on the level of fitness of the patient. According to standard stress testing protocol, the patient has continuous EKG monitoring with exercise, and blood pressure is checked every 3 minutes. With treadmill exercise, the postexercise images are obtained ideally within <1 minute.

The exercise test should be terminated if any of the following occur:

1. Severe symptoms such as chest pain or dyspnea
2. Severe ST depressions
3. Hemodynamically significant arrhythmia
4. Severe hypertensive response (BP > 220/120 mm Hg)
5. Hypotension (a decrease of >20 mm Hg)

PHARMACOLOGIC STRESS ECHOCARDIOGRAM

Alternatively for those patients who cannot exercise, dobutamine or dipyridamole stress Echos can be performed. By far, dobutamine is the most common pharmacologic agent used to provoke ischemia in stress Echos. Dobutamine is a synthetic catecholamine that binds to β_1 and β_2 receptors. The affinity of dobutamine for β_1 cardiac muscle receptors results in positive inotropic and chronotropic effects. Therefore, dobutamine induces myocardial ischemia in patients with flow-limiting coronary stenosis by increasing left ventricular contractility, heart rate, wall stress, and therefore myocardial oxygen demand. Dobutamine has a short half-life and is rapidly metabolized once the infusion is discontinued. Any adverse side effects or arrhythmias can usually be quickly terminated by discontinuation of the drip or by intravenous β-blockers.[15]

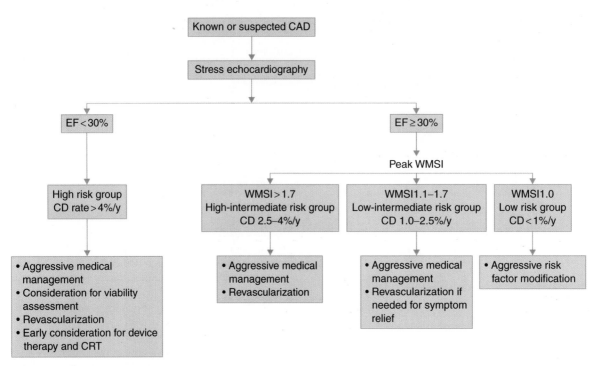

Figure 5.5. Schematic for risk stratification of patients undergoing stress echocardiography.

PATHWAY FOR MANAGEMENT OF PATIENTS BASED ON STRESS ECHO RESULTS

Risk stratification of patients undergoing stress echocardiography should be based both on peak WMSI (which includes both extent and severity of ischemia/infarction) and left ventricular ejection fraction (resting). Figure 5.5 represents a schematic for the risk stratification of patients with known or suspected CAD referred for stress echocardiography. The data for risk stratification are based on an analysis of 3,259 patients (59 ± 13 years; 48% males) followed for up to 4 years.[16]

The first step in the risk stratification process is evaluation of ejection fraction. Patients with EF <30% are a high-risk group with a cardiac death (CD) rate of >4% per year regardless of the peak WMSI. Such patients should be aggressively managed. These patients may also benefit from viability assessment and consideration for revascularization as deemed necessary. They should also be considered for early device therapy (ICD/CRT; cardiac resynchronization therapy/implantable cardioverter-defibrillator) and for cardiac transplant evaluation.

In patients with EF ≥30%, peak WMSI can further risk stratify the patient subgroup into a low-risk group (peak WMSI = 1.0) (CD <1% per year), low–intermediate (peak WMSI 1.1 to 1.7) (CD 1% to 2.5% per year) and a high–intermediate (peak WMSI >1.7) (CD 2.5% to 4.0% per year) risk groups. Patients in the low-risk category will benefit from aggressive risk factor modification. Those in the low–intermediate-risk group may benefit from aggressive medical management and consideration of revascularization for symptom relief only. Patients in the high–intermediate-risk group may benefit from aggressive medical management and revascularization therapy. Such a risk stratification approach will potentially avoid unnecessary revascularization procedures for low-risk individuals and at the same time give a framework for the management of intermediate- and high-risk subgroups.

REFERENCES

1. Panjrath GS, Herzog E, Chaudhry FA. Introduction: acute coronary syndrome and echocardiography. In: Herzog E, Chaudhry FA, eds. *Echocardiography in ACS from Prevention to Diagnosis and Treatment.* London: Springer-Verlag; 2009:Chap 1:1–4.
2. Saric M. Echo assessment of systolic and diastolic function in acute coronary syndrome. In: Herzog E, Chaudhry FA, eds. *Echocardiography in ACS from Prevention to Diagnosis and Treatment.* London: Springer-Verlag; 2009:Chap 4:37–57.
3. Multicenter Postinfarction Research Group. Risk stratification and survival after myocardial infarction. *N Engl J Med.* 1983;309(6):331–336.
4. Carlson MD, Krishen A. Risk assessment for ventricular arrhythmias after extensive myocardial infarction: what should I do? *ACC Curr J Rev.* 2003;12(2):90–93.
5. Curtis JP, Sokol SI, Wang Y, et al. The association of left ventricular ejection fraction, mortality, and cause of death in stable outpatients with heart failure. *J Am Coll Cardiol.* 2003;42(4):736–742.
6. Lang RM, Bierig M, Devereux RB, et al. Recommendations for chamber quantification: a report from the American Society of Echocardiography's Guidelines and Standards Committee and the Chamber Quantification Writing Group, developed in conjunction with the European Association of Echocardiography, a branch of the European Society of Cardiology. *J Am Soc Echocardiogr.* 2005;18(12):1440–1463.
7. Otterstad JE. Measuring left ventricular volume and ejection fraction with the biplane Simpson's method. *Heart.* 2002;88(6):559–560.
8. Ansari A, Puthumana J. The "ischemic cascade." In: Herzog E, Chaudhry FA, eds. *Echocardiography in ACS from Prevention to Diagnosis and Treatment.* London: Springer-Verlag; 2009:Chap 11:149–160.
9. Feigenbaum H, Armstrong WF, Ryan T. *Feigenbaum's Echocardiography.* Philadelphia, PA: Lippincott Williams & Wilkins; 2005.
10. Hauser AM, Vellappillil G, Ramos RG, et al. Sequence of mechanical, electrocardiographic and clinical effects of repeated coronary artery occlusion in human beings: echocardiographic observations during coronary angioplasty. *J Am Coll Cardiol.* 1985;5:193–197.
11. Nesto RW, Kowalchuk MD. The ischemic cascade: temporal sequence of hemodynamic, electrocardiographic and symptomatic expressions of ischemia. *Am J Cardiol.* 1987;57: 23C–30C.
12. Harbinson M, Anagnostopoulos CD. *Noninvasive Imaging of Myocardial Ischemia. Principles of Pathophysiology Related to Noninvasive Cardiac Imaging.* London: Springer; 2006.
13. Lewis WR. Echocardiography in the evaluation of patients in chest pain units. *Cardiol Clin.* 2005;23:531–539.
14. Kim B, Chaudhry FA. How to perform stress echocardiography. In: Herzog E, Chaudhry FA, eds. *Echocardiography in ACS from Prevention to Diagnosis and Treatment.* London: Springer-Verlag; 2009:Chap 12:161–166.
15. Valentini V, Greenfield S, McDermott E, et al. Principles and techniques of pharmacologic stress echocardiography. *Video J Echocardiogr.* 1993;3:82–89.
16. Bangalore S, Chaudhry FA. Pathway for the management of patients based on stress echo results. In: Herzog E, Chaudhry FA, eds. *Echocardiography in ACS from Prevention to Diagnosis and Treatment.* London: Springer-Verlag; 2009:Chap 14:193–200.

PATIENT AND FAMILY INFORMATION FOR:

Echocardiography in Acute Coronary Syndrome

ECHOCARDIOGRAPHY IN THE CCU

The Echocardiogram (Echo) is an ultrasound device that visualizes the heart and surrounding structures in a real-time fashion and in turn provides important anatomical and physiological information to the cardiologist. The Echo, like a radar, emits and receives ultrasound waves and constructs an image by employing the differences in the signal properties. At the end of this sophisticated and fast process, an impressive and informative animation of the heart moving in the chest is displayed for further interpretation. In the CCU, echocardiography has become an essential tool for real-time bedside heart disease diagnostics, especially in critical times. Furthermore, echocardiography lacks any major side effects and is mostly noninvasive.

THE DEVICE STRUCTURE

The Echo itself is made of two major components: the first is the transducer, that is, the "radar dish" that relays the ultrasounds waves and is in touch with the patient's body; and the second is a computer console that functions as the "brain" performing the computation. The transducer is filled with multiple crystals (called piezoelectric crystals) that have the natural property of sending and receiving ultrasound waves. Different transducers have different properties. Lower-frequency transducers can emit ultrasound waves deeper into the body but lack the picture quality of the higher-frequency ones. When placing the transducer over the chest (this common procedure is referred to as trans-thoracic Echo or TTE), a real-time moving image of the heart appears. By rotating and manipulating the transducer over the chest, different areas of the heart are seen; those are referred to as windows. Gel is used to improve the connection between the transducer and the skin. In TTE, four major areas over the chest are used to create heart images. These include the left chest area between the third and fourth ribs (parasternal), heart's tip (apical), under the ribs (subcostal), and above the chest (suprasternal). Several views of the heart are created in each location by rotating the transducer.

THE ECHOCARDIOGRAM ROLE IN THE CCU

In the CCU, echocardiography studies are performed to answer complex clinical questions. Of greater concern in the CCU are the function and integrity of the heart muscle walls (myocardium), the valves and the heart sac (pericardium). The Echo can provide information about the chamber of the heart that is involved in the disease, the hearts squeezing efficiency (ejection fraction), the amount of fluid in the heart's sac, and the presence of clots in the heart chambers.

In the case where there is fluid in the heart sac that compresses the heart (condition called pericardial tamponade), the Echo can detect this acute life-threatening situation promptly and guide an immediate draining procedure.

"HEART ATTACKS" AND ECHOCARDIOGRAPHY

The major disease treated in the CCU is of coronary origin. The coronary arteries are the vessels that feed blood to the heart muscle itself. "Heart attack" or acute MI is the condition where the coronary vessel is blocked. As the heart muscle does not receive oxygenated blood from the coronary artery, it starts dying, losing its ability to contract and pump blood. In contrast to a complete blockage, partial blockage of the coronary artery may result in symptoms such as chest pressure on exertion (referred to as angina), but no impairment in the heart squeezing function. Of note, the patient's symptoms are the last to develop in the cascade of coronary artery blockage. After complete cessation of blood supply to the heart muscle, a sequence of event occurs referred to as the ischemic cascade, where the heart muscle wall motion is affected before any EKG changes and before the patient develops symptoms. Therefore, the Echo potentially can detect in a noninvasive way heart wall motion contraction impairments in situations where the EKG is nondiagnostic and the patient's symptoms are unclear. During the complete coronary occlusion, the Echo is able to show which wall of heart is not contracting and is thus affected directly by the occlusion. The degree of muscle contraction impairment has a scoring system that provides information about the extent of occlusion and function of the muscle. The walls of the heart are divided to 17 segments. Normal wall motion gets a score of 1; hypokinesis is the term used to describe decreased contractility and receives a score of 2; Akinesis is when no wall motion is seen with a score of 3; and dyskinesis is when the wall motion direction is occurring in the opposite direction with a score of 4. The sum of the scores of each segment is then divided by 17. A normal score would be 1 (17 divided by the 17 segments) and a score above 1.7 represents a significant wall motion abnormality.

There are three major coronary arteries in the heart, and each of them provides blood supply to a certain muscle wall of the heart (with some overlapping). The Echo is able to pinpoint the culprit vessel that is occluded. The occluded coronary artery is represented in the Echo study by a specific area of impaired contraction. The assessment of the heart muscle contraction is also assessed as a whole; that is, what is the heart's global pumping efficiency? This is referred to as ejection fraction. The EF denotes the percentage of blood squeezed from the heart in one heartbeat to the rest of the body (normal value is 55%). It is known from numerous studies that the lower the ejection fraction is, the outcome of the patient is the worst. Accuracy in the calculation of the ejection fraction is getting better as three-dimensional echocardiography is being employed.

For example. A patient with an acute myocardial infarction is admitted to the CCU with an LAD occlusion; the LAD feeds the front side of the left heart chamber (main pumping chamber); during the performance of the Echo study the cardiologist notices that the front portion of the left heart chamber is not squeezing (hypokinesis) with an EF of 30%, and there is also some valve leak. Occlusion of an artery can influence the function of a heart valve as its movement relies on muscles derived from the heart wall as well. The patient is sent thereafter for a cardiac catheterization where the occluded coronary artery is opened. An Echo performed 2 days after the procedure shows some recovery in the wall motion of the front wall with resolution of the valve leakage, as blood supply was restored to the region. The Echo provides up-to-date functional information of various structures of the heart such as the muscle wall and the valves.

MANAGEMENT AFTER THE ACUTE EPISODE

The Echo has a role for diagnosing new or recurrent symptoms during the admission in the CCU after the primary diagnosis is made. For example, if a patient has recurrent chest pain, shortness of breath, or if the patient's blood pressure is coming down without a reason, the Echo can provide answers. New heart wall motion abnormalities can point to new or recurrent coronary vessel occlusions. A new murmur that is first detected on physical exam with a stethoscope could be the result of a new valve problem (e.g., leakage) or even a rupture between the heart chambers. These conditions require prompt interventions and at times may require surgery. The Echo can help diagnosing dehydration (the main heart pumping chamber becomes smaller), fluid overload (e.g., from heart failure or administration of too much fluids) or fluid in the heart sac that compresses the heart.

STRESS TESTING

Some patients admitted with chest pain and with a high suspicion of a CAD without an overt heart attack require more testing to confirm the diagnosis. This could be accomplished by performing an Echo while the patient's heart is being "stressed," that is, walking on a treadmill or giving the patient a medication that will make the heart beat faster. Actual stressing or exercising is not performed when the patient is suspected of an evolving heart attack (ACS). Images of the patient's heart muscle contraction are obtained before, during and after the stress—the muscle could be inspected for motion abnormalities that denote probable coronary disease.

TRANS-ESOPHAGEAL ECHOCARDIOGRAPHY

Some echocardiography information could be better acquired by using the device in a semi-invasive method called transesophageal echocardiogram (TEE)—Echo through the esophagus (food pipe); because of the short distance between the transducer and the heart while positioned in the esophagus, the quality of pictures becomes better. It is especially useful when imaging cardiac structures located at the back part of the heart (e.g., the left atrium).

LIMITATIONS

There are some limitations in performing Echo at bedside as compared to the echocardiography laboratory settings. Usually the patient is asked to lie on his left side to obtain some of the windows, and then to lie on his back for the rest of the images. In the CCU, the patient could be mechanically ventilated, sedated, and may not be able to cooperate. Thus some of the pictures may be much harder to obtain to produce high-quality images.

CONCLUSION

Echocardiography in the CCU provides important anatomical, structural, and clinical information that aids the cardiologist in the diagnosis and treatment of acute heart diseases. It helps to establish a diagnosis in a real-time fashion. It shows the heart's muscle function, and this information helps to designate the coronary artery that is occluded during heart attacks. It shows the integrity and function of the heart valves, the amount of fluid in the heart's sac, and the body's fluid balance. Echocardiography aids in managing severely sick patients in the CCU by sequential studies. Echocardiography has changed the way cardiologists treat patients in the CCU by having the ability to get live images of the heart apparatus at the bedside of the patient.

Seth Uretsky
Edgar Argulian

CHAPTER 6

Use of Radionuclide Imaging in Acute Coronary Syndrome

Chest pain is a common complaint and is often the presenting symptom in patients with acute coronary syndrome (ACS).[1] The evaluation of chest pain as a presenting symptom for ACS is complicated by (1) the numerous etiologies that can cause chest pain, (2) the lack of a highly specific and sensitive test available at the time of initial evaluation, (3) poor clinical outcomes of patients in whom a diagnosis of ACS is missed, and (4) the medicolegal implications. Because patients with ACS are at a high risk for poor outcomes, the ability to identify these patients rapidly during the initial evaluation is critical. The initial diagnostic workup in patients presenting with symptoms suspicious of ACS include a history, physical examination, ECG, and serum troponin. The ECG is the key diagnostic test used to determine whether the patient has ongoing myocardial ischemia. Unfortunately, the ECG is often nondiagnostic in many patients who present with symptoms suspicious for ACS. Although serum troponin has been shown to be a sensitive test for myocardial damage, there are certain drawbacks to the test (i.e., the need for ischemia of sufficient time for myocardial necrosis to take place), and the initial serum troponin is often negative in patients with ACS. Based on the pathophysiology of coronary artery plaque rupture as the cause of ACS, one of the earliest signs of ACS is the decrease in blood flow to the myocardium (Figure 6.1). This decrease in myocardial blood flow can be evaluated using single photon emission computed tomography (SPECT) myocardial perfusion imaging (MPI), which images the relative amount of myocardial blood flow to all segments of the left ventricle. The use of SPECT MPI in the patient presenting with chest pain was developed over the last several decades to allow for rapid triage in chest pain patients with an eye towards initiation of the necessary medical therapy and revascularization procedures (primary angioplasty or thrombolysis) as quickly as possible, thereby reducing the amount of myocardial necrosis. However, we would also like to identify those patients in whom the chest pain symptoms are not because of ACS so that they are not unnecessarily admitted to the hospital, thus better utilizing health care resources. In this chapter, we will explore the technical, physiologic, and current outcomes data of using SPECT MPI in patients with acute chest pain.

SPECT MPI OVERVIEW

MPI was introduced in the 1970s into clinical practice as a tool to noninvasively assess for myocardial ischemia. In the 1980s planar imaging gave way to the more robust SPECT imaging most commonly used today. The theory behind SPECT MPI relies on the fact that blood flows preferentially down the path of least resistance, that is, the vessel without intracoronary thrombus versus the vessel with intracoronary thrombus (Figure 6.2). When comparing myocardial regions with each other, a decrease in tracer uptake in a region is a sign of myocardial hypoperfusion. SPECT MPI utilizes radiotracers whose activity can be detected with a special camera called a scintillation camera. The most commonly used radiotracers are thallium-201 (Tl-201) and technetium-99m (Tc-99m). Radiotracers contain atoms that undergo radioactive decay by emitting a particle that can be detected using a SPECT camera. Once injected intravenously, the radiotracer is taken up by the myocardium and the relative "amount" of tracer in each region of the myocardium can be measured and imaged.

SPECT CAMERA

The SPECT camera is designed to detect the radioactivity emitted from a patient after injection of a radiotracer. After injection of the radiotracer, patients are placed in the camera and the images are acquired.

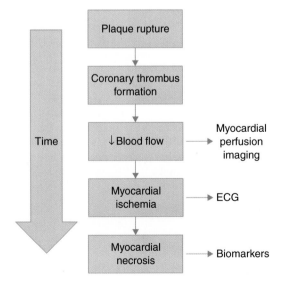

Figure 6.1. The ischemic cascade.

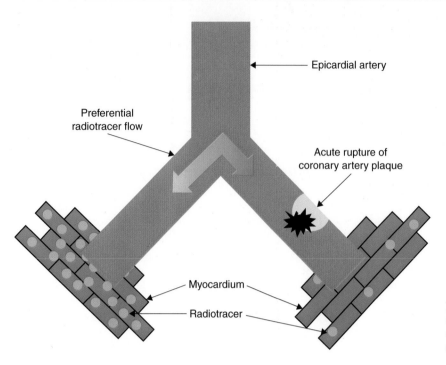

Figure 6.2. Differential myocardial radiotracer uptake in myocardium subtended by a normal coronary and a coronary with a ruptured atherosclerotic plaque.

RADIOTRACERS

Radiotracers are tagged molecules that emit radioactivity. The ideal radiotracer has several features:

1. Linear relationship between myocardial uptake and blood flow
2. High myocardial extraction rate
3. Low extra-cardiac uptake and
4. Does not decay or redistribute too rapidly.

The most commonly used radiotracers in nuclear cardiology are Tl-201 and Tc-99m. Tc-99m has several advantages over Tl-201, including a shorter half-life, higher-energy photon, poor redistribution, and it is available locally through an Mo-99 generator. The process whereby Thallium decays is called electron capture or isomeric transition (Tl-201 + e$^-$ → Hg-201 + γ), whereas Tc-99m decays by the process called gamma decay (Tc-99m → Tc-99 + γ).

MYOCARDIAL PERFUSION

MPI imaging is based on the concept that the injected radiotracer is taken up by the myocardium in proportion to the amount of blood flow that myocardial region receives. If blood flow to an area of myocardium is reduced owing to an intracoronary thrombus, this area of myocardium will receive less radiotracer in comparison with areas of myocardium in which blood flow is not reduced (Figure 6.2). The resulting SPECT images will have a decrease in tracer activity in the myocardial segments subtended by the diseased coronary artery. In patients with chest pain owing to acute coronary insufficiency, there is rupture of coronary plaque resulting in the formation of intracoronary thrombus and a subsequent decrease in myocardial blood flow to the myocardium supplied by that artery. However,

in patients without the presence of intracoronary thrombus, there will be no decrease in blood flow to the myocardium, and no decrease in tracer activity will be seen.

SPECT MPI INTERPRETATION

By convention SPECT images are displayed in three orientations: short axis, vertical long axis, and horizontal long axis (Figure 6.3). The left ventricle can be divided into the anterior wall, lateral wall, inferior wall, and septum. SPECT images are displayed with the post-stress images on the top line and the rest images below (Figure 6.4). The short-axis images are displayed apex to base, followed by the vertical long axis, and the horizontal long axis. As discussed above, SPECT MPI is measuring relative blood flow to the various segments of the myocardium. When interpreting SPECT images, one compares the amount of tracer uptake on the stress images with the amount of tracer uptake in the rest images for each myocardial segment. If the tracer uptake is homogeneous in both the rest and stress images, there is no decrease in blood flow to the myocardium, that is, no ischemia or scar (Figure 6.4). However, if there is a decrease in perfusion on the stress images in a region of normal tracer uptake on the resting images, it is termed a "reversible" defect and is indicative of ischemia (Figure 6.5). If there is a matched decrease in tracer uptake in both the stress and rest images, it is termed a "fixed" defect and is indicative of myocardial scar (Figure 6.6).

ROLE OF SPECT MPI IN PATIENTS WITH SUSPECTED ACS

The ideal test in patients with suspected ACS enables the clinician to stratify those patients who are at low risk and can be safely discharged and those who are at high risk and need

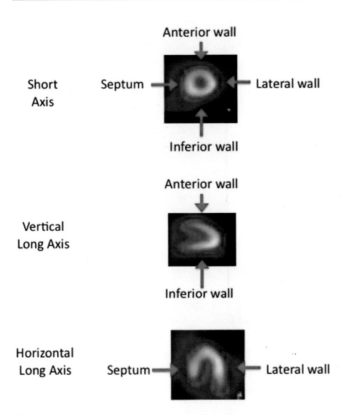

Figure 6.3. Short axis, vertical long axis, and horizontal long axis slices with labeled myocardial regions.

is experiencing an ACS. Resting SPECT MPI protocols have been developed and well studied in patients with suspected ACS. Several single center studies[2–6] and then multicenter trials[7,8] have shown that resting SPECT MPI can identify those patients undergoing ACS as well as those who can be safely discharged. Heller et al. studied 357 patients who presented with chest pain suspicious for myocardial ischemia with a non-diagnostic ECG who underwent rest SPECT MPI with Tc-99m. Among the 20 patients with myocardial infarction, 18 (90%) had abnormal SPECT images, whereas 2 had normal SPECT images, for a negative predictive value of 99%. In this study, SPECT MPI gave incremental diagnostic value over clinical and ECG variables alone, and an abnormal SPECT was the strongest predictor of myocardial infarction. The emergency room assessment of sestamibi (ERASE) for evaluation of chest pain [3] trial was a prospective multicenter randomized trial of 2,475 patients who presented with chest pain and a normal or nondiagnostic ECG. Patients were randomized to usual care or usual care plus rest SPECT MPI. The authors report that there was no difference in the rate of hospitalization between the study arms among patients with myocardial infarction. However, among patients without ACS, fewer patients were hospitalized in the rest SPECT strategy compared to standard care (42% vs. 52%).

ROLE OF SPECT IN RISK STRATIFICATION POST MYOCARDIAL INFARCTION

Risk stratification is an important clinical tool in patients who have had a myocardial infarction. The two most common scenarios in which stress SPECT is useful are in patients who (1) have not undergone revascularization and (2) those who have

further workup. As stated above, the combination of history, physical examination, ECG, and serum troponin will often be indeterminate at the time of initial evaluation, and the clinician cannot confidently determine whether the patient

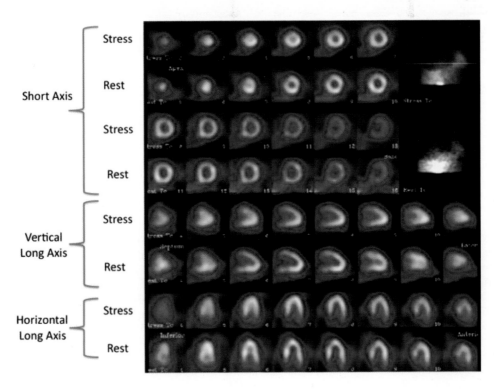

Figure 6.4. Normal SPECT MPI with homogeneous tracer uptake.

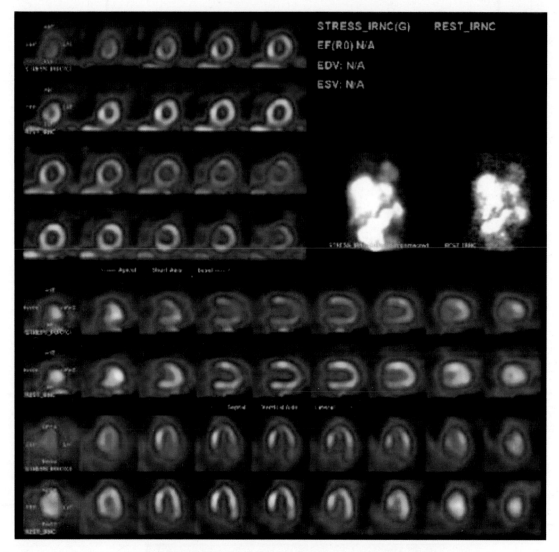

Figure 6.5. An example of a reversible perfusion defect. A decrease in tracer uptake is noted in the anteroseptal region of the apex that reverses on the resting images. This is a reversible perfusion image and is indicative of ischemia in the distribution of the left anterior descending artery.

had revascularization procedures but have ongoing symptoms. Myocardial perfusion SPECT using adenosine or dipyridamole infusion can be safely performed 48 hours post-myocardial infarction once the patient is hemodynamically stable. Prior studies have shown that the extent and severity of inducible ischemia is highly prognostic of future cardiac events and can be used to determine the patients who would benefit from revascularization. Treat angina with aggrastat and determine cost of therapy with an invasive or conservative strategy (TACTICS-TIMI18) showed that in patients with unstable angina (UA) or non-ST-elevation myocardial infarction (NSTEMI), risk stratification with SPECT MPI properly triaged patients who would benefit from revascularization and those who would not.[9] In a randomized controlled trial in patients with troponin positive ACS, there was no difference in outcomes in patients who went directly for invasive coronary angiography compared with patients who went to invasive coronary angiography based on inducible ischemia with SPECT MPI.[10]

ROLE OF RADIONUCLIDE IMAGING IN ASSESSING MYOCARDIAL VIABILITY

In patients with ischemic cardiomyopathy, the mechanism of myocardial death is the lack of blood flow. In patients who have had a myocardial infarction, the dead tissue is akinetic and does not contract during systole. However, noncontractile myocardium is not synonymous with infarcted myocardium. Myocardium can remain viable but noncontractile owing to limited resting blood flow and is considered to be in a state of hibernation. With the restoration of blood flow, the myocardium can return to its contractile state and improve systolic heart function. SPECT imaging can discern viable myocardial tissue from myocardial scar by taking advantage of the redistributive properties of Tl-201. When Tl-201 is injected, it is initially distributed and taken up by the myocardium with good blood flow. Myocardial segments with limited blood flow but are viable and myocardial segments that are dead do not take

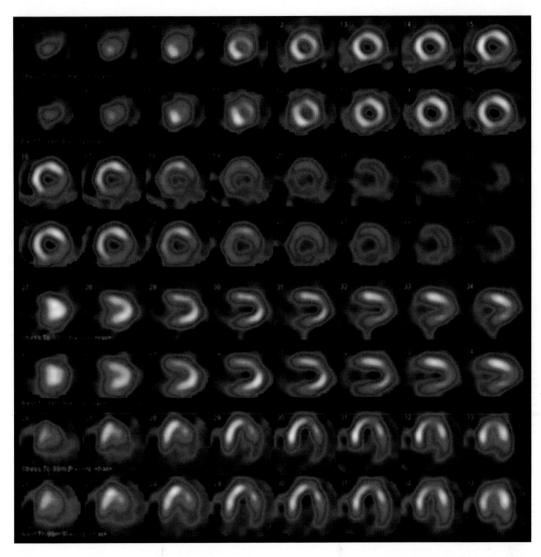

Figure 6.6. An example of a fixed perfusion defect. There is a decrease in tracer uptake noted in the lateral and inferior walls at the mid ventricle and at the base on the stress images. This finding is also noted in the rest images and is termed a fixed defect indicative of myocardial scar.

up Tl-201 initially. Over several hours, Tl-201 will redistribute and will be taken up by myocardium that is alive but has limited blood flow, that is, viable myocardium. Initial defects on imaging study may show reversibility upon redistribution imaging and the extent of viable myocardium can be assessed. Accumulating evidence suggests that heart failure patients with a significant burden of viable hibernating myocardium benefit from revascularization compared with medical therapy in terms of both left ventricular systolic function and mortality.[11,12] Other tests that are used to distinguish hibernating viable myocardium from irreversible injury include positron emission tomography (PET), dobutamine echocardiography, and cardiac magnetic resonance (CMR).

CONCLUSION

SPECT MPI is an excellent tool to image the physiologic changes that occur in ACS in patients presenting with chest pain, nondiagnostic ECGs, and negative troponin. SPECT MPI allows the clinician to triage patients safely, admitting patients at high risk, and sending home patients deemed to be low risk. Furthermore, in patients with ACS, SPECT MPI is an excellent tool to identify those who would benefit from revascularization therapy.

REFERENCES

1. Niska R, Bhuiya F, Xu J. National Hospital Ambulatory Medical Care Survey: 2007 Emergency Department Summary. http://www.cdc.gov/nchs/data/nhsr/nhsr026.pdf. Published 2010.
2. Hilton TC, Fulmer H, Abuan T, et al. Ninety-day follow-up of patients in the emergency department with chest pain who undergo initial single-photon emission computed tomographic perfusion scintigraphy with technetium 99m-labeled sestamibi. *J Nucl Cardiol.* 1996;3:308–311.
3. Hilton TC, Thompson RC, Williams HJ, et al. Technetium-99 m sestamibi myocardial perfusion imaging in the emergency room evaluation of chest pain. *J Am Coll Cardiol.* 1994;23:1016–1022.
4. Varetto T, Cantalupi D, Altieri A, et al. Emergency room technetium-99m sestamibi imaging to rule out acute myocardial ischemic events in patients with nondiagnostic electrocardiograms. *J Am Coll Cardiol.* 1993;22:1804–1808.
5. Bilodeau L, Theroux P, Gregoire J, et al. Technetium-99m sestamibi tomography in patients with spontaneous chest pain: correlations with clinical, electrocardiographic and angiographic findings. *J Am Coll Cardiol.* 1991;18:1684–1691.
6. Kontos MC, Jesse RL, Anderson FP, et al. Comparison of myocardial perfusion imaging and cardiac troponin I in patients admitted to the emergency department with chest pain. *Circulation.* 1999;99:2073–2078.

7. Heller GV, Stowers SA, Hendel RC, et al. Clinical value of acute rest technetium-99m tetrofosmin tomographic myocardial perfusion imaging in patients with acute chest pain and nondiagnostic electrocardiograms. *J Am Coll Cardiol.* 1998;31:1011–1017.

8. Udelson JE, Beshansky JR, Ballin DS, et al. Myocardial perfusion imaging for evaluation and triage of patients with suspected acute cardiac ischemia: a randomized controlled trial. *JAMA.* 2002;288:2693–2700.

9. Cannon CP, Weintraub WS, Demopoulos LA, et al. Comparison of early invasive and conservative strategies in patients with unstable coronary syndromes treated with the glycoprotein IIb/IIIa inhibitor tirofiban. *N Engl J Med.* 2001;344:1879–1887.

10. de Winter RJ, Windhausen F, Cornel JH, et al. Early invasive versus selectively invasive management for acute coronary syndromes. *N Engl J Med.* 2005;353:1095–1104.

11. Allman KC, Shaw LJ, Hachamovitch R, et al. Myocardial viability testing and impact of revascularization on prognosis in patients with coronary artery disease and left ventricular dysfunction: a meta-analysis. *J Am Coll Cardiol.* 2002;39:1151–1158.

12. Underwood SR, Bax JJ, vom Dahl J, et al. Imaging techniques for the assessment of myocardial hibernation. Report of a Study Group of the European Society of Cardiology. *Eur Heart J.* 2004;25:815–836.

PATIENT AND FAMILY INFORMATION FOR:

Radionuclide Imaging in Acute Coronary Syndrome

Radionuclide imaging, often called nuclear imaging, has been used since the 1970s to image the heart. Radionuclide imaging uses radiopharmaceuticals that are given through intravenous injection. One component of a radiopharmaceutical is a tracer, a substance that is taken up from the blood by the heart muscle. The amount of the tracer extracted from the blood by the heart muscle is proportional to the amount of the blood flow to the heart muscle. The radiopharmaceutical is a radioactive substance that emits photons that can be captured by a special camera. The information from the camera allows physicians to make pictures of the heart muscle. Essentially, these pictures represent "the map" of blood flow to the heart muscle and identify the areas where the blood flow is compromised owing to a blockage in the blood vessels supplying the heart.

Although nuclear imaging employs radioactive substances the dosage given to an individual patient is relatively small. Mostly, it is in the range of radioactivity comparable to other imaging procedures such as a CT scan and is considered safe. The dosage of the radioactive tracer is calculated based on the patient's weight. The injection is given by a technician or a doctor. After the injection, the patient is imaged by the camera that detects the photons emitted by the radiotracer. This part of the test is crucial: The technician explains to the patient the position they need to maintain and the necessity of staying still while the pictures are obtained. The patient needs to follow the instructions carefully so that high-quality images can be obtained.

Heart attacks are caused by a decrease in the blood flow that nourishes the heart muscle. If blood flow to a part of the heart muscle is blocked, the patient will have a heart attack and the heart muscle can die. In patients who experience chest pain, it is often difficult to determine whether the pain is a sign of heart disease. The initial tests for patients with chest pain include an ECG and blood tests. If these tests are inconclusive the physician may opt to perform radionuclide imaging. Radionuclide imaging maps the blood flow to the heart and is useful in identifying a blood vessel blockage that may signify a heart attack. In patients who have experienced a heart attack, radionuclide imaging enables physicians to determine who will benefit from procedures that restore blood flow to the heart muscle.

The idea behind the stress test is to compare resting images of the heart with those obtained after the stress test. The stress portion can be performed either with exercise or with medication. During an exercise stress test, the patient is asked to exercise on a treadmill or a stationary bicycle. If the patient cannot exercise or the physician thinks it is unsafe for the patient to exercise, medication can be used. The physician or a trained health care professional is always present in the room for the stress test. In general, stress testing is safe and well tolerated, although some patients may experience brief side effects from the medication. Serious events including chest pain and heart rhythm disturbances are rare.

During radionuclide stress testing two sets of heart images are usually obtained as described above: the rest images and the stress images. By comparing the two sets of images the physician can determine whether there is an impairment of blood flow to the heart. If significant blood flow impairment is identified by the stress test the patient may be referred for an invasive procedure called cardiac catheterization.

Michael Jolly
A. Michael Lincoff

Medications Used in the Management of Acute Coronary Syndrome

The pharmacologic management of an acute coronary syndrome (ACS) has evolved dramatically over the past two decades into a heavily evidence-based discipline. Contemporary treatment strategies have become more targeted, focusing on the unique pathophysiologic underpinnings of this disorder. In addition, new therapeutic approaches are rigorously tested and proven in large clinical trials before becoming standard therapy. As our armamentarium of new therapeutics continues to grow, our diagnostic and management strategies will necessarily change over time. As such, practitioners caring for patients with ACS must become lifelong students of this exciting and dynamic field to provide the best care for their patients in the years to come.

Appropriate medical therapy is indicated for all patients presenting with or suspected of having ACS. The goals of initial medical therapy are 4-fold: to relieve pain, to halt the progression of disease, to reduce morbidity, and to improve survival. Because the term ACS encompasses a spectrum of severity with a common pathophysiology, the difficulty in the pharmacologic management comes in determining where in the spectrum a particular patient falls and to balance the risks and benefits in treating that patient to achieve the desired goals.

Once the diagnosis of ACS is established, the patient should be quickly stratified by risk into one of several treatment strategies. Medical therapy should be immediately started in a rational manner to achieve the initial goals of treatment, namely, to interrupt platelet activation/aggregation, thrombus formation, and to relieve pain. Patients diagnosed with ST-segment elevation myocardial infarction (STEMI) should be emergently strategized to primary PCI or fibrinolytic therapy, whereas those with UA/NSTEMI should be risk-stratified into either an early invasive or an initial conservative approach. Regardless of what treatment strategy is initiated, patients should be continuously evaluated for high-risk features of disease, adverse hemodynamic consequences, and treatment failure. Such features often mandate deviation from the initial management strategy to a more aggressive one. It is important to note that as a patient transitions from one treatment strategy to another, the pharmacologic approach can vary substantially.

In general, the pharmacologic approach to managing ACS should be prioritized with an emphasis on rapid treatment with medications known to provide morbidity and mortality benefit. Guidelines for treatment are useful; however, they cannot address every possible nuance experienced in clinical practice. Health care providers must have a thorough understanding of their institutional capabilities and preferences as well as familiarity with the drugs, doses, indications, and side effects to provide patients with optimal benefit and minimal harm.

ANTI-ISCHEMIC AND ANALGESIC THERAPY

ß-ADRENERGIC BLOCKERS

Rationale: β-Blockers are used to inhibit the actions of catecholamines on the β_1 adrenergic receptors located in the myocardium. Inhibition of these receptors leads to a reduction in myocardial contractility, AV node conduction, sinus node rate, and an overall reduction in systolic blood pressure. The net effect of these actions results in a decrease in cardiac work and myocardial oxygen demand. In addition, β-blockers increase diastolic pressure time, which may be important in increasing coronary blood flow. In patients with ACS undergoing PCI, a large meta-analysis showed a significant reduction in mortality at 30 days and 6 months for patients who received β-blocker therapy.[1] However, the Clopidogrel and Metoprolol in Myocardial Infarction (COMMIT) failed to demonstrate a mortality benefit with the early use of β-blockers in patients with myocardial infarction.[2] This finding has been attributed to injudicious use of β-blockers in patients with heart failure or other risk factors for cardiogenic shock and has been instructive in the most recent guidelines involving recommendations for β-blocker usage in ACS. However, in contrast to the early aggressive use of β-blockers for acute MI, the Carvedilol Post-Infarct Survival Control in left ventricular dysfunction (CAPRICORN) trial demonstrated a reduction in all-cause mortality, cardiovascular mortality, and nonfatal MI when 1,959 patients with acute MI and LV dysfunction were randomized to receive to low-dose carvedilol versus placebo and treated with a more gradual up-titration strategy.[3]

Indications: ACS (without contraindications), stable angina, compensated chronic heart failure.

Dosing: Multiple preparations available including intravenous and oral, β_1 and nonselective, short and long acting (Table 7.1).

Side effects: Hypotension, bradycardia, AV block, congestive heart failure (CHF), bronchospasm, paradoxical Hypertention in setting of active cocaine use.

Contraindications: High-grade AV block, active bronchoconstriction, hypotension, bradycardia, severe LV dysfunction or heart failure (rales, S3 gallop), or in patients with MI at high risk for cardiogenic shock (older age, female sex, relative hypotension, high Killip class, and reflexive tachycardia).

TABLE 7.1	ß-Blockers Used in ACS		
Drugs	*Selectivity*	*Dose*	*Comment*
Metoprolol tartrate	β_1	50–200 mg twice daily	Often initiated with 12.5–25 mg every 6–8 h
Metoprolol succinate	β_1	12.5–200 mg daily	Short-acting tartrate preferred for ACS, however, mortality benefit shown for stable patients with CHF
Carvedilol	$\beta_1, \beta_2, \alpha_1$	3.125–25 mg twice daily	Started low and titrate up; mortality benefit for LV dysfunction
Atenolol	β_1	25–200 mg daily	
Labetalol	$\beta_1, \beta_2, \alpha_1$	200–600 mg twice daily	
Propranolol	β_1, β_2	20–80 mg twice daily	
Esmolol	β_1	50–300 mcg/kg/min	

Adapted from Gibbons RJ, Abrams J, Chatterjee K, et al.; American College of Cardiology; American Heart Association Task Force on Practice Guidelines (Committee on the Management of Patients With Chronic Stable Angina). ACC/AHA 2002 guideline update for the management of patients with chronic stable angina—summary article: a report of the American College of Cardiology/American Heart Association Task Force on Practice Guidelines (Committee on the Management of Patients With Chronic Stable Angina). *J Am Coll Cardiol.* 2003;41:159–168.

Recommendations: The acute use of β-blockers in ACS is recommended in all patients without contraindications, especially in patients with ongoing angina and hypertension. Short-acting, β_1 selective agents are typically used to minimize side effects and allow for dose titration. A typical regimen would include metoprolol 5 mg IV, repeated every 5 minutes, up to a total of 15 mg. Oral therapy can be started at metoprolol 25 to 50 mg every 6 hours and titrated to achieve the desired heart rate (HR) or BP. Frequent HR and BP checks, continuous ECG monitoring, and routine auscultation for rales and bronchospasm should be performed (preferably in an ICU setting). Once stabilized, patients should receive maintenance doses up to 100 mg twice daily. In patients with LV dysfunction, β-blockers with proven mortality benefit such as bisoprolol, carvedilol, and metoprolol succinate should be utilized for long-term management.

CALCIUM CHANNEL BLOCKERS

Rationale: Calcium channel blockers (CCBs) inhibit myocardial and vascular smooth muscle contraction by reducing transmembrane inward calcium flux. In ACS, CCBs are useful in decreasing myocardial oxygen demand (by decreasing afterload, contractility, and HR) and in coronary vasodilatation. Meta-analyses of UA/NSTEMI trials involving CCBs have suggested no overall benefit in death or nonfatal MI.[4] Retrospective studies of verapamil and diltiazem have shown increased mortality in patients with LV dysfunction.[5,6] In addition, a trial using nifedipine was stopped early because of concern for harm when taken without concomitant β-blockers.[7]

Indications: In ACS, considered second-line therapy in β-blocker-intolerant patients for relief of angina, blood pressure control, and rate control of supraventricular arrhythmias. CCBs are considered adjuncts to β-blockers and nitrates for the relief of ischemic symptoms. They are generally the preferred treatment for patients with cocaine-induced myocardial ischemia or variant angina.

Dosing: Multiple preparations both intravenous and oral, short and long acting (Table 7.2).

Side effects: Hypotension, bradycardia, myocardial depression (diltiazem and verapamil), flushing, edema, or headache.

Contraindications: Hypotension, AV conduction abnormalities, LV dysfunction or CHF (especially diltiazem and verapamil).

TABLE 7.2	Calcium Channel Blockers Used in ACS		
Drug	*Dose*	*Duration of Action*	*Comment*
NON DIHYDROPYRIDINES			
Diltiazem	Immediate release: 30–90 mg every 6 h	Short	Avoid with known or suspected LV dysfunction
	Slow release: 120–360 mg three times daily	Long	
Verapamil	Immediate release: 80–160 mg every 8 h	Short	Avoid with known or suspected LV dysfunction
	Slow release: 120–480 mg daily	Long	
DIHYDROPYRIDINES			
Amlodipine	5–10 mg daily	Long	
Felodipine	5–10 mg daily	Long	
Nisoldipine	20–40 mg daily	Short	

Recommendations: In patients with contraindications to β-blockers or in those where β-blockers and nitrates have failed to achieve relief of ischemia or rate control with supraventricular arrhythmias, CCBs can be used to further reduce blood pressure and chest pain. Caution should be exercised when CCBs and β-blockers are used concomitantly because of depressed AV nodal conduction. Diltiazem and verapamil should be avoided in patients with LV dysfunction. Use of dihydropyridines such as amlodipine and felodipine appear to be safe with LV dysfunction, although their benefit remains undefined in the treatment of ACS; nifedipine should be avoided altogether.

NITRATES

Rationale: Despite a paucity of rigorous clinical trial data, nitrates continue to remain important in the treatment of hypertension and chest pain in patients with ACS. Nitrates cause a reduction of myocardial oxygen demand while enhancing myocardial oxygen delivery and affect both peripheral and coronary vascular beds. Nitroglycerin increases venous capacitance thereby decreasing preload and reducing ventricular wall tension. Furthermore, nitroglycerin promotes the dilation of the coronary arteries and possibly has a mild inhibitory effect on platelet aggregation (although the clinical significance of this is not known).

Indications: Angina, hypertension, CHF, variant angina.

Dosing: Nitroglycerine (NTG) is available in multiple preparations including sublingual tablets and spray, transdermal, and intravenously (Table 7.3).

Side effects: Headaches, hypotension, and tachyphylaxis are common with NTG usage.

Contraindications: NTG is contraindicated after the use of phosphodiesterase inhibitors used for the treatment of erectile dysfunction such as sildenafil, tadalafil, and vardenafil as concomitant use can induce profound hypotension. In addition, nitrates should be avoided in patients suspected of having an RV infarct as its usage can result in severe hypotension even with low doses.

Recommendations: NTG use is typically initiated with three 0.4 mg sublingual NTG tablets taken 5 minutes apart with the concomitant administration of either an oral or an intravenous β-blocker. For patients with ongoing chest pain, hypertension, or decompensated heart failure, it is appropriate to switch to intravenous NTG. This is given at 10 mcg per minute through continuous infusion via nonabsorbing tubing and can be uptitrated by 10 mcg per minute every 3 to 5 minutes to achieve symptomatic relief or desired blood pressure response. Although there is no published maximal ceiling dose, 200 mcg per minute is typically used as there is unlikely to be measurable clinical benefit beyond this rate. For blood pressure titrations, NTG should not be titrated to <110 mm Hg in previously normotensive patients or to >25% lower than the starting mean arterial blood pressure (MAP) in hypertensive patients. NTG should generally be avoided in patients with starting systolic blood pressures of <90 mm Hg, in patients with marked bradycardia or tachycardia, or in patients who present with systolic blood pressures 30 mm Hg or more below their baseline. After a patient has been stable or chest pain free for 12 to 24 hours, it is prudent to attempt weaning intravenous NTG or transitioning to an oral preparation if still indicated.

MORPHINE

Rationale: Although there is a lack of randomized clinical trials, morphine sulfate provides analgesic and anxiolytic effects that might partially counteract the adrenergic drive associated with ACS. In addition, it causes mild venodilation, a modest reduction in HR through increased vagal tone, and decreased BP that lowers myocardial oxygen demand.

Dosing: Morphine sulfate 1 to 5 mg IV PRN.

Side effects: Nausea, vomiting, respiratory depression, and hypotension.

Recommendations: Morphine should be considered for anginal relief in patients not sufficiently controlled with nitrates, β-blockers, or CCBs and is often given in preparation for further invasive testing.

ANCILLARY THERAPIES

ACE INHIBITORS AND ANGIOTENSIN II RECEPTOR BLOCKERS

Rationale: Inhibition of the renin–angiotensin–aldosterone system has salutary effects on BP, afterload reduction, and LV remodeling associated with MI-induced LV dysfunction. ACE inhibitors have a proven track record in multiple clinical trials for decreasing mortality particularly in patients with depressed ejection fractions, chronic coronary artery disease (CAD), and

TABLE 7.3	Nitrate Preparations Used in ACS		
Compound	*Route*	*Dose*	*Duration of Effect*
Nitroglycerin	Sublingual tablets	0.3–0.6 mg up to 1.5 mg	1 to 7 min
	Spray	0.4 mg as needed	Similar to sublingual tablets however has a longer shelf life
	Transdermal	0.2–0.8 mg per h every 12 h	8 to 12 h with intermittent therapy, efficacy improved with 12 h off period
	Intravenous	5–200 mcg per min	Tolerance in 7 to 8 h
Isosorbide dinitrate	Oral	5–80 mg, every 8–12 h	Up to 8 h
	Oral, slow release	40 mg, every 12–24 h	Up to 8 h
Isosorbide mononitrate	Oral	20 mg twice daily	12 to 24 h
	Oral, slow release	60–240 mg daily	

diabetes.[8–12] In addition, the VALsartan In Acute myocardial iNfarcTion (VALIANT) trial demonstrated that valsartan was as effective as captopril in the reduction of death following MI in patients with demonstrable LV dysfunction or clinical heart failure.[13] Therefore, in addition to their proven clinical role in stable CHF, angiotensin II receptor blockers (ARBs) appear to also offer benefit in the ACS setting.

Indications: ACS with concurrent pulmonary congestion or LVEF ≤40%, in absence of contraindications. ARBs should be given to patients intolerant of ACE inhibitors.

Dosing: Multiple preparations both short and long acting. Intravenous forms not recommended for ACS (Table 7.4).

Side effects: Hypotension, hyperkalemia, angioedema and cough (ACE inhibitors).

Contraindications: Hemodynamic instability, renal failure, hyperkalemia.

Recommendations: Typically initiated early, within the first 24 hours of hospital stay, in patients without contraindications. Use of short-acting formulations (i.e., captopril 12.5 mg every 8 hours) allows for dose titration. Once stable, once-daily dosing can be initiated. Intravenous ACE inhibitors should be avoided in the management of ACS.

ALDOSTERONE RECEPTOR ANTAGONISTS

Rationale: Aldosterone receptor antagonists have been shown to prevent deleterious ventricular remodeling after acute MI, decrease the rate of death, and reduce hospitalizations in patients with chronic severe heart failure. The Eplerenone Post-Acute Myocardial Infarction Heart Failure Efficacy and Survival Study (EPHESUS) trial further expanded the beneficial role in renin–angiotensin–aldosterone blockade by demonstrating a reduction in morbidity and mortality for patients presenting with acute MI complicated by LV dysfunction when treated with eplerenone.

Indications: ACS with concurrent pulmonary congestion or LVEF ≤40%, in absence of contraindications.

Dosing: Eplerenone 25 mg PO daily with gradual up-titration to a maximum of 50 mg PO daily. Frequent monitoring of electrolytes, especially potassium and creatinine, is essential.

Side effects: Hypotension, hyperkalemia, and renal dysfunction.

Contraindications: Hemodynamic instability, and renal failure, hyperkalemia.

Recommendations: Given the totality of evidence to date, ACE inhibitors and ARBs remain preferred first-line therapy agents for renin–angiotensin–aldosterone blockade for patients with ACS and concurrent LV dysfunction. However, the addition of an aldosterone receptor blocker such as eplerenone may be considered in patients already receiving optimal medical treatment in the absence of contraindications.

HMG-COA REDUCTASE INHIBITORS (STATINS)

Rationale: Statins have been widely studied in both primary and secondary preventions for CAD. The "pleiotropic" effects of statins include not only their well-established ability to lower

TABLE 7.4	ACE Inhibitors and ARBs Used in ACS			
Drug	*Starting Dose*	*Typical Dose*	*Maximum Dose*	*Comments*
ACE INHIBITORS				
Benazepril	10 mg	20–40 mg	80 mg	May use BID dosing
Captopril	6.25–12 mg BID-TID	25–50 mg BID-TID	450 mg daily	Target dose in HF: 50 mg TID
Enalapril	2.5–5 mg daily-BID	10–40 mg	40 mg	Target dose in HF: 10 mg BID
Fosinopril	10 mg	20–40 mg	80 mg	
Lisinopril	2.5–5 mg	10–40 mg	80 mg	Target dose in HF: 20 mg daily
Moexipril	7.5 mg	7.5–30 mg	30 mg	
Perindopril	4 mg	4–8 mg	16 mg	
Quinapril	10 mg	20–80 mg	80 mg	Target dose in HF: 20 mg daily
Ramipril	2.5 mg	2.5–20 mg	20 mg	
Trandolapril	1 mg	2–4 mg	8mg	Reduce dose in hepatic dysfunction
ARBs				
Candesartan	8–16 mg	16–32 mg	32 mg	
Eprosartan	600 mg	600–800 mg	800 mg	
Irbesartan	75–150 mg	150–300 mg	300 mg	
Losartan	25–50 mg	50–100 mg	100 mg	Reduce dose in hepatic dysfunction
Valsartan	20 mg	160 mg	320 mg	
Olmesartan	20 mg	20–40 mg	40 mg	
Telmisartan	20–40 mg	40–80 mg	80 mg	

LDL but also their anti-inflammatory, antioxidant, and anti-thrombotic properties. In the setting of ACS, PROVE IT-TIMI 22 showed a significant 16% reduction in the hazard ratio for death, MI, UA, revascularization, and stroke in patients treated with intensive lipid-lowering therapy (atorvastatin 80 mg) compared with standard therapy (pravastatin 40 mg).[14]

Indications: STEMI and UA/NSTEMI

Dosing: Multiple agents, however, atorvastatin most studied for ACS. Typically given at 40 to 80 mg PO daily (Table 7.5).

Side effects: Dyspepsia, rash/pruritis, myalgias, hepatotoxicity, and rhabdomyolysis (rare).

Contraindications: Caution when used with cytochrome P450 inhibitors and in the setting of elevated transaminases.

Recommendations: Statins at high doses should be considered early in the course of patients presenting with ACS. LDL target goals for the ACS population should be <100 mg per dl and probably <70 mg per dl in high-risk patients and diabetics. Statins should be considered standard therapy for secondary prevention in the absence of contraindications.

ANTIPLATELET MEDICATIONS

ASPIRIN

Rationale: Aspirin (ASA) is a potent, irreversible platelet COX-1 inhibitor that inhibits the production of thromboxane A2 and resultantly decreases platelet aggregation at the site of intimal injury and thrombus formation. Although it is a relatively weak inhibitor of overall platelet aggregation, ASA confers a significant reduction in mortality.[15–19]

Indications: ACS (diagnosed or suspected), chronic CAD.

Dosing: Initial dosing should be 162 to 325 mg given orally as a nonenteric coated, chewable tablet to allow for rapid buccal absorption. In case of active nausea or vomiting, a 300 mg rectal suppository should be promptly administered.

Side effects: Nausea, vomiting, dyspepsia, gastrointestinal/genitourinary and bleeding.

Contraindications: The only contraindication is patients with true ASA allergy (anaphylaxis, hives, nasal polyps, or bronchospasm). Such patients should be given a thienopyridine such as clopidogrel, with strong consideration given for ASA desensitization treatment.

Recommendations: Aspirin 325 mg should be administered to all persons as soon as ACS is diagnosed or suspected, typically in the ambulance or the emergency department. In general, therapy with ASA should be continued indefinitely after the first presentation with ACS at a low dose of 75 to 81 mg daily. Patients who are treated with PCI should typically remain on

325 mg dosing for the first month for bare-metal stent (BMS) or 3 to 6 months for drug-eluting stent (DES) before converting to a low-dose regimen.

THIENOPYRIDINES AND ADP RECEPTOR INHIBITORS

Thienopyridines are inhibitors of ADP-induced platelet aggregation and along with ASA have become important therapies in the treatment of ACS. Three thienopyridines have received FDA approval in the United States for use in ACS: ticlopidine, clopidogrel, and prasugrel. Ticagrelor, a novel ADP receptor inhibitor, had recently been approved by the FDA. Each of these drugs works by inhibiting the $P2Y_{12}$ ADP receptor on platelets, with ticagrelor being the only one with reversible inhibition. They differ importantly with respect to their onset of action, side effect profile, and overall potency. Ticlopidine is limited by a long onset of action, more frequent dosing, and an unfavorable side-effect profile including gastrointestinal effects, neutropenia, and thrombotic thrombocytopenic purpura (TTP). Since the introduction of clopidogrel, and more recently prasugrel and ticagrelor, the clinical use of ticlopidine has decreased and is no longer recommended in the treatment of ACS. Evidence for the beneficial use of thienopyridines comes from multiple, large-scale randomized trials. Because thienopyridines exert more robust platelet inhibition than ASA alone, the risk of subsequent bleeding is higher and therefore appropriate thienopyridine selection should be tailored to a patient's individual bleeding risk.

CLOPIDOGREL

Rationale: Clopidogrel, an irreversible $P2Y_{12}$ receptor inhibitor, remains the most studied and most used thienopyridine today. In the clopidogrel in unstable angina to prevent recurrent events (CURE) trial, patients with UA or NSTEMI were found to have a lower rate of cardiovascular death, nonfatal MI, or stroke when treated with ASA and clopidogrel than ASA alone (9.3% vs. 11.4%, $P < .001$), however, this came at the expense of major bleeding, particularly in patients who subsequently underwent CABG.[20] In STEMI patients, the COMMIT-CCS-2 study demonstrated a significant reduction in the composite endpoint of death, reinfarction, and stroke (9.2% clopidogrel vs. 10.1% placebo, $P = .002$) in 45,852 patients treated with clopidogrel, 93% of whom had ST elevation.[21] The addition of clopidogrel to fibrinolytic therapy was proven beneficial in the clopidogrel as adjunctive reperfusion therapy–thrombolysis in myocardial infarction (CLARITY-TIMI 28) trial where 3,491 patients with STEMI had a significant reduction in occluded infarct artery on angiography, death, or recurrent MI when treated with clopidogrel (15% clopidogrel vs. 21.7% placebo, $P < .001$).[22] This was felt to be driven by the prevention of infarct-related reocclusion.

For clopidogrel, maximal therapeutic platelet inhibition takes 3 to 7 days to reach; however, this is typically overcome with the administration of a loading dose of 300 to 600 mg that results in substantial inhibition within approximately 2 hours.

Indications: STEMI, UA/NSTEMI, alternative to ASA in patients with true ASA intolerance.

Dosing: Loading dose of 300 to 600 mg followed by 75 mg daily. When combined with fibrinolytics, a 300-mg loading dose

TABLE 7.5	Statins Used in ACS
Drug	*Dose*
Atorvastatin	10–80 mg daily
Fluvastatin	20–80 mg daily
Lovastatin	10–80 mg daily
Pravastatin	10–80 mg daily
Rosuvastatin	5–40 mg daily
Simvastatin	10–80 mg daily

should be used for patients under 75 years of age and no loading dose for patients over 75 years of age.

Side effects: Bleeding, GI intolerance, rash, and TTP (rare).

Contraindications: High risk for intracranial/GI/GU bleeding, anticipated CABG within 5 days, high suspicion for diminished clopidogrel response (e.g., CYP2C19 variant, stent thrombosis).

Special note on clopidogrel responsiveness: It has become increasingly recognized that there is considerable interindividual variability in platelet inhibition from clopidogrel, often leading to adverse clinical events. This is thought to be primarily related to genetic polymorphisms involving the metabolism of clopidogrel and other drugs by the hepatic CYP450 system, specifically the CYP2C19 isoenzyme, and has led to an FDA warning for the use of clopidogrel. Omeprazole, commonly given to patients on thienopyridines, is a moderate CYP2C19 inhibitor and has been shown to affect the pharmacological activity of clopidogrel. Pantoprazole, a weak CYP2C19 inhibitor, appears to have milder effects on the pharmacologic activity; however, the clinical significance remains undefined. Although genetic and platelet function testing are available, routine use is not specifically recommended at this time. However, patients deemed to be at moderate to high risk (previous history of stent thrombosis, recurrent ischemic events, planned complex interventions) should be considered for platelet function testing or alternative antiplatelet strategies. This may include higher-loading doses (clopidogrel 600 mg × 2 over 2 hours), higher-maintenance dosing (clopidogrel 150 mg daily), or switching to prasugrel, which does not appear to have similar limitations.

Recommendations: Clopidogrel is indicated early in the treatment of UA/NSTEMI (both early invasive and initial conservative strategy) and STEMI, typically given with a 300- to 600-mg loading dose followed by 75 mg daily. When used with fibrinolytics, a 300-mg loading dose is recommended for patients <75 years; however, no loading dose is currently recommended for patients ≥75 years. Its use is recommended in conjunction with ASA and a GP IIb/IIIa inhibitor when indicated. Clopidogrel should be continued for at least 1 month but preferably for 1 year or longer. Following PCI with stent placement, duration of treatment is dictated by type of stent placed. For BMS, its recommended duration is at least 1 month but ideally 1 year. For DES, treatment for at least 1 year or longer is recommended to reduce the incidence of late-stent thrombosis. Because of the increased bleeding associated with CABG, clopidogrel should be held for at least 5 days and up to 7 days prior to elective CABG. In patients with a high likelihood of needing bypass, some centers opt to delay clopidogrel loading until coronary anatomy has been defined if angiography can be done in a timely manner. If a loading dose is given and a patient is subsequently found to need urgent surgical revascularization, centers with experienced surgeons can often operate with an acceptable incremental bleeding risk.

PRASUGREL

Rationale: Prasugrel is a newer irreversible $P2Y_{12}$ ADP receptor inhibitor that offers distinct advantages over clopidogrel. Like clopidogrel, prasugrel is a prodrug that requires hepatic metabolism to its active metabolite. However, its metabolism is not affected by the CYP2C19 allele and does not appear to have the same interpatient variability found with clopidogrel. In addition, its pharmacodynamic properties result in more rapid and consistent platelet inhibition when compared with clopidogrel. The TRITON-TIMI 38 study is the largest trial to date for prasugrel, comparing it with clopidogrel in ACS patients scheduled to undergo PCI. Prasugrel was found to significantly reduce the combined rates of death, nonfatal MI, and stroke when compared with clopidogrel (9.9% prasugrel vs. 12.1% clopidogrel, $P < .001$). In addition, significant reductions in MI, urgent target vessel revascularization, and stent thrombosis were shown. However, the benefit of prasugrel came at the expense of significantly increased major bleeding, including fatal bleeding.[23] Patients with prior stroke or transient ischemic attack (TIA) had worse outcome with prasugrel, and bleeding rates were noted to be particularly high in patients with body weight <60 kg or age >75 years.

Indications: STEMI and UA/NSTEMI.

Dosing: Loading dose of 60 mg followed by 10 mg daily.

Side effects: Bleeding.

Contraindications: Age ≥75 years, body weight <60 kg (or use maintenance dose of 5 mg daily), history of stroke/TIA, high risk for intracranial/GI/GU bleeding, active bleeding, CABG planned within 5 to 7 days.

Recommendations: Prasugrel is currently recommended for the treatment of STEMI in patients undergoing primary PCI. For patients undergoing nonprimary PCI, prasugrel should not be given if the patient has received a fibrinolytic. Ideally, prasugrel should be avoided for at least 7 days prior to CABG unless surgical revascularization outweighs the increased bleeding risk. For UA/NSTEMI, prasugrel is a reasonable alternative thienopyridine in patients without the aforementioned contraindications and in whom clopidogrel would otherwise be indicated. Patients with diminished clopidogrel responsiveness and those with high-risk features (recurrent ischemia, diabetes, and complex interventions) may be particularly well suited. However, it must be noted that in TRITON-TIMI 38, patients with UA/NSTEMI treated with prasugrel were given the loading dose only *after* coronary anatomy was defined. Injudicious upstream loading in patients at high risk for surgical disease prior to knowledge of coronary anatomy may lead to excessive bleeding. Prasugrel has not been studied in the early conservative management strategy.

TICAGRELOR

Rationale: Ticagrelor is a *reversible* $P2Y_{12}$ ADP receptor inhibitor and had recently been approved by the FDA for use in the treatment of ACS. Like prasugrel, it offers several potential advantages over clopidogrel: It provides more rapid and consistent platelet inhibition. In addition, because it is a reversible inhibitor, its antiplatelet effects dissipate more rapidly than other thienopyridines. The PLATelet inhibition and patient Outcomes (PLATO) trial compared ticagrelor with clopidogrel in the treatment of patients presenting with ACS both with and without STEMI. Ticagrelor was associated with a significant reduction in the primary composite endpoint of death, MI, and stroke compared with clopidogrel (9.8% vs. 11.7%, $P < .001$). There was no significant difference in the rates of major bleeding between the two groups; however, the ticagrelor group did have a higher incidence of major bleeding not related to CABG, including more intracranial bleeding.[24]

Indications: STEMI and UA/NSTEMI (both early invasive or initial conservative strategy).

Dosing: Initial loading dose of 180 mg followed by 90 mg twice daily.

Side effects: Bleeding, dyspnea, and ventricular pauses.

Contraindications: High risk for intracranial/GI/GU bleeding, active bleeding.

Recommendations: Although current guidelines have not had sufficient time to propose formal recommendations, ticagrelor, will likely be indicated for the treatment of STEMI and UA/NSTEMI. Particularly advantageous is ticagrelor's reversible pharmacokinetic properties and short half-life that make upstream loading possible irrespective of the patient's risk for surgical CAD.

PLATELET GP IIB/IIIA RECEPTOR ANTAGONISTS

GP IIb/IIIa inhibitors decrease platelet aggregation and thrombus formation by inhibiting the ability of fibrinogen to cross-link platelets. Three GP IIb/IIIa medications currently approved for use in the United States include abciximab, eptifibatide, and tirofiban. The benefit of GP IIb/IIIa medications seems to be predominantly in patients managed invasively with PCI and with high-risk clinical features (positive troponins, diabetics). However, in the modern era of dual antiplatelet therapy with aspirin plus a thienopyridine, the benefit of upstream use prior to PCI in the ACS population has become less apparent. For patients with STEMI, the Facilitated Intervention with Enhanced Reperfusion Speed to Stop Events (FINESSE) and Bavarian Reperfusion AlternatiVes Evaluation (BRAVE-3) studies showed no benefit with regard to infarct size or ischemic events in patients treated upstream with abciximab, as compared with GP IIb/IIIa blockade administered during primary PCI.[25,26] For UA/NSTEMI, the EARLY-ACS trial compared routine upstream use of eptifibatide in addition to standard dual antiplatelet therapy versus delayed use at the time of angiography. No significant reduction in ischemic complications was observed with early upstream use of GP IIb/IIIa, even though eptifibatide was used in only approximately 25% of patients in the "delayed" arm.[27] Similarly, the acute catheterization and urgent intervention triage strategy (ACUITY) trial failed to show benefit of the strategy of upstream GP IIb/IIIa inhibitors when compared with provisional use at the time of PCI. For patients treated with upstream use, increased major bleeding was observed at 30 days.[28] As such, the routine *upstream* use of GP IIb/IIIa inhibitors is not recommended in STEMI; in UA/NSTEMI, guidelines recommend dual antiplatelet therapy with ASA plus *either* a thienopyridine *or* a GP IIb/IIIa, but not routine triple antiplatelet therapy with all three class of agents. GP IIb/IIIa inhibitors should be used in addition to ASA and a thienopyridine in the setting of recurrent ischemic discomfort (see below). All GP IIb/IIIa inhibitors should be used in conjunction with ASA and heparin or enoxaparin. Benefit must be weighed against increased incidence of bleeding, especially in patients at a higher risk for this adverse outcome.

ABCIXIMAB

Rationale. Abciximab is a Fab fragment of a humanized murine antibody that inhibits the GP IIb/IIIa receptor, endothelial cell vitronectin receptors, and leukocyte MAC-1 receptors. Although it has a short half-life, its binding to GP IIb/IIIa receptors can persist for weeks although platelet aggregation gradually returns to normal 24 to 48 hours after discontinuation of the infusion. The role of abciximab in ACS was first established with the Evaluation of 7E3 for the Prevention of Ischemic Complications (EPIC) trial that demonstrated a significant reduction in the rate of death, MI, or emergent revascularization in the group treated with a bolus and infusion of the drug prior to undergoing PCI.[29] In the contemporary era, the intracoronary stenting with antithrombotic regimen- rapid early action for coronary treatment (ISAR-REACT 2) trial demonstrated a significant reduction in death, MI, or urgent revascularization in high-risk (troponin positive) UA/NSTEMI patients treated with abciximab who underwent PCI (8.9% abciximab vs. 11.9% placebo, P = 0.03).[30] However, for UA/NSTEMI patients risk stratified to the early conservative strategy, the Global Use of Strategies To Open Occluded Coronary Arteries IV–Acute Coronary Syndrome (GUSTO IV–ACS) trial showed abciximab to be of no additional benefit.[31]

Indications: UA/NSTEMI as adjunct to PCI or when PCI is planned within 24 hours, STEMI during primary PCI.

Dosing: 0.25 mg per kg 10 to 60 minutes before PCI followed by 0.125 μg/kg per minute for 12 hours (maximum rate 10 μg per minute).

Side effects: Bleeding, thrombocytopenia, hypersensitivity reactions.

Contraindications: Prior hypersensitivity, high risk for intracranial/GI/GU bleeding.

Recommendations: Useful in patients with UA/NSTEMI being treated with early invasive strategy when PCI is likely to be performed. It can be given upstream of angiography if there is no appreciable delay to angiography. Abciximab should not be used in the treatment of UA/NSTEMI when PCI is not planned. For STEMI, it should be initiated at the time of primary PCI.

EPTIFIBATIDE

Rationale. A heptapeptide antagonist that reversibly inhibits GP IIb/IIIa. In the Platelet Glycoprotein IIb/IIIa in Unstable Angina: Receptor Suppression Using Integrilin Therapy (PURSUIT) trial, patients with UA/NSTEMI treated eptifibatide in addition to ASA and heparin had reduced rates of death and nonfatal MI at 96 hours and 6 months, particularly in those who underwent PCI.[32]

Indication: UA/NSTEMI treated medically or with PCI, STEMI during primary PCI.

Dosing: Upstream ACS: loading dose 180 μg per kg bolus followed by 2 μg/kg/minute for 96 hours. If CrCl ≤50 ml per minute, reduce to 1 μg/kg/min.

Primary PCI: Loading dose of 180 μg per kg bolus twice, separated by 10 minutes, followed by 2 μg/kg/minute for 18 to 24 hours. If CrCl ≤50 ml per minute, reduce to 1 μg/kg/min.

Side effects: Bleeding, thrombocytopenia (rarely severe).

Contraindications: Renal dialysis, severe thrombocytopenia, high risk for intracranial/GI/GU bleeding.

Recommendations: Eptifibatide use is acceptable in the management of UA/NSTEMI for patients treated with PCI or medically. Typically, its addition to other standard antiplatelet medications is reserved for patients with high-risk features or recurrent ischemia. Daily monitoring of hemoglobin and platelets is recommended. For STEMI, eptifibatide should be initiated at the time of primary PCI.

TIROFIBAN

Rationale. Tirofiban is a nonpeptide antagonist that reversibly inhibits the GP IIb/IIIa receptor. When combined with Unfractionated heparin (UFH), has been shown to reduce death, MI, and refractory ischemia up to 30 days in patients with high-risk presentations (ischemic ECG features, elevated cardiac biomarkers).[33]

Indications: UA/NSTEMI treated medically or with PCI, STEMI.

Dosing: High dose—25 μg per kg bolus, followed by 0.15 μg/kg/minute infusion for 18 to 24 hours; Standard dose—0.4 μg/kg/minute for 30 minutes, then 0.1 μg/kg/minute for 96 hours. Dose should be reduced by half for patients with CrCl <30 ml per minute.

Side effects: Bleeding or thrombocytopenia (rarely severe).

Contraindications: High risk for intracranial/GI/GU bleeding, severe thrombocytopenia.

Recommendations: Tirofiban use is acceptable in the management of UA/NSTEMI for patients treated with PCI or medically. Typically, its addition to other standard antiplatelet medications is reserved for patients with high-risk features or recurrent ischemia. Most contemporary trials utilize the high-dose regimen for patients undergoing PCI owing to more robust platelet inhibition. Daily monitoring of hemoglobin and platelets is recommended.

ANTICOAGULANTS

UNFRACTIONATED HEPARIN

Rationale: Heparin accelerates the action of circulating antithrombin that leads to inactivation of factor IIa (thrombin), factor IXa, and factor Xa. Ultimately, this prevents further clot propagation but not lysis of existing thrombus. A meta-analysis involving six trials showed a nonsignificant RR reduction of 33% ($P = .06$) in death or MI when combined with ASA.[34]

Indications: ACS (both STEMI and UA/NSTEMI).

Dosing: Weight-based nomogram preferred over fixed-dose regimens. Bolus: 60 U per kg (max 4,000 U) with initial infusion at 12 U/kg/hour (max 1,000 U per hour). The activated partial thromboplastin time (aPTT) should be monitored every 6 hours until dosing is therapeutic (aPTT 50 to 70).

Side effects: Mild thrombocytopenia, bleeding, and heparin-induced thrombocytopenia (HIT).

Contraindications: Severe thrombocytopenia, previously documented HIT.

Recommendations: UFH is recommended early in the management of STEMI and UA/STEMI (for both conservative and early invasive strategies). A weight-based dosing regimen should be utilized with frequent monitoring of aPTT, hemoglobin, and platelets. For conservative management strategy, UFH should be continued for at least 48 hours or until discharge (up to 8 days). For CABG or PCI, continue up until the time of procedure (holding according to institutional practices).

LOW-MOLECULAR WEIGHT HEPARIN—ENOXAPARIN

Rationale: Enoxaparin is a low-molecular weight heparin (LMWH) that is more selective than UFH at inhibition of factor Xa. When compared with UFH, LMWHs have decreased binding to plasma proteins and endothelial cells, dose-independent clearance, a longer half-life, and more sustained and predictable anticoagulation. Multiple clinical trials have shown a reduction in death, MI, and recurrent angina up to 40 days when compared with UFH.[35–37] For patients with STEMI treated with fibrinolysis, the ExTRACT TIMI 25 study showed that enoxaparin was superior to UFH with regard to death, nonfatal reinfarction, and urgent revascularization but with increased rates of major bleeding.[38]

Advantages over UFH: More predictable anticoagulation, more cost-effective (less monitoring), less occurrence of HIT, twice-daily subcutaneous dosing, better reduction of nonfatal MI, death, or recurrent angina.

Disadvantages compared with UFH: Not possible to administer in a setting of severe renal impairment, not reversible with protamine, increased major bleeding,[39] inability to reliably monitor ACT during PCI.

Indications: UA/NSTEMI and STEMI.

Dosing: Enoxaparin 30 mg IV × 1 may be given early. Then, 1 mg per kg every 12 hours for 2 to 8 days. Avoid in patients with CrCl <30 (or consider reducing to every 24 hours). Unclear dosing strategy for morbidly obese patients; however, an anti-Xa level is often measured with a commonly accepted therapeutic target of 0.5 to 1.0 anti-Xa units per ml. For patients >75 years, no IV bolus should be given and dose at 0.75 mg per kg every 12 hours.

Side effects: Bleeding, HIT (rare), injection site complications.

Contraindications: CrCl <30 ml per minute.

Recommendations: In patients with UA/NSTEMI use of enoxaparin is considered an acceptable alternative to UFH, especially in those being managed conservatively. Duration of treatment is at least 48 hours and typically until discharge (up to 8 days). If CABG is pursued, enoxaparin should be discontinued 12 to 24 hours prior and bridged with UFH according to institutional practice. Although there are limited data for the use of dalteparin for this indication, enoxaparin remains the preferred LMWH. For STEMI patients treated with fibrinolysis, enoxaparin has proven efficacy, albeit at increased risk for bleeding, and can be used throughout the index hospitalization up to 8 days.

DIRECT THROMBIN INHIBITORS—BIVALIRUDIN

Rationale: Direct thrombin inhibitors (DTIS) bind reversibly to thrombin and inhibit clot-bound thrombin more effectively than UFH. Bivalirudin is a synthetic derivative of hirudin (older DTI no longer used clinically) with a shorter half-life. The ACUITY trial studied UA/NSTEMI patients undergoing PCI and showed noninferiority of bivalirudin monotherapy as compared with UFH or LMWH plus GP IIb/IIIa with respect to ischemia (9% vs. 8%, $P = .45$), but more important a significant reduction in major bleeding (4% vs. 7%, $P < .0001$).[40] The HORIZONS-AMI trial showed that STEMI patients undergoing primary PCI treated with bivalirudin alone compared with UFH plus GP IIb/IIIa had significantly reduced 30 days rates of death from cardiac causes (1.8% vs. 2.9%, $P = .03$) and a lower rate of major bleeding (4.9% vs. 8.3%, $P < .001$).[41] When followed out to 1 year, patients classified as high risk had a decreased mortality (8.4% vs. 15.9%, $P = .01$) and a decreased rate of recurrent MI (3.6% vs. 7.9%, $P = .04$).[42]

Indications: UA/NSTEMI (early invasive strategy only); STEMI undergoing primary PCI.

Dosing: Bolus 0.75 mg per kg followed by infusion of 1.75 mg/kg/hour up to 4 hours, then decrease to 0.2 mg/kg/hour for up to 20 hours.

Side effects: Bleeding.

Contraindications: Dosing adjustments for renal impairment.

Recommendations: Bivalirudin is an acceptable alternative for treatment of UA/NSTEMI in patients undergoing early invasive strategy when used with thienopyridine given upstream of PCI. It is not recommended for UA/NSTEMI patients being treated with an initial conservative strategy. For STEMI, bivalirudin can be used during primary PCI with or without prior treatment with UFH.

FACTOR XA INHIBITORS—FONDAPARINUX

Rationale: Fondaparinux is a synthetic pentasaccharide that selectively binds and inhibits antithrombin with less binding to plasma proteins. Its dose-independent clearance and long half-life allow for once daily administration and predictable and sustained anticoagulation effects. The OASIS-5 study compared fondaparinux with enoxaparin in the treatment of UA/NSTEMI. Patients treated with fondaparinux had similar rates of death, MI, and refractory ischemia at 9 days but significantly less major bleeding. At 180 days, fondaparinux was associated with a significant reduction in all major endpoints.[43] However, there was an increased incidence of catheter-associated thrombus formation during PCI, which led to the open-labeled use of UFH. The OASIS-6 study found that patients with STEMI treated with fondaparinux and fibrinolysis had reduced mortality and rates of reinfarction without increased bleeding or strokes,[44] although again there was evidence of increased thrombotic complications during coronary intervention.

Indications: UA/NSTEMI and STEMI.

Dosing: Initial dose of 2.5 mg IV followed by 2.5 mg subcutaneous injection daily (maximum antifactor Xa activity is reached in 3 hours).

Side effects: Bleeding, rash/pruritis at injection site, mild elevation of aminotransferases, and thrombocytopenia.

Contraindications: CrCl <30 ml per minute, caution if body weight <50 kg.

Recommendations: Fondaparinux is an alternative anticoagulant for the treatment of UA/NSTEMI patients being managed conservatively and should be continued for up to 8 days. Its use is preferred in the treatment of those with an increased bleeding risk. In the event of PCI, coadministration of UFH or bivalirudin is recommended to decrease the incidence of catheter-associated thrombosis. Fondaparinux should be avoided in patients with planned CABG within 24 hours owing to its long half-life. For STEMI, fondaparinux is an acceptable alternative to UFH in patients undergoing fibrinolysis and should be continued for up to 8 days. The incidence of catheter-associated thrombosis has limited its use for primary PCI; therefore fondaparinux should not be used in this setting. Additional anticoagulants with anti-IIa activity (UFH or bivalirudin) should be used during angiography if fondaparinux was initiated upstream.

WARFARIN

Rationale: Warfarin exerts its anticoagulant effect by inhibiting the hepatic synthesis of the vitamin K-dependent coagulation factors II, VII, IX, and X as well as the anticoagulant proteins C and S. Although older, small studies found limited benefit when used in the post-MI setting, the role of warfarin for ACS in the modern era primarily relegates to the treatment of LV thrombus, atrial fibrillation, or mechanical heart valves. Given the role of dual antiplatelet therapy for ACS, the addition of warfarin (triple antithrombotic therapy) for other indications introduces a greater overall risk of bleeding and can often be challenging to manage in clinical practice.

Indications: Atrial fibrillation, LV thrombus, mechanical heart valve, and venous thromboembolism.

Dosing: Start 2 to 5 mg PO daily and adjust according to INR. Standard nomograms or genotype-specific dosing strategies available. Consider starting lower dose in elderly or debilitated patients. Target INR varies with indication.

Side effects: Bleeding, hypersensitivity reactions, and skin/tissue necrosis (rarely).

Contraindications: Active bleeding or unacceptable bleeding risk, unsupervised patient with high nonadherence risk, or pregnancy.

Recommendations: The use of warfarin during or after ACS is predominately guided by expert opinion with limited evidence in the current literature. Warfarin should be started or continued in high-risk patients with a clear indication for its use (atrial fibrillation, LV thrombus, mechanical heart valve, or venous thromboembolism). When used in combination with ASA and a thienopyridine, the benefit of warfarin should outweigh the incremental risk of bleeding, and it should be given for the minimal time necessary to achieve the desired protection. Patients on triple antithrombotic therapy should be closely monitored for bleeding with strict attention paid to maintaining a therapeutic INR.

FIBRINOLYTICS

All fibrinolytic agents are plasminogen activators and work by catalyzing the cleavage of endogenous plasminogen to generate plasmin. Their thrombolytic action is derived from the ability to plasmin to degrade the fibrin matrix of the thrombus. Although contemporary practice favors the use of a catheter-based reperfusion strategy when available, fibrinolytic reperfusion still remains an important component in the treatment of STEMI in the United States and worldwide. The mortality benefit of fibrinolytic therapy is well proven and, when compared with control, fibrinolysis has been estimated to confer a significant 18% relative reduction in 35 days mortality.[45] Similar to primary PCI, fibrinolytic reperfusion offers the greatest benefit when given early, ideally within the 30 minutes of diagnosis. As a thrombus becomes more organized over time, the efficacy of fibrinolytic therapy decreases. Patients at higher risk for adverse consequences (anterior MI, diabetes, hypotension, left bundle branch block [LBBB]) seem to derive the most benefit when pharmacologic reperfusion is initiated early in the course.

Fibrinolytic agents differ substantially with regard to their antigenicity, specificity for clot-bound fibrin, dosing, and cost. There is not a preferred fibrinolytic agent currently recommended by ACC/AHA guidelines. Instead, the choice of fibrinolytic agent should be based on physician familiarity, timely availability, and, in the case of streptokinase, past exposure. The most feared and catastrophic adverse consequence of fibrinolytic therapy is intracranial hemorrhage, which is estimated to occur in 0.5% to 0.7% of patients. As such, the absolute contraindications for fibrinolytic therapy include patients with increased risk for intracerebral hemorrhage (ICH; prior hemorrhagic stroke, prior ischemic stroke within 3 months, intracranial neoplasm or vascular lesions, or closed-head injury within 3 months). Fibrinolytic reperfusion is contraindicated in the treatment of UA/NSTEMI.

Concominant use of anticoagulants in patients treated with fibrinolytics. All patients receiving fibrinolytic reperfusion should receive anticoagulant therapy for a minimum of 48 hours and preferably for the duration of the hospitalization, up to 8 days. UFH, enoxaparin, and fondaparinux have established efficacy when used with fibrinolytics and are the recommended anticoagulants. UFH should be dosed according to recommended ACS weight-based dosing guidelines. However, use for >48 hours is discouraged owing to the increased risk of developing HIT and therefore should be changed to enoxaparin or fondaparinux. Enoxaparin should be dosed with specific attention to age, weight, and CrCl. In patients <75 years with normal creatinine, an initial 30 mg IV bolus is given followed by 1 mg per kg SC every 12 hours. If ≥75 years the IV bolus is eliminated and 0.75 mg per kg SC every 12 hours is given. For all patients with CrCl <30 ml per minute, give 1 mg per kg SC daily. Fondaparinux is dosed with an initial 2.5 mg IV followed by 2.5 mg SC daily. It should be avoided in patients with creatinine <3.0 mg per dl.

STREPTOKINASE

Rationale. Streptokinase (SK) is a first-generation nonfibrin-specific lytic that exerts its effects both on clot-bound and circulating plasminogen. Although inexpensive by comparison, SK is limited by the possible development of neutralizing antibody titers in previously treated patients. In addition, SK results in systemic fibrinolysis.

Indication: STEMI.

Dosing: 1.5 million IU over 60 minutes.

Side effects: Bleeding, bronchospasm, anaphylaxis, hypotension, angioedema, periorbital swelling, fever, and urticaria.

Contraindications: Table 7.6.

ALTEPLASE

Rationale. A second-generation fibrinolytic considered to be more specific for clot-bound fibrin. Compared to SK, alteplase (TPA) was shown to confer a significant 30 days mortality reduction (15%) when administered with UFH.[46] However, TPA is associated with a slightly higher risk of ICH than SK.

Indications: STEMI.

Dosing: Accelerated protocol—(for patients >67 kg) 15 mg IV bolus, then 50 mg over 30 minutes, and 35 mg over 60 minutes (Total dose = 100 mg). For patients ≤67 kg, 15 mg IV bolus, then 0.75 mg per kg (50 mg max) over 30 minutes, and 0.5 mg per kg (35 mg max) over 60 minutes (Total dose ≤100 mg).

Side effects: Bleeding, hypotension, nausea/vomiting.

Contraindications: Table 7.6.

RETEPLASE

Rationale. Reteplase (rPA) is a third-generation fibrinolytic similar to TPA but with less high-affinity fibrin binding and increased potency. Although no increased mortality was shown over TPA in GUSTO III, its ability to be given as a double bolus may confer a theoretical advantage related to it timely administration and less dosing errors.

Indications: STEMI.

Dosing: 10 units IV bolus followed by a second 10 units IV bolus in 30 minutes.

Side effects: Bleeding.

Contraindications: Table 7.6.

TENECTEPLASE

Rationale. Tenecteplase (TNK) is a third-generation fibrinolytic that, compared to TPA, has increased fibrin specificity, decreased clearance, and decreased inhibition from plasminogen activator 1. The ASsessment of the Safety and Efficacy of New Thrombolytic (ASSENT-2) trial showed similar 30 days mortality rates when compared with TPK, although fewer systemic mild-to-moderate bleeding complications and need for blood transfusions.[47]

TABLE 7.6	Contraindications for the Use of Fibrinolytic Agents in STEMI

ABSOLUTE CONTRAINDICATIONS
Any prior ICH
Known intracranial neoplasm or cerebral vascular lesion
Ischemic stroke within 3 months (EXCEPT acute ischemic stroke within 3 h)
Suspected aortic dissection
Active bleeding or bleeding diathesis (excluding menopause) such as active peptic ulcer
Significant closed head or facial trauma within 3 months

RELATIVE CONTRAINDICATIONS
Severe, uncontrolled HTN on presentation (SBP > 180 mm Hg or DBP > 110 mm Hg)
History of ischemic stroke > 3 months, dementia, or intracranial pathology not specified above
Traumatic or prolonged (> 10 min) CPR
Noncompressible vascular punctures
Pregnancy
Recent (2–4 weeks) internal bleeding
Major surgery within past 3 weeks

Adapted from Antman EM, Anbe DT, Armstrong PW, et al. ACC/AHA guidelines for the management of patients with ST-elevation myocardial infarction: a report of the American College of Cardiology/American Heart Association Task Force on Practice Guidelines (Committee to Revise the 1999 Guidelines for the Management of Patients with Acute Myocardial Infarction). *J Am Coll Cardiol.* 2004;44:E1–E211.

Indications: STEMI.

Dosing: Single 30 to 50 mg IV bolus given over 5 seconds, dosed by body weight. For <60 kg give 30 mg, 60 to 70 kg give 35 mg, 70 to 80 kg give 40 mg, 80 to 90 kg give 45 mg, ≥90 kg give 50 mg.

Side effects: Bleeding, hypotension.

Contraindications: Table 7.6.

REFERENCES

1. Ellis K, Tcheng JE, Sapp S, et al. Mortality benefit of β-blockade in patients with acute coronary syndromes undergoing coronary intervention: pooled results from the Epic, Epilog, Epistent, Capture and Rapport Trials. *J Interv Cardiol.* 2003;16(4):299–305.
2. Chen ZM, Pan HC, Chen YP, et al.; COMMIT (ClOpidogrel and Metoprolol in Myocardial Infarction Trial) Collaborative Group. Early intravenous then oral metoprolol in 45,852 patients with acute myocardial infarction: randomised placebo-controlled trial. *Lancet.* 2005;366(9497):1622–1632.
3. Dargie HJ. Effect of carvedilol on outcome after myocardial infarction in patients with left-ventricular dysfunction: the CAPRICORN randomised trial. *Lancet.* 2001;357(9266): 1385–1390.
4. Held PH, Yusuf S, Furberg CD. Calcium channel blockers in acute myocardial infarction and unstable angina: an overview. *BMJ.* 1989;299(6709):1187–1192.
5. Hansen JF, Hagerup L, Sigurd B, et al. Cardiac event rates after acute myocardial infarction in patients treated with verapamil and trandolapril versus trandolapril alone. Danish Verapamil Infarction Trial (DAVIT) Study Group. *Am J Cardiol.* 1997;79(6):738–741.
6. Gibson RS, Boden WE, Theroux P, et al. Diltiazem and reinfarction in patients with non-Q-wave myocardial infarction. Results of a double-blind, randomized, multicenter trial. *N Engl J Med.* 1986;315(7):423–429.
7. Lubsen J, Tijssen JG. Efficacy of nifedipine and metoprolol in the early treatment of unstable angina in the coronary care unit: findings from the Holland Interuniversity Nifedipine/metoprolol Trial (HINT). *Am J Cardiol.* 1987;60(2):18A–25A.
8. Yusuf S, Pepine CJ, Garces C, et al. Effect of enalapril on myocardial infarction and unstable angina in patients with low ejection fractions. *Lancet.* 1992;340(8829):1173–1178.
9. Rutherford JD, Pfeffer MA, Moyé LA, et al. Effects of captopril on ischemic events after myocardial infarction. Results of the Survival and Ventricular Enlargement trial. SAVE Investigators. *Circulation.* 1994;90(4):1731–1738.
10. Indications for ACE inhibitors in the early treatment of acute myocardial infarction: systematic overview of individual data from 100,000 patients in randomized trials. ACE Inhibitor Myocardial Infarction Collaborative Group. *Circulation.* 1998;97(22):2202–2212.
11. Gustafsson I, Torp-Pedersen C, Køber L, et al. Effect of the angiotensin-converting enzyme inhibitor trandolapril on mortality and morbidity in diabetic patients with left ventricular dysfunction after acute myocardial infarction. Trace Study Group. *J Am Coll Cardiol.* 1999;34(1):83–89.
12. Buch P, Rasmussen S, Abildstrom SZ, et al.; TRACE Investigators. The long-term impact of the angiotensin-converting enzyme inhibitor trandolapril on mortality and hospital admissions in patients with left ventricular dysfunction after a myocardial infarction: follow-up to 12 years. *Eur Heart J.* 2005;26(2):145–152.
13. Pfeffer MA, McMurray JJ, Velazquez EJ, et al.; Valsartan in Acute Myocardial Infarction Trial Investigators. Valsartan, captopril, or both in myocardial infarction complicated by heart failure, left ventricular dysfunction, or both. *N Engl J Med.* 2003;349(20):1893–1906.
14. Cannon CP, Braunwald E, McCabe CH, et al.; Pravastatin or Atorvastatin Evaluation and Infection Therapy-Thrombolysis in Myocardial Infarction 22 Investigators. Intensive versus moderate lipid lowering with statins after acute coronary syndromes. *N Engl J Med.* 2004;350(15):1495–1504.
15. Collaborative overview of randomised trials of antiplatelet therapy—I: Prevention of death, myocardial infarction, and stroke by prolonged antiplatelet therapy in various categories of patients. Antiplatelet Trialists' Collaboration. *BMJ.* 1994;308(6921):81–106.
16. Lewis HD Jr, Davis JW, Archibald DG, et al. Protective effects of aspirin against acute myocardial infarction and death in men with unstable angina. Results of a Veterans Administration Cooperative Study. *N Engl J Med.* 1983;309(7):396–403.
17. Cairns JA, Gent M, Singer J, et al. Aspirin, sulfinpyrazone, or both in unstable angina. Results of a Canadian Multicenter Trial. *N Engl J Med.* 1985;313(22):1369–1375.
18. Theroux P, Ouimet H, McCans J, et al. Aspirin, heparin, or both to treat acute unstable angina. *N Engl J Med.* 1988;319(17):1105–1111.
19. Risk of myocardial infarction and death during treatment with low dose aspirin and intravenous heparin in men with unstable coronary artery disease. The RISC Group. *Lancet.* 1990;336(8719):827–830.
20. Yusuf S, Zhao F, Mehta SR, et al.; Clopidogrel in Unstable Angina to Prevent Recurrent Events Trial Investigators. Effects of clopidogrel in addition to aspirin in patients with acute coronary syndromes without ST-segment elevation. *N Engl J Med.* 2001;345(7): 494–502.
21. Chen ZM, Jiang LX, Chen YP, et al.; COMMIT (ClOpidogrel and Metoprolol in Myocardial Infarction Trial) Collaborative Group. Addition of clopidogrel to aspirin in 45,852 patients with acute myocardial infarction: randomised placebo-controlled trial. *Lancet.* 2005;366(9497):1607–1621.
22. Scirica BM, Sabatine MS, Morrow DA, et al. The role of clopidogrel in early and sustained arterial patency after fibrinolysis for ST-segment elevation myocardial infarction: the ECG CLARITY-TIMI 28 Study. *J Am Coll Cardiol.* 2006;48(1):37–42.
23. Wiviott SD, Braunwald E, McCabe CH, et al.; TRITON-TIMI 38 Investigators. Prasugrel versus clopidogrel in patients with acute coronary syndromes. *N Engl J Med.* 2007;357(20):2001–2015.
24. Wallentin L, Becker RC, Budaj A, et al. Ticagrelor versus clopidogrel in patients with acute coronary syndromes. *N Engl J Med.* 2009;361(11):1045–1057.
25. Mehilli J, Kastrati A, Schulz S, et al.; Bavarian Reperfusion Alternatives Evaluation-3 (BRAVE-3) Study Investigators. Abciximab in patients with acute ST-segment-elevation myocardial infarction undergoing primary percutaneous coronary intervention after clopidogrel loading: a randomized double-blind trial. *Circulation.* 2009;119(14):1933–1940.
26. Ellis SG, Tendera M, de Belder MA, et al.; FINESSE Investigators. Facilitated PCI in patients with ST-elevation myocardial infarction. *N Engl J Med.* 2008;358(21):2205–2217.
27. Giugliano RP, White JA, Bode C, et al.; EARLY ACS Investigators. Early versus delayed, provisional eptifibatide in acute coronary syndromes. *N Engl J Med.* 2009;360(21):2176–2190.
28. Stone GW, Bertrand ME, Moses JW, et al.; ACUITY Investigators. Routine upstream initiation vs deferred selective use of glycoprotein IIb/IIIa inhibitors in acute coronary syndromes: the ACUITY Timing Trial. *JAMA.* 2007;297(6):591–602.
29. Use of a monoclonal antibody directed against the platelet glycoprotein IIb/IIIa receptor in high-risk coronary angioplasty. The EPIC Investigation. *N Engl J Med.* 1994;330(14):956–961.
30. Kastrati A, Mehilli J, Neumann FJ, et al.; Intracoronary Stenting and Antithrombotic: Regimen Rapid Early Action for Coronary Treatment 2 (ISAR-REACT 2) Trial Investigators. Abciximab in patients with acute coronary syndromes undergoing percutaneous coronary intervention after clopidogrel pretreatment: the ISAR-REACT 2 randomized trial. *JAMA.* 2006;295(13):1531–1538.
31. Simoons ML; GUSTO IV-ACS Investigators. Effect of glycoprotein IIb/IIIa receptor blocker abciximab on outcome in patients with acute coronary syndromes without early coronary revascularisation: the GUSTO IV-ACS randomised trial. *Lancet.* 2001;357(9272):1915–1924.
32. Inhibition of platelet glycoprotein IIb/IIIa with eptifibatide in patients with acute coronary syndromes. The PURSUIT Trial Investigators. Platelet Glycoprotein IIb/IIIa in Unstable Angina: Receptor Suppression Using Integrilin Therapy. *N Engl J Med.* 1998;339(7):436–443.
33. Inhibition of the platelet glycoprotein IIb/IIIa receptor with tirofiban in unstable angina and non-Q-wave myocardial infarction. Platelet Receptor Inhibition in Ischemic Syndrome Management in Patients Limited by Unstable Signs and Symptoms (PRISM-PLUS) Study Investigators. *N Engl J Med.* 1998;338(21):1488–1497.
34. Oler A, Whooley MA, Oler J, et al. Adding heparin to aspirin reduces the incidence of myocardial infarction and death in patients with unstable angina. A meta-analysis. *JAMA.* 1996;276(10):811–815.
35. Low-molecular-weight heparin during instability in coronary artery disease, Fragmin during Instability in Coronary Artery Disease (FRISC) study group. *Lancet.* 1996;347(9001):561–568.
36. Antman EM, McCabe CH, Gurfinkel EP, et al. Enoxaparin prevents death and cardiac ischemic events in unstable angina/non-Q-wave myocardial infarction. Results of the thrombolysis in myocardial infarction (TIMI) 11B trial. *Circulation.* 1999;100(15):1593–1601.
37. Cohen M, Demers C, Gurfinkel EP, et al. A comparison of low-molecular-weight heparin with unfractionated heparin for unstable coronary artery disease. Efficacy and Safety of Subcutaneous Enoxaparin in Non-Q-Wave Coronary Events Study Group. *N Engl J Med.* 1997;337(7):447–452.
38. Antman EM, Morrow DA, McCabe CH, et al.; ExTRACT-TIMI 25 Investigators. Enoxaparin versus unfractionated heparin with fibrinolysis for ST-elevation myocardial infarction. *N Engl J Med.* 2006;354(14):1477–1488.
39. Ferguson JJ, Califf RM, Antman EM, et al.; SYNERGY Trial Investigators. Enoxaparin vs unfractionated heparin in high-risk patients with non-ST-segment elevation acute coronary syndromes managed with an intended early invasive strategy: primary results of the SYNERGY randomized trial. *JAMA.* 2004;292(1):45–54.
40. Stone GW, McLaurin BT, Cox DA, et al.; for the ACUITY Investigators. Bivalirudin for patients with acute coronary syndromes. *N Engl J Med.* 2006;355(21):2203–2216.
41. Stone GW, Witzenbichler B, Guagliumi G, et al.; for the HORIZONS-AMI Trial Investigators. Bivalirudin during primary PCI in acute myocardial infarction. *N Engl J Med.* 2008;358(21):2218–2230.
42. Parodi G, Antoniucci D, Nikolsky E, et al. Impact of bivalirudin therapy in high-risk patients with acute myocardial infarction: 1-year results from the HORIZONS-AMI (Harmonizing Outcomes with RevasculariZatiON and Stents in Acute Myocardial Infarction) Trial. *JACC Cardiovasc Interv.* 2010;3(8):796–802.
43. Yusuf S, Mehta SR, Chrolavicius S, et al.; Fifth Organization to Assess Strategies in Acute Ischemic Syndromes Investigators. Comparison of fondaparinux and enoxaparin in acute coronary syndromes. *N Engl J Med.* 2006;354(14):1464–1476.
44. Yusuf S, Mehta SR, Chrolavicius S, et al.; OASIS-6 Trial Group. Effects of fondaparinux on mortality and reinfarction in patients with acute ST-segment elevation myocardial infarction: the OASIS-6 randomized trial. *JAMA.* 2006;295(13):1519–1530.
45. Indications for fibrinolytic therapy in suspected acute myocardial infarction: collaborative overview of early mortality and major morbidity results from all randomised trials of more than 1000 patients. Fibrinolytic Therapy Trialists' (FTT) Collaborative Group. *Lancet.* 1994;343(8893):311–322.
46. An international randomized trial comparing four thrombolytic strategies for acute myocardial infarction. The GUSTO Investigators. *N Engl J Med.* 1993;329(10):673–682.
47. Van De Werf F, Adgey J, Ardissino D, et al.; Assessment of the Safety and Efficacy of a New Thrombolytic (ASSENT-2) Investigators. Single-bolus tenecteplase compared with front-loaded alteplase in acute myocardial infarction: the ASSENT-2 double-blind randomised trial. *Lancet.* 1999;354(9180):716–722.

PATIENT AND FAMILY INFORMATION FOR:

Medications in the Management of Acute Coronary Syndrome

The medicines used to treat heart attacks in the modern day era stem from decades of laboratory and clinical trial research. As more and more is learned about coronary artery disease (CAD), the drugs used to treat heart attack victims will hopefully become even more safe and effective. Today, medical therapy forms the cornerstone of heart attack care. Early after diagnosis, much emphasis is placed on controlling chest pain, interrupting further heart damage, and maintaining a safe blood pressure and heart rate (HR). Powerful blood thinners, pain medications, blood pressure and cholesterol lowering drugs, catheterization procedures, and sometimes even bypass surgery are used to varying degrees in the early treatment of heart attacks. Alongside these therapies, other medicines may be added to treat cardiac arrhythmias, congestive heart failure (CHF), diabetes, or tobacco addiction. The decisions underlying the medicines to be used to treat a specific patient are complex and often change depending on one's age, cardiac risk factors, medical history, and type of heart attack encountered.

The following sections are divided into the various classes and types of medications routinely used in the treatment of heart attacks. Many of the medicines described are also used to treat other conditions, both related and unrelated to the heart. The rationale behind each medication's use, both generic and commonly used trade names, potential side effects, and important details are provided. It is important to emphasize that the following pages should be used only as a general guide. Specific details about each drug, doses, and potential interactions with other medications should always be discussed with a physician and pharmacist.

TREATING THE PAIN OF A HEART ATTACK

A heart attack results from the interruption of blood flow to the muscle of the heart, most commonly by a small blood clot known as a thrombus. Because the heart muscle is dependent on the oxygen and nutrients carried by the blood, it quickly becomes starved in a process known as ischemia. Ischemia in most patients results in chest pain, or angina. It is classically described as a chest pressure or tightness, often moving to the shoulder, neck, jaw, or arms. Other symptoms may include nausea, vomiting, or shortness of breath. For patients who have experienced chest

pain or pressure in the past, the discomfort associated with a heart attack is usually more intense, more frequent, and even occurring at rest. In some patients, particularly diabetics and the elderly, symptoms may be more subtle and present only as mild stomach pain or indigestion, occasional palpitations, or there may be no symptoms at all. The onset of chest pain is often the first sign of a heart attack, and it provides warning that the heart muscle is threatened. Although the primary goal in treating all heart attacks is to restore blood flow within the jeopardized coronary artery, the adequate treatment of pain is of paramount importance to all patients.

Medications used to specifically treat a heart attack pain are called "antianginals" and include nitrates, ß-blockers, and calcium channel blockers (CCBs). For pain unrelieved with these classes of drugs, various forms of narcotic medications, known as opioids, are commonly used.

NITRATES

Names: Nitroglycerin (*Minitran, Nitro-Bid, Nitro-Dur, Nitro-Time, Nitrolingual, NitroQuick, Nitrostat*).

Related medications: Isosorbide mononitrate (*Imdur, Ismo, Monoket*), isosorbide dinitrate (*Isordil, Dilatrate-SR, Isochron*).

Nitroglycerin is one of the most commonly used medicines for the treatment of chest pain. It is a "vasodilator" and primarily works by dilating, or expanding, the size of coronary arteries. The net effect is that more blood can get to the heart muscle. Even in patients with a completely blocked coronary artery, nitroglycerin is useful because it recruits blood flow to other, less diseased arteries. Nitroglycerin lowers blood pressure, a property that is helpful in relieving pain and decreasing the amount of strain placed on the heart. Nitroglycerin can be administered in a variety of forms, a feature that makes it particularly useful when treating someone with ongoing nausea and vomiting.

Preparations: Sublingual (dissolved under the tongue), translingual (sprayed into the mouth), oral, transcutaneous (absorbed through the skin), and intravenous.

Side effects: Headache (most common), flushing, dizziness, lightheadedness, nausea, vomiting, blurred vision, and swelling.

Important information: Patients who use medications to treat erectile dysfunction such as sildenafil (*Viagra*), tadalafil (*Cialis*), or vardenafil (*Levitra*) *should not* use nitroglycerin because combined use may result in a severe, rapid reduction in blood pressure or even death. The prior or ongoing use of any of these medications should immediately be reported to a physician.

ß-BLOCKERS

Names: Metoprolol (*Lopressor, Toprol-XL*), carvedilol (*Coreg*), atenolol (*Tenormin*), labetalol (*Trandate*), propranolol (*Inderal*),esmolol (*Brevibloc*).

ß-Blockers are a class of blood pressure medications commonly used in the treatment of heart attacks, abnormal heart rhythms, and CHF. They work to relieve angina by both lowering blood pressure and reducing the HR. When the heart is forced to pump blood against a high blood pressure or beat at a fast rate, it requires greater amounts of oxygen and thus greater coronary blood flow. During exercise and especially during a heart attack, blood flow to the heart muscle is jeopardized and is unable to meet the demands required. By lowering both the blood pressure and HR, ß-blockers are useful at reducing this strain on the heart and often result in reduced levels of chest pain.

Preparations: Oral, intravenous.

Side effects: Dizziness, fatigue, lightheadedness, change in sexual ability or desire, depression, diarrhea, and slow heartbeat.

Important information: Some patients with asthma, emphysema, bronchitis, or related diseases of the lungs may experience excessive wheezing or shortness of breath while taking ß-blockers. Such reactions should be reported to a physician. In addition, abruptly discontinuing ß-blockers has been reported to sometimes result in worsening of chest pain.

CALCIUM CHANNEL BLOCKERS

Names: Diltiazem (*Cardizem, Cartia, Dilacor, Dilt, Diltia, Diltzac, Taztia, Tiazac*), verapamil (*Calan, Covera, Isoptin, Verelan*), amlodipine (*Norvasc*), felodipine (*Plendil*), nisoldipine (*Sular*).

CCBs, a class of blood pressure medications, are also used to treat heart attacks, angina, and abnormal heart rhythms. Like ß-blockers, they work by reducing the HR and blood pressure, thus reducing strain on the heart. CCBs are often used as a substitute for ß-blockers in certain patients or sometimes in combination. They are the preferred treatment for a rare form of angina caused by spasm of the coronary arteries.

Preparations: Oral, intravenous.

Side effects: Dizziness, lightheadedness, headache, nausea or vomiting, constipation, swelling, and slow heartbeat.

NARCOTICS (OPIOIDS)

Names: Morphine (*Avinza, MS Contin, Roxanol*), fentanyl (*Sublimaze*), oxycodone (*OxyContin, OxyFast, Percocet, Endocet, Magnacet*), hydrocodone (*Lortab, Norco,*

Vicodin, Zydone), hydromorphone (*Dilaudid*), meperidine (*Demerol*).

Narcotics such as morphine do not specifically treat angina. Rather, they act more generally to block pain signals in the body from reaching the brain. Narcotics are often prescribed for heart attack patients when other antianginal medications have failed to completely control pain. In addition, they have several beneficial side effects, one of which is to help slow the HR. Like ß-blockers and CCB, this helps to reduce the workload exerted by the heart. Although narcotics come in many different preparations, only very few patients require narcotics at discharge; therefore they are most commonly administered intravenously when used in the treatment of heart attacks as this provides the most rapid relief of symptoms.

Preparations: Oral, intravenous, transdermal (through the skin).

Side effects: Nausea, vomiting, constipation, dizziness, flushing, slow heartbeat, and shallow breathing.

ANTIPLATELET MEDICATIONS

Platelets are specialized blood cells that constantly survey the body for areas of injury. In blood vessels, and in the coronary arteries in particular, platelets are responsible for identifying damaged areas of vessel wall and then sealing off these areas before further harm ensues. Most blood vessel injuries occur in places where cholesterol deposits have caused significant hardening of the arteries, which are usually flexible and elastic. When platelets recognize damage, they quickly change shape, become sticky, and along with other platelets form a small blood clot (thrombus) to plug the injured area of vessel wall. Unfortunately, this small blood clot may often grow large enough to impede flow completely or incompletely through the entire artery. This, most simply, is the cause of a heart attack. Antiplatelet drugs are special medications that interfere with the ability of platelets to form clots, particularly large obstructive clots. Antiplatelet medications work particularly well at reducing heart attacks caused from blood clots in the coronary arteries. However, because they block the natural actions of platelets throughout the body they can also increase the risk of unintended bleeding.

ASPIRIN

Names: Aspirin (*Bayer Aspirin, Ecotrin, Anacin*).

Aspirin is one of the oldest, most widely used, cheap, and effective antiplatelet medicines around. Even today, it remains an essential component in the treatment of heart attacks both during hospitalization and after discharge. With very few exceptions, aspirin therapy should be taken for life in individuals who suffer a heart attack.

Preparations: Oral, rectal.

Side effects: Upset stomach, heartburn, stomach bleeding, and easy bruising.

Important information: Because aspirin remains such an important medicine in the treatment and prevention of heart attacks, patients should take it daily. This is especially important if a stent is used in the treatment of one's heart disease. Although a true aspirin allergy exists, fortunately, it is rare and most side effects from aspirin can be overcome with the use of coated formulations and certain medicines to reduce stomach acid. Consultation with a cardiologist is recommended prior to stopping aspirin, even temporarily, for situations such as elective surgery.

THIENOPYRIDINES AND ADP RECEPTOR INHIBITORS

Names: Clopidogrel (*Plavix*), prasugrel (*Effient*), ticagrelor (*Brilinta*).

Each of these medications works as potent antiplatelet medication, most commonly taken in addition to aspirin, and works to greatly reduce the body's ability to form blood clots in the coronary arteries and elsewhere. Studies of patients with heart attacks have consistently proven that these drugs help to reduce the incidence of future heart attacks and prolong one's lifespan. In addition to their role in the treatment of heart attacks, they are critically important in patients treated with coronary stents.

Preparations: Oral.

Side effects: Easy bruising or bleeding, nausea, and dizziness.

Important information: As in the case of aspirin, patients prescribed medications from this class should strive to take them exactly as requested by a physician. In patients with coronary stents, this becomes of even greater importance because the abrupt discontinuation can result in new blood clots forming within the stent itself. Although such events are rare, they often lead to a second heart attack and have even been fatal. As with aspirin, consultation with a cardiologist is recommended prior to electively stopping these medications for upcoming surgeries. Patients should avoid missing doses or running out before a prescription can be renewed.

PLATELET GLYCOPROTEIN IIB/IIIA RECEPTOR ANTAGONISTS

Names: Abciximab (*Reopro*), eptifibatide (*Integrilin*), tirofiban (*Aggrastat*).

Glycoprotein IIb/IIIa receptor antagonists are small molecules named for the specific platelet receptor they bind. As with other antiplatelet medications, they work to decrease the ability of platelets to form clots within the coronary arteries. However, this class of medications is given only intravenously. Although these drugs are often used in addition to aspirin for the early treatment of heart attacks, they are most commonly used during coronary stent implantation. Their highly potent platelet-blocking effects make them particularly well suited to prevent clot formation within stents, thereby increasing stent durability. Like with other antiplatelet medications, drugs from this class have been proven in thousands of heart attack patients to prolong life and reduce future heart attacks.

Preparation: Intravenous.

Side effects: Easy bruising or bleeding, nausea, and stomach aches.

ANTICOAGULANTS

A blood clot, or thrombus, is not formed by platelets alone. Within the circulating blood exist a multitude of microscopic proteins that work alongside platelets to assist in the formation of blood clots at sites of vessel injury. When damage is detected, these proteins form long, thin threads call fibrin. In turn, these fibrin threads create a mesh-like plug that helps to stabilize blood clots. Whereas antiplatelet medications block the actions of platelets, anticoagulants block the body's ability to form fibrin. Because they work to prevent blood clot formation, they are often referred to as "blood thinners."

HEPARIN AND RELATED MEDICATIONS

Names: Heparin.

Related medications: Enoxaparin (*Lovenox*), bivalirudin (*Angiomax*), fondaparinux (*Arixtra*), dalteparin (*Fragmin*).

Heparin and its related medicines comprise a central role in the treatment of heart attacks. They are given early in the course of a heart attack and often continued throughout the duration of a hospital stay. In addition to preventing blood clots associated with heart attacks, heparin or similar drugs are routinely used in the prevention of clots associated with other disorders. Typical uses may include the prevention of blood clots in the legs (DVT; deep vein thrombosis), those associated with mechanical heart valves, and those that may form with certain abnormal heart rhythms.

Preparations: Intravenous, subcutaneous (under the skin) injections.

Side effects: Easy bruising or bleeding, pain at injection site, abnormal blood counts (especially platelets), and rash.

Important information: A rare condition known as HIT can occur in some patients who have had previous exposure to heparin. This condition causes a dramatic drop in platelets and can lead to both excessive bleeding and clotting. Patients with a history of heparin-induced thrombocytopenia (HIT) should promptly notify their physicians during any hospital admission or office visit.

WARFARIN

Names: Warfarin (*Coumadin, Jantoven*).

Related medications: Dabigatran (*Pradaxa*).

Warfarin is a blood thinner that has been used for decades to treat a multitude of conditions associated with blood clotting. Inherited clotting disorders, mechanical heart valves, abnormal heart rhythms, and prior blood clots in the legs or lungs are all common reasons for warfarin to be prescribed. Although it is seldom used to specifically treat or prevent heart attacks, warfarin deserves special mention because it is often used in addition to the antiplatelet and anticoagulant medications commonly prescribed for heart attack patients. A unique and often frustrating feature of warfarin is that it requires frequent monitoring of blood levels. Newer medications such as dabigatran (*Pradaxa*) are increasingly being approved for use in place of warfarin and do not require blood level monitoring.

Preparations: Oral.

Side effects: Easy bruising or bleeding, nausea, vomiting, and altered sense of taste.

Important information: Each blood thinner added to a patient's list of medications introduces an incremental risk of unintended bleeding. In properly selected patients, these drug combinations can be safely followed but often require more aggressive monitoring and physician visits. It is not uncommon for warfarin dosing, even if stable for years, to need adjusting after the initiation of new medications. Patients should pay close attention to early signs of bleeding, especially bleeding related to the stomach or intestines, and report these to their physician.

FIBRINOLYTICS, OR "CLOT BUSTERS"

Names: Streptokinase (*Streptase*), TPA (*Activase*), reteplase (*Retavase*), tenecteplase (*TNKase*).

Fibrinolytics, also called "thrombolytics" or "clot busters," are a class of medications used to treat a specific type of heart attack where blood flow through a coronary artery is completely obstructed. Unlike antiplatelet and anticoagulant drugs that prevent blood clots from forming or expanding, fibrinolytics actually target and destroy clots that have already formed. These extremely potent medications work best when given very early in the course of a heart attack, and are used in areas where a cardiac catheterization laboratory is not immediately available. Unfortunately, they have not proven to be useful in treating heart attacks caused by only partially obstructive clots.

Preparations: Intravenous.

Side effects: Easy bruising or bleeding, stroke (rare).

OTHER IMPORTANT MEDICATIONS USED IN TREATING HEART ATTACKS

The immediate control of chest pain, addition of antiplatelet and anticoagulant medications, and often cardiac catheterization are crucially important during the early stages of a heart attack. These therapies are largely targeted at aborting further damage and salvaging heart muscle from permanent damage. Aggressive and early control of blood pressure, fluid volume, and cholesterol levels are equally important in achieving these goals. In many cases, additional blood pressure medications may be added to more closely control one's hypertension. In other cases, they may be added simply for the unique and beneficial properties they provide to patients with heart disease.

ACE INHIBITORS AND ANGIOTENSIN RECEPTOR BLOCKERS

Names: **ACE inhibitors**—benazepril (*Lotensin*), captopril (*Capoten*), enalapril (*Vasotec*), fosinopril (*Monopril*), lisinopril (*Prinivil, Zestril*), moexipril (*Univasc*), perindopril (*Aceon*), quinapril (*Accupril*), ramipril (*Altace*), **ARBs**—trandolapril (*Mavik*); cadesartan (*Atacand*), eprosartan

(*Teveten*), irbesartan (*Avapro*), losartan (*Cozaar*), olmesartan (*Benicar*), valsartan (*Diovan*), telmisartan (*Micardis*).

Medications from these two classes of blood pressure drugs are commonly used alongside other therapies to treat specific consequences of heart attacks. This is particularly true for patients who develop CHF, that is, a weakened heart muscle resulting from a heart attack. Apart from being blood pressure lowering drugs, these medications have shown to be beneficial in prolonging life, reducing the incidence of CHF, and protecting the kidneys in diabetic patients.

Preparations: Oral.

Side effects: Dizziness, lightheadedness, cough (ACE inhibitors), abnormal electrolyte levels, and swelling.

DIURETICS

Names: Furosemide (*Lasix*), bumetanide (*Bumex*), torsemide (*Demadex*), hydrochlorothiazide (*Esidrix, Microzide*), chlorothiazide (*Diuril*), metolazone (*Zaroxolyn*), amiloride (*Midamor*), triamterene (*Dyrenium*), spironolactone (*Aldactone*), eplerenone (*Inspra*).

Diuretics, commonly referred to as "water pills," are routinely used in the care of heart attack patients who suffer from CHF or any condition characterized by increased fluid in the body, most often in the lower extremities or lungs. They work to remove excess fluid by stimulating urine production in the kidneys. Furosemide (*Lasix*) remains the most prescribed drug used in the hospital for this purpose. Some weaker diuretics are often added for their blood pressure–lowering properties, whereas others such as spironolactone (*Aldactone*) and eplerenone (*Inspra*) may be added in special circumstances characterized by severe CHF.

Preparations: Oral, intravenous.

Side effects: Dizziness, lightheadedness, dry mouth, thirst, hearing difficulty, and abnormal electrolyte levels.

CHOLESTEROL LOWERING MEDICATIONS

Names: Atorvastatin (*Lipitor*), fluvastatin (*Lescol*), lovastatin (*Mevacor, Altoprev*), pravastatin (*Pravachol*), rosuvastatin (*Crestor*), simvastatin (*Zocor*).

Related medications: Niacin (*Niaspan, Niacor*), gemfibrozil (*Lopid*), fenofibrate (*Tricor*), cholestyramine (*Questran*), colestipol (*Colestid*), colesevelam (*Welchol*), and ezetimibe (*Zetia*).

Cholesterol-lowering medications, most notably the statins, have emerged as some of the most important drugs used in the treatment CAD in the past quarter century. Stringent cholesterol control helps prevent both future heart attacks and strokes. In patients suffering from a heart attack, powerful statins such as atorvastatin (*Lipitor*), simvastatin (*Zocor*), or rosuvastatin (*Crestor*) are often prescribed. The related medications listed above are sometimes added to better control certain types of cholesterol or triglycerides abnormalities, most often in addition to statins.

Preparations: Oral.

Side effects: Muscle aches or pains, nausea, stomach aches, flushing or itching (niacin), insomnia (niacin), gas, and diarrhea.

Ronald E. Ross
Sandhya K. Balaram

CHAPTER 8

Coronary Artery Bypass Surgery and Postoperative Care

BACKGROUND

Coronary artery bypass surgery (CABG) has been proven in multiple clinical trials as a safe and effective treatment for coronary artery disease.[1–3] Current American College of Cardiology (ACC) and American Heart Association (AHA) guidelines recommend CABG in specific patients with coronary disease (Table 8.1).[4] Additional indications exist for those patients who present with acute myocardial infarction (MI) (Table 8.2).[4] Specific clinical scenarios, such as an acute right coronary artery (RCA) infarction, support early percutaneous revascularization to prevent the severe right ventricular (RV) dysfunction that may occur postoperatively.[4,5]

Multiple factors affect surgical outcome (Table 8.3), and various risk stratification scores have been developed to evaluate their impact.[6–8] It is important to determine how comorbidities affect patients to adequately discuss risks and benefits prior to surgery. Optimization of renal function and respiratory status, smoking cessation, and glucose control are the methods by which surgical risk can be improved prior to proceeding with revascularization.

SURGICAL TECHNIQUE

CABG is performed under general anesthesia. All patients receive prophylactic preoperative antibiotics within 30 to 60 minutes of incision and this is redosed if the operation exceeds 3 hours. A cephalosporin, usually cefazolin, is used as the first-line agent, with vancomycin being used for patients who are penicillin and/or cephalosporin allergic, or in areas where methicillin-resistant *Staphylococcus* species prevalence is high.[9,10]

Intraoperative monitoring includes placement of a radial or femoral arterial catheter, a central venous catheter, a Swan-Ganz pulmonary arterial (PA) catheter (often used but may be omitted in uncomplicated low-risk cases), a Foley catheter, a bladder or rectal temperature probe, and a transesophageal echocardiography (TEE) probe. Intraoperative TEE provides assessment of cardiac anatomy and function, qualifies the presence and severity of aortic plaque, assists in placement of intracardiac catheters and vents, aids in the evaluation of intracardiac air or thrombus, and provides vital data regarding valve and cardiac function.

Cardiopulmonary bypass (CPB) is often used for CABG. This is an extracorporeal circuit that completely replaces the function of the heart and lungs, allowing the surgeon to work with a motionless and bloodless heart. In its simplest form, it consists of a venous cannula that drains blood by gravity from the right atrium or vena cava to a venous reservoir. A pump then pushes the blood through a membrane oxygenator (oxygenates the blood and removes carbon dioxide), a filter (removes particulate matter and prevents embolism), and then back into the patient through an arterial cannula into the aorta (common femoral or axillary artery if the aorta is unsuitable). There are additional catheters that allow for delivery of cardioplegia, venting of the heart, and suctioning blood from the operative field. A heat exchanger that allows systemic cooling and rewarming regulates the blood temperature. The CPB circuit is usually primed with balanced crystalloid solution such as lactated Ringers that is about 30% of the patient's blood volume.[11]

Prior to cannulation and initiating CPB, the patient is systemically anticoagulated with intravenous heparin (300 to 400 units per kg) to achieve an activated clotting time (ACT) of >400 to 480 seconds. The ACT is checked every 30 minutes and more heparin given as necessary. After institution of CPB and aortic cross-clamping, cold cardioplegia solution is given antegrade through the coronary arteries and sometimes retrograde through the coronary sinus to stop the heart and provide myocardial protection. The patient is then cooled to 28°C or up to 32°C to reduce cellular metabolism and offer some organ protection.[11]

TABLE 8.1	ACC/AHA Guidelines for CABG in Patients with Coronary Artery Disease

1. Greater than 50% stenosis of the left main coronary artery (LMCA).

2. Equivalent LMCA stenosis, that is, >70% stenosis of the proximal left anterior descending artery (LAD) and the proximal left circumflex artery (LCX).

3. Three-vessel disease, that is, >50% stenosis of the LAD, LCX and the right coronary artery (RCA). Survival benefit in this group is greater when the left ventricular ejection fraction (LVEF) is <0.50.

4. One-or two-vessel disease (with or without significant proximal LAD stenosis) with LVEF <0.50 and/or significant demonstrable myocardial ischemia on non-invasive testing.

5. Sustained ventricular tachycardia or after resuscitation from cardiac death with LMCA or proximal LAD stenosis.

Adapted from Eagle KA, Guyton RA, Davidoff R, et al.; American College of Cardiology; American Heart Association. ACC/AHA 2004 guideline update for coronary artery bypass graft surgery: a report of the American College of Cardiology/American Heart Association Task Force on Practice Guidelines (Committee to Update the 1999 Guidelines for Coronary Artery Bypass Graft Surgery). *Circulation.* 2004;110(14):e340–e437.

TABLE 8.2	ACC/AHA Guidelines for CABG After Acute MI

1. Cardiogenic shock
2. Failed percutaneous revascularization with persistent or recurrent ischemia refractory to medical therapy, and with significant area of myocardium at risk
3. Failed percutaneous revascularization with ongoing angina or hemodymanic instability.
4. Concurrent postinfarction ventricular septal rupture or mitral valve insufficiency
5. Life-threatening ventricular arrhythmias in the presence of >50% LMCA stenosis or three-vessel disease

Adapted from Eagle KA, Guyton RA, Davidoff R, et al.; American College of Cardiology; American Heart Association. ACC/AHA 2004 guideline update for coronary artery bypass graft surgery: a report of the American College of Cardiology/American Heart Association Task Force on Practice Guidelines (Committee to Update the 1999 Guidelines for Coronary Artery Bypass Graft Surgery). *Circulation.* 2004;110(14):e340–e437.

Conduits used for CABG include the left and right internal mammary arteries (IMA), the greater saphenous vein (GSV), and less frequently, the radial artery. The mammary arteries are frequently left in situ with the proximal end left connected to the subclavian artery and the distal end anastomosed to the target coronary. Segments of GSV or radial artery are used as free grafts and anastomosed in an aorta-to-coronary fashion. Patency rates of IMA grafts are usually >90% at 10 years, whereas that of GSV are 70% to 80% at 5 years and 40% to 60% at 10 years. The GSV grafts have a higher rate of formation of neointimal hyperplasia and atherosclerosis that compromise long-term patency.[4] Radial artery grafts have approximately 84% patency at 5 years.[12]

At the completion of the procedure, patients are rewarmed and weaned off CPB once they are hemodynamically stable

TABLE 8.3	Factors Associated with Increased CABG Perioperative Mortality

- Increased age
- Female sex
- Unstable hemodynamics
- Decreased ejection fraction
- Preprocedural MI
- Chronic obstructive pulmonary disease
- Extensively calcified ascending aorta
- Peripheral vascular disease
- Renal failure, particularly requiring dialysis
- Previous open heart surgery

Adapted from Higgins TL, Estafanous FG, Loop FD, et al. Stratification of morbidity and mortality outcome by preoperative risk factors in coronary artery bypass patients. A clinical severity score. *JAMA.* 1992;267(17):2344–2348; Hannan EL, Wu C, Bennett EV, et al. Risk stratification of in-hospital mortality for coronary artery bypass graft surgery. *J Am Coll Cardiol.* 2006;47(3):661–668; Nashef SA, Roques F, Michel P, et al. European system for cardiac operative risk evaluation (EuroSCORE). *Eur J Cardiothorac Surg.* 1999;16(1):9–13.

with adequate cardiac output (CO). Acid–base, electrolyte, and oxygenation parameters must also be satisfactory. Protamine, 1 mg for every 100 units of heparin given, is administered to reverse anticoagulation and allow for hemostasis (ACT should normalize; 107 ± 13 seconds). Protamine is given slowly as it can activate the complement cascade and lead to hypotension, anaphylaxis, or right heart failure, particularly in patients who have been presensitized from previous administration of protamine or protamine insulin.[11]

A number of physiologic changes occur because of CPB. Contact of the patient's blood with the extracorporeal circuit leads to activation of the coagulation, fibrinolytic, complement, and cytokine cascades. This occasionally results in coagulopathy, a systemic inflammatory response, and varying degrees of multiorgan dysfunction. The CPB circulation is relatively hypotensive (usually mean arterial pressure of 40 to 60 mm Hg) and nonpulsatile, and this stimulates sympathetic activation with resultant increased arrhythmias. It can also lead to end-organ hypoperfusion with resultant prerenal azotemia, stroke, or mesenteric ischemia. Required clamps placed on the aorta may put the patient at risk for embolic stroke, particularly in the setting of an atherosclerotic aorta.[11]

In some cases, CABG can be performed without the use of CPB, termed "off-pump" CABG. Mechanical cardiac stabilizers along with various anesthetic and surgical techniques allow the surgeon to operate on coronary arteries while the heart is beating. Off-pump CABG aims to avoid the possible complications of CABG that are directly because of CPB. Benefits are seen in terms of decreased hospital cost and length of stay. Decreased operative mortality and postoperative morbidity in terms of renal failure, myocardial dysfunction, atrial fibrillation, gastrointestinal complications, pulmonary dysfunction, blood loss, and transfusion requirements have been reported.[13–15] Significant benefits for female patients in particular have been documented.[16] Multiple factors are considered in the recommendation of off-pump surgery including the skill and experience of the surgeon, stability of the patient, presence of LV dysfunction, target vessels, and concomitant valve disease.

INITIAL CRITICAL CARE MANAGEMENT

The first phase of critical care management begins at the completion of surgery with the safe and expedient transfer of the patient from the operating room to the cardiac care unit (CCU) (Table 8.4). The patient should be completely stable and transported with continuous EKG, pulse oximetry, and blood pressure tracings on a portable monitor. All necessary drug infusions to maintain hemodynamic stability are continued through fully charged battery-powered infusions pumps. Additional medications that may be necessary in case of an emergency should also be available. The patient should be adequately hand-ventilated with 100% oxygen.

On arrival to the CCU, the patient is reconnected to the ventilator at appropriate settings. A standard ventilator setting is the use of a volume-cycled mode in which the ventilator is programmed to deliver a set tidal volume and fixed minute ventilation. This can be in the form of assist-control ventilation (A/C) in which every breath, whether ventilator- or patient-initiated, is fully ventilator-delivered. Another common mode is synchronous intermittent mandatory ventilation (SIMV) in

TABLE 8.4	Guideline for Initial Critical Care Management After CABG
Transfer patient from OR to ICU	– Portable monitor for EKG, pulse oximetry, arterial blood pressure. – Check drug infusions – Check emergency medications – Ventilate with 100% oxygen
Set ventilator	See Table 8.5
Connect to monitors	– Ensure correct calibration – Monitor continuous EKG, BP, pulse oximetry, and CVP – Use PA catheter if present to monitor PA pressures, PAWP, SvO_2, CO/CI, and SVR
Sign out from anesthesia	– Patient past history – Indication for CABG – Pertinent intraoperative details – Current postoperative status
Complete physical examination	– Check core temperature and actively rewarm to ~37°C – Check end-organ perfusion: mental status, UOP, skin color, peripheral pulses – Check all lines and tubings: ensure secured and not occluded or kinked – Check labeling and dosage of medications – Check adequate capture of pacing wires
CXR, EKG, laboratory studies	– Check correct placement of chest lines and tubes – Check for intrathoracic pathology – Address abnormalities in heart rate/rhythm – Replete electrolytes, correct acid–base abnormalities – Correct coagulopathy, transfuse blood products as indicated – Check blood glucose and control within range of 80–110mg/dl
Pain control and sedation	– Tailor to suit patient needs – Two-point wrist restraints for sedated patients

which a preset number of breaths are fully ventilator-delivered, but the patient is also allowed additional spontaneous breaths that can be supported to varying degrees. Ventilator settings should be tailored to suit the patient (Table 8.5). A pressure-cycled mode in which a peak inspiratory pressure is set can be used to avoid barotrauma in a chronically ventilated patient, but this mode can result in varying tidal volumes and minute ventilation based on pulmonary compliance and is not commonly used immediately after cardiac surgery.[17]

The patient is connected to CCU monitors that follow continuous EKG, pulse oximetry, arterial blood pressure, and central venous pressure (CVP) readings. A PA catheter, if present, can be used to monitor core temperature, PA pressures, left heart filling pressures measurements, mixed-venous oxygen saturation, and CO. Other continuous CO monitors are also available. Hypothermic patients should be actively rewarmed to 37°C using forced-air warming devices. The CCU clinician

then checks to ensure that all intravenous lines and tubing are in place (not occluded or kinked), and that all medications are correctly labeled and being infused at the appropriate dosage.

At this point, a full "sign-out" between the surgeon, the anesthesiologist, and the CCU clinician should take place. This should include the patient's past medical history, intraoperative course, details of the bypass surgery, CPB and aortic cross-clamp times, and blood loss and products transfused, and pre- and postoperative cardiac function. A complete physical examination should then be performed. Note should be taken of the adequacy of the CO and end-organ perfusion as evidenced clinically by the following parameters:

- *Mental status.* Although the effects of residual anesthesia are present immediately postoperatively, the patient's mental status should be assessed as soon as they become conscious. Specific neurologic changes such as lack of spontaneous movement or lack of movement to command should be documented.

TABLE 8.5	Suggested Initial Ventilator Settings After CABG

1. Tidal volume of 6–8 ml/kg of ideal body weight, and adjusted to keep plateau pressures <35 cm H_2O.

2. Fraction of inspired oxygen (FiO_2) of 100% and adjusted downwards to keep the arterial oxygen saturation (SaO_2) >90% and arterial oxygen tension (PaO_2) >60 mm Hg.

3. Positive end-expiratory pressure (PEEP) set at a "physiologic" value of 5 cm H_2O. Higher levels of PEEP can be used to increase oxygenation and to limit FiO_2 to nontoxic levels (< 50%), but increased PEEP causes decreased venous return to the heart and can also worsen cardiac tamponade. Brief periods of increased PEEP can be used in cases of postoperative bleeding with increased chest tube drainage. Increased PEEP causes higher pulmonary artery wedge pressure (PAWP) readings on the PA catheter which can be falsely interpreted as elevated left heart filling pressures.

4. Pressure support (PS) if in SIMV of 5–10 cm H_2O, adjusted to patient comfort

5. Respiratory rate of 12–16 breaths per minute.

- *Urine output* (UOP) measured via an indwelling Foley catheter. At least 0.5 cc/kg/hour indicates satisfactory renal perfusion in the adult patient. Hypothermia or diuretics such as furosemide or mannitol received during CPB can cause the UOP to be relatively high initially.
- *Skin perfusion and peripheral pulses.* Many CABG patients also have concurrent peripheral arterial disease in the lower extremities. Warm skin with good capillary refill and palpable pulses indicate good peripheral perfusion.

All patients receive a postoperative chest X-ray to evaluate for any intrathoracic pathology such as hemothorax, pneumothorax, pulmonary edema, atelectasis, widened mediastinum, or enlarged cardiac silhouette. The X-ray also confirms the correct position of all catheters and tubes including the endotracheal tube (2 to 4 cm above the carina), the central venous catheter (at the junction between the superior vena cava (SVC) and the right atrium), the PA catheter (no more than 2 cm from the hilum), the intraaortic balloon pump (IABP; tip in descending aorta just distal to the left subclavian artery), and the pleural and mediastinal tubes.[18]

Immediate laboratory studies on admission to the CCU include arterial blood gas, hemoglobin (Hb) and hematocrit (Hct) levels, prothrombin time and international normalized ratio (PT/INR), activated partial thromboplastin time (aPTT), basic metabolic panel, magnesium, and blood glucose. Necessary labs are then repeated every 4 to 6 hours depending on the clinical circumstances. All abnormalities should be corrected with the necessary ventilator adjustment, blood product transfusion, and/or electrolyte repletion. Blood glucose should be strictly controlled within a range of 80 to 110 mg per dl within 24 hours of CCU admission using adequate insulin coverage, as tight glucose control has been associated with decreased rates of sepsis, renal failure, and death.[19]

A 12-lead EKG is performed on admission to the CCU and each day thereafter to assess for myocardial ischemia and arrhythmia. Continuous telemetric EKG monitoring is mandatory to monitor for the development of arrhythmias. Patients with epicardial pacing wires should have these checked to ensure adequate capture.

Pain control and adequate sedation with intravenous narcotics, benzodiazepines, and/or propofol should be titrated to individual patient needs. Pain and anxiety can stimulate catecholamine release and lead to tachycardia, arrhythmia, hypertension, elevated systemic vascular resistance (SVR), and increased myocardial oxygen consumption.

MANAGEMENT OF SPECIFIC POSTOPERATIVE ISSUES

CARDIOVASCULAR SYSTEM

Postoperative hemodynamic monitoring is critical after CABG. This starts with the surgical team prior to closing the chest. Direct observation and TEE examination allow assessment of wall motion, right and left ventricular function, and the volume status of the patient. The various cardiovascular issues after CABG can be subdivided into problems with cardiac rate and rhythm, preload, afterload, cardiac contractility, or various combinations of these. All these areas should be monitored and managed appropriately to ensure adequate end-organ perfusion and oxygenation.

Cardiac rate and rhythm. Disturbances in cardiac rate and rhythm can be the result of many different etiologies including electrolyte abnormalities (especially calcium, magnesium, and potassium), hypoxemia, hypercarbia, myocardial and nodal ischemia, acid–base abnormalities, hypothermia, pain, medications (e.g., β-blockers, narcotics, catecholamines), drug-withdrawal (e.g., alcohol), postpericardiotomy inflammation, CPB-induced sympathetic activation, the presence of central venous or PA catheters, and complications such as pericardial tamponade and pneumothorax. Both bradyarrhythmia (including conduction blocks) and tachyarrhythmia can result in diminished CO and hypotension and should be treated by correcting the underlying cause while temporizing with pacing and/or medications.

In the initial postoperative period, bradycardia and conduction blocks resulting in heart rates <60 beats per minute with inadequate CO should be managed with pacing using intraoperatively placed temporary epicardial pacing wires, or through transvenous or transcutaneous pacing methods. Using atrioventricular (AV) sequential pacing for conduction blocks and atrial pacing for other bradyarrhythmias are preferred over just ventricular pacing as the latter does not allow for the contribution of the atrial contraction to increase ventricular preload. In the absence of pacing, atropine may be used to increase the heart rate. Patients with persistent second and third degree AV conduction block may eventually need a permanent pacemaker.[20]

Besides correcting any of the causative abnormalities mentioned above, tachycardias are managed using medications such as β-blockers, calcium channel blockers (CCBs), or digoxin to decrease the heart rate to <100 beats per minute. Some tachyarrhythmias that develop after cardiac surgery can also be terminated by overdrive pacing. These include atrial flutter, paroxysmal supraventricular tachycardia (SVT), ventricular tachycardia, and torsades de pointes. Torsades patients should also receive intravenous magnesium.[20]

Atrial fibrillation (AF) is very common after CABG with an incidence of 15% to 40%, and is associated with higher hospital costs, length of stay, and postoperative morbidity (renal dysfunction, cognitive changes, and infection) and mortality.[21] It usually occurs within the first 5 days, with a peak incidence on postoperative day 2. Advanced age, a history of AF, chronic obstructive pulmonary disease (COPD), obesity, concurrent valve surgery, withdrawal of β-blocker or ACE inhibitor preoperatively, failure to institute β-blocker, ACE inhibitor and nonsteroidal anti-inflammatory drugs (NSAID) postoperatively, CPB, and longer CPB times are risk factors for AF after CABG.[21,22] Preoperative and early postoperative β-blockers are given to reduce the incidence of postoperative AF. Patients who cannot be given β-blockers may receive amiodarone pre- and postoperatively.[23] At present, digoxin and CCBs have no role for prophylaxis, and their use to control ventricular rate in postoperative AF is less effective than β-blockers because of increased CPB-induced sympathetic activity.[24] Amiodarone not only helps with chemical cardioversion of AF but also has sympatholytic and β-Blockade properties and helps to control ventricular rate.[23,25] Electrical cardioversion of AF in post-CABG patients is usually not necessary unless the patient is hemodynamically compromised by the arrhythmia. Patients who develop postoperative AF that is recurrent or persistent should be anticoagulated with heparin within 48 hours of onset and continued on warfarin (target INR of 2.0 to 3.0) for at least 4 weeks.[23,26]

Preload. Preload is the actual stretch experienced by a left ventricular myocyte just prior to ventricular contraction and gives an idea of volume status. In keeping with the Starling law, increasing preload causes an increase in cardiac stroke volume until a point is reached where the ventricle becomes overdistended and stroke volume decreases. Preload should therefore be optimized to allow the best possible CO.

The left ventricular end-diastolic pressure (LVEDP) gives the best estimate of preload, but this can be measured only through trans-arterial cardiac catheterization. As a surrogate, the PA catheter measures the PAWP that approximates the left atrial mean pressure (provided the lungs are normal and there is no pulmonary vascular hypertension), which in turn approximates the LVEDP (the LVEDP is transmitted through the open mitral valve to the LA at the end of ventricular diastole).[27] Normal LVEDP is 5 to 15 mm Hg. An LV that requires pressures of 15 to 20 mm Hg to pump is somewhat dysfunctional, and that it requires LVEDP of >20 mm Hg implies severe dysfunction.[28]

Normal PAWP is 6 to 15 mm Hg, with values less then these indicating inadequate preload. In cases of low CO, the PAWP can be increased to 18 and up to 20 mm Hg. Other parameters such as afterload and contractility should be optimized before increasing the preload further. Checking a PAWP requires inflating the PA catheter's balloon, which can lead to PA rupture if the balloon tip is located too far distal into the pulmonary artery. Some clinicians will observe the relationship of the PAWP with the PA diastolic pressure (usually 2 to 5 mm Hg higher than the PAWP), and thereafter, use the PA diastolic pressure to estimate the left-sided pressures. This, however, can be done only in cases where there is no pulmonary hypertension and/or pulmonary valve incompetence. The same principle applies to patients with only a central venous catheter, in which the CVP can be used to estimate volume status, provided that there is no pulmonary hypertension, RV failure, or right-sided valve incompetence (normal CVP is 7 ± 2 mm Hg).[27,28]

Preload can be decreased from inadequate volume replacement at the end of CPB, ongoing blood loss with significant chest tube drainage, or third-space fluid loss from CPB-induced systemic inflammatory syndrome (SIRS) and capillary leak. Management should be aimed at replacing circulating volume and red cell mass and definitively treating any ongoing bleeding. Boluses of crystalloid or noncellular colloid can be given initially, and if the Hb is low (usually <7 g per dl), the patient may require immediate blood transfusion. Inotropic and/or vasopressor agents may be needed temporarily to maintain adequate CO and blood pressure.

Pericardial tamponade can also cause decreased preload owing to cardiac underfilling. Tamponade occurring acutely after CABG is owing to blood collecting in the pericardial sac causing compression of the myocardium. The right-sided heart chambers with their relatively lower pressures are more susceptible to external compression. Patients present with tachycardia, hypotension, and increased need for vasopressors. Table 8.6 shows other findings on clinical evaluation. Definitive management requires operative evacuation, but until this can be accomplished, the patient should be temporized with volume loading to increase preload, and with inotropic and vasopressor support.[28,29]

Afterload. Afterload refers to the pressure a cardiac chamber must generate to empty the blood. For the LV, this would be

TABLE 8.6	**Clinical Findings of Pericardial Tamponade**

1. Tachycardia and hypotension.

2. Distended neck veins and elevated CVP (only if patient not concurrently hypovolemic).

3. Equalization (usually within 5 mm Hg) of the central venous, RA mean, RV diastolic, PA diastolic and pulmonary artery wedge pressures.

4. Low-voltage EKG tracing. Sometimes electrical alternans may be present from the heart swinging in the pericardial fluid.

5. Mediastinal and cardiac silhouette widening on the CXR

6. TEE showing pericardial fluid, RA and/or RV diastolic compression, and IVC distension.

the pressure needed to overcome the resistance offered by the systemic vasculature, the SVR (normal range 900 to 1,200 dynes·seconds per m[5]).[27] Increased SVR after CABG can be because of excess sympathetic activity from pain, anxiety, hypothermia, or CPB.

After CABG, it is vital in most cases to keep the systolic BP between 100 and 130 mm Hg. A higher BP may be needed in patients with significant atherosclerotic disease to improve end-organ perfusion. However, hypertension in this setting may exacerbate postoperative bleeding and cause disruption of suture lines. The BP should not be maintained at the expense of a supranormal SVR as this could lead to end-organ ischemia. An elevated SVR leads to increased afterload, which in turn leads to increased myocardial oxygen consumption with possible worsening in myocardial dysfunction.[28]

An elevated BP and/or SVR can be decreased post-CABG with continuous infusions of nitroglycerine and/or nitroprusside, both of which also increase venous capacitance and can also decrease preload. Both agents can induce some degree of reflex tachycardia and prolonged use of nitroprusside can lead to accumulation of toxic cyanide radicals. Infusion of short-acting β-blockers such as esmolol or labetalol can be used in the patient with elevated BP in the setting of normal or near normal ventricular function.

A low SVR is also not desirable as this may increase CO to maintain peripheral perfusion, thereby increasing myocardial oxygen consumption. A low SVR after CABG is often because of the CPB-induced systemic inflammation causing decreased peripheral vasomotor tone, but it may also be owing to adrenocortical insufficiency, allergic reaction, or septic shock. Treatment includes ensuring an adequate preload with volume repletion and using a peripheral vasoconstrictor such as norepinephrine, vasopressin (typically added as a second agent in patients with moderate norepinephrine requirements), or phenylephrine (a pure α_1-agonist that causes peripheral vasoconstriction and some reflex bradycardia).

Cardiac contractility. Some post-CABG patients have a degree of myocardial dysfunction and diminished cardiac contractility. This is usually the result of preexisting MI or ventricular failure, or from the actual CABG procedure that causes some degree of myocardial ischemia and reperfusion injury (myocardial "stunning"). Cardiac contractility can be estimated with a TEE intraoperatively. Postoperatively, the PA catheter that measures CO through thermodilution is used. Cold saline solution is injected into the right atrial (RA) port and a thermistor near the tip of the PA catheter measures the blood temperature curve of the cold bolus. The slower the decay of the temperature, the lower the CO; this is calculated and displayed by the monitor in liters per minute (normal 4.5 to 6 L per minute). Three to four measurements are made and averaged to improve accuracy. To allow for comparison between different patients with different body habitus, the CO is divided by the body surface area to provide a cardiac index (CI; normal is 2.5 to 4.5 $L/minute/m^2$). Acceptable post-CABG CI is >2 $L/minute/m^2$, with values less than this requiring inotropic support with various medications (Figure 8.1). A CI <1.5 $L/minute/m^2$ represents a heart with severely depressed CO.[27,28]

The PA catheter can also estimate CO using mixed venous blood drawn from its PA port. A sample from the PA is used because blood returning to the RA through the SVC, inferior vena cava (IVC), and coronary sinus has different oxygen saturations. The blood returning through the coronary sinus has the lowest oxygen saturation in the body (approximately 30%) because the myocardium extracts a relatively greater amount of oxygen from the blood flowing into it than any other tissue. Blood in the PA has been sufficiently mixed to give an accurate assessment of the overall saturation of blood that has returned to the heart from systemic circulation. Normal mixed venous oxygen saturation (SvO_2) levels range from 60% to 80%. In patients with poor CO, tissues extract a relatively greater amount

of oxygen from the systemic circulation and the SvO_2 is lower. SvO_2 is also dependent on the fraction of inspired oxygen (FiO_2) levels and the oxygen carrying capacity (total red cell mass) of the blood, so the ICU clinician should ensure that these are also appropriate.[27,28]

Post-CABG myocardial dysfunction is usually temporary and resolves within 12 to 48 hours. If the patient's CO continues to be low (<1.5 to 2.0 $L/minute/m^2$) despite adequate preload and afterload control, and with moderate-to-high doses of inotropic support, mechanical support with an IABP may be necessary Figure 8.1. With persistent low CO, one should also consider technical issues with the surgery such as an occluded bypass conduit, embolization of a coronary vessel, inadequate revascularization, or inadequate myocardial protection during CPB.

Mention should be made of low CO as a result of RV failure. Predisposing factors include RV infarction, pulmonary hypertension with preexistent RV dysfunction, right coronary or right bypass conduit embolism, and inadequate RV protection during CPB. These patients have elevated right-sided filling pressures (CVP, RA pressure) with normal to low left-sided filling pressures (PAWP). Echocardiography shows a poorly contracting RV, dilated RA and RV, and tricuspid regurgitation. Management requires careful volume loading to increase the RV preload, inotropic support, and reduction of the RV afterload (Table 8.7). Suitable medications include milrinone, dobutamine, and isoproterenol (Figure 8.1). Inhaled nitric oxide or prostacycline have also been used in some centers to

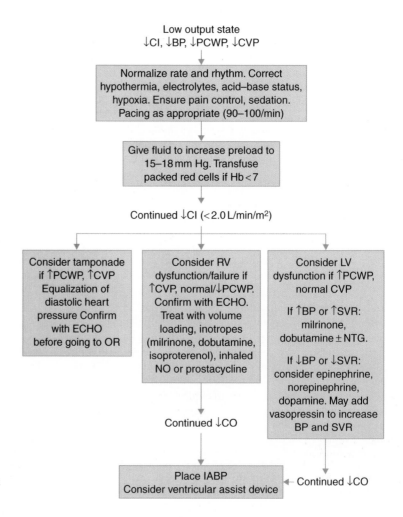

Figure 8.1. Algorithm for the management of a low output state after CABG.

TABLE 8.7	Commonly Used Inotropes and Their Characteristics[11,28]
Dobutamine	Catecholamine with $ß_1$ and $ß_2$ activity. Increases inotropy and causes decreased systemic and pulmonary vascular resistance. A good first line drug for mild to moderate low CO. Starting dose is 2–5 µg/kg/min, and can be increased up to 20 µg/kg/min. Can cause reflex tachycardia and is tachyarrhythmogenic.
Dopamine	Catecholamine in which doses 2–10 µg/kg/min causes predominantly ß-agonism. Higher doses have more α_1 activity which can lead to increased SVR, tachycardia, and increased myocardial oxygen consumption. In general, it is not a very strong inotropic agent and can be arrhythmogenic.
Epinephrine	Catecholamine with mixed $ß_1$, $ß_2$ and, α_1 activity. Used as a first-line agent. Doses < 0.02 µg/kg/min has mostly $ß_1$ and $ß_2$ activity with resultant increased inotropy and decreased SVR. Higher doses have more α_1 activity causing resultant increased SVR, tachycardia, and increased myocardial oxygen consumption. These effects can be lessened if given with nitroglycerine. It is arrhythmogenic, but causes less tachycardia than dobutamine. Standard dose: 0.5–20 µg/min.
Norepinephrine	Catecholamine similar to epinephrine but with minimal $ß_2$ activity. Increase in SVR can overshadow inotropy, so more useful when given with milrinone or nitroglycerine. It is less arrhythmogenic than epinephrine. Standard dose: 1–20 µg/min.
Isoproterenol	Catecholamine with $ß_1$ and $ß_2$ activity. Increases inotropy and decreases vascular resistance. Usefulness limited by increased tachycardia, increased myocardial oxygen consumption and increased arrhymogenicity. Standard dose 2–10 µg/min.
Milrinone	Phosphodiesterase inhibitor that increases inotropy and causes a decrease in the SVR and the pulmonary vascular resistance. There is little effect on myocardial oxygen consumption. Useful as a second agent with a catecholamine in patients with decreased CO and increased afterload. Loading dose 50 µg/kg followed by infusion of 0.375–0.75 µg/kg/min.

decrease pulmonary hypertension.[30,31] A decrease of the mean airway pressure, by adjusting tidal volume and pressure support, may also help to decrease RV afterload.

Intraaortic balloon pump. The IABP is an inflatable balloon placed in the descending aorta via the common femoral artery using the Seldinger technique. Inflation during ventricular diastole provides a counterpulsation that improves coronary blood flow and myocardial perfusion. Deflation just prior to ventricular systole decreases afterload and helps to decrease myocardial oxygen consumption and increase CO. Indications for use include severe ongoing myocardial ischemia and/or refractory anginal pain, cardiogenic shock despite maximal inotropic therapy, and postinfarction ventricular septal rupture or acute mitral regurgitation. IABP use is contraindicated in patients with aortic regurgitation, as this can overwhelm the LV with increased regurgitation during diastole. It is also contraindicated in patients with aortic dissection, aortic aneurysm, or severe aorto-iliac disease.[28,32,33]

The balloon is cyclically inflated (to 40 ml in the adult) and deflated using helium. Helium has a low viscosity and allows for rapid inflation/deflation cycles and, in case of balloon rupture, there is a low risk of harmful embolization. Preoperative use requires anticoagulation with heparin to prevent thrombus from forming on the surface of the balloon. Immediately postoperatively anticoagulation is held, but with extended use, usually >48 hours, anticoagulation is restarted.

Inflation should be programmed to coincide with the peak of the T-wave on the EKG or the beginning of the dicrotic notch on the arterial pressure waveform. This produces an augmented pressure during ventricular diastole that appears as the second spike after the dicrotic notch on the arterial waveform. The spike before the dicrotic notch is the pressure generated by the LV during ventricular systole. Deflation should be set to occur just prior to the QRS complex on the EKG as this coincides to the instant just prior to ventricular systole.

Complications of IABP use include arterial dissection or perforation during placement, thromboembolism, traumatic lysis of blood cells (especially platelets), and renal, gastrointestinal, or lower extremity ischemia.[28]

Before removal, the IABP should be weaned to minimal support by gradually decreasing the ratio of balloon inflation to ventricular contraction from 1:1 to 1:2 to 1:3, or by decreasing the amount of helium in the balloon. Myocardial function as determined by CI and SvO_2 should be checked at each stage of weaning. If the function remains satisfactory on minimal support, anticoagulation is held, and the IABP is removed and pressure held on the femoral artery entry site for about 20 to 30 minutes.[28]

POSTOPERATIVE BLEEDING

Of all patients undergoing cardiac surgery, up to 50% require transfusion of blood products and 10% to 20% will consume about 80% of the products transfused.[34] Postoperative bleeding may occur after CABG and up to 4% of patients will require surgical reexploration.[35,36] CPB can lead to postoperative coagulopathy from residual systemic heparinization, hypothermia, CPB-induced platelet dysfunction, and hemodilution, and consumption of platelets and clotting factors. Adequate hemostasis is critical at the completion of each procedure, and the presence of obvious coagulopathy should be addressed prior to leaving the operating room.

Risk factors for bleeding or blood transfusion during or after CABG include increased age, small body habitus, preoperative anemia, preoperative antithrombotic or antiplatelet therapy, heredity or acquired bleeding diatheses (e.g., hemophilia, von Willebrand disease, antiphospholipid antibody syndrome, cirrhosis, renal failure), emergency surgery, reoperative or complex surgery (e.g., concurrent valve surgery), prolonged CPB time, postoperative hypothermia, and lack of a transfusion algorithm.[34]

In high-risk patients, measures to minimize allogenic blood product transfusion include preoperative use of erythropoietin and iron supplements, intraoperative acute normovolemic hemodilution (AHN; 1 to 2 units of blood is removed intraoperatively, replaced with crystalloid, and later transfused back into the patient after heparin reversal), use of cell saver device, off-pump CABG, use of minimized CPB circuits (results in less hemodilution), retrograde autologous priming of the CBP circuit (the patient's blood is used to partially prime the CPB circuit), and use of antifibrinolytic agents such as epsilon-aminocaproic acid and tranexamic acid.[34] Medications such as warfarin, GP-IIb/IIIa antagonists, and platelet ADP-receptor blockers (e.g., clopidogrel and prasugrel) should be discontinued prior to surgery, optimally for at least 4 days to prevent excessive bleeding.[34,37]

Chest tube output is measured carefully to evaluate postoperative bleeding. Excessive bleeding is generally considered as any chest tube output >200 ml per hour for 1 hour, >150 ml per hour for 2 consecutive hours, or >100 ml per hour for 3 consecutive hours.[29] The quality of the chest tube drainage should be noted. Brisk bleeding, but with visible clot formation, may indicate a problem with surgical bleeding necessitating surgical exploration in the operating room.

In all cases of postoperative bleeding, the goal of the clinician is to first treat supportively by maintaining adequate circulating volume and red cell mass to ensure tissue oxygenation, and then to expeditiously correct any coagulopathy. The patient's core temperature should be checked, and active rewarming should be done to keep the temperature near 37°C. All cold blood products should also be warmed prior to transfusion. A chest X-ray should also be done to evaluate for retained blood in the pleural space or mediastinum.

Transfusion of blood products may be required. Frequent laboratory studies should be obtained to monitor Hb, hematocrit, PT/INR, aPTT, and platelet count. Although no true "transfusion trigger" exists, red cells may be transfused to keep Hb >6 g per dl while on CPB, and >7 g per dl postoperatively. For older patients, and patients with severe ongoing bleeding and/or cardiovascular instability, the Hb can be kept >8 to 9 g per dl. Patient with critical end-organ ischemia (e.g., bowel, central nervous system) can be transfused to Hb of 10 g per dl.[34] Generally, in an adult, the Hb can be multiplied by 3 to get the equivalent Hct value, and 1 unit of packed red blood cells will increase the Hb by 1 g per dl and the Hct by 3%. Fresh frozen plasma is used if INR >1.5.[38,39] If the aPTT is >1.5 times normal but the PT is normal, residual systemic heparin should be considered and additional 50 to 100 mg doses of protamine (should not surpass total of 1.3 mg per 100 unit heparin given during CPB) may be given. Platelet counts <10,000 per μl may lead to spontaneous bleeding in nonsurgical patients, but owing to platelet dysfunction after CBP, platelet levels should be kept >100,000 per μl in a bleeding patient.[39] In an adult, 1 platelet apheresis unit will generally increase the platelet count by 30,000 to 40,000 per μl. Fibrinogen levels (normal 150 to 400 mg per dl) may also be helpful. Cryoprecipitate may be transfused to keep levels >100 mg per dl.[38,39] One unit of cryoprecipitate per 10 kg body weight increases the fibrinogen levels by about 50 mg per dl.

The routine prophylactic use of desmopressin acetate (DDAVP), 0.3 μg per kg, to prevent bleeding after CPB-induced platelet dysfunction is not recommended, but in cases of excessive bleeding its use is acceptable.[34,40] It causes a release of von Willebrand factor and factor VIII from endothelial cells and is also useful in bleeding patients with renal failure, or type I von Willebrand disease. Activated factor VII is also utilized in cases of persistent bleeding despite routine hemostatic therapy.[34] This produce stimulates the extrinsic pathway's production of thrombin.

Increasing positive end-expiratory pressure (PEEP) may be beneficial in reducing postoperative bleeding by increasing mechanical forces against the bleeding surfaces, but it can also reduce venous return and CO.[41] If bleeding continues despite aggressive hemostatic measures, the patient may have true surgical bleeding that requires surgical exploration. Absolute indications for reoperation include 300 to 500 ml per hour for 1 hour, 200 to 300 ml per hour for 2 hours, or >100 ml per hour for 6 to 8 hours (Figure 8.2).

RENAL SYSTEM

Fluid management after CABG can be divided into an initial volume loading phase followed by a diuresis phase. Initial volume loading is needed to maintain intravascular volume lost to third spacing (from CPB-induced systemic inflammation and capillary leak), and transient postoperative increased UOP (from hypothermia, diuretics given during CPB, and sometimes uncontrolled hyperglycemia). Over the first or second day, the SIRS response of CPB resolves and third-spaced fluid starts to return to the intravascular space. However, UOP may be insufficient to eliminate the excess total body water because CPB also activates the renin–aldosterone pathway and stimulates antidiuretic hormone production, both of which reduce UOP. It is often necessary, therefore, to aid diuresis starting with the second postoperative day with loop diuretics such as furosemide.

Some 1.1% to 7.9% of patients develop acute renal failure (ARF) and 0.2% to 0.7% require dialysis after CABG. More than 85% of those who develop ARF after CABG will not need dialysis. Mortality, however, for those with ARF is about 14%, and twice as much for those who require dialysis.[42,43] Patients at increased risk for ARF include those with advanced age, preoperative comorbidities (renal insufficiency, diabetes mellitus, peripheral arterial disease, hypertension, reduced LV function, obesity, COPD), concurrent valve and CABG surgery, and prolonged CPB time.[43,44] Nephrotoxic agents should be avoided in high-risk patients, and hemodynamics should always be optimized to ensure adequate CO and peripheral perfusion. Use of diuretics, N-acetyl cysteine and low-dose dopamine (1 to 2 μg/kg/minute) may offer renal protection.[45,46] Fenoldopam (a dopamine$_1$-receptor agonist, 0.1 μg/kg/minute for $\geq$24 hours) has been shown to increase renal blood flow without decreasing SVR, decrease the need for hemodialysis, and decrease mortality.[46]

RESPIRATORY SYSTEM

Most patients can be successfully weaned from the ventilator within 6 to 8 hours after cardiac surgery; however, 3% to 5% of patients will require prolonged mechanical ventilation for 7 or more days, with resultant higher morbidity and mortality. Risk factors for prolonged mechanical ventilation include increasing age, smoking, female gender, preoperative renal failure on dialysis, emergency surgery, and postoperative complications, such as low output state and cerebrovascular accidents.[47,48] Patients who are hemodynamically stable, alert and following commands, and are warm with a core temperature

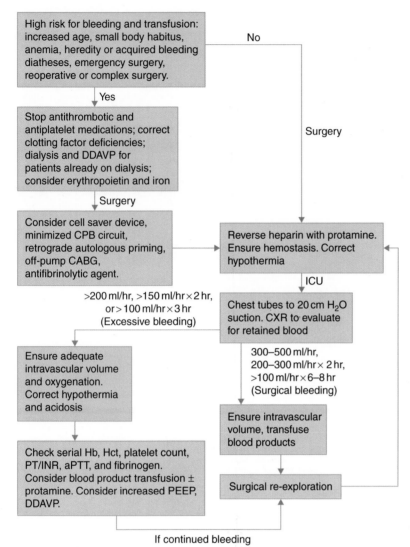

Figure 8.2. Management of postoperative bleeding.

of approximately 37°C, may be weaned from the ventilator. Although a variety of weaning methods exist, one technique is to place the patient on a spontaneous breathing trial with continuous positive airway pressure (CPAP) of 5 cm H_2O, and PS of zero (can give PS of 8 cm H_2O if endotracheal tube ≤7.0). Final decisions about extubation are made based on the absence of increased work of breathing, diaphoresis, and agitation, along with adequate oxygen saturations in a setting of hemodynamic stability. After 30 minutes of CPAP, an arterial blood gas is sent and the PaO_2 should be ≥60 mm Hg and the PCO_2 ≤45 mm Hg, with pH ≥7.32. If the patient meets the above criteria, the ICU clinician can proceed with extubation.[11,49]

After extubation, patients should be given humidified supplemental oxygen through face mask, and this can later be weaned once SaO_2 remains ≥90%. Patients should receive frequent chest physical therapy and be encouraged to use an incentive spirometer hourly.

Mediastinal and pleural tubes should be removed as soon as the total drainage is <100 ml per 8 hours.[28] To prevent air from going into the chest, tubes are pulled briskly with the patient in forced expiration, or if on mechanical ventilation, during positive pressure inspiration. If a purse-string suture was left in place at the time of surgery, it is tied to occlude the tube site incision, followed by a petroleum-based occlusive dressing.

GASTROINTESTINAL SYSTEM

Gastrointestinal complications after CABG are relatively rare with a 2% incidence but have been shown in multiple studies to result in high mortality.[50] Common complications include acute cholecystitis (sometimes acalculous), intestinal ischemia, paralytic ileus, and upper gastrointestinal bleeding. Acute pancreatitis, hepatic failure, perforated viscus, and esophagitis are rarer conditions. Visceral hypoperfusion and/or embolism from aortic/myocardial manipulation are thought to be the underlying causes. Patients at high risk include those with advanced age, hypertension, perioperative MI, emergency surgery, reoperative surgery, low preoperative LVEF, prolonged CBP time, low output state postoperatively, and IABP use.[50–52] Many patients may not have any abdominal signs or symptoms thus making the diagnosis clinically challenging. Thorough examinations of the abdomen should be performed looking for abdominal distension, decreased bowel sounds, tenderness, signs of peritoneal irritation (e.g., guarding and rebound tenderness), and melena or heme-positive stools. Liver function tests, pancreatic amylase and lipase, abdominal X-ray, abdominal sonogram, upper and lower endoscopies, and abdominal computed tomogram are all studies that should be utilized depending on clinical suspicion. Early diagnosis and treatment is essential to decrease mortality.

Enteral feeding is usually resumed on postoperative day 1. Intubated patients can be fed via a nasogastric feeding tube. Nausea, vomiting, excessive belching, decreased bowel sounds, and abdominal distension are signs that the patient may have a paralytic ileus, in which case, feeding can be temporarily held until these signs and symptoms improve. Continuous nasogastric suctioning may also be required. It is advisable to use postoperative acid reducing agents such as proton-pump inhibitors on all patients to reduce the incidence of gastrointestinal bleeding.[11]

REFERENCES

1. Takaro T, Hultgren HN, Lipton MJ, et al. The VA cooperative randomized study of surgery for coronary arterial occlusive disease II. Subgroup with significant left main lesions. *Circulation.* 1976;54(6)(suppl):III107–III117.
2. Rogers WJ, Coggin CJ, Gersh BJ, et al. Ten-year follow-up of quality of life in patients randomized to receive medical therapy or coronary artery bypass graft surgery. The Coronary Artery Surgery Study (CASS). *Circulation.* 1990;82(5):1647–1658.
3. Williams DO, Vasaiwala SC, Boden WE. Is optimal medical therapy "optimal therapy" for multivessel coronary artery disease? Optimal management of multivessel coronary artery disease. *Circulation.* 2010;122(10):943–945.
4. Eagle KA, Guyton RA, Davidoff R, et al.; American College of Cardiology; American Heart Association. ACC/AHA 2004 guideline update for coronary artery bypass graft surgery: a report of the American College of Cardiology/American Heart Association Task Force on Practice Guidelines (Committee to Update the 1999 Guidelines for Coronary Artery Bypass Graft Surgery). *Circulation.* 2004;110(14):e340–e437.
5. Bowers TR, O'Neill WW, Grines C, et al. Effect of reperfusion on biventricular function and survival after right ventricular infarction. *N Engl J Med.* 1998;338(14):933–940.
6. Higgins TL, Estafanous FG, Loop FD, et al. Stratification of morbidity and mortality outcome by preoperative risk factors in coronary artery bypass patients. A clinical severity score. *JAMA.* 1992;267(17):2344–2348.
7. Hannan EL, Wu C, Bennett EV, et al. Risk stratification of in-hospital mortality for coronary artery bypass graft surgery. *J Am Coll Cardiol.* 2006;47(3):661–668.
8. Nashef SA, Roques F, Michel P, et al. European system for cardiac operative risk evaluation (EuroSCORE). *Eur J Cardiothorac Surg.* 1999;16(1):9–13.
9. Ariano RE, Zhanel GG. Antimicrobial prophylaxis in coronary bypass surgery: a critical appraisal. *DICP.* 1991;25(5):478–484.
10. Vuorisalo S, Pokela R, Syrjala H. Comparison of vancomycin and cefuroxime for infection prophylaxis in coronary artery bypass surgery. *Infect Control Hosp Epidemiol.* 1998;19(4):234–239.
11. Yuh DD, Vricella LA, Baumgartner WA. *The Johns Hopkins Manual of Cardiothoracic Surgery.* New York, NY: McGraw-Hill Medical Pub.; 2007:369–408, 496–497.
12. Acar C, Ramsheyi A, Pagny JY, et al. The radial artery for coronary artery bypass grafting: clinical and angiographic results at five years. *J Thorac Cardiovasc Surg.* 1998;116(6):981–989.
13. Cleveland JC Jr, Shroyer AL, Chen AY, et al. Off-pump coronary artery bypass grafting decreases risk-adjusted mortality and morbidity. *Ann Thorac Surg.* 2001;72(4):1282–1288; discussion 1288–1289.
14. Raja SG, Dreyfus GD. Current status of off-pump coronary artery bypass surgery. *Asian Cardiovasc Thorac Ann.* 2008;16(2):164–178.
15. Puskas JD, Thourani VH, Kilgo P, et al. Off-pump coronary artery bypass disproportionately benefits high-risk patients. *Ann Thorac Surg.* 2009;88(4):1142–1147.
16. Puskas JD, Kilgo PD, Kutner M, et al. Off-pump techniques disproportionately benefit women and narrow the gender disparity in outcomes after coronary artery bypass surgery. *Circulation.* 2007;116(11)(suppl):I192–I199.
17. George RB. *Chest Medicine: Essentials of Pulmonary and Critical Care Medicine.* 5th ed. Philadelphia, PA: Lippincott Williams & Wilkins; 2005:525–527.
18. Batra P. Radiology for monitoring devices. Syllabus for Thoracic Imaging, The Annual Meeting of the Society of Thoracic Radiology Boca Raton Resort & Club, Boca Raton, Florida, Apr 4–8, 2001; 2001:202–204.
19. Van den Berghe G, Wouters P, Weekers F, et al. Intensive insulin therapy in the critically ill patients. *N Engl J Med.* 2001;345(19):1359–1367.
20. Epstein AE, DiMarco JP, Ellenbogen KA, et al. ACC/AHA/HRS 2008 guidelines for device-based therapy of cardiac rhythm abnormalities. *Heart Rhythm.* 2008;5(6):e1–e62.
21. Mathew JP, Fontes ML, Tudor IC, et al.; Investigators of the Ischemia Research and Education Foundation; Multicenter Study of Perioperative Ischemia Research Group. A multicenter risk index for atrial fibrillation after cardiac surgery. *JAMA.* 2004;291(14):1720–1729.
22. Zacharias A, Schwann TA, Riordan CJ, et al. Obesity and risk of new-onset atrial fibrillation after cardiac surgery. *Circulation.* 2005;112(21):3247–3255.
23. Fuster V, Rydén LE, Cannom DS, et al. ACC/AHA/ESC 2006 Guidelines for the management of patients with atrial fibrillation: a report of the American College of Cardiology/American Heart Association Task Force on Practice Guidelines and the European Society of Cardiology Committee for Practice Guidelines (Writing Committee to Revise the 2001 Guidelines for the Management of Patients with Atrial Fibrillation): developed in collaboration with the European Heart Rhythm Association and the Heart Rhythm Society. *Circulation.* 2006;114(7):e257–e354.
24. Andrews TC, Reimold SC, Berlin JA, et al. Prevention of supraventricular arrhythmias after coronary artery bypass surgery. A meta-analysis of randomized control trials. *Circulation.* 1991;84(5)(suppl):III236–III244.
25. Clemo HF, Wood MA, Gilligan DM, et al. Intravenous amiodarone for acute heart rate control in the critically ill patient with atrial tachyarrhythmias. *Am J Cardiol.* 1998;81(5):594–598.
26. Dunning J, Nagarajan DV, Amanullah M, et al. What is the optimal anticoagulation management of patients post-cardiac surgery who go into atrial fibrillation? *Interact Cardiovasc Thorac Surg.* 2004;3(3):503–509.
27. O'Leary JP, Tabuenca A,Capote LR. *The Physiologic Basis of Surgery.* 4th ed. Philadelphia, PA: Wolters Kluwer Health/Lippincott Williams & Wilkins; 2008:418–421.
28. Elefteriades JA, Geha AS, Cohen LS. *House Officer Guide to ICU Care: Fundamentals of Management of the Heart and Lungs.* 2nd ed. New York, NY: Raven Press; 1994:57–109.
29. Conte JV. *The Johns Hopkins Manual of Cardiac Surgical Care.* 2nd ed. Philadelphia, PA: Mosby/Elsevier; 2008:237–253. *Mobile Medicine.*
30. Oz MC, Ardehali A. Collective review: perioperative uses of inhaled nitric oxide in adults. *Heart Surg Forum.* 2004;7(6):E584–E589.
31. De Wet CJ, Affleck DG, Jacobsohn E, et al. Inhaled prostacyclin is safe, effective, and affordable in patients with pulmonary hypertension, right heart dysfunction, and refractory hypoxemia after cardiothoracic surgery. *J Thorac Cardiovasc Surg.* 2004;127(4):1058–1067.
32. Davidson J, Baumgartner F, Omari B, et al. Intra-aortic balloon pump: indications and complications. *J Natl Med Assoc.* 1998;90(3):137–140.
33. Lewis PA, Mullany DV, Townsend S, et al. Trends in intra-aortic balloon counterpulsation: comparison of a 669 record Australian dataset with the multinational Benchmark Counterpulsation Outcomes Registry. *Anaesth Intensive Care.* 2007;35(1):13–19.
34. Ferraris VA, Ferraris SP, Saha SP, et al. Perioperative blood transfusion and blood conservation in cardiac surgery: the Society of Thoracic Surgeons and the Society of Cardiovascular Anesthesiologists clinical practice guideline. *Ann Thorac Surg.* 2007;83(5)(suppl):S27–S86.
35. Karthik S, Grayson AD, McCarron EE, et al. Reexploration for bleeding after coronary artery bypass surgery: risk factors, outcomes, and the effect of time delay. *Ann Thorac Surg.* 2004;78(2):527–534; discussion 534.
36. Sellman M, Intonti MA, Ivert T. Reoperations for bleeding after coronary artery bypass procedures during 25 years. *Eur J Cardiothorac Surg.* 1997;11(3):521–527.
37. Ferraris VA, Ferraris SP, Moliterno DJ, et al. The Society of Thoracic Surgeons practice guideline series: aspirin and other antiplatelet agents during operative coronary revascularization (executive summary). *Ann Thorac Surg.* 2005;79(4):1454–1461.
38. Practice parameter for the use of fresh-frozen plasma, cryoprecipitate, and platelets. Fresh-Frozen Plasma, Cryoprecipitate, and Platelets Administration Practice Guidelines Development Task Force of the College of American Pathologists. *JAMA.* 1994;271(10):777–781.
39. Practice Guidelines for blood component therapy: a report by the American Society of Anesthesiologists Task Force on Blood Component Therapy. *Anesthesiology.* 1996;84(3):732–747.
40. Fremes SE, Wong BI, Lee E, et al. Metaanalysis of prophylactic drug treatment in the prevention of postoperative bleeding. *Ann Thorac Surg.* 1994;58(6):1580–1588.
41. Ilabaca PA, Ochsner JL, Mills NL. Positive end-expiratory pressure in the management of the patient with a postoperative bleeding heart. *Ann Thorac Surg.* 1980;30(3):281–284.
42. Swaminathan M, Shaw AD, Phillips-Bute BG, et al. Trends in acute renal failure associated with coronary artery bypass graft surgery in the United States. *Crit Care Med.* 2007;35(10):2286–2291.
43. Conlon PJ, Stafford-Smith M, White WD, et al. Acute renal failure following cardiac surgery. *Nephrol Dial Transplant.* 1999;14(5):1158–1162.
44. Shaw A, Swaminathan M, Stafford-Smith M. Cardiac surgery-associated acute kidney injury: putting together the pieces of the puzzle. *Nephron Physiol.* 2008;109(4):55–60.
45. Schetz M, Bove T, Morelli A, et al. Prevention of cardiac surgery-associated acute kidney injury. *Int J Artif Organs.* 2008;31(2):179–189.
46. Landoni G, Biondi-Zoccai GG, Marino G, et al. Fenoldopam reduces the need for renal replacement therapy and in-hospital death in cardiovascular surgery: a meta-analysis. *J Cardiothorac Vasc Anesth.* 2008;22(1):27–33.
47. Herlihy JP, Koch SM, Jackson R, et al. Course of weaning from prolonged mechanical ventilation after cardiac surgery. *Tex Heart Inst J.* 2006;33(2):122–129.
48. Pappalardo F, Franco A, Landoni G, et al. Long-term outcome and quality of life of patients requiring prolonged mechanical ventilation after cardiac surgery. *Eur J Cardiothorac Surg.* 2004;25(4):548–552.
49. Kollef MH, Bedient TJ, Isakow W, et al. *The Washington Manual of Critical Care.* 1st ed. Philadelphia, PA: Wolters Kluwer Health/Lippincott Williams & Wilkins; 2008:101–103.
50. Christenson JT, Schmuziger M, Maurice J, et al. Gastrointestinal complications after coronary artery bypass grafting. *J Thorac Cardiovasc Surg.* 1994;108(5):899–906.
51. Hanks JB, Curtis SE, Hanks BB, et al. Gastrointestinal complications after cardiopulmonary bypass. *Surgery.* 1982;92(2):394–400.
52. Krasna MJ, Flancbaum L, Trooskin SZ, et al. Gastrointestinal complications after cardiac surgery. *Surgery.* 1988;104(4):773–780.

PATIENT AND FAMILY INFORMATION FOR:

Coronary Artery Bypass Surgery and Postoperative Care

BACKGROUND

Coronary artery bypass surgery, or CABG, is required when patients have significant atherosclerotic lesions, commonly referred to as blockages, in the coronary arteries that supply blood to the heart. These lesions are caused by atherosclerosis—a disease that occurs in patients over many years. The end result is the accumulation of abnormal cells that eventually form a plaque within the artery. Certain specific risk factors are associated with this disease including smoking, hypertension, high cholesterol, diabetes mellitus, and family history.

Once a patient is diagnosed with coronary artery disease, treatment can be medical, percutaneous (using catheters and stents) or surgical. Surgery is reserved for those patients who have left main coronary disease, disease in multiple vessels, diabetic patients who have had some loss of function of the heart, complex lesions, or those who also have valvular abnormalities.

Sometimes patients require heart surgery emergently or urgently after a large heart attack. Those patients are at higher risk for surgery, but surgery is required to help protect the heart muscle at risk from the acute blockage.

PROCEDURE

The patient is put to sleep under general anesthesia during the entire procedure. Typically, these surgeries take between 3 and 6 hours to perform, depending on the number of bypass grafts and any additional procedures that may be required. Multiple tubes and lines are used for monitoring. During the surgery, the patient is usually placed on the CPB circuit, also known as the heart–lung machine. This machine takes over the work of the heart and lungs during the time the surgeon is operating and provides oxygenated blood flow to the body and vital organs.

The technical aspects of CABG involve the placement of a graft, either an artery taken from the chest wall or arm, or a vein most often harvested from the leg. These vessels are used as conduits to bypass the blockage. The original lesion is not removed. The blood is "rerouted" from the aorta to the diseased vessel beyond the lesion to increase the blood supply to the heart muscle. After the bypasses are completed, the patient is weaned from the CPB machine, and the heart resumes beating on its own and takes over the function of pumping blood to the lungs and body.

After the completion of the procedure, prior to closing the chest, temporary pacing wires are placed on the surface of the heart in case they are needed for a slow heart rhythm after surgery. Drainage chest tubes are left within the chest to remove any blood and fluid that may collect.

INITIAL CRITICAL CARE MANAGEMENT

After the surgery, the patient is brought directly to the cardiac care unit for monitoring. There is a special line in the neck, the Swan–Ganz catheter, which measures pressures in the heart and lungs and has the ability to provide immediate information about how well the heart is pumping. The patient is often on multiple medications immediately after surgery through intravenous lines that are carefully regulated and monitored. Mechanical ventilation, or a breathing machine, is required after surgery to assist patients until they wake up from anesthesia and are strong enough to breathe on their own.

Some of the parameters that are monitored include the ability of the heart to pump, the heart rate, blood pressure, oxygen content in the blood, urine output, chest tube output, temperature, and laboratory values such as blood counts and electrolyte measurements. Chest X-rays and ECG are performed immediately after the procedure and daily thereafter.

Pain control is a very important part of postoperative management. Patients receive intravenous medications until they are extubated (taken off the breathing machine) and slowly transitioned to oral medications. Most patients are put out of bed into a chair on the first or second postoperative day. Breathing deeply and coughing are important to keep the airways expanded and prevent pneumonia and collapse of the lungs. All patients should use their incentive spirometer to keep their lungs well expanded until after they leave the hospital.

POSSIBLE COMPLICATIONS

The first 24 to 48 hours are the most critical time after heart surgery. During this time, all the organ systems are carefully assessed in the intensive care unit. The most serious complications after heart surgery are stroke and death. The risk for either one of these complication is <2% for the majority of patients. The risk can be increased depending on age, cardiac function, urgency of the procedure, and underlying medical problems.

Other risks after surgery include bleeding and infection. Bleeding after heart surgery occurs because patients require anticoagulation while on the heart–lung machine and this causes their blood to clot abnormally. Some patients are on aspirin or other "blood thinners" prior to surgery, which can also impair their clotting ability. The output from the chest tubes are carefully measured every hour or every few hours to make sure that it is not too high. If the drainage is excessive, sometimes the surgeon will elect to take the patient back to the operating room to evacuate clot and ensure there is no surgical site of bleeding.

Some patients have heart rhythm abnormalities immediately after surgery. One common abnormality is called atrial fibrillation, which can occur in up to 30% of cases. Although this rhythm is not dangerous, it may require the addition of medications or in some cases, cardioversion (a controlled electrical shock to the heart) to control the disturbance. Another benign rhythm is sinus tachycardia, which is simply a fast heart rate owing to some underlying cause. The treatment of this is to determine the cause of the fast rate, which may be related to pain. Other more serious rhythm changes such as ventricular tachycardia or ventricular fibrillation seldom occur. These are considered emergencies and are treated with immediate cardioversion.

RECOVERY

Most patients are discharged from the CCU after 48 hours of observation. The average length of stay for a CABG patient is 5 days in the hospital. The patient continues to be monitored for arrhythmias, fever, and other complications. The remaining days are spent on the ward where a normal diet is resumed, the patient ambulates, and daily physical therapy is begun.

SECTION II

Heart Failure

Edgar Argulian
Eyal Herzog
Emad F. Aziz
Marrick L. Kukin

CHAPTER

9

Pathway for the Management of Acute Heart Failure

EPIDEMIOLOGY AND IMPACT

Heart failure is a common and growing problem in the United States with estimated prevalence of almost 6 million patients. Acute decompensated heart failure accounts for more than a million hospital admissions per year with numbers expected to rise owing to an aging population.[1] The current chapter is intended to outline a simple, yet comprehensive approach to the diagnosis and management of acute decompensated heart failure by synthesizing the evidence from multiple studies and major cardiology society recommendations.[2,3] It is based on the initial acute heart failure management pathway published by our heart failure team (Figure 9.1).[4]

DEFINITIONS

Acute decompensated heart failure refers to the acute onset of dyspnea owing to elevated cardiac filling pressures. It can be newly diagnosed heart failure or exacerbation of preexisting chronic heart failure condition. Despite major advances in laboratory and diagnostic modalities, heart failure remains a clinical diagnosis of a constellation of signs and symptoms. Careful history taking and focused physical examination are the cornerstones of the diagnosis. The diagnosis is established by the combination of symptoms of heart failure (such as dyspnea and orthopnea), signs of fluid overload (such as jugular venous distention, pulmonary crackles, and peripheral edema) and objective evidence of structural heart disease (such as third heart sounds, cardiac murmurs, and echocardiographic findings). Acute decompensated heart failure is a continuum of clinical presentations ranging from mild dyspnea to florid pulmonary edema to cardiogenic shock. Although initially described for patients with myocardial infarction, the Forrester classification can be applied to patients with acute decompensated heart failure to guide the management.[5] It assigns patients to groups based on estimation of left-sided filling pressures ("wet" meaning pulmonary congestion and high pulmonary capillary wedge pressures) and perfusion state ("cold" meaning low perfusion state and low systemic blood pressure). Most patients with acute decompensated heart failure fall into the "wet" and "warm" category: They have evidence of pulmonary congestion/pulmonary edema with normal or high blood pressure. Patients with pulmonary edema and low systemic pressures are in cardiogenic shock, which typically signifies bad prognosis unless a reversible cause is rapidly identified and corrected (e.g., reperfusion therapy in a patient with acute myocardial

infarction or a corrective surgery in a patient with acute valvular dysfunction). Sometimes patients with cardiogenic shock ("cold" state) have no evidence of pulmonary congestion and systemic hypoperfusion dominates the clinical picture. Patients with right ventricular infarction are a classic example in this category.

ETIOLOGY AND PREDISPOSING FACTORS

There is a long list of possible heart failure etiologies but in reality a few causes account for most of the cases. From long-term heart failure management perspective, the causes can be broadly divided into heart failure with low left ventricular ejection fraction (LVEF) and heart failure with preserved LVEF. Coronary artery disease is the most common cause of heart failure with low LVEF.[6] Dilated cardiomyopathy that can be idiopathic or associated with other conditions (infections, toxins, peripartum, etc.) is a less common cause. The prevalence of heart failure with preserved LVEF increases with age and overall accounts for almost 50% of heart failure cases.[7] Diastolic heart failure is the largest category within the heart failure with preserved LVEF, and hypertension is the most important etiologic factor. Some valvular diseases (such as aortic stenosis and mitral regurgitation), hypertrophic cardiomyopathy, and restrictive cardiomyopathy also present as heart failure with preserved LVEF.[8]

In any patient who presents with new-onset acute decompensated heart failure or chronic heart failure exacerbation, the precipitating cause should be identified and adequately addressed. Myocardial ischemia is a common precipitating factor and should be considered in the differential diagnosis. Valvular pathology can cause acute heart failure if it develops suddenly: typical examples include flail mitral valve with chordal rupture or aortic valve perforation in infectious endocarditis. Myocarditis and postpartum cardiomyopathy can present as acute heart failure. VAMP (Valvular disease, Acute coronary syndromes, Myocarditis, and Peripartum/Postpartum cardiomyopathy) is a useful mnemonic in evaluating a patient with new-onset acute heart failure (Figure 9.2).[4] Severe hypertension is another common condition typically associated with preserved LVEF and better in-hospital outcomes. Both supraventricular and ventricular arrhythmias can precipitate heart failure. It is important to know that patients with diastolic dysfunction are highly dependent on preload for left ventricular filling. Certain arrhythmias such as atrial fibrillation decrease

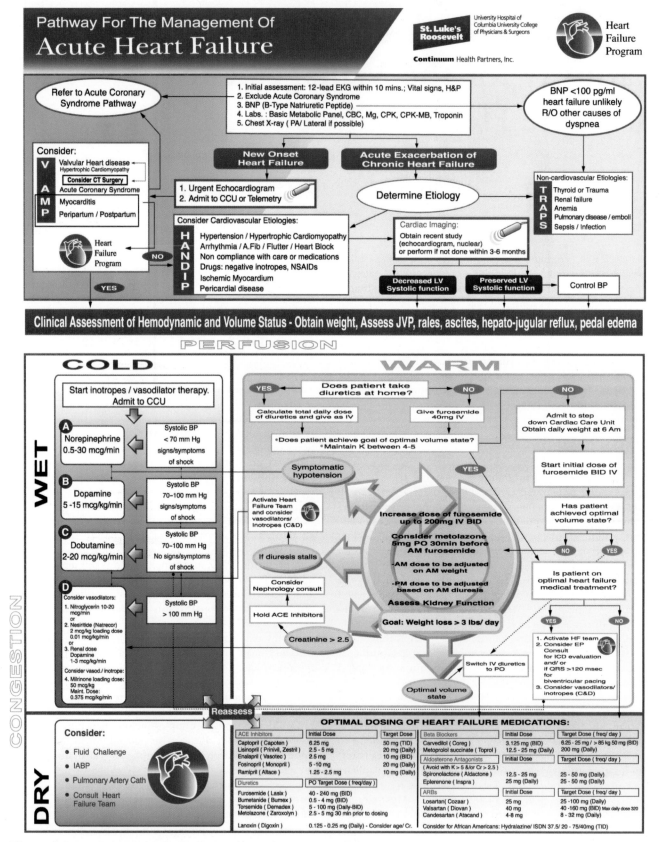

Figure 9.1. Pathway for the evaluation and management of acute heart failure.

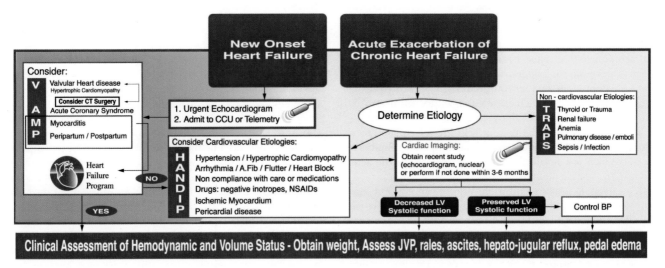

Figure 9.2. Differential diagnosis between new onset heart failure and acute exacerbation of chronic heart failure with timing of imaging and consideration of precipitating pathophysiology.

diastolic filling by increasing heart rate and eliminating atrial kick, and therefore they can provoke florid heart failure in an otherwise stable patient. Interestingly, frequent ventricular premature beats and right ventricular pacing can create dyssynchrony contributing to heart failure.[9] Medication along with diet noncompliance is one of the most common factors that precipitates acute exacerbation in patients with chronic heart failure. HANDIP (hypertension, arrhythmias, noncompliance with care, drugs, ischemic myocardium, and pericardial disease) is another useful mnemonic in evaluating patients with heart failure exacerbation from cardiac causes (Figure 9.2).[4]

Noncardiac factors can precipitate heart failure in otherwise stable patients by creating high oxygen demand and inducing tachycardia (such as anemia, thyroid diseases, drugs, fever and infection, and pulmonary emboli), causing fluid overload (in-hospital IV fluid administration, renal failure, and nonsteroidal anti-inflammatory drugs or NSAIDs) or decreasing myocardial contractility (negative inotropes such as verapamil). TRAPS (thyroid, renal failure, anemia, pulmonary disease, and sepsis) is a mnemonic to help categorize noncardiac precipitants of heart failure exacerbation (Figure 9.2).[4]

DIAGNOSIS AND WORKUP

Once the history and physical examination findings consistent with heart failure are ascertained, further workup is directed towards confirming the diagnosis, establishing the cause of the heart failure, addressing the precipitating factor(s), and identifying prognostic indicators. Physical examination should specifically focus on the degree of respiratory failure (tachypnea, accessory respiratory muscle use), vital signs, and signs of fluid overload (pulmonary crackles, jugular venous distension, and peripheral edema). Cardiac assessment may provide important clues to the diagnosis (e.g., a new murmur). Bedside rapid assessment of left-sided filling pressures and systemic perfusion helps to assign the patient to one of the Forrester categories as described above. The essential set of initial tests includes EKG, laboratory workup (electrolytes, renal function and liver function test, and coagulation profile), cardiac enzymes and

chest X-ray. It is important to remember that up to one-third of patients with Acute Coronary Syndrome (ACS) have no chest pain upon presentation.[10] Therefore, serial EKGs and cardiac enzymes are an essential part of the initial workup. Of note, some repolarization abnormalities and QTc interval prolongation can be caused by acute heart failure per se, not necessarily myocardial ischemia.[11] Similarly, small increase in cardiac biomarkers is often seen in acute decompensated heart failure.[12] Other important findings on EKG include arrhythmias, conduction delays, and hypertrophy. Chest X-ray helps to assess the degree of fluid overload, and it can demonstrate some other relevant pathology (large pleural effusion, infiltrates, and cardiomegaly). Arterial blood gases provide information about oxygenation, ventilation, and acid–base status; arterial blood gases should be obtained in every patient with significant respiratory distress as well as low perfusion ("cold") state.

B-type natriuretic peptides (BNP and proBNP) are released from myocardial cells in response to increase in the wall stress. Their levels are elevated in systolic as well as diastolic heart failure.[13] Measuring BNP level can supplement the evaluation of patients with suspected acute decompensated heart failure if used in the appropriate clinical context. Low BNP levels (<100 pg per ml) have a high negative predictive value, which makes the diagnosis of heart failure unlikely in a patient who presents to the emergency department with dyspnea.[14] Values >400 pg per ml are consistent with heart failure, whereas intermediate values (100 to 400 pg per ml) are in the gray zone.[2] Studies showed linear correlation between the admission BNP levels in patients with acute decompensated heart failure and in-hospital mortality.[15] Of note, obese patients with heart failure have lower BNP levels that should be factored in during clinical decision making. Sudden, "flash" pulmonary edema can sometimes be associated with falsely low BNP levels. At the same time, the positive predictive value of elevated BNP levels (especially gray zone values) is not very high as they can be elevated in patients with left ventricular hypertrophy, pulmonary hypertension, sepsis, renal dysfunction, and liver disease.[16] For example, in a septic patient with possible heart failure elevated BNP levels add little information to clinical judgment. In patients with preexisting chronic heart failure who come with acute exacerbation, one-time elevated BNP level conveys little information.

Echocardiography is an essential tool in evaluating patients with acute decompensated heart failure.[3] The urgency of getting echocardiogram is determined by the clinical presentation: for example, in a patient suspected to have acute valvular pathology or an acute mechanical complication of myocardial infarction, a bedside echocardiogram can immediately confirm the diagnosis whereas in a patient with known chronic heart failure, subacute symptoms, and medication noncompliance, the immediate test would add little information. In the acute settings, an echocardiogram helps to assess the presence and degree of systolic dysfunction, right ventricular size and function, valvular and pericardial pathology. It can assess the diastolic dysfunction and give the estimate of right-sided pressures as well as left-sided filling pressures. Regional wall motion abnormalities and dyssynchrony can provide clues to the possible causes of the symptoms. Determination of LVEF (heart failure with decreased LVEF versus preserved LVEF) is fundamental in long-term management of heart failure patients.

The routine insertion of a pulmonary artery catheter in patients with acute decompensated heart failure is not recommended as it has not been shown to improve major clinical outcomes.[17] It can be considered under specific circumstances to estimate left-sided filling pressures and cardiac output. Possible scenarios include complex patients with cardiac and pulmonary disease, persistent hypotension, worsening renal function, and so on. The benefits of getting important hemodynamic information should be weighed in each patient against the complications of the invasive monitoring and limitations of the technique.

Coronary angiography is indicated in patients with acute decompensated heart failure believed to be precipitated by myocardial ischemia. Successful reperfusion in these settings has been shown to improve survival.[2]

Comprehensive assessment of patients admitted for acute decompensated heart failure includes identification of prognostic indicators. The indicators of poor prognosis include clinical variables (age, poor functional status at baseline, low admission blood pressure, etc.), laboratory factors (wide QRS complex, certain arrhythmias, hyponatremia, positive cardiac biomarkers, marked elevation of BNP, etc.) and imaging findings (low LVEF, restrictive mitral inflow pattern, abnormal RV function, etc.).[2]

MANAGEMENT

The management of acute decompensated heart failure should be approached in systematic manner and tailored to each individual patient. Figure 9.1 outlines the general approach to the management of acute decompensated heart failure.[4] The following components of the therapy should be addressed: (1) oxygenation, (2) hemodynamics, (3) fluid overload, and (4) precipitating factors.

OXYGENATION

The range of respiratory distress varies along the spectrum of presentations in acute decompensated heart failure. Rapid assessment of oxygenation and ventilation is an important initial step. Mild respiratory distress might require oxygen supplementation through nasal canula or a mask with the goal of keeping the patient comfortable and maintaining oxygen saturation above 90% to 92%. Caution should be exercised in chronic CO_2 retainers because high-flow oxygen delivery in those patients can result in acute CO_2 retention and respiratory acidosis.[18] Patients with significant respiratory distress need arterial blood gas analysis to access oxygenation, ventilation, and acid–base status. Patients with pulmonary edema have been shown to benefit from noninvasive positive pressure ventilation provided they do not have contraindications (e.g., impaired level of consciousness, agitation, inability to protect airways, high risk of aspiration, etc.).[19] The benefits of noninvasive positive pressure ventilation result from improved V/Q mismatch and decreased cardiac preload. Meta-analyses of randomized clinical trials in patients with pulmonary edema suggest a decrease in the need of intubation and improvement in respiratory signs and symptoms. Mortality benefit from noninvasive positive pressure ventilation in those patients has not been consistently demonstrated.[19] Patients in significant respiratory distress and those who have contraindications to noninvasive positive pressure ventilation should be intubated and mechanical ventilation should be initiated.

HEMODYNAMICS

Rapid bedside assessment of hemodynamics as described above is important in initial management of acute decompensated heart failure. Most heart failure patients are in "warm" and "wet" category and need treatment with diuretics and vasodilators. Patients with borderline or low blood pressure, poor perfusion, and pulmonary edema ("cold" and "wet") are in cardiogenic shock and generally carry poor prognosis. Rapid correction of precipitating factors may improve their condition (e.g., revascularization in ACS). Vasopressor agents such as norepinephrine or dopamine are used in such patients to maintain blood pressure. Patients with borderline systolic blood pressure (90 to 100 mm Hg) and poor perfusion (cold and clammy), and patients who are resistant to diuretic therapy experience symptomatic improvement from inotropic agents. Dobutamine, a β-adrenergic agonist, can be used in these settings. Phosphodiesterase inhibitors (such as milrinone) are potent inotropes and can also provide significant symptomatic relief. It is important to remember that inotropic agents should be used only as temporary measure and withdrawn as early as possible once adequate perfusion is restored and congestion has been relieved. Symptomatic relief provided by these agents comes at the expense of increased risk of ischemia, arrhythmias, and myocardial damage. Moreover, vasodilator effect of inotropic agents may cause hypotension. They have been shown to increase short-term and long-term mortality in patients with congestive heart failure.[20,21] Their use should be restricted to patients with known severe systolic left ventricular dysfunction. Finally, patients with hypotension and no signs of significant pulmonary congestion ("cold" and "dry" state) can receive a fluid challenge. In patients who develop symptomatic hypotension during aggressive diuresis, the diuretics should be held and careful fluid challenge might be considered if the blood pressure does not rapidly stabilize. Patients who are highly preload-dependant (e.g., severe aortic stenosis or severe concentric left ventricular hypertrophy and normal LVEF) are at a higher risk of hypotension with aggressive diuresis.

FLUID OVERLOAD

Symptoms of dyspnea in acute decompensated heart failure are attributed to elevated left-sided filling pressures. Most patients with decompensated heart failure are fluid overloaded owing to renal retention of sodium and water, whereas some patients with acute, especially precipitous heart failure are normovolemic. Early diuresis and manipulation of preload are the most effective ways to bring symptomatic relief to those patients. Most patients with acute decompensated heart failure require intravenous loop diuretic therapy except for those with hypotension and shock. Patients with hypotension, severe acidosis, renal failure and hyponatremia are less likely to respond to loop diuretics. The dosing of the intravenous loop diuretic (e.g., furosemide) used in patients with acute decompensated heart failure should be based on the degree of fluid overload, renal function, and preadmission loop diuretic use (Figure 9.3).[4] It of interest to note that loop diuretics improve symptoms even before the diuretic effect by venodilation and decrease in preload. Parameters that need to be monitored during diuretic therapy include volume status, intake and output (commonly by placing urinary catheter), blood pressure, electrolytes, and renal function. Patients with decreasing renal function upon diuresis (labeled as "cardiorenal syndrome") carry a worse prognosis.[22] In patients who show suboptimal response to escalating doses of loop diuretics the following options should be considered: addition of a thiazide diuretic, addition of an, inotropic therapy, and continuous infusion of a loop diuretic. In patients with renal dysfunction, metholazone added to loop diuretics might be used.[23] Dopamine in low doses has been shown to improve renal perfusion, but the clinical implications of this finding needs to be further explored.[24] Ultrafiltration is the last-resort therapy, especially in patients with severe renal dysfunction.[25]

Preload reduction brings significant symptomatic relief in patients with acute decompensated heart failure by decreasing left-sided filling pressures. It can be achieved by using venodilators such as nitroglycerine and nitroprusside. Nitroglycerin, in the form of intravenous infusion should be used as add-on therapy to diuretics if systolic blood pressure is >110 mm Hg. In patients with systolic blood pressure <90 mm Hg vasodilators should be avoided, whereas in patients with systolic blood pressure of 90 to 110 mm Hg they should be used with caution. Hypotension is the main side effect of nitroglycerine, especially in patients who are significantly preload-dependant (e.g., severe aortic stenosis, right ventricular infarction). Nitrates should be avoided in patients using phosphodiesterase inhibitors (e.g., sildenafil). Headache is a common complaint and tachyphylaxis develops with continuous use. Nitroprusside is a potent vasodilator that achieves significant afterload reduction along with preload reduction. This property is important in certain situations such as hypertensive emergencies and acute valvular pathology such as acute mitral regurgitation. Accumulation of cyanide is a potential side effect with continuous infusion. Neseritide is an analog of brain natriuretic peptide. It produces vasodilation, reduces preload and brings symptomatic relief to patients with pulmonary congestion. The major concern with the use of neseritide is worsening renal function and possible increase in mortality; it can be used as a second-line agent in patients who are poorly responsive to loop diuretics.[26] Morphine reduces anxiety and sense of dyspnea and produces vasodilation in patients with pulmonary edema.

However, retrospective studies raised some concerns regarding the use of morphine in such patients owing to its association with increased in-hospital mortality.[27] In patients with ACS and chest pain morphine should not be withheld.

OTHER THERAPIES

Angiotensin converting enzyme (ACE) inhibitors reduce morbidity and mortality in patients with chronic heart failure and decreased LVEF, but their role in managing patients with acute decompensated heart failure is limited. They are generally avoided in those patients until they are stable because of the following concerns: ACE inhibitors can precipitate hypotension and worsening renal function in patients who are aggressively diuresed. Similarly, β-blockers are the mainstay of chronic heart failure treatment in patients with systolic left ventricular dysfunction but they should be avoided in the settings of acute exacerbation. In patients already taking β-blockers they can be cautiously resumed once the patients are stable.[2,3]

PRECIPITANTS

Identifying the precipitating factors for acute decompensated heart failure should be the part of the initial thought process. The common precipitating factors are described above and some of them should be actively considered and corrected such as myocardial ischemia, hypertensive crisis, arrhythmias, and acute valvular pathology. Medication and diet noncompliance is a common precipitant, and it should be specifically inquired. Other precipitating factors such as infection, medications (e.g., NSAIDs), and pulmonary disease could be more subtle and their identification requires a systematic approach to history taking, physical examination, and laboratory workup.

END-STAGE HEART FAILURE

Patients with severe, "end-stage" heart failure that are resistant to optimal medical therapy often have symptoms at rest (NYHA functional class IV). They have frequent hospitalizations, long hospital stays, and poor quality of life. Options for those patients are limited to continuous inotrope infusion as palliative measure, ultrafiltration, and mechanical support as "bridge" therapy to transplantation or as "destination" therapy.[3]

OPTIMAL DISCHARGE PLANNING

Optimal discharge planning involves patient education, proper follow-up, identification and correction of precipitants, and evidence-based therapy for heart failure. Patient education should include information about the nature of the disease, importance of diet- and medication compliance, self-monitoring (e.g., weight, edema) and early recognition of decompensation symptoms. Precipitating factors should be addressed, which in specific circumstances might include ischemic workup, valvular disease surgery, long-term control of arrhythmias, control of hypertension, and so on. Chronic management of heart failure is based on the estimation of LVEF. Patients with systolic LV dysfunction should be placed on a β-blocker and an ACE inhibitor (or angiotensin receptor blocker), and optimal dosing of the agents should be achieved by slow uptitration during outpatient follow-up. Other therapies for those patients

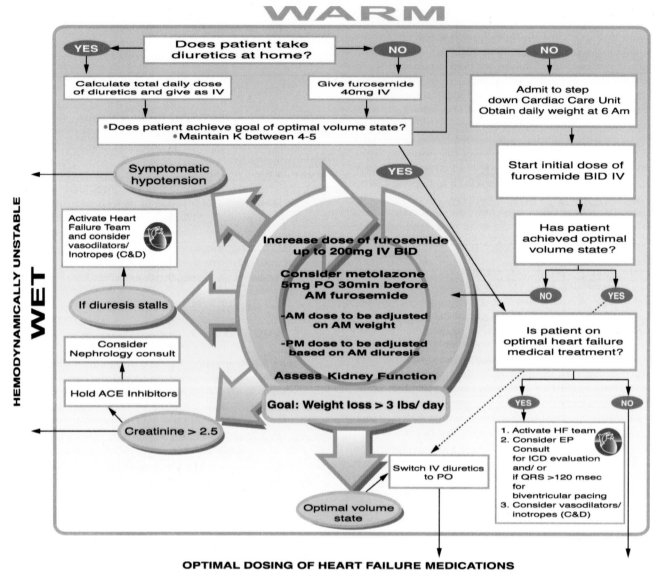

Figure 9.3. The "loop" concept of aggressive usage of loop diuretics to rapidly and safely diurese patients, shorten length of stay, and transition to oral therapy upon successful completion of diuresis.

include aldosterone antagonists, hydralazine and isosorbide dinitrate combination and digoxin. The evidence for chronic management of diastolic heart failure is more limited; optimal volume control and treatment of hypertension seem to be the best strategy at this point.

REFERENCES

1. Lloyd-Jones D, Adams RJ, Brown TM, et al. Executive summary: heart disease and stroke statistics—2010 update: a report from the American Heart Association. *Circulation.* 2010;121:948–954.

2. Dickstein K, Cohen-Solal A, Filippatos G, et al. ESC guidelines for the diagnosis and treatment of acute and chronic heart failure 2008: the Task Force for the diagnosis and treatment of acute and chronic heart failure 2008 of the European Society of Cardiology. Developed in collaboration with the Heart Failure Association of the ESC (HFA) and endorsed by the European Society of Intensive Care Medicine (ESICM). *Eur J Heart Fail.* 2008;10:933–989.

3. Hunt SA, Abraham WT, Chin MH, et al. 2009 focused update incorporated into the ACC/AHA 2005 Guidelines for the diagnosis and management of heart failure in adults: a report of the American College of Cardiology Foundation/American Heart Association Task Force on Practice Guidelines: developed in collaboration with the International Society for Heart and Lung Transplantation. *Circulation.* 2009;119:e391–e479.

4. Herzog E, Varley C, Kukin M. Pathway for the management of acute heart failure. *Crit Pathw Cardiol.* 2005;4:37–42.

5. Forrester JS, Diamond GA, Swan HJ. Correlative classification of clinical and hemodynamic function after acute myocardial infarction. *Am J Cardiol.* 1977;39:137–145.

6. He J, Ogden LG, Bazzano LA, et al. Risk factors for congestive heart failure in US men and women: NHANES I epidemiologic follow-up study. *Arch Intern Med.* 2001;161:996–1002.

7. Bursi F, Weston SA, Redfield MM, et al. Systolic and diastolic heart failure in the community. *JAMA.* 2006;296:2209–2216.

8. Oh JK, Hatle L, Tajik AJ, et al. Diastolic heart failure can be diagnosed by comprehensive two-dimensional and Doppler echocardiography. *J Am Coll Cardiol.* 2006;47:500–506.

9. Sweeney MO, Prinzen FW. A new paradigm for physiologic ventricular pacing. *J Am Coll Cardiol.* 2006;47:282–288.

10. Canto JG, Shlipak MG, Rogers WJ, et al. Prevalence, clinical characteristics, and mortality among patients with myocardial infarction presenting without chest pain. *JAMA.* 2000;283:3223–3229.

11. Littmann L. Large T wave inversion and QT prolongation associated with pulmonary edema: a report of nine cases. *J Am Coll Cardiol.* 1999;34:1106–1110.

12. Horwich TB, Patel J, MacLellan WR, et al. Cardiac troponin I is associated with impaired hemodynamics, progressive left ventricular dysfunction, and increased mortality rates in advanced heart failure. *Circulation.* 2003;108:833–838.

13. Lubien E, DeMaria A, Krishnaswamy P, et al. Utility of B-natriuretic peptide in detecting diastolic dysfunction: comparison with Doppler velocity recordings. *Circulation.* 2002;105:595–601.

14. Maisel AS, Krishnaswamy P, Nowak RM, et al. Rapid measurement of B-type natriuretic peptide in the emergency diagnosis of heart failure. *N Engl J Med.* 2002;347:161–167.

15. Fonarow GC, Peacock WF, Phillips CO, et al. Admission B-type natriuretic peptide levels and in-hospital mortality in acute decompensated heart failure. *J Am Coll Cardiol.* 2007;49:1943–1950.
16. De Lemos JA, McGuire DK, Drazner MH. B-type natriuretic peptide in cardiovascular disease. *Lancet.* 2003;362:316–322.
17. Binanay C, Califf RM, Hasselblad V, et al. Evaluation study of congestive heart failure and pulmonary artery catheterization effectiveness: the ESCAPE trial. *JAMA.* 2005;294:1625–1633.
18. Aubier M, Murciano D, Milic-Emili J, et al. Effects of the administration of O2 on ventilation and blood gases in patients with chronic obstructive pulmonary disease during acute respiratory failure. *Am Rev Respir Dis.* 1980;122:747–754.
19. Weng CL, Zhao YT, Liu QH, et al. Meta-analysis: noninvasive ventilation in acute cardiogenic pulmonary edema. *Ann Intern Med.* 2010;152:590–600.
20. Cuffe MS, Califf RM, Adams KF Jr, et al. Short-term intravenous milrinone for acute exacerbation of chronic heart failure: a randomized controlled trial. *JAMA.* 2002;287:1541–1547.
21. Abraham WT, Adams KF, Fonarow GC, et al. In-hospital mortality in patients with acute decompensated heart failure requiring intravenous vasoactive medications: an analysis from the Acute Decompensated Heart Failure National Registry (ADHERE). *J Am Coll Cardiol.* 2005;46:57–64.
22. Shlipak MG, Massie BM. The clinical challenge of cardiorenal syndrome. *Circulation.* 2004;110:1514–1517.
23. Ellison DH. Diuretic drugs and the treatment of edema: from clinic to bench and back again. *Am J Kidney Dis.* 1994;23:623–643.
24. Elkayam U, Ng TM, Hatamizadeh P, et al. Renal vasodilatory action of dopamine in patients with heart failure: magnitude of effect and site of action. *Circulation.* 2008;117:200–205.
25. Rogers HL, Marshall J, Bock J, et al. A randomized, controlled trial of the renal effects of ultrafiltration as compared to furosemide in patients with acute decompensated heart failure. *J Card Fail.* 2008;14:1–5.
26. Sackner-Bernstein JD, Kowalski M, Fox M, et al. Short-term risk of death after treatment with nesiritide for decompensated heart failure: a pooled analysis of randomized controlled trials. *JAMA.* 2005;293:1900–1905.
27. Peacock WF, Hollander JE, Diercks DB, et al. Morphine and outcomes in acute decompensated heart failure: an ADHERE analysis. *Emerg Med J.* 2008;25:205–209.

PATIENT AND FAMILY INFORMATION FOR:

The Management of Acute Heart Failure

DEFINITION AND CAUSES

Heart failure is a common problem in the United States, especially in the elderly population. Each year more than one million patients are admitted to the hospital with diagnosis of heart failure. Heart failure is a clinical syndrome and not a specific disease. It can have many causes. It results from decreased pumping function of the heart and its inability to propagate adequate amounts of blood to the tissues. Acute heart failure is a serious, life-threatening condition; it can be the presentation of newly diagnosed illness or an exacerbation of a preexisting disease. Shortness of breath is the most common presentation of acute heart failure. It results from fluid accumulation in the lungs. Other manifestations of heart failure include cough, swelling of the legs, fatigue, tiredness, and poor appetite. Some patients experience nighttime episodes of breathlessness and find it difficult to sleep flat in bed. Patients with preexisting chronic heart failure often experience slow and progressive shortness of breath on exertion, leg swelling, and weight gain—all symptoms of fluid accumulation in the body before they present to the hospital with breathlessness at rest. Acute heart failure is not synonymous to "heart attack," but it can sometimes be precipitated by heart attack. In that case it is common for patients to have chest pain, chest discomfort, or pressure-like sensation in the chest. The severe form of acute heart failure is called "pulmonary edema"; it causes significant distress and breathing difficulty owing to rapid build-up of the fluid in the lungs. Another extreme form of heart failure is called "cardiogenic shock"; it causes poor perfusion of the tissues owing to significant impairment of heart function. Patients appear cold and clammy, their blood pressure is low, and their thinking can be impaired. Those patients are at a high risk of dying and often need drastic measures to correct the underlying problem and support the circulation.

Heart failure is not a single disease; it is a manifestation of a big variety of structural heart disorders. The most common disorder that results in heart failure is coronary artery disease. Blockage of the blood vessels that supply the heart muscle can result in a significant heart muscle damage causing the heart to fail. High blood pressure, if unrecognized or untreated, causes pathologic changes in the heart muscle over months to years and can eventually result in heart failure. The heart valve narrowing or leakage is a relatively common cause of heart failure. Diseases of the heart muscle itself termed "cardiomyopathy" manifest

as heart failure. Some causes of cardiomyopathy are known (such as infection, alcohol, and illegal drugs) and some are genetically inherited. A well-described form of cardiomyopathy is associated with pregnancy. Sometimes, there is no obvious cause for the heart muscle weakness, and in medical literature it is referred to as "idiopathic." Besides the structural heart disease that results in heart failure it is important to realize that a variety of conditions can provoke an acute exacerbation of heart failure. Those conditions are called "precipitating factors." Precipitating factors superimposed on the underlying structural heart disease are responsible for acute onset of symptoms in an otherwise stable patient. A "heart attack" or inadequate blood supply to the heart muscle called "ischemia" is a common precipitating factor. Poorly controlled blood pressure exerts excessive strain on the heart and precipitates heart failure. Noncompliance with the diet and medications is among the most common precipitating factors for acute heart failure. Other conditions that can precipitate or worsen heart failure include infection, certain medications (including painkillers), low blood count, heart rhythm disturbances (called "arrhythmias"), kidney disease, and so on.

DIAGNOSIS AND TREATMENT

The physician establishes the diagnosis of acute heart failure by taking history (asking questions about the patient's symptoms), performing physical examination, and ordering appropriate tests. Besides confirming the diagnosis, the physician needs to determine the underlying structural heart disease that causes heart failure and also the precipitating factor for the current acute exacerbation. Blood tests are commonly sent and electrocardiogram and chest X-ray are also typically performed. Ultrasound examination of the heart (also known as echocardiogram) helps to visualize cardiac chambers and it is the most commonly used tool to evaluate the structure and function of the heart. Other tests are performed as deemed necessary by the physician. Cardiac catheterization is an invasive test that includes placing catheters into the heart chambers and major vessels to diagnose vessel blockage or get important pressure readings from various heart chambers. It is also used for interventions if vessel blockage seems to be causing patient's symptoms.

Treatment of heart failure has several important components. Patients are given oxygen by nasal prongs or a mask to ensure adequate oxygen delivery to the tissues. In patients with significant breathing difficulty, assisted ventilation through special mask is employed (commonly called "CPAP"). Occasionally, a breathing tube is placed in the airway and mechanical ventilation is initiated. In patients with low blood pressure and poor perfusion, medications are used to maintain blood pressure. In severe cases, medications that enhance heart muscle contractility are used; unfortunately, these medications are associated with significant adverse effects and therefore their use is limited to refractory cases. As explained above, fluid overload underlies many symptoms of heart failure; therefore, diuretic medications are commonly administered to increase water and sodium excretion from the body. Other medications that help to relieve the symptoms include vasodilators; these medications dilate the blood vessels in the body decreasing the workload on the heart, and they are commonly administered as intravenous drips. Precipitating factors are also addressed. These could include controlling abnormal heart rhythm, lowering blood pressure, treating infection, and so on.

FOLLOW-UP AND PREVENTION

Once the acute phase is over the long-term management plan should be discussed in detail. Medications used to treat chronic heart failure are often different from those used to treat acute exacerbation. ß-Blockers (such as metoprolol or carvedilol) and ACE inhibitors (such as lisinopril and enalapril) are commonly used in the treatment of chronic heart failure. They help to maintain heart function and prevent acute exacerbation. They have also been shown to decrease the risk of death in certain patients with heart failure. Proper education of the patient includes teaching them about the appropriate medication regimen, necessity of taking the medications daily, and compliance with low-salt diet. Sodium contained in salt retains fluid in the body and causes heart failure exacerbations. Moreover, it commonly elevates blood pressure by exerting excessive strain on the heart. Patients should not only follow appropriate diet but should also be able to recognize early signs and symptoms of heart failure such as exertional shortness of breath, fatigue, inability to lie flat in bed, awakening from sleep short of breath, using several pillows to elevate the head and thereby making breathing at night easier, gradual weight gain, and ankle swelling. Weight gain is commonly the first manifestation of fluid built up in the body; therefore, the patients should know their "dry weight" and try to follow their weight regularly. Proper follow-up after discharge is necessary to ensure stability of clinical symptoms and proper adjustment of medications doses. Some of the medications (such as ß-blockers) need to be titrated up slowly during follow-up visits to avoid adverse effects. In case of coronary artery disease and valvular heart disease certain interventions or surgery can fix the problem. Implantations of certain devices such as a pacemaker or defibrillator might be beneficial in certain groups of patients.

Gregory Janis
Sandeep Joshi
Eyal Herzog

Mechanical Complications of Myocardial Infarction

Acute myocardial infarction (AMI) affects 1.7 million people in the United States. Mechanical complications of AMI result in some of the deadliest outcomes. It is difficult to assess the true incidence of these complications as both clinical and autopsy series differ considerably. Nevertheless, they are thought to be responsible for about 15% of all AMI deaths.[1] It is important to realize that these catastrophic events can occur within minutes to hours after the inciting event or even days to weeks later. Mechanical complications of AMI can be subdivided into two major categories: acute phase and chronic phase. These phases are further broken down into the seven major topics of this chapter (Table 10.1).

LEFT VENTRICULAR FREE WALL RUPTURE

Left ventricular free wall rupture (LVFWR) is almost a fatal complication of myocardial infarction (MI). Despite great progress in the reduction of both mortality and morbidity from AMI, death related to LVFWR has been high.

In patients who die after an AMI many large studies have found a 14% to 26% incidence of cardiac rupture.[2] According to the National Registry of Myocardial Infarction, which reviewed data from 350,755 patients, the incidence of cardiac rupture was <1%.[3] Approximately 50% of the time, myocardial rupture occurs within the first 5 days after MI and within 2 weeks in >90% of cases.[4,5] Regardless, acute or subacute myocardial rupture is a serious and predominantly fatal complication of acute MI.[6]

Studies have also suggested a higher mortality from free wall rupture with thrombolytics, as cardiac rupture was responsible

for 7.3% of all deaths and 12.1% with thrombolytic agents. Thrombolytic therapy does not necessarily increase the risk of rupture but it may accelerate occurrence, often within the first 24 hours of drug administration.[7] In contrast, the incidence of cardiac rupture may be lower in patients treated with percutaneous coronary intervention. In an observational study of 1,375 patients who received a thrombolytic agent or underwent primary angioplasty, the incidence of rupture was 3.3% and 1.8%, respectively.[8] It is well known that myocardial rupture after MI is less common in patients with successful reperfusion.[9]

One study found that myocardial rupture was 9.2 times more likely to occur in patients who had no prior history of angina or MI, ST-segment elevation or Q-wave development on the initial ECG, and peak MB-creatine kinase was >150 IU per L.[4] The absence of collateral blood flow, demonstrated by the lack of prior ischemic symptoms, and the greater the infarct territory correlate with a higher risk of myocardial rupture. Other risk factors for rupture include anterior location of the infarction, age >70, and female sex.[8,10]

PATHOPHYSIOLOGY

Myocardial rupture more frequently involves the left ventricle than the right ventricle and seldom involves the atria.[3] The infarct commonly affects the anterior and lateral walls of the left ventricle near the junction of the infarct and normal myocardium. Ventricular free wall rupture is defined as an acute, traumatic perforation of the ventricles, which may include pericardial rupture.[6] With unsuccessful or no reperfusion, coagulation necrosis develops within the first 3 to 5 days.[5] As the necrosis progresses, neutrophils infiltrate the myocardial space and release lytic enzymes that disintegrate the necrotic myocardium leading to perforation. The rupture thus is a result of transmural infarction, and the actual perforation can range in size from millimeters to centimeters depending on infarct size.[5] Early phase rupture is defined as within 72 hours post-MI and late rupture is >4 days.

The hallmark of rapid deterioration is primarily because of the extravasation of blood into the pericardial space with resultant instantaneous, acute pericardial tamponade. Because these events occur so quickly, patients usually deteriorate before any therapeutic intervention. Less commonly, subacute rupture can provide a longer therapeutic window as the acute rupture may be temporarily contained by pericardial adhesions or by thrombosis at the rupture site. It is in these patients that immediate, lifesaving, cardiovascular surgery is possible (Figure 10.1).[11]

TABLE 10.1	Acute Phase vs. Chronic Phase Complications of Acute Myocardial Infarction	
Acute Phase	**Chronic Phase**	
Left Ventricular Free Wall Rupture	True Ventricular Pseudaneurysm	
Ventricular Septal Rupture	Ventricular Aneurysm	
Right Ventricular Infarction	Left Ventricular Thrombus	
Acute Mitral Regurgitation		

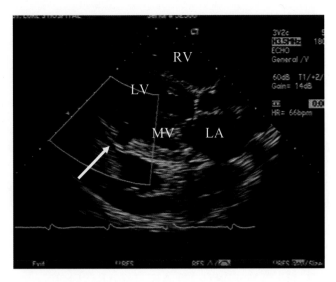

Figure 10.1. Transthoracic Echocardiogram Demonstrating a Posterior Free Wall Rupture (arrow); RV=right ventricle; LV=left ventricle; LA=left atrium; MV=mitral Valve

CLINICAL PRESENTATION

The clinical course of myocardial rupture is variable and challenging to diagnose, as patients may rapidly decompensate. Their clinical course parallels that of any patient suffering from pericardial tamponade. Thus, rupture can present as sudden death in an undetected or silent MI or as incomplete/subacute rupture in those with known MI.[12]

Complete rupture of the left ventricular free wall usually leads to hemopericardium and death from cardiac tamponade. Patients may complain of transient chest pain or dyspnea. Acute tamponade can cause tachypnea, tachycardia, muffled heart sounds, elevated jugular venous pressure, and pulsus paradoxus. The presence of rupture is first suggested by the development of sudden profound right heart failure and shock, often progressing rapidly to pulseless electrical activity and death. Emergent transthoracic echocardiography (TTE) will confirm the diagnosis and emergent pericardiocentesis can transiently relieve the tamponade.[12]

Incomplete/subacute rupture of the left ventricular free wall can occur when organized thrombus and the pericardium seal the ventricular perforation. Patients may present with persistent or recurrent chest pain (particularly pericardial pain), nausea, restlessness, agitation, abrupt hypotension, and/or electrocardiographic features of localized or regional pericarditis.[4,5] The diagnosis of incomplete/subacute rupture is again confirmed by TTE.[12]

TREATMENT

As mentioned, the mortality for acute and subacute free wall rupture is high owing to rapid clinical deterioration. Survival depends primarily on the prompt recognition of myocardial rupture and provision of immediate therapy. Patients displaying suggestive symptoms, signs, and ECG changes require emergent bedside echocardiogram and echocardiographically guided pericardiocentesis if fluid is visualized. Immediate surgical intervention is indicated if the pericardiocentesis identifies the fluid as blood. Medical therapy aimed at hemodynamic stabilization should also be instituted. In addition to pericardiocentesis this includes fluids, inotropic support, vasopressors, and even intra-aortic balloon pump (IABP) counterpulsation and percutaneous cardiopulmonary bypass when available and indicated.[4]

With rapid recognition and initiation of both medical and surgical therapies, the potential for survival, particularly with subacute rupture, can improve dramatically. In one study 25 of 33 patients (76%) with subacute ventricular rupture survived the surgical procedure and 16 (48%) were long-term survivors.[13]

VENTRICULAR SEPTAL RUPTURE

Another deadly complication of AMI involves rupture of the interventricular septum. The need for rapid diagnosis, aggressive medical therapy, and prompt surgical intervention is essential to increase the possibility of survival. As medical therapy has advanced, the incidence and timing of ventricular septal rupture has been up for debate.

In the era before reperfusion therapy, rupture of the interventricular septum is thought to have occurred in 1% to 2% of patients with AMI and accounts for approximately 5% of deaths in this setting.[14] It typically occurs in the first week after infarction, with a mean-time from symptom onset of 3 to 5 days.[15] The classic risk factors for septal rupture in the pre-reperfusion era include hypertension, advanced age, female sex, and the absence of a history of MI or angina.[16] Prognosis for ventricular septal rupture in the pre-reperfusion era was very poor, with an in-hospital mortality of about 45% in those treated surgically and about 90% in those treated medically.[15] With the advent of thrombolysis and percutaneous intervention, outcomes have changed.

In the reperfusion era, studies show a much lower incidence and an accelerated time to diagnosis of interventricular septal rupture than had been previously reported. Today, 0.2% of the population experiences this complication. Early reperfusion therapy may prevent the extensive myocardial necrosis that is associated with ventricular rupture.[15] Patients generally have a meantime of 1 day from infarction to development of a ventricular septal defect (VSD). Many have postulated that this acceleration of rupture may be because of thrombolysis causing hemorrhage during the "lytic state," so that if a ventricular septal rupture occurs, its time course may be accelerated.[15] In the reperfusion era, advanced age, anterior infarct location, female sex, and no current smoking were found to be the most potent predictors of a VSD.[15]

PATHOPHYSIOLOGY

The pathophysiology of interventricular septal rupture is similar to that of free wall rupture. Without reperfusion, coagulation necrosis develops within the first 3 to 5 days. The septum that becomes necrotic is infiltrated by neutrophils, which release lytic enzymes and thus disintegrate the necrotic myocardium.[16] A transmural septal infarction underlies rupture of the interventricular septum, with the tear ranging in size from millimeters to centimeters.[14]

The ventricular septum is very vascular. The rarity of septal rupture and the variable infarct location relate to the fact that the interventricular septum has a dual blood supply. The anterior two-thirds is supplied by the left anterior descending (LAD)

coronary artery and its branches. The posterior one-third is supplied by branches of the posterior descending artery, which come from the right coronary or the left circumflex artery, depending on the dominance of the circulation.[17] Studies have conflicted in determining the artery that is predominantly responsible for septal rupture, but anterior MI is most frequently followed by inferior infarction. Similar to free wall rupture, interventricular septal rupture occurs most frequently with a first MI when there is less likely to be collateral blood flow. In this setting, with an abrupt cessation of flow in the infarct-related artery, no collateral flow exists to support the infracted zone, thereby making the septum prone to rupture (Figure 10.2).

CLINICAL PRESENTATION

Whether in the pre-reperfusion era or post-, it is generally agreed upon that the clinical presentation and examination of a patient with a ventricular septal rupture has remained constant. Symptoms of rupture include shortness of breath, chest pain, and signs of low cardiac output and shock.[16] In 1934, Sager proposed a set of clinical criteria for suspecting a ruptured septum. The sudden onset of a systolic murmur, often accompanied by a thrill, in a patient with rapid hemodynamic decompensation is highly suggestive of a ruptured interventricular septum.[18] The rupture produces a harsh, loud, holosystolic murmur along the left sternal border, radiating toward the base, apex, and right parasternal area with a palpable thrill present in half of patients. Compared with acute mitral regurgitation (MR), initially there is often right ventricular failure and absence of severe pulmonary edema before left ventricular failure ensues. As the disease progresses complete biventricular failure invariably occurs.[16]

In the setting of cardiogenic shock, the thrill and murmur may be difficult to appreciate because turbulent flow across the defect is reduced. Pulmonary hypertension may cause the pulmonic component of the second heart sound to be accentuated. Right and left ventricular S3 gallops are often heard. Tricuspid regurgitation may be present and biventricular failure generally occurs within hours to days.[16]

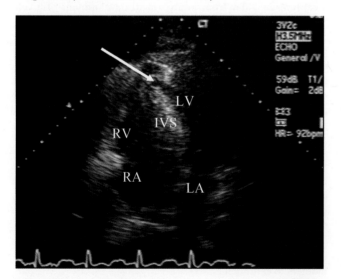

Figure 10.2. Transthoracic echocardiogram demonstrating a ventricular septal defect in the distal portion of the interventricular septum (arrow). LV=left ventricle; RV=right ventricle; RA=right atrium; LA=left atrium; IVS=interventricular septum

TREATMENT

In the correct clinical setting, immediate echocardiogram is crucial to confirm the diagnosis. After the diagnosis is made, medical therapy may consist of mechanical support with an IABP, afterload reduction, diuretics, and inotropic agents.[16] Prompt surgical intervention is essential as most patients have a rapid deterioration and die. It was previously believed that shortly after an AMI, the myocardium was too fragile for safe repair of the rupture. A waiting period of 3 to 6 weeks, to allow the margins of the infracted muscle to develop a firm scar to facilitate surgical repair, was standard before surgical intervention.[19] Medical therapy carries close to a 100% mortality. Although surgical therapy results are poor as well, about 13% survival, it is still considered the primary therapy.[20] Surgical therapy consists of placing a myocardial patch across the ruptured septum with concomitant coronary artery bypass as needed.

RIGHT VENTRICULAR INFARCTION

Right ventricular infarction (RVI) had been described more than 60 years ago, but for decades it was not considered important because it showed no hemodynamic consequence in animal models.[21] Over time, it has become important to diagnose as it defines a specific clinical entity that is associated with considerable, immediate morbidity and mortality.[22] RVI complicates up to half of inferior wall left ventricular infarctions.[21] Prompt recognition of this mechanical complication of AMI is crucial as its initial management differs from that of other types of infarction.

PATHOPHYSIOLOGY

The physiology of right side of the heart varies considerably from that of the left. It is a low-pressure system that has one-sixth of the muscle mass of the left ventricle and performs one-fourth of the stroke work. Despite this, both ventricles have the same cardiac output.[21] This is owing to the fact that the pulmonary vascular resistance is one-tenth that of the peripheral systemic resistance.[23] These factors are important in the hemodynamic consequences of RVI.

Coronary blood flow to the right ventricle is unique in that it occurs in both systole and diastole.[21] The right coronary artery (RCA) supplies the right ventricle through the acute marginal branches in most patients. The inferior wall and posterior interventricular septum are perfused via the posterior descending artery. Typically, RVI occurs when there is occlusion of the RCA proximal to the acute marginal branches. It can also occur with an occlusion of the left circumflex in those who have a left dominant system. Although quite rare, occlusion of the LAD artery may result in infarction of the anterior right ventricle.[21]

The incidence of RVI in association with left ventricular infarction ranges from 14% to 84%, depending on the study preformed. Incidence of isolated RVI accounts for <3% of all cases of infarction.[21] When isolated to the right ventricle, the occlusion is usually in the acute marginal vessels or of a nondominant RCA.[23] Many RCA occlusions do not result in right ventricular necrosis.[22] Up to half of inferior MIs involve the right ventricle. This may be owing to the lesser right ventricular myocardial oxygen demand as a result of its smaller muscle mass, or from its improved oxygen delivery from the biphasic nature of the coronary blood flow during both systole and diastole. A rich left-to-right collateral system is also thought to play a part.[21]

Acute underperfusion of the right ventricular free wall and adjacent interventricular septum leads to a stunned and noncompliant right ventricle. Loss of right ventricular contractility results in a serious deficit in left ventricular preload with a resultant drop in cardiac output, thereby causing systemic hypotension.[24] Augmented atrial contractility is necessary to overcome the increased myocardial stiffness associated with RVI.[25] Factors that impair filling of the noncompliant right ventricle and cause decreased preload are likely to have profound adverse effects on hemodynamics in patients with large RVIs. These factors include volume depletion owing to the use of diuretics and nitrates or any diminution in atrial function caused by concomitant atrial infarction or the loss of atrioventricular synchrony.[21]

To complicate matters, acute right ventricular dilatation causes a leftward shift of the interventricular septum, increasing left ventricular end-diastolic pressure with a resultant decrease in left ventricular compliance and cardiac output. Left ventricular compliance is further aggravated by increased intrapericardial pressure as a result of right ventricular dilatation (Figure 10.3). As a consequence, the left ventricular filling and systolic function may be below normal.[22] If significant left ventricular dysfunction complicates RVI, the results can be disastrous.

CLINICAL PRESENTATION

Given that management of RVI is quite different from left ventricular infarction, recognizing its clinical presentation is paramount. A patient presenting an inferior MI and the triad of hypotension, clear lung fields, and elevated jugular venous pressure, is virtually pathognomonic for RVI.[21] This triad is very specific but has a sensitivity of <25%.[26] Auscultation may reveal a right-sided S3 and S4.[27] Tricuspid regurgitation may also be noted if the right ventricle is sufficiently dilated.

Pulsus paradoxus (decreased systolic blood pressure with inspiration) and Kussmal's sign (elevated jugular venous distention with inspiration) have also been reported in RVI.[27] Careful examination of neck veins in the setting of an inferior

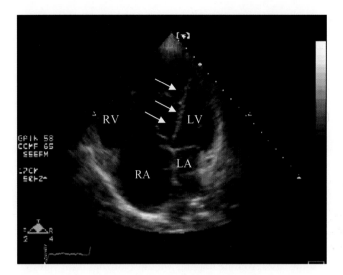

Figure 10.3. Transthoracic echocardiogram demonstrating a dilated and severely hypokinetic right ventricle with compression of the left ventricle (arrows); RV=right ventricle; RA=right atrium; LV=left ventricle; LA=left atrium

MI should alert the physician to the drastic consequences that use of nitrates, diuretics, and morphine can have. These agents should be avoided as they reduce preload and can promote or exacerbate hypotension.

The ECG is crucial for the diagnosis of RVI. The most frequent finding is any degree of ST elevation in leads II, III, and aVF with or without q waves. Occlusion sufficiently proximal in the RCA to cause right ventricular free wall injury also frequently compromises the blood supply to the sinoatrial node, atrium, and atrioventricular node, producing such effects as sinus bradycardia, atrial infarction, atrial fibrillation, and atrioventricular (AV) block.[24] Involvement of the right ventricular free wall may be suspected with the presence of ST depression in precordial leads V2 and V3 when compared with V1. Confirmation of RV ischemia can be quickly obtained when right-sided leads V4R through V6R show ST segment elevations >1 mm (Figure 10.4).[24] A 1-mm ST elevation in V4R is 70% sensitive and 100% specific for RVI.[21] ST-segment elevation in V4R has been shown to be

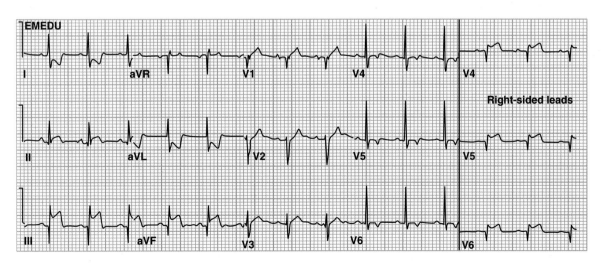

Figure 10.4. Electrocardiogram showing an inferior wall myocardial infarction with right-sided leads showing significant ST elevation in RV4 through RV6

a strong independent predictor of major complications and in-hospital mortality.[22] When EKG shows signs of RVI, echocardiography can aid in the diagnosis.

TREATMENT

The treatment strategy of RVI includes early maintenance of right ventricular preload, reduction of right ventricular afterload, inotropic support of the dysfunctional right ventricle, and early reperfusion.[21] When the right ventricle is ischemic, use of drugs such as nitrates and diuretics will reduce preload and may reduce cardiac output and cause severe hypotension. Volume loading with normal saline alone will often increase filling of the right ventricle and in turn increase filling of the underfilled left ventricle and increase cardiac output.[22]

Excessive fluid administration can further elevate right-sided filling pressures without improvement in cardiac output. In some cases, volume loading will cause further right ventricular dilatation, which in turn further compromises left ventricular output through pericardial restraining effects.[21] Inotropic support with dobutamine should be initiated if the cardiac output fails to improve with up to 1 L of fluid administration.[22]

Often inferior MI can result in bradyarrhythmias and atrioventricular dyssynchrony. When stroke volume is impaired cardiac output depends on heart rate; therefore bradycardia can be deleterious. The development of high-degree atrioventricular block has been reported in as many as 48% of patients with RVI.[28] Atrioventricular dyssynchrony causes loss of right atrial contribution to preload and can lead to further hemodynamic compromise. Several investigators have shown that atrioventricular sequential pacing in patients with complete heart block leads to significant increase in cardiac output and reversal of shock when ventricular pacing alone has no benefit.[29] Prompt cardioversion for atrial fibrillation should be considered to restore atrioventricular synchrony at the earliest signs of hemodynamic compromise.[21]

Reperfusion should be considered in the initial management of RVI. Recent studies have shown that patients with predominant right ventricular failure who underwent revascularization with either percutaneous angioplasty or coronary artery bypass grafting (CABG) had much better outcomes. Mortality was 42% for those revascularized versus 65% for those not revascularized. These numbers were similar for those with predominant left ventricular failure (40% and 73%). The conclusion was made that right ventricular failure complicating AMI carries a very high mortality risk similar to that for left ventricular failure. Revascularization helps to improve these numbers and should be considered immediately.[30]

Long-term prognostic data for those suffering from RVI is conflicting. It is generally thought that when patients survive to discharge, prognosis is favorable but large-scale studies are needed to confirm this theory.[21]

ACUTE MITRAL REGURGITATION

Acute MR is another major fatal mechanical complication of AMI. As with the other complications of AMI, the rapid recognition, diagnosis, and treatment can result in significant improvement in survival. The three main causes of MR in the setting of an AMI include ischemic papillary muscle dysfunction, papillary muscle or chordal rupture, and left ventricular dilatation.[31]

MR of mild-to-moderate severity occurs in 14% to 45% of patients following an AMI. Most MR is transient in nature but sudden papillary muscle rupture can be a life-threatening event. Fibrinolysis may decrease the incidence of rupture; however, when administered, rupture may occur earlier in the post-MI period than in the absence of reperfusion. In the prefibrinolytic era papillary muscle rupture was reported to occur between days 2 and 7 post-AMI. However, it is now thought that a median time to papillary muscle rupture is 13 hours.[32] Papillary muscle rupture is found in 7% of patients in cardiogenic shock and contributes to 5% of the mortality after acute MI.[33]

Studies have shown that the risk factors for acute MR with papillary muscle rupture include advanced age, female sex, and absence of previous angina, inferoposterior AMI, single vessel disease, and no history of diabetes. When considering acute MR without papillary muscle rupture, the risk factors also include female sex and advanced age; however, these patients are likely to have had a prior MI, recurrent ischemia and multivessel coronary artery disease.[34]

PATHOPHYSIOLOGY

The mitral valve is located retrosternally at the fourth costal space and consists of an anterior and posterior leaflet. Any portion of the mitral apparatus can become anatomically disrupted and result in a portion of the mitral valve becoming flail and dysfunctional. The degree of resultant regurgitation is directly related to the extent of anatomic disruption. Most of the time in the setting of acute MI, the rupture of an entire papillary muscle or muscle head typically results in acute severe MR.[35] In most patients, the anterolateral papillary muscle receives dual blood supply from the LAD and circumflex coronary arteries and is less likely to be involved by the ischemic process than the posteromedial papillary muscle, which is supplied solely by the posterior descending artery. Because of its singe vessel blood supply the posteromedial papillary muscle is 6 to 12 times more vulnerable to vascular compromise and rupture than the anterolateral papillary muscle. Often, the infarct expansion is relatively small with poor collaterals, and up to 50% of patients have single vessel disease, with many of them being a consequence of a first-time MI.[6,36] Several studies support that acute MR is not only a common complication post-acute MI but that the degree of MR is predictive of patient survival. Many studies calculate the mortality of patients with moderately severe to severe MR during an acute MI to be 24% at 30 days and 52% at 1 year.[37] Mild MR in the setting of acute MI, however, is not associated with clinically adverse events as it is likely reversible and secondary to the acute ischemic insult.

Of note, select patients with moderate to severe MR, but without papillary muscle rupture, are hemodynamically stable. In this setting patients respond well to medical therapy and revascularization with or without eventual surgical intervention (mitral valve repair or replacement or CABG).[38]

TREATMENT

As with all of the acute phase complications of AMI the proper treatment of acute, severe MR is emergent surgical correction of the mitral valve and CABG when indicated. Prompt diagnosis with echocardiogram and aggressive medical therapy prior to surgery markedly improve patient outcomes (see Figure 10.5). When considering hemodynamic compromise second-

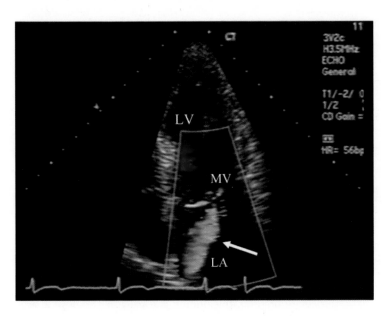

Figure 10.5. Transthoracic echocardiogram showing mitral regurgitation as a result of an inferior wall myocardial infarction (arrow). MV=mitral valve; LA=left atrium; LV=left ventricle.

ary to significant and acute MR, aggressive medical resuscitation involves improving forward flow by afterload reduction and thus improving the regurgitant fraction. Afterload reduction is accomplished with the use of nitrates, sodium nitroprusside, diuretics, and IABP counterpulsation.

The operative mortality for these patients is an estimated 20% to 25% and heavily dependent on the timing of diagnosis and treatment. Despite such a high mortality, survival in patients restricted to medical therapy alone is significantly lower. Thus, emergent surgical intervention remains the treatment of choice for papillary muscle rupture.[39] Of note, mitral valve repair rather than replacement should be attempted in centers experienced in performing this procedure,[37,38] and patients must meet the strict criteria for mitral valve repair, which includes the preserved integrity of the mitral apparatus (i.e., intact papillary muscles, and chordae). Interestingly, long-term results in one small study of 22 patients revealed a perioperative mortality of 27% and a 7-year survival for the survivors of surgery of 64% (the overall 7-year survival was 47%).[39] The only factor that improved both immediate and long-term survival was the concomitant performance of CABG.

TRUE VENTRICULAR ANEURYSM

In contrast to the acute complications of MI, the chronic complications of AMI, are not immediately life-threatening. They have very different presentations and require different treatments. True left ventricular aneurysm (LVA) is a common chronic complication of AMI that is important to diagnose.

LVA is a common mechanical complication following an AMI, often occurring between 10% and 15% of patients. Prior to the era of current management, strategies such as thrombolytic therapy, percutaneous coronary intervention, and the administration of afterload reducing agents, the incidence was approaching 40%.[40,41] A recent analysis of 350 patients has shown that the incidence of LVA among 350 successive patients with ST-segment AMI, treated with thrombolytic therapy, was significantly lower in those with a patent infarct-related artery (7.2% vs. 18.8%).[42] LVA of the apex and anterior wall are ap-

proximately four times more common than those of the inferior or inferoposterior walls.

Approximately 70% to 85% of LVAs are located in the anterior or apical walls, and in most cases are owing to complete occlusion of the LAD coronary artery and the absence of collateralization. However, 10% to 15% of cases involve the inferior-basal walls owing to RCA occlusion. A rare finding is a lateral LVA, which is the result of an occluded left circumflex coronary artery. Among patients with multivessel disease, LVA is uncommon if there is extensive collateralization or a nonoccluded LAD artery.

PATHOPHYSIOLOGY

LVA has been described as a well-delineated and distinct break ("hinge point") in the LV geometry and contour present in both systole and diastole. The walls consist of thin, scarred, or fibrotic myocardium, completely devoid of muscle, a resultant of a healed transmural AMI. The pathognomonic features include a wide mouth that enables communication with the aneurysmal cavity. Often this is evident at 4 to 6 weeks following an AMI. The involved wall segment is either akinetic or dyskinetic during systole and collapses inward when the ventricle is fully vented during surgery (Figures 10.6 and 10.7).

Although the size of an aneurysm varies widely, most are within 1 to 8 cm in diameter. The wall of the aneurysm typically consists of a hybrid of necrotic myocardium and white fibrous scar tissue. This wall is extremely thin and delicate and may calcify over an extended period. Of note, it is imperative to distinguish between an LVA and a pseudoaneurysm, which is characterized by a narrow neck and a distinct "shelf-like" opening.

The endocardial surface is smooth and nontrabeculated. The aneurysm is filled with organized thrombus in >50% of cases, which has the tendency to calcify over time.[43] Dense adhesions between the aneurysm and the overlying pericardium are common phenomena. At a molecular level, initially, the ventricular wall is characterized by myocardial muscle necrosis and a concomitant intense inflammatory reaction, which eventually is replaced with scar tissue formation, and a mature aneurysm consists mostly of hyalinized fibrous tissue. The "border

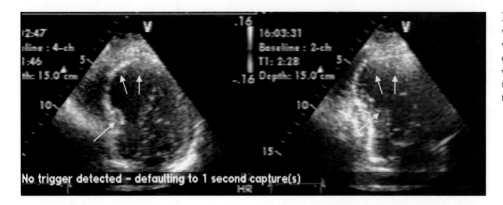

Figure 10.6. Apical four-chamber view (left) and two-chamber (right) views obtained during stress echocardiography depicting a large apical AMI with a large aneurysm (arrows). Notice the distinct break in wall thickness and function (arrows).

zone," that is, the layer between the aneurysm and the healthy myocardium, is characterized by patchy fibrosis and abnormal alignment of the muscle fibers.

CLINICAL PRESENTATION

A prior history of AMI is almost universally present in patients with an LVA that is not associated with other etiologies such as hypertrophic cardiomyopathy or Chagas' disease. The physical examination may reveal one or more of the following findings, although it may prove to be somewhat difficult to diagnose an LVA as the physical exam findings are nonspecific.

- Cardiac enlargement with a diffuse apical impulse located to the left of the midclavicular line.
- An area of dyskinesis can be occasionally appreciated with palpation of the apex or left lateral chest wall, in the area of the anterior wall of the LV.
- A third and/or fourth heart sound (S3 or S4) is often heard, which heralds the onset of coronary blood flow into a dilated and stiffened LV chamber.
- A MR like systolic murmur may be appreciated owing to the distortion of LV geometry that results in the absence of leaflet apposition, papillary muscle dysfunction, and/or annular dilatation.

The presence of an LVA should be suspected in a patient with a history of a large, predominantly, anterior AMI develops one of the aforementioned complications. The ECG usually reveals evidence of a large AMI and there may be persistent ST-segment elevation; however, this finding is usually the result of a large area of scar and does not necessarily imply an aneurysm (see Figure 10.8).

Although limited and seldom used today, chest radiography may aid in the diagnosis of an LVA; however, given the extreme limitations of chest radiography, the diagnosis is definitively made through two-dimensional echocardiography. A simple definition of an LVA on echocardiography imaging is the presence of a dyskinetic wall motion abnormality with the feature of diastolic deformity.[44,45] TTE is most often used and has globally emerged as the diagnostic tool of choice. Even before the diagnosis is made, a number of serious complications can result from an LVA, such as heart failure, ventricular arrhythmias, and thrombus formation.

During ventricular systole, the paradoxical bulging of the aneurysmal segment results in "stealing" part of the LV stroke volume, resulting in decreasing cardiac output and predisposing to LV volume overload. Left ventricular dilatation and increase in wall stiffness can increase oxygen demand. In the setting of underlying coronary artery disease, the increase in

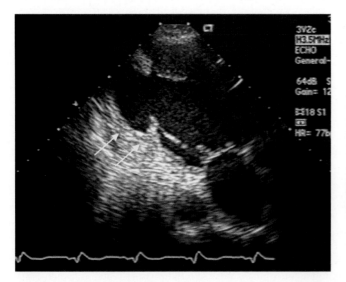

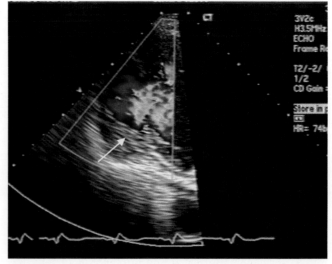

Figure 10.7. Left: Apical three chamber view obtained from transthoracic echocardiogram revealing a large left ventricular aneurysm enhanced with color flow Doppler (right) establishing an area of communication between the normal left ventricle and the aneurysmal portion.

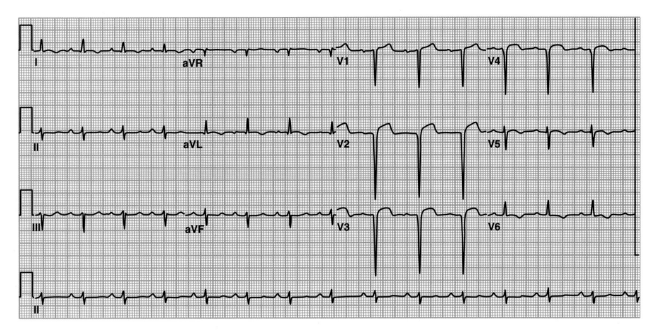

Figure 10.8. EKG of a patient with a true left ventricular aneurysm displaying persistent ST elevation with q waves in V1 through V4

oxygen demand may lead to myocardial ischemia with subsequent angina. The end result of long-standing volume overload and prolonged ischemia is a globally dilated, failing left ventricle. Heart failure symptoms are common.

The myocardial scarring present in LVA is a substrate for ventricular arrhythmias. Two mechanisms contribute to this possible deadly outcome. First, myocardial ischemia and increased myocardial stretch can lead to enhanced cardiac automaticity. Second, the myocardium located at the border zone is made up of a mix of fibrotic tissue, inflammatory cells, and damaged muscle fibers, which is a suitable substrate for a reentrant tachycardia. Ventricular arrhythmias often result in sudden cardiac death.

As previously mentioned, a mural thrombus is identified in autopsy or surgery in >50% of patients with LVA. A possible fatal consequence of thrombus formation is possible systemic embolization that can result in stroke, ischemic colitis, ischemic limbs, and a variety of other disastrous complication.

It is important to note that true LVA may enlarge over time. However, unlike false aneurysms, a true LVA seldom ruptures because of the dense fibrosis that comprises the walls.[46,47]

TREATMENT

Mild-to-moderate size asymptomatic aneurysms can be safely treated medically with an anticipated 5-year survival of up to 90%. Therapy is aimed at reduction of afterload of the LV enlargement through angiotensin-converting enzyme inhibitors, nitrates, and anticoagulation in the setting of significant LV dysfunction or evidence of thrombus within the aneurysm or LV. The optimal approach to the patient with a large, asymptomatic LVA remains a clinical dilemma. Concomitant repair of the aneurysm has been advocated when CABG surgery or valve surgery is performed. In the absence of such indications for surgery, these patients should otherwise be treated with the same regimen as those with a small LVA; they should also be followed closely for progressive left ventricular dilation. Similar

to other settings of chronic volume overload, a progressive increase in LV diameter and/or decrease in LV ejection fraction are a clear indication for surgery even prior to the presence of advanced heart failure or other symptoms.

As per the 2004 American College of Cardiology/American Heart Association (ACC/AHA) guidelines on ST-elevation MI, aneurysmectomy, accompanied by CABG—in patients with an LVA who have repetitive ventricular arrhythmias and/or heart failure unresponsive to medical and catheter-based therapy—is a Class IIa recommendation and is therefore reasonable.[48] Surgical repair should be considered for symptomatic patients with either akinetic or dyskinetic segments, as they represent variants in the spectrum of the same disease. Surgical repair of an LVA is very effective and results in a significant improvement in patient survival, symptoms, and functional class compared with medical treatment.[49,51] Furthermore, a marked decrease in surgical mortality has been achieved in the past 25 years, resulting in an expansion of indications for surgery. Endocardial mapping with subsequent endocardial resection and possible cryoablation are performed in patients with malignant ventricular arrhythmias.

LEFT VENTRICULAR PSEUDOANEURYSM

A left ventricular pseudoaneurysm (LVPA) or false aneurysm is a less common form of a ventricular aneurysm present in <1% of patients post-MI.

PATHOPHYSIOLOGY

An LVPA forms when cardiac rupture is contained by adherent pericardium or scar tissue. Unlike a true aneurysm, an LVPA is devoid of endocardium or myocardium and because these aneurysms are prone to rupture, a quick and accurate diagnosis is of extreme importance. Unlike a true LVA where the walls consist of dense fibrous tissue with excellent tensile strength, the wall of an LVPA comprises varying portions of the pericardium. It is the result of an AMI (typically an inferior or posterolateral wall AMI) with myocardial rupture and hemorrhage into the pericardial space, becoming progressively compressive. Cardiac tamponade occurs, thereby preventing further hemorrhage into the pericardium. Over time, thrombus organizes with overall poor structural integrity and thus is prone to inevitable rupture, which is a fatal event.[52]

CLINICAL PRESENTATION

It has been suggested that the most frequent symptoms associated with LVPA include chest pain and dyspnea. However, symptoms can be often somewhat vague and nonspecific. The other symptomatology includes tamponade, heart failure, syncope, arrhythmia, or systemic embolism. Cardiac murmurs are present in about two-thirds of patients. The murmur is often indistinguishable from that of MR. Almost all patients have some degree of underlying ECG changes, which include ST segment elevation and nonspecific T-wave changes. Evidence of a mass on chest X-ray is seen in more than one-half of patients; however, as previously mentioned this is not specific or sensitive for the diagnosis of an LVPA.[53,54]

The most reliable method for diagnosis of an LVPA is through echocardiography. A TTE is a reasonable first step, but a definitive diagnosis is made in only a fraction of patients. Echocardiography can usually distinguish a pseudoaneurysm from a true aneurysm by the appearance of the connection between the aneurysm and ventricular cavity. LVPA has a narrow neck, typically <40% of the maximal aneurysm diameter, which causes an abrupt interruption in the ventricular wall contour (Figures 10.9 and 10.10). In contrast, true aneurysms are nearly as wide at the neck as they are at the apex.

TREATMENT

Untreated LVPAs have a 30% to 45% risk of rupture and, with medical therapy, a mortality of almost 50%. Thus, surgery is the preferred therapeutic option. With current techniques, the perioperative mortality is <10%, although the risk is greater

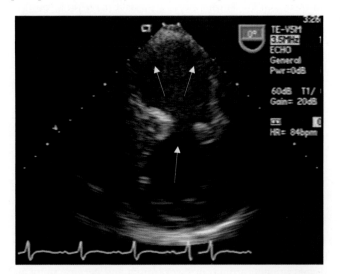

Figure 10.9. Short axis view of the left ventricle (lower cavity) during transesophogeal echocardiography. Large pseudoaneurysm (higher cavity). Notice the narrow "bottleneck" opening (arrow).

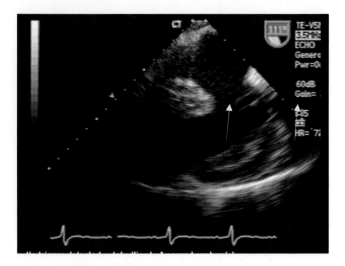

Figure 10.10. Short axis view from transesophogeal echocardiogram depicting a large pseudouaneurysm. Notice the narrow "shelf-like" opening into the aneurysmal cavity.

among patients with severe MR requiring concomitant mitral valve replacement.

LEFT VENTRICULAR THROMBUS

A mural LV thrombus is a common sequel of an AMI and most commonly develops in the presence of a large infarction. Although its formation is prone to originate in regions of stasis, it is most commonly noted to occur in the apex but may also occur in lateral and inferior aneurysms. With extensive transmural infarction, mural thrombi may overlie the infracted myocardium. Prior to current conventional medical therapy, the incidence ranged between 25% and 40%.[53] The initiation of heparin and perhaps thrombolysis can reduce the development of a left ventricular thrombus by 50%. The major risk of a thrombus is subsequent distal embolization, which is highest during the first 2 weeks following an AMI with eventual reduction of risk by 6 to 8 weeks. This is attributed to a relative endothelialization of the thrombus with reduction in its embolic potential. Echocardiography has high sensitivity (95%) and high specificity (85%) for identification of a left ventricular thrombus and has emerged as the diagnostic modality of choice. Characteristically, a thrombus has a nonhomogeneous echo density with a margin distinct from the underlying wall, which is akinetic to dyskinetic (Figure 10.11a and 10.11b). A thrombus is more likely to occur following an AMI in the LAD artery distribution (up to 33%) versus the right coronary or circumflex (<1%) coronary arteries.

Current data on the correct treatment of left ventricular thrombi are lacking. There are no large-scale trials that direct treatment; however it is generally recommended that patients who have already embolized or have a large anterior infarction receive full anticoagulation. They should be initiated with heparin and converted to full dose warfarin for 3 to 6 months with a goal international normalized ratio (INR) between 2 and 3.[1]

In summary mechanical complications of an AMI are important to recognize, diagnose, and especially to treat. Having an understanding of the most important signs and symptoms should prompt an immediate echocardiogram and in most

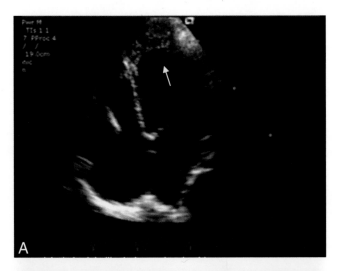

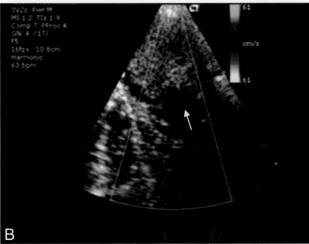

Figure 10.11: Apical four chamber transthoracic view (A) and two chamber view (B) from a 74 year old patient three months following AMI. Notice the large protruding apical thrombus (arrow). Color flow imaging may be used to demonstrate abnormal swirling patterns of blood.

cases, surgical intervention. Most therapies carry with them a poor prognosis, but surgery is clearly a better option with improved survival than medical therapy alone. Physicians in the cardiac care unit must grasp all of these concepts to provide proper medical care.

REFERENCES

1. Antman EM. ST elevation myocardial infarction. In: Libby P, Bonow R, Mann D, et al., eds. *Braunwald's Heart Disease: A Textbook of Cardiovascular Medicine*. 8th ed. Philadelphia, PA: Elsevier Saunders; 2008:1233–1299.
2. Pohjola-Sintonen S, Muller JE, Stone PH, et al. Ventricular septal and free wall rupture complicating acute myocardial infarction: experience in the Multicenter Investigation of Limitation of Infarct Size. *Am Heart J.* 1989;117:809.
3. Becker RC, Gore JM, Lambrew C, et al.; for the National Registry of Myocardial Infarction Participants. A composite view of cardiac rupture in the United States National Registry of Myocardial Infarction. *J Am Coll Cardiol.* 1996;27:1321.
4. Purcaro A, Costantini C, Ciampani N, et al. Diagnostic criteria and management of subacute ventricular free wall rupture complicating acute myocardial infarction. *Am J Cardiol.* 1997;80:397.
5. Batts KP, Ackerman DM, Edwards WD. Postinfarction rupture of the left ventricular free wall: clinicopathologic correlates in 100 consecutive autopsy cases. *Hum Pathol.* 1990;21:530.
6. Reeder GS. Identification and treatment of complications of myocardial infarction. *Mayo Clin Proc.* 1995;70:880.
7. Becker RC, Charlesworth A, Wilcox RG, et al. Cardiac rupture associated with thrombolytic therapy: impact of time to treatment in the Late Assessment of Thrombolytic Efficacy (LATE) study. *J Am Coll Cardiol.* 1995;25:1063.
8. Moreno R, Lopez-Sendon J, Garcia E, et al. Primary angioplasty reduces the risk of left ventricular free wall rupture compared with thrombolysis in patients with acute myocardial infarction. *J Am Coll Cardiol.* 2002;39:598.
9. Cheriex EC, de Swart H, Dijkman LW, et al. Myocardial rupture after myocardial infarction is related to the perfusion status of the infarct-related coronary artery. *Am Heart J.* 1995;129:644.
10. Becker RC, Hochman JS, Cannon CP, et al.; for the TIMI 9 Investigators. Fatal cardiac rupture among patients treated with thrombolytic agents and adjunctive thrombin antagonists. Observations from the Thrombolysis and Thrombin Inhibition in Myocardial Infarction 9 study. *J Am Coll Cardiol.* 1999;33:479.
11. Ivor L. Gerber, MD, MBChB, Elyse Foster, MD Otto C. *The Practice of Clinical Echocardiography*. Chapter 12: Echocardiography in the coronary care unit. Philadelphia, PA: WB Saunders; 2002.
12. McMullan MH, Maples MD, Kilgore TL Jr, et al. Surgical experience with left ventricular free wall rupture. *Ann Thorac Surg.* 2001;71:1894.
13. Lopez-Sendon J, Gonzalez A, Lopez de Sa E, et al. Diagnosis of subacute ventricular wall rupture after acute myocardial infarction: sensitivity and specificity of clinical, hemodynamic and echocardiographic criteria. *J Am Coll Cardiol.* 1992;19:1145–1153.
14. Topaz O, Taylor AL. Interventricular septal rupture complicating acute myocardial infarction: from pathophysiologic features to the role of invasive and noninvasive diagnostic modalities in current management. *Am J Med.* 1992;93:683–688.
15. Crenshaw BS, Granger CB, Birnbaum Y, et al. Risk factors, angiographic patterns, and outcomes in patients with ventricular septal defect complicating acute myocardial infarction. *Circulation.* 2000;101:27–32.
16. Birnbaum Y, Fishbein MC, Blanche C, et al. Ventricular septal rupture after acute myocardial infarction. *N Engl J Med.* 2002;347(18):1426–1432.
17. Buda AJ. The role of echocardiography in the evaluation of mechanical complications of acute myocardial infarction. *Circulation.* 1991;84(3)(suppl I):109–121.
18. Sager RV. Coronary thrombosis; perforation of the infracted interventricular septum. *Arch Intern Med.* 1934;53:140–148.
19. Giuliani ER, Danielson GK, Pluth JR, et al. Postinfarction ventricular septal rupture: surgical considerations and results. *Circulation.* 1974;49:455–459.
20. Menon V, Webb JG, Hillis LD, et al. Outcome and profile of ventricular septal rupture with cardiogenic shock after myocardial infarction: a report from the SHOCK Trial Registry. *J Am Coll Cardiol.* 2000;36(suppl A):1110–1116.
21. Kinch JW, Ryan TJ. Right ventricular infarction. *N Engl J Med.* 1994;330:1211–1219.
22. Haji SA, Movahed A. Right ventricular infarction—diagnosis and treatment. *Clin Cardiol.* 2000;23:473–482.
23. Lee FA. Hemodynamics of the right ventricle in normal and disease states. *Clin Cardiol.* 1992;10:59–67.
24. Horan LG, Flowers NC. Right ventricular infarction: specific requirements of management. *Am Fam Physician.* 1999;60(6):1727–1734.
25. Goldstein JA, Barzilai B, Rosamond TL, et al. Determinants of hemodynamic compromise with severe right ventricular infarction. *Circulation.* 1990;82:359–368.
26. Dell'Italia LJ, Starling MR, O'Rourke RA. Physical examination for exclusion of hemodynamically important right ventricular infarction. *Ann Intern Med.* 1983;99:608–611.
27. Cintron GB, Hernandez E, Linares E, et al. Bedside recognition, incidence and clinical course of right ventricular infarction. *Am J Cardiol.* 1981;47:224–227.
28. Braat SH, de Zwann C, Brugada P, et al. Right ventricular involvement with acute inferior wall myocardial infarction identifies high risk of developing atrioventricular nodal conduction disturbances. *Am Heart J.* 1984;107:1183–1187.
29. Love JC, Haffajee CI, Gore JM, et al. Reversibility of hypotension and shock by atrial or atrioventricular sequential pacing in patients with right ventricular infarction. *Am Heart J.* 1984;108:5–13.
30. Jacobs AK, Leopold JA, Bates E, et al. Cardiogenic shock caused by right ventricular infarction: a report from the SHOCK registry. *J Am Coll Cardiol.* 2003;41:1273–1279.
31. Tcheng JE, Jackman JD, Nelson CL, et al. Outcome of patients sustaining acute ischemic mitral regurgitation during myocardial infarction. *Ann Intern Med.* 1992;117:18.
32. Thompson CR, Buller CE, Sleeper LA, et al.; for the SHOCK Investigators. Cardiogenic shock due to acute severe mitral regurgitation complicating acute myocardial infarction: a report from the SHOCK Trial Registry. *J Am Coll Cardiol.* 2000;36:1104–1109.
33. Thompson CR, Buller CE, Sleeper LA, et al.; for the SHOCK Investigators. Cardiogenic shock complicating acute myocardial infarction—etiologies, management and outcome: a report from the SHOCK Trial Registry. *J Am Coll Cardiol.* 2000;36:1063–1070.
34. Birnbaum Y, Chamoun AJ, Conti VR, et al. Mitral regurgitation following acute myocardial infarction. *Coron Artery Dis.* 2002;13:337–344.
35. Feigenbaum H, Armstrong W, Ryan T. *Feigenbaum's Echocardiography*. 6th ed. Chapter 15: Coronary artery disease. Philadelphia, PA: Lippincott Williams and Wilkins; 2005.
36. Feigenbaum H, Armstrong W, Ryan T. *Feigenbaum's Echocardiography*. 6th ed. Chapter 11: Mitral valve disease. Philadelphia, PA: Lippincott Williams and Wilkins; 2005.
37. Lavie CJ, Gersh BJ. Mechanical and electrical complications of acute myocardial infarction. *Mayo Clin Proc.* 1990;65:709.
38. David TE. Techniques and results of mitral valve repair for ischemic mitral regurgitation. *J Card Surg.* 1994;9:274.
39. Kishon Y, Oh JK, Schaff HV, et al. Mitral valve operation in postinfarction rupture of a papillary muscle: immediate results and long-term follow-up of 22 patients. *Mayo Clin Proc.* 1992;67:1023.
40. Friedman BM, Dunn MI. Postinfarction ventricular aneurysms. *Clin Cardiol.* 1995;18(9):505–511.
41. Glower DG, Lowe EL. Left ventricular aneurysm. In: Edmunds LH, ed. *Cardiac Surgery in the Adult*. New York, NY: McGraw-Hill; 1997:677.

42. Tikiz H, Balbay Y, Atak R, et al. The effect of thrombolytic therapy on left ventricular aneurysm formation in acute myocardial infarction: relationship to successful reperfusion and vessel patency. *Clin Cardiol.* 2001;24:656.

43. Feigenbaum H, Armstrong WF, Ryan T. *Feigenbaum's Echocardiography.* Philadelphia, PA: Lippincott Williams & Wilkins; 2005:469–473.

44. Nicolosi AC, Spotnitz HM. Quantitative analysis of regional systolic function with left ventricular aneurysm. *Circulation.* chapter 15: Philadelphia, PA: 1988;78:856.

45. Matsumoto M, Watanabe F, Goto A, et al. Left ventricular aneurysm and the prediction of left ventricular enlargement studied by two-dimensional echocardiography: quantitative assessment of aneurysm size in relation to clinical course. *Circulation.* 1985;72:280.

46. Vlodaver Z, Coe JL, Edwards JE. True and false left ventricular aneurysms: propensity for the latter to rupture. *Circulation.* 1975;51:567.

47. Dubnow MH, Burchell HB, Titus JL. Postinfarction ventricular aneurysm. A clinicomorphologic and electrocardiographic study of 80 cases. *Am Heart J.* 1965;70:753.

48. Antman EM, Anbe DT, Armstrong PW, et al. ACC/AHA guidelines for the management of patients with ST-elevation myocardial infarction. September 1st, 2010. www.acc.org/qualityandscience/clinical/statements.htm.

49. Rao G, Zikria EA, Miller WH, et al. Experience with sixty consecutive ventricular aneurysm resections. *Circulation.* 1974;50:II149.

50. Antunes PE, Silva R, Ferrão de Oliveira J, et al. Left ventricular aneurysms: early and long-term results of two types of repair. *Eur J Cardiothorac Surg.* 2005;27(2):210–215.

51. Shapira OM, Davidoff R, Hilkert RJ, et al. Repair of left ventricular aneurysm: long-term results of linear repair versus endoaneurysmorrhaphy. *Ann Thorac Surg.* 1997;63:701.

52. Frances C, Romero A, Grady D. Left ventricular pseudoaneurysm. *J Am Coll Cardiol.* 1998;32:557.

53. Dachman AH, Spindola-Franco H, Solomon N. Left ventricular pseudoaneurysm: its recognition and significance. *JAMA.* 1981;246:1951.

54. Yeo TC, Malouf JF, Oh JK, et al. Clinical profile and outcome in 52 patients with cardiac pseudoaneurysm. *Ann Intern Med.* 1998;128:299.

PATIENT AND FAMILY INFORMATION FOR:

Mechanical Complications of Myocardial Infarction

For decades heart disease has consistently been the number one killer in the world. When a family member or loved one has a heart attack, it can be a terrifying experience for everyone involved. Most of the time, everything goes smoothly, and that family member or loved one walks out of the hospital with a new outlook on life. However, there are occasions when a patient's condition can rapidly deteriorate and circumstances drastically change. These potential complications can happen at home, in transit to the hospital, in the emergency room, or even in the cardiac care unit. An understanding of the complications that go hand in hand with an acute heart attack is crucial for comprehending the nature of the disease.

The heart is the most important muscle in the human body. Like all muscles, it needs oxygen to live. However, unlike all muscles, it continuously beats around 100,000 times a day. A heart attack is the result of the blockage of blood flow to that muscle, therefore cutting off its oxygen supply, and for all intensive purposes, suffocating that muscle. Without oxygen, the heart muscle will die. The intense chest pain that a patient senses during an acute heart attack is mostly because of thrombosis in one of the main arteries that supplies oxygen to the cardiac muscle, thereby causing it to suffocate and die rapidly. Relieving that blockage will restore blood flow to the damaged muscle, replenish its oxygen supply, and hopefully allow it to live. The timely nature of this intervention is paramount to the heart's survival.

Prompt recognition and initiation of therapy for an acute heart attack is the most important factor in that patient's survival. The longer the heart muscle goes without oxygen, the faster it dies, and the worse the prognosis. The medical conditions and risk factors that one may have include high blood pressure, high cholesterol, smoking, diabetes, and a family history of heart attacks. The signs and symptoms of a heart attack include a left-sided chest pressure accompanied by any combination of shortness of breath, nausea, vomiting, sweating, or a sensation of left arm pain or neck pain. The moment these symptoms commence, one should seek immediate medical attention.

Doctors have various methods to relieve the obstruction, whether with medications or direct intervention. Medical therapy involves the administration of an intravenous (IV) medication called a thrombolytic. This medicine will rapidly break up the blood clot in the blocked coronary artery, thereby thwarting the heart attack. Interventional therapy involves the placement of a tube or "catheter" into one of several arteries in the arms or the legs that lead to the heart. These catheters are inserted directly into the coronary arteries, and through the use of a moving X-ray, the thrombus can be directly visualized and extracted. Subsequently, a little piece of metal, called a stent, can be inserted in the artery and allow blood to freely flow to the dying heart muscle. The faster the therapy is delivered, the better. There are times when a substantial amount of irreversible damage has been done, causing the muscle to die and possibly tear, leading to life-threatening complications. There are other times when the muscle does not tear, but simply dies, and causes more chronic complications. In this chapter we discuss the disastrous complications of a heart attack.

When the heart muscle dies, it can eventually tear and cause sudden clinical deterioration and possibly death. If there is a delay in a patient's presentation to the emergency room, therapy cannot be initiated and the heart muscle will die. This delay can be from hours to days. If there is no delay and therapy is administered immediately, there is always a possibility that the therapy may not be completely successful, the artery will remain blocked, and the heart muscle will die anyway. This is an unfortunate reality as not all treatments are successful. In rare occasions, the area of the heart muscle between the dead and viable tissue will completely sever. This will result in free communication between the two areas of the heart, causing brisk bleeding and inevitable death. There are three such scenarios that must be promptly recognized because surgical therapy usually provides the only means for survival. These three scenarios include ventricular free wall rupture, interventricular septal rupture, and papillary muscle rupture.

It is not as important to know the intricate details of these complications as it is important to understand their deadly potential. Any sudden deterioration in clinical condition should prompt suspicion of myocardial rupture. Development of increased chest pain or shortness of breath accompanied by a new murmur on physical exam, accelerated heart rate, and drop in blood pressure must be followed by an immediate echocardiogram which is an ultrasound examination of the heart. This will provide visualization of the cardiac muscle and diagnosis of a myocardial tear. If the situation arises, intravenous medications can be administered to temporarily stabilize the patient, but emergent surgical intervention is paramount to provide any chance of survival.

Emergent surgery should be performed within a number of hours. IV medications will support the patient's blood pressure and heart rate until the operating room is ready for patient transfer. The surgical procedure will involve opening the chest wall, directly visualizing the heart, and repairing the torn tissue. Often, bypass of any blocked arteries will accompany repair of the damaged cardiac muscle. The procedure will take many hours to complete, and even if successful, the probability of eventual death is still very high. When the ruptured myocardium is repaired and bypass complete, the patient still has a long and dangerous road ahead.

The postoperative period is every bit as important as the procedure itself. Making it out of the operating room does not mean that long-term survival is guaranteed. There are many factors such as age and comorbidities that complicate both the surgical procedure and the recovery period. The older a person is, the more unlikely it is for him or her to survive such a difficult surgery and the more difficult it is to recover. Coexisting medical conditions such as asthma, emphysema, kidney disease, cancer, and diabetes, among others, increase mortality. Friends and family must be realistic about the severity of the situation and expectations for survival. Most studies quote far less than 50% survival with the actual numbers being <25%.

The left ventricle is the most important of the four heart chambers for survival. Most of what has been discussed involves damage to this all important chamber. The right ventricle is a less muscular part of the heart that can also be damaged during a heart attack. It is important to recognize right ventricular injury, (RVI) as its treatment is very different from that of garden variety left ventricular injury. There are specific clinical signs and EKG findings that will lead to the diagnosis of an RVI. When present, a physician must be careful not to administer certain medications, such as nitroglycerine or diuretics, as they can lead to clinical deterioration. The astute medical professional can easily diagnose this situation and provide appropriate therapy. As with all heart attacks, restoring blood flow to the right ventricle will prevent poor clinical outcomes and improve survival. Surgical intervention is generally not necessary, and if the patient survives to discharge, outlook is favorable.

Chronic complications of a heart attack are probably more common than the acute ones. Depending on the timing of the revascularization, a certain amount of heart muscle invariably dies. As described earlier, the longer the muscle goes without oxygen, more of it dies. The commonest phrase used is, "Time is muscle." Patients who suffer large heart attacks and do not receive adequate therapy, lose large amounts of muscle forever. The heart weakens, blood is not pumped forward as it should, and over the following weeks an aneurysm can form. Aneurysms are described as a weakening of the muscle to the point that it forms a pocket within or outside the walls of the heart. To either side of the aneurysm is living tissue, and within the aneurysm is dead tissue. Aneurysms are divided into two categories that require different therapies: true aneurysms and pseudoaneurysms.

The more common and less dangerous of the two types of aneurysms are the true aneurysms. The entire aneurysm forms a pocket that is made of dead cardiac tissue. An indentation is created in the myocardium with a wide neck that contains the aneurysm. True aneurysms are entirely made of dead myocardial tissue. See Figure 10.6 for an echocardiographic representation of a true aneurysm. As the muscle does not contract, there is invariably stasis of blood flow within the pocket, making it prone to forming blood clots. Often, a piece of the blood clot can break off and result in many complications including stroke. True aneurysms should be treated with the same aggressive medical therapy that all heart attack patients receive. This includes but is not limited to ß-blockers, ACE inhibitors, statin and aspirin. If a blood clot is present, patients should be administered blood thinners to prevent stroke. Seldom is surgical intervention necessary to excise the aneurysm when there is evidence of deadly arrhythmias that are resistant to medical therapy.

Pseudoaneurysms are extremely rare and are very dangerous. A pseudoaneurysm represents a contained rupture of the cardiac tissue. As has been described previously, tearing of the heart muscle results in brisk bleeding and often death. Occasionally, this bleeding can be contained by the thin layer of tissue surrounding the heart called the pericardium. The pericardium is a rigid layer of tissue that encases the heart and at times will seal off a myocardial rupture, thereby preventing certain death. A pseudoaneurysm forms when the pericardium bubbles outward and contains a rupture during a heart attack. See Figures 10.9 and 10.10 for an echocardiographic demonstration of a psudoaneurysm.

Instead of the wide neck seen in true aneurysms, a pseudoaneurysm has a narrow neck that communicates with the left ventricle. There is no dead myocardium in the psuedoaneurysm as it is entirely made of pericardium. Invariably, the pocket of the pseudoaneurysm contains a blood clot, as there is complete stasis of blood flow. A pseudoaneurysm is prone to rupture because it consists of only the thin pericardium that has sealed off the prior rupture. Surgical excision of the pseudoaneurysm is the only treatment that can be offered to prevent rupture and certain death.

Both acute and chronic complications of a heart attack have become less common as medical therapy has advanced. The development of thrombolytics and interventional procedures have improved survival and drastically reduced the number of disastrous complications that can occur. In the unfortunate cases when they do occur, advancements in surgical technology and techniques have further improved the chance of survival. Even with all the advancements in therapy, the prompt recognition, timely diagnosis and eventual initiation of treatment can be the difference between life and death. Survival to hospital discharge is a rare occurrence, and family members must realize that there is a long road ahead.

When a patient does survive a complication of an AMI, he or she must realize that great care must be taken to improve the likelihood of long-term survival. Outpatient follow-up with a cardiologist, surgeon, and a primary care physician should be in place before discharge. The patient will invariably be on a new regimen of medications that can be extremely complicated. Survivors will often need a significant amount of rehabilitation before they can return to their preheart attack state. Social support and family encouragement increase the likelihood of recovery. Patients should not leave the hospital without a strict understanding of the medications they are to take and who they are to follow-up with. A structured regimen of medication compliance, physician follow-up, and cardiac rehabilitation can turn a life-threatening situation into a rewarding experience for patients, families, and all medical professionals involved.

Matthew A. Cavender
Venu Menon

Cardiogenic Shock Complicating Acute Myocardial Infarction

The overall rates of myocardial infarction and the incidence of cardiogenic shock in patients with myocardial infarction have declined over time owing to advances in medical, surgical, and interventional treatments.[1,2] However, mortality rates in acute myocardial infarction (AMI) complicated by cardiogenic shock remain high. Cardiogenic shock in the setting of myocardial infarction is a heterogeneous clinical entity that most commonly occurs with the sudden onset of left ventricular dysfunction owing to a large area of dysfunctional myocardium because of acute ischemia and ensuing cardiac necrosis. In this setting, the heart attempts to maintain cardiac output despite the marked reduction in stroke volume by increasing the heart rate. When this compensatory mechanism is inadequate, end-organ hypoperfusion and circulatory collapse result.

There is no universally accepted definition of cardiogenic shock as it is a subjective and clinical diagnosis best made by the clinician at the bedside. Its occurrence is characterized by inadequate end-organ tissue perfusion secondary to decreased cardiac output despite adequate or elevated left ventricular filling pressures. The SHOCK (SHould we emergently revascularize Occluded Coronaries for cardiogenic shocK) trial utilized these core principles to create a definition for cardiogenic shock that could be applied objectively in the setting of a randomized clinical trial.[3] To be included in the SHOCK trial (Table 11.1), patients with AMI had to manifest hypotension (systolic blood pressure <90 mm Hg sustained for at least 30 minutes or the use of hemodynamic support measures to maintain blood pressure >90 mm Hg) and have evidence of end-organ hypoperfusion (<30 ml of urine output per hour, heart rate >60 beats per minute, cool extremities). Hemodynamic confirmation was mandatory in this trial and patients had to have a cardiac index of <2.2 L per m^2 and pulmonary capillary wedge pressure of ≥15 mm Hg on right heart catheterization unless there was overt evidence of pulmonary congestion on chest radiography.

ETIOLOGY OF CARDIOGENIC SHOCK IN THE SETTING OF ACUTE MYOCARDIAL INFARCTION

Most of the patients with cardiogenic shock have left ventricular failure owing to an ongoing or recently completed AMI.[4] Prior necropsy studies have found that most of the patients who die from cardiogenic shock have lost >40% of their myocardium.[5] In this condition, the culprit artery is almost always either left anterior descending or right coronary artery (RCA). The left circumflex is the culprit artery only 13% of the time.[6] Isolated right ventricular involvement in the absence of an overt inferoposterior infarction is rare and occurs in only 2% of cases.[4] Patients with non–ST-elevation myocardial infarction (NSTEMI) can also develop cardiogenic shock but represent <20% of overall patients and are typically older with more medical comorbidities.[6]

In addition to the myocardial dysfunction as a result of ischemia, myocardial infarction can also result in mechanical complications such as acute mitral regurgitation owing to loss of the integrity of the mitral valve, ventricular septal rupture (VSR), or ventricular wall rupture. These complications of myocardial infarction are fairly uncommon resulting in <15% of all cases of cardiogenic shock. Hemodynamic instability resulting from β-blockers or occult blood loss can also present in a similar manner. Other acute cardiac emergencies such as acute aortic dissection, acute pulmonary embolism, myocarditis, and pneumothorax and cardiac tamponade can also have similar presentations and should to be considered by the astute clinician. Seldom is dynamic left ventricular outflow tract obstruction in the setting of an anterior myocardial infarction or hypertrophic obstructive cardiomyopathy encountered. Critical aortic stenosis and stress-induced cardiomyopathy can also be encountered in patients with circulatory collapse. Recognition

TABLE 11.1	Criteria for Cardiogenic Shock Complicating AMI
Clinical Criteria	*Hemodynamic Criteria*

• Hypotension—systolic blood pressure <90 mm Hg sustained for at least 30 min or the use of hemodynamic support measures to maintain blood pressure >90 mm Hg
• End-organ hypoperfusion
  ◆ <30 cc urine output/h
  ◆ Heart rate >60 beats/min
  ◆ Cool extremities
	• Cardiac index of <2.2
	• Pulmonary capillary wedge pressure of ≥15 mm Hg
	  Or evidence of pulmonary congestion on chest X-ray in patients with anterior myocardial infarction

of the causative etiology of shock is pivotal to directing appropriate interventions.

PATHOPHYSIOLOGY

Cardiac myocytes need oxygen to generate energy and maintain integrity of the contractile apparatus. Although the body as a whole extracts between 30% and 50% of the oxygen delivered through arterial blood flow, myocytes extract approximately 70% of oxygen delivered to them. The amount of oxygen required by cardiac myocytes, known as myocardial oxygen demand, is predominately dependent on myocardial wall stress, contractility, and the heart rate.[7,8] Thus, in the setting of an AMI, when blood supply is abruptly diminished there is immediate loss of contractility in the area at risk. When compensatory mechanisms are inadequate, hemodynamic instability and cardiogenic shock can ensue.

Coronary artery blood flow, especially to the left coronary artery occurs primarily during diastole and is dependent on a pressure gradient that exists between mean central aortic pressure and the left ventricular end diastolic pressure.[9] Cardiogenic shock results in decreased mean arterial blood pressure and elevations in the left ventricular end diastolic pressure so that the pressure gradient driving coronary perfusion decreases. As a result, coronary blood flow is further diminished and ischemia is worsened in the myocardium supplied by both the culprit and nonculprit blood vessels.

Decreased cardiac output, regardless of the etiology, significant enough to cause end-organ hypoperfusion activates the compensatory mechanisms of the body in an attempt to restore tissue perfusion.[10] Catecholamine release through activation of the sympathetic nervous system increases heart rate and causes systemic vasocontriction. The decreased renal perfusion causes activation of the renin–angiotensin system, increased angiotensin II, and further systemic vasocontriction. All of these compensatory mechanisms increase myocardial oxygen demand because vasoconstriction increases wall stress, catecholamines increase heart rate and contractility, and increased left ventricular filling pressure from cardiac dysfunction increases wall stress. This results in a self-perpetuating deterioration in hemodynamic status that can ultimately result in death. Large myocardial infarctions can also result in increased levels of nitric oxide and cytokine-release–mediated vasodilation. These agents also have a negative inotropic impact and may manifest in a shock state that closely resembles sepsis. The clinical presentation of this variant of cardiogenic shock is quite heterogeneous although elderly patients with large anterior myocardial infarction appear to be at greatest risk.[10]

INCIDENCE

Cardiogenic shock is an infrequent complication of AMI. Analyses of large national databases, such as the National Registry of Myocardial Infarction (NRMI) have estimated that the incidence of cardiogenic shock is between 5% and 9%.[11] Recent data suggest that the incidence has been decreasing in conjunction with the widespread utilization of primary angioplasty.[12,13] Shock on presentation remains unchanged but definitive revascularization and salvage of myocardium appear to have decreased the incidence of shock after presentation.[12,14]

MANAGEMENT

DIAGNOSIS

The management of patients with cardiogenic shock requires prompt recognition of the severity of illness and rapid identification of the etiology of shock (Figure 11.1). All patients should be initially evaluated with a history that is focused on the determination of risk factors, comorbidities, and potential etiologies of shock. Early identification of patients at high risk for the development of shock is crucial as these patients benefit from early revascularization and aggressive medical therapy.[15] The physical exam should focus on identifying potential etiologies of shock (murmur consistent with a ventricular septal defect/mitral insufficiency) and signs of end-organ hypoperfusion (decreased mentation, increased lethargy, cool peripheries, rapid low-volume pulse, and decreased urine output). In addition, patients with cardiogenic shock will also frequently have elevated jugular venous pressure, rales consistent with pulmonary edema and tachypnea. Patients with cardiogenic shock will frequently have cyanosis and extremities that are cool to the touch. In contrast, patients with distributive shock will typically have extremities that are warm with adequate capillary refill and no signs of peripheral cyanosis.

In patients with cardiogenic shock of uncertain etiology, obtaining a transthoracic echocardiogram (TTE) can be helpful. A well-performed echo can rule out the presence of mechanical complications, tamponade, or right ventricular infarct physiology. It can also provide the clinician with initial clues needed to diagnose a pulmonary embolism or dissection and provide and immediate assessment of both the amount of myocardium at risk and the function of the remote myocardium. Pulmonary arterial catheter placement can be used to evaluate SVR and cardiac output. The information obtained from pulmonary artery catheters is often confirmatory but can be especially useful in patients with renal failure and with acute respiratory distress syndrome complicating shock or in monitoring the impact of treatment.

REVASCULARIZATION

Patients with cardiogenic shock in the setting of STEMI should undergo prompt coronary angiography with intent to perform urgent revascularization. This is a class I indication for patients aged <75 years of age and is based on findings from the landmark SHOCK trial.[3,16] Patients aged >75 with reasonable premorbid status should also be considered for this strategy. The SHOCK trial randomized 302 patients between 1993 and 1998 with cardiogenic shock within 30 hours of an index myocardial infarction to either emergency revascularization (intra-aortic balloon pump (IABP) and percutaneous coronary intervention (PCI) or coronary artery bypass graft (CABG) within 6 hours of randomization) or initial medical stabilization followed by delayed revascularization if needed (intensive medical therapy with IABP and fibrinolytic therapy were recommended). At 30 days, patients treated with emergent revascularization had a 9.3% lower mortality than patients treated with initial medical stabilization that was statistically nonsignificant (46.7% vs. 56%, *P* = .11). The differences in mortality between the two groups increased over time such that at 6 months patients treated with emergent revascularization had 12.8% lower mortality rate than patients treated with medical stabilization (50.3% vs. 63.1%, *P* = .027).[3] In patients with a clear culprit lesion, patients who

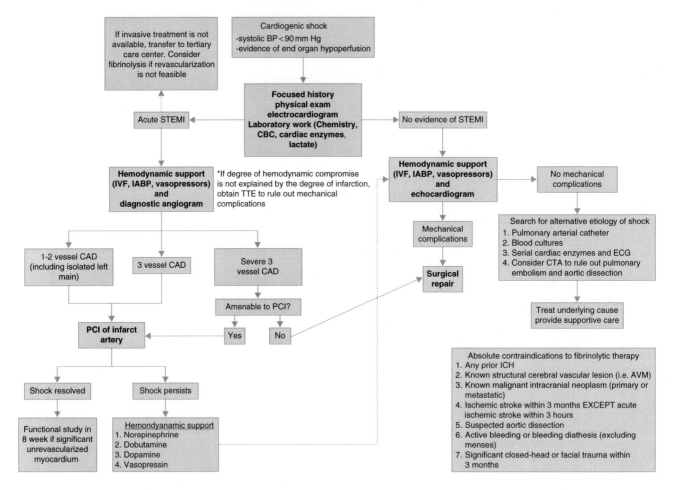

Figure 11.1. Algorithm for the approach and treatment of cardiogenic shock. (Adapted from Antman EM, Anbe DT, Armstrong PW, et al. ACC/AHA guidelines for the management of patients with ST-elevation myocardial infarction—executive summary: a report of the American College of Cardiology/American Heart Association Task Force on Practice Guidelines (Writing Committee to Revise the 1999 Guidelines for the Management of Patients With Acute Myocardial Infarction). *Circulation.* 2004;110:588–636.)

have only one- to two-vessel coronary artery disease or isolated left main disease, PCI of the infarct-related artery can be performed efficiently and effectively at the time of angiography. The optimal revascularization strategy for the nonculprit arteries in subjects with multivessel disease is unclear. Although current treatment guidelines recommend against the treatment of the non–infarct-related artery in patients without hemodynamic compromise they do support consideration of revascularization of the non–infarct-related artery in cardiogenic shock. This strategy of percutaneous multivessel revascularization has been called into question by recent data that have shown patients in cardiogenic shock treated with multivessel PCI including PCI to the non–infarct-related artery are at higher risk of mortality even after adjusting for potential confounders.[17] This is also supported by observational evidence from the SHOCK trial that showed similar outcomes for patients regardless of whether they were treated with revascularization of the infarct-related artery alone or with multivessel PCI.[18]

ROLE OF CABG

Emergent CABG provides a number of theoretical benefits for patients with AMI complicated by cardiogenic shock. Prompt cardiopulmonary bypass may protect against end-organ hypoperfusion and allow for complete revascularization. Among patients randomized to the early intervention arm of the SHOCK trial, the method of revascularization was left to the discretion on the treating physician. CABG was recommended for patients with left main stenosis of ≥50%, ≥2 total or subtotal occlusions, or stenoses of >90% in two non-infarct major epicardial vessels. Consequently, 64% of patients in the emergent revascularization arm of the SHOCK trial were treated with PCI and 36% received CABG. Despite being a higher risk population (higher incidence of diabetes, three-vessel disease, and left main disease), patients treated with CABG had similar survival as patients treated with percutaneous revascularization.[18]

The high rate of CABG for patients with cardiogenic shock seen in the SHOCK trial is not indicative of current treatment patterns. Owing to the widespread availability of percutaneous therapy, efficiency of proceeding with PCI instead of CABG after diagnostic angiography and high mortality of patients in cardiogenic shock, <5% of patients with cardiogenic shock are treated with emergent/immediate CABG.[11] In patients with complex left main disease, isolated lesions not amenable to PCI, severe three-vessel coronary artery disease or mechanical complications, emergent cardiac surgery remains the treatment of choice.

HEMODYNAMIC SUPPORT AND STABILIZATION

Placement of an IABP was an integral component of the early revascularization strategy in the SHOCK (Table 11.2) trial. IABP support will improve hemodynamics and may mitigate ischemia. IABP placement is contraindicated in patients with severe aortic regurgitation, peripheral vascular disease or coagulopathy. IABP placement should be performed by an experienced operator under fluoroscopic guidance but can be placed at the bedside under emergency conditions. Arterial access is first obtained through the femoral artery and a guidewire is placed into the aorta. The balloon pump is then advanced over this wire and placed in the descending aorta just distal to the takeoff of the left subclavian artery.[19] Once in the proper position, the IABP uses either the ECG or a pressure transducer located in the tip of the balloon to time inflation of the balloon so that it inflates during diastole and actively deflates during systole. Because coronary artery perfusion is dependent on the pressure difference between diastolic blood pressure in the aorta and the left ventricular end diastolic pressure, the increase in diastolic blood pressure improves coronary artery perfusion. The active deflation of the IABP during systole effectively reduces the pressure against which the heart must overcome when pumping (afterload), which may increase cardiac output and reduce myocardial oxygen demand.[20]

Adequate intravascular status should be confirmed in all patients. In the setting of hypotension, pharmacologic agents are also frequently used for additional hemodynamic support. In the setting of severe hypotension, intravenous norepineprine should be initiated as a recent trial has provided data showing that norepinephrine is superior to dopamine in this setting.[21] Vasopressin may be useful especially in settings of low systemic vascular resistance (SVR) but published experience in this setting is limited.

Pulmonary arterial catheters have not been shown to improve mortality in patients with chronic heart failure that has resulted in some providers moving away from its routine use.[22] Pulmonary arterial catheters can be helpful to monitor the response of patients with cardiogenic shock (Table 11.2) and this is reflected in the American College of Cardiology, American Heart Association (ACC/AHA) guidelines for the treatment of STEMI (which give a class I indication for placement in patients with hypotension that is unresponsive to IV fluid or if IV fluid is contraindicated).[16] Invasive arterial blood pressure monitoring is also indicated if there is significant hypotension that requires hemodynamic support or vasopressors.

PERSISTANT SHOCK

Cardiogenic shock may not resolve despite PCI and patency of the infarct-related artery. Patients with this clinical scenario have a grim prognosis and advanced ventricular support options should be considered in this group of subjects until there is resolution of shock (Figure 11.2).[23] These therapies are available only at large volume centers; therefore, consideration of transfer to centers that specialize in advanced heart therapies should be considered for all patients with refractory shock after revascularization. Short-term options available in the catheterization laboratory at the time of revascularization include the percutaneous TandemHeart and Impella devices. Surgical options

TABLE 11.2	Pulmonary Artery Catheter Findings in Shock	
	Pulmonary Capillary Wedge Pressure	*Cardiac Index*
Cardiogenic shock	High	Low
Distributive shock	Low	High

in this setting include extracorporeal membrane oxygenation (ECMO); however, these options are designed to provide only temporary support.

Definitive therapies for eligible patients with persistent shock are becoming more refined and available. Cardiac transplantation is a long-term option; however, the scarcity of available donor organs and the significant pretransplant evaluation necessary prior to listing prevent emergent transplantation from being a viable option under most circumstances. Left ventricular and biventricular assist devices are now available that can provide more hemodynamic support both as destination therapy and a bridge to transplantation. Although these therapies do offer promise, they are limited by the number of centers at which they are available, the high cost of implantation, and the difficulty in patient selection in this acute care setting.[19]

DISCHARGE PLANNING

Survivors of cardiogenic shock complicating myocardial infarction appear to have a reasonable long-term prognosis and an acceptable quality of life. They should be treated with appropriate evidence-based therapy for patients following an MI. Measures to prevent recurrent events such as smoking cessation, weight loss, and control of hypercholesterolemia with HMG Co-A reductase inhibitors (statins) should be emphasized. Cardiac rehabilitation has been shown to be beneficial after MI and should be utilized by all patients.[16] Finally, patients with AMI who are in NHYA class II–III heart failure with a left ventricular ejection fraction (LVEF) ≤35%, 40 days after the myocardial infarction benefit from an implantable cardiac defibrillator (ICD). In addition, current guidelines also recommend ICD placement in patients with AMI and no heart failure symptoms if the LVEF is ≤30%.[24]

SUMMARY

Cardiogenic shock occurs when cardiac output is insufficient to provide adequate perfusion for the body. Cardiogenic shock is most commonly seen in patients with AMI and is diagnosed using a definition that includes both clinical and hemodynamic criteria. The treatment of cardiogenic shock is based on reversal of the underlying cause (most commonly through revascularization and restoration of coronary blood flow) while providing hemodynamic support with an IABP and vasopressor medications. With prompt treatment and early revascularization, outcomes in this high-risk condition can be improved.

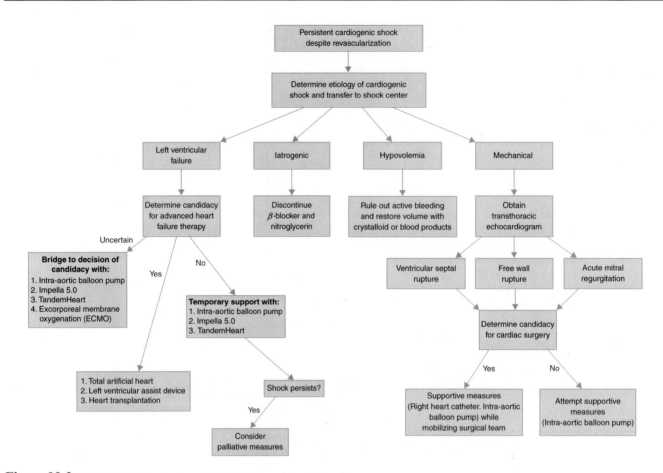

Figure 11.2. Algorithm for the treatment of persistent cardiogenic shock.

REFERENCES

1. Gruppo Italiano per lo Studio della Streptochinasi nell'Infarto Miocardico (GISSI). Effectiveness of intravenous thrombolytic treatment in acute myocardial infarction. *Lancet.* 1986;1:397–402.

2. Fox KA, Steg PG, Eagle KA, et al. Decline in rates of death and heart failure in acute coronary syndromes, 1999–2006. *JAMA.* 2007;297:1892–1900.

3. Hochman JS, Sleeper LA, Webb JG, et al. Early revascularization in acute myocardial infarction complicated by cardiogenic shock. SHOCK Investigators. Should We Emergently Revascularize Occluded Coronaries for Cardiogenic Shock. *N Engl J Med.* 1999;341:625–634.

4. Hochman JS, Boland J, Sleeper LA, et al. Current spectrum of cardiogenic shock and effect of early revascularization on mortality. Results of an International Registry. SHOCK Registry Investigators. *Circulation.* 1995;91:873–881.

5. Page DL, Caulfield JB, Kastor JA, et al. Myocardial changes associated with cardiogenic shock. *N Engl J Med.* 1971;285:133–137.

6. Jacobs AK, French JK, Col J, et al. Cardiogenic shock with non-ST-segment elevation myocardial infarction: a report from the SHOCK Trial Registry. SHould we emergently revascularize Occluded coronaries for Cardiogenic shocK? *J Am Coll Cardiol.* 2000;36:1091–1096.

7. Libby P, Braunwald E. *Braunwald's Heart Disease: A Textbook of Cardiovascular Medicine.* 8th ed. Philadelphia, PA: Saunders/Elsevier; 2008.

8. Guyton AC, Hall JE. *Textbook of Medical Physiology.* 11th ed. Philadelphia, PA: Elsevier Saunders; 2006.

9. Khouri EM, Gregg DE, Rayford CR. Effect of exercise on cardiac output, left coronary flow and myocardial metabolism in the unanesthetized dog. *Circ Res.* 1965;17:427–437.

10. Aymong ED, Ramanathan K, Buller CE. Pathophysiology of cardiogenic shock complicating acute myocardial infarction. *Med Clin North Am.* 2007;91:701–712; xii.

11. Babaev A, Frederick PD, Pasta DJ, et al. Trends in management and outcomes of patients with acute myocardial infarction complicated by cardiogenic shock. *JAMA.* 2005;294:448–454.

12. Goldberg RJ, Spencer FA, Gore JM, et al. Thirty-year trends (1975 to 2005) in the magnitude of, management of, and hospital death rates associated with cardiogenic shock in patients with acute myocardial infarction: a population-based perspective. *Circulation.* 2009;119:1211–1219.

13. Fang J, Mensah GA, Alderman MH, et al. Trends in acute myocardial infarction complicated by cardiogenic shock, 1979–2003, United States. *Am Heart J.* 2006;152:1035–1041.

14. Hochman JS, Sleeper LA, Webb JG, et al. Early revascularization and long-term survival in cardiogenic shock complicating acute myocardial infarction. *JAMA.* 2006;295:2511–2515.

15. Ortolani P, Marzocchi A, Marrozzini C, et al. Usefulness of prehospital triage in patients with cardiogenic shock complicating ST-elevation myocardial infarction treated with primary percutaneous coronary intervention. *Am J Cardiol.* 2007;100:787–792.

16. Antman EM, Anbe DT, Armstrong PW, et al. ACC/AHA guidelines for the management of patients with ST-elevation myocardial infarction—executive summary: a report of the American College of Cardiology/American Heart Association Task Force on Practice Guidelines (Writing Committee to Revise the 1999 Guidelines for the Management of Patients With Acute Myocardial Infarction). *Circulation.* 2004;110:588–636.

17. Cavender MA, Milford-Beland S, Weintraub WS, et al. Prevalence and in-hospital outcomes of multivessel PCI during primary PCI for ST-segment elevation myocardial infarction: results from the American College of Cardiology National Cardiovascular Data Registry (ACC-NCDR). *J Am Coll Cardiol.* 2008;51:A236.

18. White HD, Assmann SF, Sanborn TA, et al. Comparison of percutaneous coronary intervention and coronary artery bypass grafting after acute myocardial infarction complicated by cardiogenic shock: results from the Should We Emergently Revascularize Occluded Coronaries for Cardiogenic Shock (SHOCK) trial. *Circulation.* 2005;112:1992–2001.

19. Baim DS, Grossman W. *Grossman's Cardiac Catheterization, Angiography, and Intervention.* 7th ed. Philadelphia, PA: Lippincott Williams & Wilkins; 2006.

20. Santa-Cruz RA, Cohen MG, et al. Aortic counterpulsation: a review of the hemodynamic effects and indications for use. *Catheter Cardiovasc Interv.* 2006;67:68–77.

21. De Backer D, Biston P, Devriendt J, et al. Comparison of dopamine and norepinephrine in the treatment of shock. *N Engl J Med.* 2010;362:779–789.

22. Binanay C, Califf RM, Hasselblad V, et al. Evaluation study of congestive heart failure and pulmonary artery catheterization effectiveness: the ESCAPE trial. *JAMA.* 2005;294:1625–1633.

23. Kiernan MS, Krishnamurthy B, Kapur NK. Percutaneous right ventricular assist via the internal jugular vein in cardiogenic shock complicating an acute inferior myocardial infarction. *J Invasive Cardiol.* 2010;22:E23–E26.

24. Epstein AE, DiMarco JP, Ellenbogen KA, et al. ACC/AHA/HRS 2008 guidelines for device-based therapy of cardiac rhythm abnormalities: executive summary: a report of the American College of Cardiology/American Heart Association Task Force on Practice Guidelines (Writing Committee to Revise the ACC/AHA/NASPE 2002 Guideline Update for Implantation of Cardiac Pacemakers and Antiarrhythmia Devices) Developed in Collaboration With the American Association for Thoracic Surgery and Society of Thoracic Surgeons. *J Am Coll Cardiol.* 2008;51:2085–2105.

PATIENT AND FAMILY INFORMATION FOR:

Cardiogenic Shock Complicating Acute Myocardial Infarction

DEFINITION

The body requires a continuous supply of oxygen to properly function. Blood, pumped by the heart, carries the necessary oxygen to all parts of the body. If the pumping function of the heart becomes weak enough that it is unable to provide sufficient blood flow to the organs of the body, the body begins to shut down resulting in *cardiogenic shock*. Many different conditions can cause cardiogenic shock, but it is most commonly caused by a *myocardial infarction*, also known as a heart attack.

Like the rest of the body, human hearts also require a constant supply of oxygen. The *coronary arteries* carry the oxygen-carrying blood to the heart tissue. If this blood flow is interrupted by a blockage in one or more of the coronary arteries, a heart attack ensues. The heart tissue stops functioning properly when blood flow is disrupted, and it can die if it lacks blood flow for long. Large heart attacks can cause such significant damage to the heart that it is unable to pump enough blood to meet the needs of the body. When this occurs, it is known as cardiogenic shock.

SIGNS AND SYMPTOMS OF CARDIOGENIC SHOCK

Patients with cardiogenic shock will often complain of shortness of breath and appear to be unable to catch their breath. Chest, neck/jaw, or arm pain is also common in patients with cardiogenic shock caused by a heart attack. As a result of the weak condition of the heart, patients with cardiogenic shock will often have low blood pressures and high heart rates. It is also common for patients to be confused, have cool skin and make only minimal amounts of urine.

MANAGEMENT AND TREATMENT

Cardiogenic shock is a medical emergency, and patients with this condition need urgent care. When physicians are concerned that cardiogenic shock is present they will act quickly in an attempt to figure out the cause. Blood work will be obtained to determine the amount of red blood cells in the body, how well the kidneys are functioning, and if a patient is having a heart attack. Patients will have IV placed in their blood vessels so that medicines that act quickly can be given. At times it may even be necessary to place a large intravenous line, known as a central venous line, so that numerous medications can be given at the same time.

Patients who have evidence of an ongoing heart attack need blood flow to the heart restored quickly to minimize the amount of heart damage. Some hospitals have the ability to perform cardiac catheterization that allows for identification of the blocked artery. Using balloons and *stents*, special devices that prop the blood vessel open, blood flow can be restored to the heart. Some patients have such severe blockages that they require emergency *coronary artery bypass surgery* to restore blood flow or fix defects in the heart caused by the heart attack. In the event that the nearest hospital that performs catheterization is too far away or not available in a timely manner, some patients may be treated with medications designed to dissolve the blood clot in the coronary artery.

Patients who have blood flow restored through one of these methods (or in patients with cardiogenic shock owing to a cause other than a myocardial infarction) may require a device that improves the hearts ability to pump blood to the remainder of the body. The most common of these devices is an *balloon pump*. The balloon pump sits in a large blood vessel near the heart and inflates and deflates in such a way that maximizes blood flow to both the heart and the rest of the body. In addition, patients with cardiogenic shock are often treated with *mechanical ventilators* to assist with breathing, have *pulmonary artery catheters* placed to measure blood pressures and are given medications that improve the function of the heart. Physicians will also use an ultrasound machine, known as a *cardiac echocardiogram*, to evaluate the function and structure of the heart.

OUTCOMES/QUALITY OF LIFE

Cardiogenic shock is a serious problem that results in the death of one out of every two patients; however, survival in patients with heart attacks can be improved with the rapid restoration of blood flow to the heart. The amount of time, size, and area of the heart that is without blood flow are the most important factors in determining whether patients will survive heart attacks complicated by cardiogenic shock. Poor heart function, older age, and poor kidney function increase the odds that patients will not survive.

Although patients with cardiogenic shock are at high risk of death, about half of all patients will survive. Patients who had a normally functioning heart prior to the event that caused them to develop cardiac shock and survive their hospitalization have good outcomes and can live for long periods. In fact, most of the patients who survive cardiogenic shock and are discharged home will have minimal signs of heart failure 1 year after their hospitalization.

SUMMARY

Cardiogenic shock is serious problem that results in the death of half of affected patients. The most common cause of cardiogenic shock is a major heart attack. The treatment of patients with heart attacks begins with rapid restoration of blood flow to the heart. After blood flow is restored, patients are treated supportively with an IABP and medicines to improve the function of the heart. Despite the high risk of death, patients who were healthy prior their illness and can survive the hospitalization have a good chance of resuming a normal life.

Rajeev Joshi
Mark Sherrid

CHAPTER 12

Hypertrophic Cardiomyopathy

Hypertrophic cardiomyopathy (HCM) is characterized by hypertrophy of the left ventricle that occurs without clinical causes such as hypertension or aortic valve disease and is marked by variable morphologic, clinical, and hemodynamic abnormalities. HCM is the great masquerader of cardiology. It often masquerades as coronary artery disease as it presents with anginal chest pain owing to myocardial ischemia—although in the absence of epicardial coronary narrowings. It is particularly confusing when HCM presents with ST depressions, T-wave inversions, or pathologic Q waves. It often masquerades as dilated or ischemic cardiomyopathy, with congestive heart failure and cardiomegaly on X-ray. It may masquerade as mitral or aortic valve disease with systolic murmur and heart failure symptoms. Sometimes, tragically, HCM can masquerade as normal, when young adults die suddenly, sometimes at rest and sometimes on the athletic playing field. With this great diversity of presenting syndromes, HCM patients are admitted to the cardiac care unit (CCU) not infrequently, where it is vital to rapidly diagnose them and initiate disease-specific therapy. Missing the diagnosis of HCM in the CCU can lead to disastrous outcomes.

Its pathophysiology, diagnosis, and treatment span the gamut of cardiologic disciplines. The pathophysiology includes understanding of left ventricular (LV) outflow obstruction, mitral regurgitation, ischemia, atrial fibrillation, sudden death, diastolic dysfunction, aspects of molecular biology and genetics. Diagnostic testing with echocardiography, nuclear scintigraphy, stress testing, catheterization, 24-hour ECG, and MRI may be applied. Treatment may involve pharmacologic agents, the implanted defibrillator, surgical septal myectomy, transcoronary intervention in the form of alcohol septal ablation (ASA), or pacing. However, when these lists are examined, one recognizes that this is identical to the spectrum encountered in more common cardiac diseases. The challenge in HCM is learning the disease-specific pathophysiology and treatment indications.

GENETICS

HCM is inherited as an autosomal dominant trait; approximately half of patients have another family member with HCM. Unexplained hypertrophy occurs in 1:500 in the general population, making it the most common inherited cardiac disorder. Sarcomeric mutations of 18 genes that code for myofilaments or their supporting proteins have been identified as a cause of HCM.[1,2] In a cohort of referred, unrelated patients with HCM, approximately 50% of the patients were found to have sarcomeric mutations. In the remaining 50%, none of the known genotype abnormalities was found. Younger age at diagnosis, marked wall thickness, and a family history of HCM increase the frequency that a patient will be gene positive.

Echocardiographic appearance also appears to predict a high likelihood of sarcomeric protein mutation HCM; a reversed septal curvature causing a crescent-shaped LV cavity predicts gene-positive patients as compared with those with localized subaortic bulge and preserved septal curvature.[3] The most common mutations found are in the ß-myosin heavy chain and in myosin-binding protein C. Although most of genetically determined HCM occur on eight genes, many hundreds of HCM-causing mutations are dispersed over the many loci of the 18 genes. These genes may cause different phenotypes and may have different prognoses. Even among families with the same mutation on a particular locus, individuals vary with respect to phenotype and prognosis. This has markedly delayed genotype–phenotype correlation. The pathophysiologic linkage between mutations and hypertrophy appears to be mediated by mutation-induced functional abnormalities, most often because of increased contractile function. Recent theories about cause of hypertrophy have focused on inefficient utilization of ATP.

PATHOPHYSIOLOGY

On light microscopy individual myocyte hypertrophy is noted. Myocardial fiber disarray is the pathognomonic abnormality. In normal individuals, myocytes are arranged in linear parallel arrays. In HCM with fiber disarray, myocytes form chaotic intersecting bundles. With electron microscopy myofilament disarray is noted as well. Although fiber disarray is noted in other diseases, the percentage of the myocardium occupied by disarray is higher in patients with HCM. Fiber disarray is thought to predispose to electrical reentry and sudden death.

Fibrosis is also a prominent feature on light microscopy. Interstitial and perivascular fibrosis may occupy as much as 14% of the myocardium in patients who die suddenly. Fibrosis and hypertrophy decrease LV chamber compliance and cause diastolic dysfunction and exercise intolerance. Fibrosis appears to predispose to complex ventricular arrhythmia. Although the epicardial coronary arteries are dilated, narrowings of the intramural penetrating coronary arteries are noted, owing to arteriolar intimal and medial hyperplasia. These narrowings are thought to contribute to ischemia, well documented in HCM. Figure 12.1 shows such narrowings in myectomy resections.

DIAGNOSIS

HCM is diagnosed when LV hypertrophy occurs in the absence of a clinical condition that would cause the degree of hypertrophy noted.[4,5] Thus, to make the diagnosis of HCM it is important to evaluate for other cardiac or systemic conditions capable of

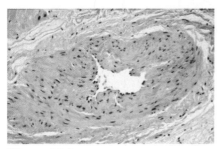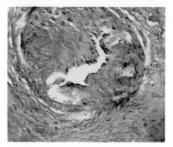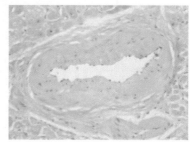

Figure 12.1. Histopathology from surgical specimens of three patients with obstructive HCM who underwent surgical septal myectomy for progressive heart failure symptoms. All three patients had intimal and medial hypertrophy of the intramural septal branches with luminal narrowing. Dense perivascular fibrosis is present in the middle frame. **Left** and **right**: Hematoxylin and eosin. **Middle**: Masson's trichrome stain.

producing the magnitude of hypertrophy evident (e.g., aortic valve stenosis, systemic hypertension, athlete's heart. Athlete's heart occurs only in elite highly trained competitive athletes where wall thickness up to 15 mm occurs.) Wall thickness >14 mm is the criteria used for diagnosis. Most of the patients who reach clinical attention have wall thicknesses between 20 and 30 mm. The location of the abnormal hypertrophy is most often the anterior septum, although the posterior septum and anterior wall are frequently hypertrophied as well. Typical of the heterogeneity of HCM is that hypertrophy can occur in any segment, even among relatives known to have the same genotype. Apical hypertrophy that spares the basilar and mid segments is a variant that occurs more frequently in East Asian patients with HCM. However, it is a relatively common variant in North American and European patients as well, occurring in 7%. This variant generally has a better prognosis. Truly atypical HCM variants include thickening just of the lateral wall or posterior wall. Wall thickening is most often assessed by two-dimensional echocardiography. Particular attention should be paid to the septum and also to the thickness of the anterior wall. The anterior wall is more difficult to visualize clearly than the septum because of poorer lateral resolution compared with the axial resolution of echocardiography systems. Magnetic resonance imaging may be useful in selected cases.

In a subset of patients, the site and extent of cardiac hypertrophy and abnormalities of the mitral valve result in obstruction to LV outflow. LV outflow tract (LVOT) obstruction is an important determinant of symptoms and is associated with adverse outcome. The commonest location of obstruction is in the LV outflow tract, caused by systolic anterior motion (SAM) of the mitral valve and mitral-septal contact.[6] The phenomenon of dynamic SAM is caused by a crucial anatomic overlap between the inflow and outflow portions of the left ventricle. Figure 12.2 shows dynamic SAM as it progresses though the early moments of systole. Narrowing of the LVOT and the anterior position of the coaptation point places the protruding leaflet into the edge of the flow stream, subject to the pushing force of flow that strikes the undersurface of the leaflet as illustrated in Figure 12.3.

LEFT VENTRICULAR OUTFLOW TRACT OBSTRUCTION

LVOT obstruction is quantified by measuring the pressure drop and the gradient across the narrowing. This is most commonly done with continuous wave Doppler echocardiography.

Pulsed Doppler correlation with the two-dimensional echocardiogram allows determination of the site of obstruction, which must be ascertained in every patient, especially if intervention is contemplated. LV outflow obstruction causes a mid-systolic drop in LV ejection velocities and flow when the gradient is >60 mm Hg. This echocardiographic pattern has been termed the "lobster claw" abnormality because of its characteristic appearance (Figure 12.4). Resting obstruction is considered present when a resting gradient of 30 mm Hg is present. Reducing preload may provoke a gradient by increasing the overlap between the inflow and outflow portions of the LV. Patients who have no resting gradient but who have gradients >30 mm Hg after maneuvers have latent obstruction, and patients with mild obstruction <30 mm Hg that rises >30 mm Hg after maneuvers have provocable obstruction. Typically, Valsalva, exercise, and standing may be used to provoke obstruction[7] and, on occasion, exercise in the postprandial state. As the main reason for provoking gradient is to correlate patient symptoms with obstruction and to provide a target for therapy, one should use only physiologic maneuvers, such as standing, exercise, or Valsalva. Dobutamine and amyl nitrite are not physiologic stimuli and should not be used to provoke gradient. Furthermore, dobutamine may provoke gradients in normal individuals. Clinically, we perform treadmill stress exercise echocardiography on all patients with HCM who are

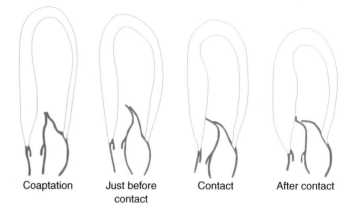

Coaptation   Just before contact   Contact   After contact

Figure 12.2. Systolic anterior motion of the mitral valve, drawn from apical five-chamber view, as it proceeds in early systole. (Adapted from Sherrid MV, Chu CK, Delia E, et al. An echocardiographic study of the fluid mechanics of obstruction in hypertrophic cardiomyopathy. *J Am Coll Cardiol.* 1993;22:816–825.)

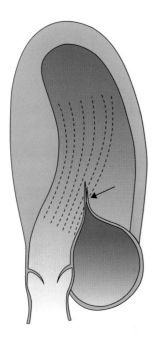

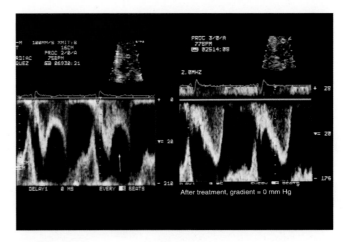

After treatment, gradient = 0 mm Hg

Figure 12.3. Left: The pushing force of flow. Intraventricular flow relative to the mitral valve in the apical five-chamber view. In obstructive HCM, the mitral leaflet coaptation point is closer to the septum than normal. The protruding leaflets extend into the edge of the flowstream and are swept by the pushing force of flow toward the septum. Flow pushes the underside of the leaflets *(arrow)*. Note that the midseptal bulge redirects flow so that it comes from a relatively lateral and posterior direction; on the five-chamber view flow comes from "right field" or "1 o'clock" direction. This contributes to the high angle of attack relative to the protruding leaflets. Also note that the posterior leaflet is shielded and separated from outflow tract flow by the cowl of the anterior leaflet. Venturi flow in the outflow tract cannot be lifting the posterior leaflet because there is little or no area of this leaflet exposed to outflow tract flow. Venturi forces cannot be causing the anterior motion of the posterior leaflet. (Adapted from Sherrid MV, Gunsburg DZ, Moldenhauer S, et al. Systolic anterior motion begins at low left ventricular outflow tract velocity in obstructive hypertrophic cardiomyopathy. *J Am Coll Cardiol.* 2000;36:1344–1354.)

Figure 12.4. Left: Mid-systolic drop in LV ejection velocity in obstructive HCM. Pulsed wave Doppler recording just apical of the entrance to the LVOT in a patient with severe dynamic obstruction due to SAM and mitral-septal contact. The pulsed wave cursor is 2 cm apical of the tips of the mitral valve leaflets. Long arrow points to the nadir of LV mid-systolic drop in LV ejection flow velocity. This drop in velocity has been called the lobster claw abnormality because of its characteristic appearance. The drop in velocity is due to the sudden imposition of afterload due to the mitral-septal contact and the gradient. **Right:** Pulsed wave Doppler in the same patient, from the same position, after pharmacologic relief of obstruction. The mid-systolic drop is no longer present.

able to exercise. An exception would be for patients with resting gradients of >80 mm Hg where little available information will be gained.

TREATMENT

There are *five aspects of care* that should be covered in the treatment of every HCM patient: (1) Risk of sudden death should be discussed and individual stratification of risk should be done. The average risk of dying suddenly is 1% per year for HCM patient populations, but the risk may be higher or lower depending on whether risk factors for sudden death are present. For patients deemed by their physicians to be at high risk, discussion of implantation of a cardioverter defibrillator should be considered. (2) Treatment of symptoms. (3) Discussion and advice to avoid athletic competition and extremes of exertion. (4) Detection and management of hypercholesterolemia (HCM and coronary disease have an adverse synergistic effect on prognosis). (5) Screening of first degree family members either through echocardiograms and EKGs, or through genetic

testing to assess who has inherited the HCM genes. Although many aspects of this evaluation can wait until a patient is stabilized after the CCU stay, it must be remembered that HCM is a lifelong condition and that these issues need discussion and management when the dust clears.

PHARMACOLOGIC TREATMENT OF SYMPTOMS

Figure 12.5 outlines an algorithm for the management of symptomatic HCM. It divided the patient into two groups of obstructed HCM and nonobstructed HCM.

NONOBSTRUCTIVE HCM

In symptomatic nonobstructive HCM symptoms are owing to diastolic dysfunction, impaired relaxation early in diastole, and decreased chamber compliance in late diastole. The pathology is small LV volumes, hypertrophy, fiber disarray, and fibrosis. Few agents are available, and they are not particularly effective in improving severe symptoms owing to diastolic dysfunction. No pharmacologic agent has been consistently shown to improve LV relaxation and chamber compliance in HCM.[8] Therefore, treatment options for symptomatic nonobstructive HCM are limited.[9] Two treatment goals are to improve LV diastolic function and to improve ischemia. Two classes of agents are currently used—β-blockade and calcium channel blockade. Neither class of agents has been shown to improve diastolic chamber compliance.[10] Verapamil's positive contribution in the pathophysiology of nonobstructive HCM appears to be relief of ischemia. Verapamil improves myocardial perfusion as

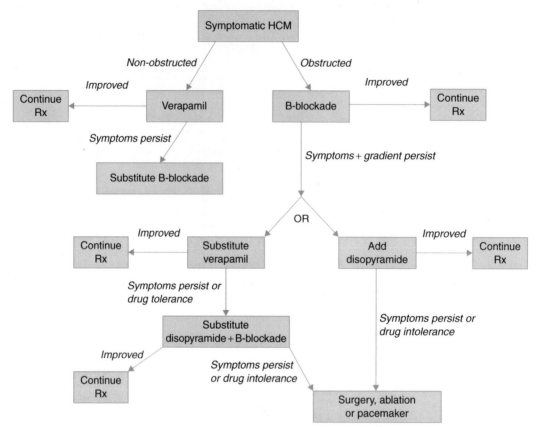

Figure 12.5. A schematic summary of the pharmacologic therapy of HCM. (Adapted from Sherrid M, Barac I. Pharmacologic treatment of symptomatic hypertrophic cardiomyopathy. In: Maron B, ed. *Diagnosis and Management of Hypertrophic Cardiomyopathy*. London: Blackwell-Futura; 2004:200–219.)

assessed by stress radionuclide perfusion imaging[11] and may thus improve symptoms.

Beta blockade, and, to a lesser degree, verapamil, may cause chronotropic incompetence in HCM.[12] As diastolic dysfunction may limit the exercise-induced increase in stroke volume, patients with HCM often rely on increased heart rate to increase cardiac output. In such patients, pharmacologic limitation of increase in heart rate may impair exercise capacity. Whereas disopyramide has been shown to improve diastolic function in obstructed patients, by decreasing gradient and systolic load,[13,14] it has not been shown to improve diastolic function in nonobstructed patients and should be avoided in this group, pending further investigation. For the patient with fluid retention, with edema or rales, diuretics may be helpful by relieving dyspnea and uncommon edema. Overdiuresis should be avoided as patients with HCM are often preload dependent for adequate cardiac output. If patients initially present with edema, another diagnosis should be sought as this is very unusual. Amyloid may be suspected in this clinical situation, especially if the ECG QRS voltage is low. In animal models of HCM, aldosterone antagonism has been shown to improve or prevent fibrosis and hypertrophy.[15] Similarly, statin therapy has been shown to prevent phenotype in genotype-positive animals.[16] As a new designation, these pharmacologic agents may be termed fibrotardive. Clinical trials would seem appropriate for these new approaches as there is currently no good pharmacologic treatment for advanced symptoms in nonobstructive HCM.

OBSTRUCTIVE HCM

Pharmacologic therapy of symptoms in obstructive HCM (OHCM) is successful in two-thirds of patients. Negatively inotropic drugs improve dynamic LV outflow obstruction by decreasing ejection acceleration.[17] Decreasing ejection acceleration decreases flow velocities early in systole, decreasing early drag forces on the mitral valve, delaying mitral-septal contact, and reducing gradient. Delaying the early trigger of SAM may allow reassertion of chordal tension by papillary muscle shortening to provide countertraction to prevent SAM—even completely.

β-Blockade is the initial treatment for symptomatic obstructed patients.[9,18] β-Blockers decrease the sympathetic-mediated rise in gradient with exercise and improve symptoms. However, β-blockade is not expected to reduce resting gradient and less than half of patients have sustained improvement in symptoms. For patients with refractory symptoms and high gradients after β-blockade, there is regional variation in the choice of the next drug trial. In many centers, the next trial selected is substitution of verapamil for β-blocker.[9,19] In other centers, disopyramide is added to β-blockade.[9,14,20,21]

Verapamil, a potent calcium channel blocker (CCB), has negative inotropic properties but is also a vasodilator. It has been shown to decrease gradient and improve symptoms. In a limited number of patients, exercise tolerance has been shown to increase as well. Verapamil is indicated for patients with mild to moderate symptoms and moderate gradients. However, it is not used in patients with severe obstruction and severe symptoms because, on occasion, vasodilating effects outweigh negatively inotropic effects: gradient may rise, and pulmonary edema and death have been reported. In addition, heart block and bradycardia may complicate its use.

Disopyramide is a type I antiarrhythmic drug, with potent negatively inotropic properties; in normal individuals, it decreases echocardiographic fractional shortening by 28%. It is a sodium channel blocker and may have calcium channel blocking properties as well; however, it is not a vasodilator. Disopyramide is generally given to patients who are refractory to β-blockade and would otherwise require intervention with surgical septal myectomy or alcohol septal ablation. In a multicenter study, two-thirds of patients with obstructed HCM treated with disopyramide combined with a β-blocker could be managed medically with amelioration of symptoms and 50% reduction in LVOT gradient when followed for 3 years. The remaining one-third of patients could not be managed successfully with disopyramide and required invasive treatments because of inadequate symptom and gradient control or vagolytic side effects. There was a trend to lower cardiac mortality and sudden death. Disopyramide therapy was not proarrhythmic in OHCM (Figures 12.6 and 12.7).

The dose of disopyramide that is most often successful is 250 mg twice a day, using the controlled release preparation to allow twice a day dosing.[9] For patients who do not respond, dose is increased to 300 mg twice a day. Disopyramide is generally given with an agent with atrioventricular (AV) nodal blocking properties, to slow exercise heart rate and to slow ventricular response, should atrial fibrillation occur. Although disopyramide has been most often used with β-blockade, it may also be used in conjunction with verapamil. Disopyramide does not cause hepatic, renal, or central nervous system toxicity. Mild vagolytic side effects, dry mouth, blurred vision, and constipation are common but generally subside. If they prove troubling, the dosage

may be reduced, or controlled-release pyridostigmine may be added, 180 mg per day (Mestinon Timespan, ICN, Costa Mesa, CA). A more serious vagolytic side effect is urinary retention. Disopyramide should not be given to patients with symptoms of prostatism. If this proscription is observed, urinary retention is rare. Vagolytic side effects cause discontinuation of disopyramide in 7% of patients. Because of its impaired elimination in renal failure, disopyramide should be administered in reduced dosage or with serum monitoring. We do not administer concomitant amiodarone, sotolol, or other antiarrhythmic drugs with disopyramide to avoid electrophysiologic drug interaction and ventricular arrhythmia. We also avoid macrolide antibiotics. Because disopyramide is a type I antiarrhythmic, and because proarrhythmia has been observed in patients with other heart diseases, we begin disopyramide in the hospital for 3 days with ECG monitoring. However, this is not the practice of the non-US centers that actively use disopyramide, and the nearly complete absence of any significant arrhythmia during our 3-day admissions would support outpatient initiation in uncomplicated cases. We routinely perform ECG surveillance of the QTc interval every 4 months at all follow-up clinic visits. We will not increase disopyramide if QTc prolongation has occurred longer than 525 milliseconds in patient with normal QRS duration, but QTc prolongation has not prompted drug discontinuation.

DRUGS TO AVOID (OR DISCONTINUE) IN OBSTRUCTIVE HYPERTROPHIC CARDIOMYOPATHY

All vasodilators are contraindicated in OHCM. These include drugs widely used in clinical cardiology and in the CCU in coronary disease patients. These include all nitrate preparations (sublingual, topical, and IV); dihydropyridine CCBs

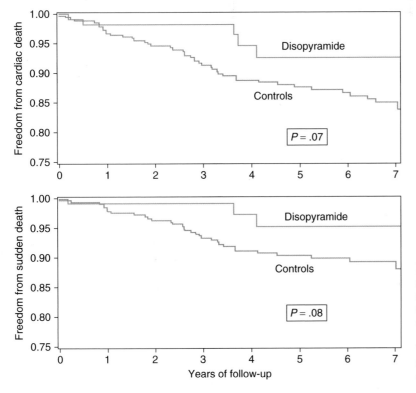

Figure 12.6. **Top:** Kaplan-Meier survival plot for all-cause cardiac mortality in disopyramide-treated and nondisopyramide patients. **Bottom:** Kaplan-Meier survival plot for sudden cardiac death mortality in disopyramide-treated and nondisopyramide patients. (Adapted from Sherrid MV, Barac I, McKenna WJ, et al. Multicenter study of the efficacy and safety of disopyramide in obstructive hypertrophic cardiomyopathy. *J Am Coll Cardiol.* 2005;45:1251–1258.)

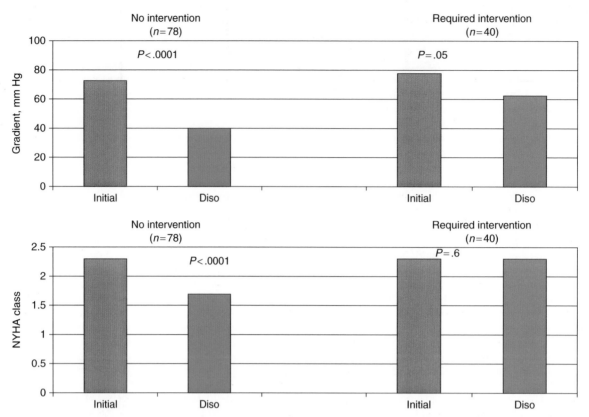

Figure 12.7. Top: Response of LV outflow tract gradient to disopyramide in 78 patients treated medically without require-ment for major nonpharmacologic intervention (such as surgical septal myectomy, alcohol septal ablation, or dual-chamber pacing), and 40 patients who required invasive intervention. **Bottom:** Response of NYHA class to disopyramide in 78 patients treated medically without requirement for non-pharmacologic intervention (such as surgical septal myectomy, alcohol septal ablation, or dual-chamber pacing), and 40 patients who ultimately had such interventions. (Adapted from Sherrid MV, Barac I, McKenna WJ, et al. Multicenter study of the efficacy and safety of disopyramide in obstructive hypertrophic cardiomyopa-thy. *J Am Coll Cardiol.* 2005;45:1251–1258.)

(amlodipine and nifedipine); angiotensin-converting enzyme in-hibitors, angiotensin receptor blockers; α-blockers that are used for prostatism. Furthermore, drugs that increase contractility should always be avoided in OHCM—including dopamine, dobu-tamine, milrinone, and digoxin. If OHCM patient is hypotensive, we should choose pure α-agonists such as phenylephrine or levo-phed, for therapy.

SURGICAL SEPTAL MYECTOMY

Myectomy is the treatment of choice for patients who fail medical therapy.[22,23] Candidates for myectomy have persistent disabling symptoms and gradients of >50 mm Hg at rest or af-ter physiologic provocation. Myectomy has been successfully performed for 30 years, and in experienced centers it can be performed with low-surgical mortality of 1%. It is uniformly successful in reducing both gradient and symptoms.

NEW METHODS TO RELIEVE OBSTRUCTION

New methods to relieve obstruction have been developed:

1. Revised surgical techniques
2. Alcohol septal ablation
3. Dual chamber pacing.

REVISED SURGICAL TECHNIQUES

Interventions are not always successful and the reason for het-erogeneity in response is not clear. Understanding the central role of flow drag in the pathogenesis of SAM may prevent treat-ment failures. Inadequate myectomy resection focused on just the subaortic septum, targeted to widen the outflow tract and to reduce Venturi forces, may result in persistent SAM and ob-struction. A limited myectomy misses the impact of the mid-ventricular septal bulge that redirects LV flow so that it comes from a relatively posterolateral direction. This sort of resec-tion results in persistent SAM and either outflow obstruction or mitral regurgitation because flow must still course around the remaining septal hypertrophy, and it still catches the mitral valve and pushes it into the septum, and causes mitral regurgi-tation. To alleviate this sort of residual SAM, investigators from Germany have popularized the extended myectomy. More ex-tensive resection redirects flow away from the mitral valve pre-cluding drag-induced SAM. A large decrease in the angle of attack of flow relative to the mitral valve has been shown after successful myectomy; flow is made more parallel to the mitral valve. The myectomy resection must be extended far enough down toward the apex to allow flow to track anteriorly along the surgically reduced septum away from the mitral valve.

Practically, preoperatively, the resection should be planned by measuring the distance on the echocardiogram from the aor-tic valve to the far side of the septal bulge, well past the contact point of the mitral valve. In our experience, in most patients with a mid-septal bulge, this distance is about 4.5 cm. These considerations also apply to site selection for percutaneous ASA procedures. Targeting the basal septum alone is unlikely to completely relieve SAM, obstruction, and mitral regurgitation.

When surgery is selected, myectomy is preferred over mitral replacement for relief of LV outflow tract obstruction in HCM patients refractory to pharmacotherapy. At our institution myectomy is selected whenever feasible with a ratio of >10:1 myectomy:mitral valve replacement.

ALCOHOL SEPTAL ABLATION

Percutaneous ASA offers the attractive promise of septal reduction without cardiopulmonary bypass and its complications. After placement of a temporary right ventricular pacing lead, a small diameter balloon catheter is placed in a selected left anterior descending (LAD) septal branch, and after inflating the balloon, angiographic contrast is injected to assure that contrast does not reflux back into the LAD septal branch. Diluted echo contrast is then injected during transthoracic or transesophageal echocardiographic imaging. In 8% of such injections, contrast is seen to flow to structures where alcohol injection would be disastrous: posterior LV wall, RV free wall, mitral papillary muscles, or the entire septum. With this information, the operator searches for a septal branch that can be demonstrated to supply just the upper septum, preferably including and extending past the point of mitral septal contact. A dose of 1 to 3 ml of absolute alcohol is instilled into the septal branch. Optimally, a controlled myocardial infarction occurs. This is accompanied by typical chest pain, enzyme elevation, and risk for potentially lethal ventricular arrhythmia. The acute gradient reduction of ASA is caused by reduced ejection acceleration from the infarct and decreased hemodynamic force on the mitral valve decreasing SAM identically as in negatively inotropic medications. Late improvement stems from septal thinning owing to septal scar.

DUAL-CHAMBER PACING

Dual-chamber pacing with complete ventricular preexcitation through a short AV delay significantly reduces outflow tract gradients.[24] However, therapeutic effect is often incomplete; SAM persists with mean gradients of 30 to 55 mm Hg after 3 months of pacing. The mechanism by which pacing benefits SAM is unclear at this time. It must be because of the dyssynchrony caused by the right ventricular pacing, or because of the short AV delay. DDD pacing helps only about half the patients; therefore it is not first line therapy for obstruction. It is usually reserved for patients with comorbid medical conditions or old age where it is given in conjunction with disopyramide and β-blocker.

IMPLANTED CARDIOVERTER DEFIBRILLATOR

Although not a decision made solely in the CCU, the implanted defibrillator has a role in the spectrum of care for HCM patients. Situations that may arise in CCU patients that may prompt recommendation of implantable cardioverter defibrillator (ICD) insertion include presentation with unexplained syncope or ventricular tachycardia—nonsustained or

persistent. Other risk factors that are associated with higher risk for SCD and may prompt ICD include massive segmental wall thickening ≥30 mm, family history of SCD from HCM in a young family member, and apical akinetic aneurysm owing to mid-LV obstruction.

MANAGEMENT OF ACUTE DECOMPENSATION OF PATIENTS WITH HCM

The most common cause of acute decompensation is the acute onset of atrial fibrillation. Loss of the atrial kick and rapid heart rate can provoke heart failure symptoms but uncommonly shock. The first consideration should be whether the patient needs acute cardioversion for severe heart failure or shock. For most other patients slowing ventricular rate with β-blockade, often IV, is generally the best first treatment option. Verapamil may be used in nonobstructed patients but not in patients with resting obstruction. Amiodarone may be used to slow ventricular rate, but in nonanticoagulated patients it should be used only in those who have recent (<48 hours) atrial fibrillation because the drug has the potential to cardiovert the patient. Anticoagulation with parenteral heparin is indicated. Systemic embolism is very common in HCM atrial fibrillation patients. For patients in atrial fibrillation >48 hours transesophageal echocardiogram (TEE) should be performed to exclude the presence of left atrial appendage thrombus. If there is no left atrial appendage thrombus, cardioversion may be performed either electrically or pharmacologically.

In patients with HCM and latent obstruction with severe LV dysfunction, pulmonary congestion and cardiogenic shock may develop acutely, in association with severe resting LV outflow obstruction. The complete reversal of these findings after relief of LV outflow tract obstruction indicates that they were caused by the dynamic obstruction caused by SAM of the mitral valve and mitral-septal contact. There are reports of OHCM with pulmonary edema and cardiogenic shock reversed by removing inciting causes and cautious pharmacotherapy. In shock from obstruction that is refractory to pharmacologic management, profound LV systolic dysfunction due to afterload mismatch has been observed. If all other measures fail, urgent surgical relief of obstruction has been associated with immediate reversal of systolic dysfunction and shock.[25]

REFERENCES

1. Seidman JG, Seidman C. The genetic basis for cardiomyopathy: from mutation identification to mechanistic paradigms. *Cell.* 2001;104:557–567.
2. Van Driest SL, Ommen SR, Tajik AJ, et al. Yield of genetic testing in hypertrophic cardiomyopathy. *Mayo Clin Proc.* 2005;80:739–744.
3. Binder J, Ommen SR, Gersh BJ, et al. Echocardiography-guided genetic testing in hypertrophic cardiomyopathy: septal morphological features predict the presence of myofilament mutations. *Mayo Clin Proc.* 2006;4:459–467.
4. Maron BJ, McKenna WJ, Danielson GK, et al. American College of Cardiology/European Society of Cardiology clinical expert consensus document on hypertrophic cardiomyopathy. A report of the American College of Cardiology Foundation Task Force on Clinical Expert Consensus Documents and the European Society of Cardiology Committee for Practice Guidelines. *J Am Coll Cardiol.* 2003;42:1687–1713.
5. Ommen SR, Nishimura RA. Hypertrophic cardiomyopathy. *Curr Probl Cardiol.* 2004;29:239–291.
6. Sherrid MV, Gunsburg DZ, Moldenhauer S, et al. Systolic anterior motion begins at low left ventricular outflow tract velocity in obstructive hypertrophic cardiomyopathy. *J Am Coll Cardiol.* 2000;36:1344–1354.
7. Sasson Z, Yock PG, Hatle LK, et al. Doppler echocardiographic determination of the pressure gradient in hypertrophic cardiomyopathy. *J Am Coll Cardiol.* 1988;11:752–756.

8. Kass DA, Wolff MR, Ting CT, et al. Diastolic compliance of hypertrophied ventricle is not acutely altered by pharmacologic agents influencing active processes. *Ann Intern Med.* 1993;119:466–473.

9. Sherrid M, Barac I. Pharmacologic treatment of symptomatic hypertrophic cardiomyopathy. In: Maron B, ed. *Diagnosis and Management of Hypertrophic Cardiomyopathy*. London: Blackwell-Futura; 2004:200–219.

10. Nishimura RA, Holmes DR, Tajik AJ. Failure of calcium channel blockers to improve ventricular relaxation in humans. *J Am Coll Cardiol.* 1993;21:182–188.

11. Udelson JE, Bonow RO, O'Gara PT, et al. Verapamil prevents silent myocardial perfusion abnormalities during exercise in asymptomatic patients with hypertrophic cardiomyopathy. *Circulation.* 1989;79:1052–1060.

12. Gilligan DM, Chan WL, Joshi J, et al. A double-blind, placebo-controlled crossover trial of nadolol and verapamil in mild and moderately symptomatic hypertrophic cardiomyopathy. *J Am Coll Cardiol.* 1993;21:1672–1679.

13. Matsubara H, Nakatani S, Nagata S, et al. Salutary effect of disopyramide on left ventricular diastolic function in hypertrophic obstructive cardiomyopathy. *J Am Coll Cardiol.* 1995;26:768–775.

14. Pollick C, Kimball B, Henderson M, et al. Disopyramide in hypertrophic cardiomyopathy. I. Hemodynamic assessment after intravenous administration. *Am J Cardiol.* 1988;62:1248–1251.

15. Tsybouleva N, Zhang L, Chen S, et al. Aldosterone, through novel signaling proteins, is a fundamental molecular bridge between the genetic defect and the cardiac phenotype of hypertrophic cardiomyopathy. *Circulation.* 2004;109:1284–1291.

16. Senthil V, Chen SN, Tsybouleva N, et al. Prevention of cardiac hypertrophy by atorvastatin in a transgenic rabbit model of human hypertrophic cardiomyopathy. *Circ Res.* 2005;97:285–292.

17. Sherrid MV, Pearle G, Gunsburg DZ. Mechanism of benefit of negative inotropes in obstructive hypertrophic cardiomyopathy. *Circulation.* 1998;97:41–47.

18. Flamm MD, Harrison DC, Hancock EW. Muscular subaortic stenosis. Prevention of outflow obstruction with propranolol. *Circulation.* 1968;38:846–858.

19. Rosing DR, Condit JR, Maron BJ, et al. Verapamil therapy: a new approach to the pharmacologic treatment of hypertrophic cardiomyopathy: III. Effects of long-term administration. *Am J Cardiol.* 1981;48:545–553.

20. Sherrid MV, Barac I, McKenna WJ, et al. Multicenter study of the efficacy and safety of disopyramide in obstructive hypertrophic cardiomyopathy. *J Am Coll Cardiol.* 2005;45: 1251–1258.

21. Sherrid M, Delia E, Dwyer E. Oral disopyramide therapy for obstructive hypertrophic cardiomyopathy. *Am J Cardiol.* 1988;62:1085–1088.

22. Williams WG, Wigle ED, Rakowski H, et al. Results of surgery for hypertrophic obstructive cardiomyopathy. *Circulation.* 1987;76:V104–V108.

23. Ommen SR, Maron BJ, Olivotto I, et al. Long-term effects of surgical septal myectomy on survival in patients with obstructive hypertrophic cardiomyopathy. *J Am Coll Cardiol.* 2005;46:470–476.

24. Fananapazir L, Epstein ND, Curiel RV, et al. Long-term results of dual-chamber (DDD) pacing in obstructive hypertrophic cardiomyopathy. Evidence for progressive symptomatic and hemodynamic improvement and reduction of left ventricular hypertrophy. *Circulation.* 1994;90:2731–2742.

25. Sherrid MV, Balaram S, Korzenieki E et al. Reversal of Acute Systolic Dysfunction and Cardiogenic Shock in Hypertrophic Cardiomyopathy by Surgical Relief of Obstruction. *Echocardiography* 2011;28:E174–E179.

PATIENT AND FAMILY INFORMATION FOR:
Hypertrophic Cardiomyopathy

HYPERTROPHIC CARDIOMYOPATHY (HCM)

HCM is characterized by thickening of the left ventricle that occurs without clinical cause such as high blood pressure or aortic valve disease. It is marked by varying symptoms and abnormalities. HCM is the great masquerader of cardiology. It often masquerades as coronary artery disease as it presents with chest pain, but in the absence of significant coronary narrowings. It is paticularly confusing when HCM may present with EKG abnormalities mimicking those found in coronary disease.

HCM is characterized by thickening of the heart muscle, most commonly at the septum between the ventricles. This leads to stiffening of the walls of the heart and abnormal mitral valve function that may obstruct normal blood flow out of the heart. Many people with HCM have no symptoms or only minor symptoms and live a normal life. Other people develop symptoms that progress and worsen as heart function worsens.

Symptoms of HCM can occur at any age and may include chest pain or pressure that can occur with exercise or physical activity or at rest as well. Shortness of breath especially with exertion and fatigue (feeling overly tired) are often experienced. Initial presenting symptom could be a fainting episode (syncope) caused by irregular heart rhythms or abnormal responses of the blood vessels. Some patients may experience palpitations (fluttering in the chest) because of abnormal heart rhythms (arrhythmias), such as atrial fibrillation or ventricular tachycardia. Sudden death may occur as the presenting symptom in a small number of patients with HCM. HCM can run in families as a dominant genetic trait, owing to a gene that is inherited in half of the first degree relatives. In other instances, the cause is unknown.

HCM is diagnosed based on medical history (symptoms and family history), a physical exam, and echocardiogram results. Additional tests may include blood tests, ECG, chest X-ray, exercise stress test, cardiac catheterization, CT scan, and MRI.

In a subset of patients, the site and extent of cardiac thickening and abnormalities of the mitral valve result in obstruction to left ventricular outflow. Left ventricular outflow tract (LVOT) obstruction is an important determinant of symptoms and is associated with adverse outcome. Obstruction is an important therapeutic target in HCM because relief of obstruction by any means leads to improved symptoms. The commonest location of obstruction is in the LV outflow tract, caused by systolic anterior motion (SAM) of the mitral valve and mitral-septal contact. The phenomenon of dynamic SAM is caused by a crucial anatomic overlap between the inflow and outflow portions of the left ventricle. Figure 12.2 shows dynamic SAM as it progresses though the early moments of cardiac contraction.

There are *five aspects of care* that should be covered in the treatment of every HCM patient: (1) Risk of sudden death should be discussed and individual stratification of risk should be done. The average risk of dying suddenly is 1% per year for HCM patient populations, but the risk may be higher or lower depending on whether risk factors for sudden death are present. For patients deemed by their physicians to be at high risk implantation of a cardioverter defibrillator should be considered. (2) Treatment of symptoms. (3) Discussion and advice to avoid athletic competition and extremes of exertion. (4) Detection and management of hypercholesterolemia (HCM and coronary disease have an adverse synergistic effect on prognosis). (5) Screening of first degree family members either through echocardiograms and EKGs, or through genetic testing to assess who has inherited the HCM genes. Gene testing is positive for a disease-causing mutation. Although many aspects of this evaluation can wait until a patient is stabilized after the CCU stay, it must be remembered that HCM is a lifelong condition and that these issues need discussion and management when the dust clears.

Lifestyle changes may alter the course of HCM. Simple things like drinking adequate amounts of fluids, and avoiding competitive sports are important. Regular visits with a cardiologist are highly important. Patients with HCM should seek at least one consultation with a cardiologist at a specialized HCM treatment center—such doctors treat many HCM patients, whereas the usual cardiologist will see few in his/her career.

Patients with HCM may find themselves in a CCU setting because of acute onset of symptoms of chest pain, shortness of breath or syncope, or the new onset of atrial fibrillation, a rapid irregular heart rhythm. Pharmacologic therapy is the first line of treatment for symptoms of HCM. Drugs are used to treat symptoms and prevent further complications of HCM. Medications are used to reduce the degree of obstruction in the heart so that it can pump more efficiently. ß-Blockers, disopyramide and calcium channel blockers are medications that may be prescribed for obstruction. If there is an arrhythmia, medications to control heart rate or decrease the occurrence of arrhythmias may be prescribed. Certain medications, such as nitrates (because they lower blood pressure and worsen obstruction in the heart) or digoxin, dopamine, and dobutamine (because they increase the force of the heart's contraction and worsen obstruction) may need to be avoided.

If pulmonary fluid collection occurs, treatment is aimed at controlling it through diuretics.

Surgical procedures are used to treat HCM when pharmacologic therapy fails to improved symptoms and obstruction. The "gold standard" is surgical septal myectomy. During this open heart surgical procedure, the surgeon removes a small amount of the thickened septal wall of the heart to widen the outflow tract (the path the blood takes) from the left ventricle to the aorta. This highly effective operation is done at specialized centers with a surgical mortality of <1%. Another important complication is the need for permanent pacing because of interruption of the normal electrical pathway of the heart.

Ethanol ablation is another approach that involves cardiac catheterization to locate the small coronary artery that supplies blood flow to the septum. Small amounts of pure alcohol are injected through the catheter, which kills the cells on contact, causing a small "controlled" heart attack. This therapy decreases the contractile force of the heart and decreases obstruction in that way acutely. Later the septum shrinks back to a more normal size over the following months, widening the passage for blood flow. Most HCM centers reserve ethanol ablation for patients who have substantial complicating medical illnesses, or old age and frailty because the procedural risks are comparable to surgical myectomy, but the results are overall not as satisfactory.

IMPLANTABLE CARDIOVERTER DEFIBRILLATORS

Implantable cardioverter defibrillators (ICD) are suggested for people at risk for life-threatening arrhythmias or sudden cardiac death. The ICD constantly monitors the heart rhythm. When it detects a very fast, abnormal heart rhythm, it delivers small electric currents or shocks to the heart muscle to cause the heart to beat in a normal rhythm again.

A small number of people with HCM have an increased risk of sudden cardiac death. People at risk include the following:

1. Patients with massive thickening of the left ventricle.

2. Those who have close family members who have had sudden cardiac death at a young age, thought to be because of HCM.

3. Young patients with HCM with fainting without cause. Generally, this is considered most important when blackout has happened within the last 6 months.

4. Adults who have a history of arrhythmia with a fast heart rate originating from the ventricles, called ventricular tachycardia.

5. Those who have an abnormal blood pressure response with exercise.

6. Those with severe symptoms and poor contractile heart function.

If a risk factor or risk factors are present, the strategy of the ICD is discussed with the patient, and the decision to implant depends on physician judgment and patient choice.

MANAGEMENT OF ACUTE DECOMPENSATION OF PATIENTS WITH HCM

Atrial fibrillation can cause an acute worsening of symptoms and may be treated with medications to slow the heart or conversion back to a regular rhythm, either with medication or with small electric shock to the chest wall after deep sedation. On occasion transesophageal echocardiogram (passing a probe down the esophagus to carefully inspect the heart chambers) is necessary to be sure there are no clots in the heart.

In patients with HCM and underlying obstruction to blood flow, severe heart failure can develop acutely with congestion in the lungs and severe decrease in the blood flow to the organs in the body (cardiogenic shock). This condition requires patients to be admitted and treated in the intensive cardiac care units as the acute decompensation can be fatal as well. Negatively inotropic medications are administered either through the veins or as pills that help relieve the obstruction to blood flow from the heart and hence improve heart function. Generally intravenous fluids are given. The blood pressure has to be continuously monitored and certain specific medications may need to be given through the veins to maintain blood pressure. Continuous monitoring of possible arrhythmias is an integral part of the cardiac care unit management.

Common medications to avoid in obstructive HCM (because they worsen heart failure symptoms) are listed Table 12.1.

TABLE 12.1	**Common Medications to Avoid in Obstructive HCM**

All nitrate preparations: sublingual, topical, or intravenous
Dihydropyridine calcium channel blockers (the "...pines"): amlodipine, nifedipine
ACE inhibitors (The "...prils"): lisinopril, enalapril, ramipril
Angiotension receptor blockers (the "...sartans"): losartan, valsartan, irbesartan
α-Blockers: tamsulosin (Flomax), terazosin (Hytrin)
Inotropic agents: dopamine, dobutamine, digoxin, milrinone

Mechanical Circulatory Support

Medical and electrical therapies have greatly improved the prognosis of patients with chronic heart failure (CHF). However, for patients with end-stage, refractory CHF (American College of Cardiology/American Heart Association Stage D CHF), medical and electrical therapies are insufficient. It is estimated that 0.2% of people aged >45 years in the United States have Stage D CHF,[1-2] meaning that approximately 200,000 people could benefit from cardiac transplantation as the treatment for their disease. Unfortunately, approximately only 2,200 cardiac transplantations are performed each year in the United States because of a huge donor shortage. Owing to the epidemiologic limitations of cardiac transplantation, mechanical circulatory support has evolved to meet the needs of patients with Stage D CHF.

Mechanical circulatory support involves the use of a left ventricular assist device (LVAD) to improve hemodynamics. There are three main situations when LVADs are implanted: bridge to recovery, bridge to transplantation (BTT), and destination therapy (DT).

Bridge to recovery encompasses a clinical setting where there is an expectation of recovery of cardiac function. Examples include acute myocarditis, acute myocardial infarction, and postcardiotomy shock after open heart surgery.

BTT involves implanting an LVAD in patients who are listed for cardiac transplantation. Owing to the extended wait times for a donor organ, BTT patients need to have hemodynamic support with an LVAD prior to transplantation.

DT refers to the long-term placement of an LVAD in patients with Stage D CHF who are ineligible for cardiac transplantation. There was initial enthusiasm for the use of LVADs in patients with severe CHF to completely unload the LV and allow the initiation of high-dose CHF medications as well as the β_2-adrenergic receptor agonist clenbuterol. In a small single-center study, this regimen led to the reversal of CHF and allowed LVAD explantation in 11 of 15 patients.[3] Unfortunately, such a degree of myocardial improvement was not seen in a multicenter study, with only 9% of patients with a degree of clinical recovery sufficient enough to allow explantation.[4]

An LVAD system consists of many components (Figure 13.1). The inflow cannula is inserted into the apex of the left ventricle (LV) and blood is removed from the LV and is pumped through the LVAD and into the outflow cannula to be returned to the aorta. The LVAD pump is positioned below the left rectus abdominis muscle or in the peritoneal cavity. A percutaneous driveline connected to the LVAD pump is tunneled outside the body and is connected to an electronic controller worn on the patient's belt. The controller is then connected to battery packs that the patient wears in a holster. Alternatively, the controller may be connected to a power base unit when the patient is at home or in the hospital.

There are several different types of LVADs. First generation LVADs were pulsatile-flow devices (Figure 13.2A). These pumps have a volume displacement chamber that fills and empties with blood every time a pusher plate moves up and down. One-way valves in the inflow and outflow cannulas assure that blood is moved from the LV into the volume displacement chamber and then pumped into the aorta. Pulsatile-flow LVADs thus operate similarly to the systolic and diastolic phases of the heart and generate a systolic and diastolic blood pressure. The Thoratec Heartmate XVE (Thoratec, Pleasanton, CA) and the WorldHeart Novacor (WorldHeart, Oakland, CA) are examples of implantable pulsatile-flow LVADs. For patients too small to allow implantation of an LVAD, the Thoratec PVAD is a pulsatile-flow paracorporeal LVAD. Because of wear in the bearings and failure of the inflow valves and motor, the pulsatile-flow LVADs have a finite lifespan, usually <2 years.[5] This led to the development of continuous-flow LVADs that are more durable because of fewer moving parts. There are two types of continuous-flow LVADs: axial-flow and centrifugal-flow. *Axial-flow* LVADs (Figure 13.2B), such as the Thoratec Heartmate II, have

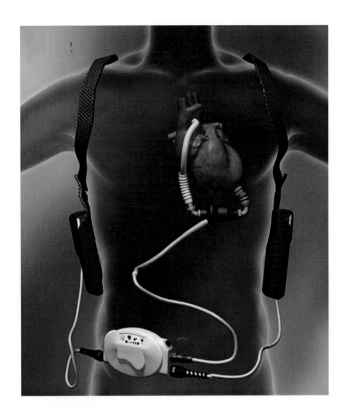

Figure 13.1. Components of an LVAD system.

A. Volume-displacement pump

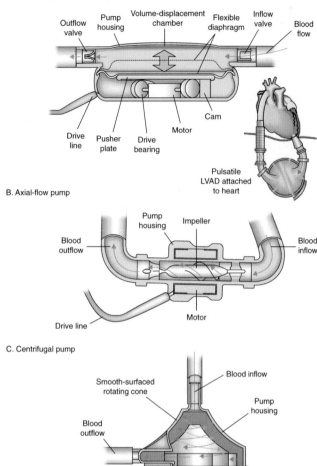

B. Axial-flow pump

C. Centrifugal pump

Figure 13.2. **Types of LVADs. A:** Pulsatile-flow LVAD. A motor moves the pusher plate up and down that causes filling and emptying of the volume displacement chamber with blood. Blood enters the LVAD from the inflow cannula and is returned to the aorta through the outflow cannula. One-way valves in the cannula prevent regurgitation of blood. **B:** Axial-flow LVAD. An impeller is the only moving part and it continuously turns drawing blood from the inflow cannula into the LVAD pump and then into the outflow cannula. **C:** Centrifugal-flow LVAD. A rotating cone draws blood from the inflow cannula to the base of the cone where it is continuously pushed into the outflow cannula.

an impeller that rotates around a central shaft. Blood is continuously drawn from the inflow cannula into the LVAD and then into the outflow cannula. The only moving part is the impeller. *Centrifugal-flow* LVADs (Figure 13.2C) have blood exit the inflow cannula at the top of the cone. Continuous spinning of the rotor causes centrifugal force, which pulls blood to the base and propels the blood into the outflow cannula. Examples of centrifugal-flow pumps are the external Thoratec CentriMag or the internal HeartWare LVAD (HeartWare International, Framingham, MA). Because of the continuous flow generated by the axial-flow and centrifugal-flow LVADs, the patient no longer has a systolic or diastolic blood pressure and pulses are no longer palpable. The ramifications of continuous-flow physiology on end-organ function will be discussed later.

CLINICAL TRIALS

The first trials looking at mechanical circulatory support with LVADs examined the BTT population. In a multicenter study of 280 patients awaiting cardiac transplantation who were unresponsive to intra-aortic balloon pump counterpulsation and inotropes, Frazier et al.[6] implanted the Heartmate VE pulsatile-flow LVAD (the forerunner of the Heartmate XVE). Average cardiac flow (expressed as pump index) improved to 2.8 L/minute/m^2 from a baseline cardiac index of 1.68 L/minute/m^2 ($P = .0001$). Creatinine improved from 1.5 mg per dl at baseline to 1.1 mg per dl with LVAD support ($P = .0001$). Sixty-seven percent of patients were successfully bridged to cardiac transplantation compared to a control group without LVAD implantation where only 33% of patients survived to cardiac transplantation. By log-rank analysis, the probability of survival to cardiac transplantation was higher for LVAD-treated patients than for control patients ($P < .001$) (Figure 13.3). Average duration of LVAD therapy lasted 112 days with 54 patients being supported for >180 days. This trial was also notable because it allowed patients who were being bridged to transplantation to be released from the hospital and await their cardiac transplant at home on LVAD support.

The use of LVADs as DT was evaluated in the landmark Randomized Evaluation of Mechanical Assistance for the Treatment of Congestive Heart Failure (REMATCH) study.[5] Patients with New York Heart Association (NYHA) class IV CHF with contraindications to cardiac transplantation were randomized to receive a Heartmate VE LVAD or optimal medical therapy. The primary endpoint was death from any cause. As might be expected from a trial involving patients with end-stage CHF who were ineligible for transplantation, the patient population was very ill. The average age was 68 years with an average left ventricular ejection fraction of 17% and an average blood pressure of only 102/62 mm Hg. Average cardiac index was 2 L/minute/m^2, average creatinine was 1.8 mg per dl, and 69% of patients needed intravenous inotropes. Survival at 1 year was

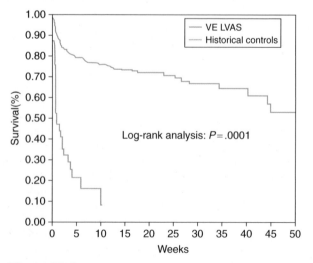

Figure 13.3. Probability of survival to transplantation for HeartMate VE LVAD-treated patients versus historical control patients by log-rank analysis.

52% in the LVAD-treated group and 25% in the medical therapy group (*P* = .002) (Figure 13.4). Relative risk reduction at 1 year was 48% for LVAD-treated patients and the absolute risk reduction of LVAD treatment was 27%. Survival declined at 2 years to 23% in the LVAD-treated group and to only 8% in the medical therapy group (*P* = .09). Cause of death was nearly universally LV failure in the medically treated group, but most commonly was sepsis or LVAD failure in the LVAD therapy group. Median NYHA class at 1 year for the LVAD group was NYHA class II and for the medical therapy group was NYHA class IV (*P* < .001). Although LVAD therapy afforded patients ineligible for cardiac transplantation an impressive survival benefit, the morbidity and mortality associated with the use of the pulsatile-flow LVAD was not inconsequential. Infection was a significant problem, particularly because of the relatively large percutaneous driveline. The rate of neurologic events in the LVAD-treated group was four times that of the medically treated group. Breakdown of the pulsatile flow LVAD owing to inflow valve regurgitation, erosion of the outflow graft, and wear of the motor and of the bearings were common, with a 2-year probability of device failure of 35%. Ten patients required device replacement. The only other published trial evaluating pulsatile-flow LVADs for DT was the nonrandomized study of the Novacor LVAD.[7] This trial also showed a survival advantage for LVAD-treated patients with end-stage CHF compared with medically managed patients. Similar to REMATCH, this trial showed high adverse events rates associated with LVAD therapy.

Although the Heartmate XVE was approved for DT in the United States by the Food and Drug Administration (FDA) in November 2002, only 451 patients received an LVAD as DT during the first 5 years after the REMATCH trial.[8] For greater adoption of mechanical circulatory support technology for the DT patients, improvements needed to be made in the durability and adverse event profile of LVADs. These improvements came in the form of the axial-flow LVADs. Axial-flow LVADs such as the Heartmate II have only one moving part (the impeller), and because blood is constantly being suctioned from the LV cavity and ejected into the aorta, there is no need for valves (which can fail) in the inflow and outflow cannulas. The driveline of the Heartmate II is smaller than that of the Heartmate XVE. The Heartmate II pump itself is much smaller than the Heartmate XVE pump (0.39 kg and 63 ml vs. 1.25 kg and

450 ml) (Figure 13.5). Before the introduction of the Heartmate II, implantable LVADs were limited to patients with a body surface area (BSA) of >1.5 m^2, restricting the use of this therapy in women and adolescents. The only option for patients with smaller BSAs was to have a paracorporeal LVAD such as the Thoratec PVAD. Furthermore, the newer continuous-flow pumps are much quieter than the pulsatile-flow LVADs.

Before testing the axial-flow technology in the long-term use DT setting, the devices were tested in the BTT population. In a prospective multicenter observational study, the Heartmate II was implanted in 133 patients awaiting cardiac transplantation with a primary endpoint of cardiac transplantation, cardiac recovery allowing device explantation, or continued mechanical support at 180 days and remaining eligible for cardiac transplant. Twenty-four hours after device implantation, cardiac index increased from 2.0 to 2.8 L/minute/m^2 (*P* < .001), whereas pulmonary capillary wedge pressure (PCWP) decreased from 26 to 16 mm Hg (*P* < .001) and mean pulmonary artery pressure (PAP) decreased from 37 to 26 mm Hg (*P* < .001). Although 100% of patients at enrollment into the study had NYHA class IV symptoms, after 3 months of continuous-flow support, only 3% of patients had NYHA class IV symptoms with 83% having NYHA classes I–II symptoms. From the 133 patients studied, 100 patients (75%) met the primary endpoint, with 56 patients being successfully bridged to cardiac transplantation, 1 patient having cardiac recovery with device explantation, and 43 patients continuing to receive mechanical circulatory support while awaiting cardiac transplantation. The commonest adverse effects were bleeding, ventricular arrhythmias, localized infections not related to the LVAD, and sepsis. A follow-up study by the same investigators reported data on the first 281 patients enrolled who had reached the clinical endpoints or had 18 months of follow-up after Heartmate II implantation.[9] Seventy-nine percent of patients received a cardiac transplant, had device explantation owing

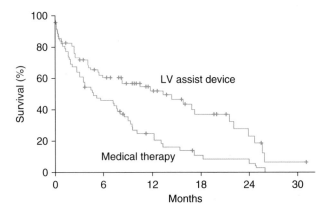

Figure 13.4. Kaplan–Meier curves for survival of patients receiving a pulsatile flow LVAD (Heartmate VE) versus optimal medical therapy.

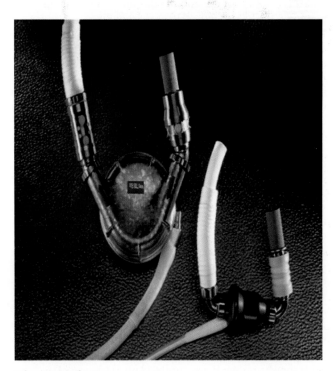

Figure 13.5. Heartmate XVE versus Heartmate II.

to cardiac recovery, or were still alive on LVAD support with 18 months follow-up. Overall survival was 82% at 6 months, 73% at 1 year, and 72% at 18 months. The longest duration of support in the study was 3.1 years with a median duration of 1.6 years. Questions arose about the effects of this degree of long-term mechanical circulatory support on end-organ function as the kidney and liver previously received pulsatile flow from the heart in vivo. Russell et al.[10] were able to demonstrate that with continuous-flow LVAD support, patients with normal blood urea nitrogen (BUN) and creatinine and aspartate transaminase (AST), alanine transaminase (ALT), and total bilirubin remained with normal values of these parameters of renal and hepatic function during LVAD support. For patients with abnormal values of renal and liver function, after 6 months of continuous-flow LVAD therapy, BUN improved from 37 to 23 mg per dl ($P < .0001$) and creatinine decreased from 1.8 to 1.4 ($P < .01$). AST and ALT decreased from 121 and 171 international units to 36 and 31 international units ($P < .001$), respectively. Total bilirubin also decreased from 2.1 to 0.9 mg per dl ($P < .0001$). Thus, long-term support with a continuous-flow LVAD was effective at providing hemodynamic support while improving end-organ perfusion in patients awaiting cardiac transplantation.

The Heartmate II continuous-flow LVAD was compared with the pulsatile-flow Heartmate XVE for DT in a randomized multicenter trial that enrolled 200 patients.[11] The primary endpoint was a composite of survival at 2 years free of a disabling stroke or reoperation to replace the LVAD. The average age of the patients was 62 years and the average LV EF was 17%. Eighty percent of patients were on intravenous inotropes and 60% of patients had a cardiac resynchronization device. Twenty-two percent of patients were on intra-aortic balloon pump support prior to LVAD placement. Forty-six percent of patients with a continuous-flow LVAD reached the primary endpoint compared to 11% of patient with a pulsatile flow LVAD ($P < .001$). Of the individual components of the primary endpoint, the hazard ratio (HR) for a disabling stroke was similar between the continuous-flow and the pulsatile-flow LVAD (HR 0.78, $P = .56$). The HRs for reoperation to repair or replace the LVAD (HR 0.18, $P < .001$) and death within 2 years after LVAD implantation (HR 0.59, $P = .048$) significantly favored the continuous-flow LVAD. Of the 59 patients who received a pulsatile-flow LVAD, 20 required 21 pump replacements. Of the 133 patients who received a continuous-flow LVAD, only 12 required 13 pump replacements. By as-treated analysis, actuarial survival was improved for patients with a continuous-flow LVAD (1- and 2-year survival rates of 68% and 58%, respectively) compared with the pulsatile-flow LVAD (1- and 2-year survival rates of 55% and 24%, respectively) ($P = .008$) (Figure 13.6). The 1- and 2-year survival rates for the pulsatile-flow patients were identical to the 1- and 2-year survival rates from the REMATCH study.[5] Despite improved experience, surgical technique, and postoperative care, the survival of the pulsatile-flow LVAD group could not be improved upon over the course of a decade. Rates of device-related infection, sepsis, right heart failure (RHF), respiratory failure, renal failure, and cardiac arrhythmia were all lower in the continuous-flow LVAD-treated group.[11] The rates of stroke and bleeding did not differ between the continuous-flow LVAD-treated group and the pulsatile-flow LVAD group. Based on the results of this study the HeartMate II was approved for DT by the FDA.[12]

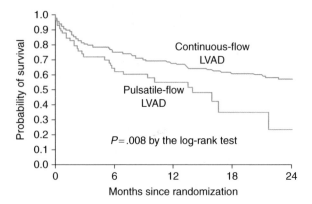

Figure 13.6. Kaplan–Meier curves of survival for patients treated with a continuous-flow LVAD versus a pulsatile-flow LVAD.

COMPLICATIONS

As experience with mechanical circulatory support has been obtained, several common complications have been noted.

INFECTIONS

Sepsis was the commonest cause of death (41%) in the LVAD-treated patients in the REMATCH study.[5] Prevention of sepsis and other infections begins prior to LVAD insertion. Preoperative bathing of patients with an antiseptic, rotation and removal of intravenous lines, dental hygiene, eradication of *Staph aureus* nasal carriage, administration of appropriate antibiotic prophylaxis based on the hospital's antibiogram, and meticulous hand hygiene are recommended to decrease the infection risk.[13] The percutaneous driveline exit site requires regular dressing changes that must be done using sterile technique including surgical mask and cap and sterile gloves. The patient's caregiver must be taught how to perform the sterile dressing changes prior to the patient's discharge from the hospital. LVAD percutaneous driveline infections occurred at a rate of 0.31 events per patient-year[9] in the HeartMate II BTT trial. All LVAD-related infections (including driveline and pump pocket infections) occurred at a rate of 0.48 events per patient-year for the HeartMate II compared to 0.90 events per patient-year for the HeartMate XVE ($P = .01$).[11] Thus, the smaller driveline and smaller pump size decreased the number of infections but did not eliminate them. Immobilization of the driveline with an abdominal binder allows tissue ingrowth and decreases tissues injury that can lead to an infection.[13] Treatment of driveline infections with antibiotics targeted at skin flora (after obtaining cultures) along with local wound care is recommended. For LVAD pocket infections, percutaneous or surgical drainage is necessary and pump exchange may be required. For LVAD intravascular infections, antibiotics and pump exchange are usually required for adequate treatment.

RIGHT HEART FAILURE

RHF, requiring the extended use of an inotrope, late use of an inotrope after LVAD implantation, or the use of an RVAD, is a serious complication of LVAD therapy. For an LVAD to function properly, the RV must be able to provide an adequate preload to the LVAD. Although the LVAD does decrease RV afterload by unloading the LV and reducing PAP, there is increased systemic venous return to a right heart, which is unable to tolerate the volume load. This can cause the interventricular septum to shift towards the LV, inducing geometric changes that cause increased tricuspid regurgitation and reduced septal contribution to RV stroke volume.[14] Twenty percent of patients in the HeartMate II BTT trial had RHF, 6% requiring an RVAD, 7% requiring extended use of inotropes, and 7% initiating an inotrope 14 days after LVAD implantation. Patients without RHF were more likely to be successfully bridged to cardiac transplantation, have cardiac recovery, or still be eligible for transplantation on LVAD support at day 180 compared with patients with RHF (89% vs. 71%, $P < .001$).[15] The right ventricular stroke work index (RVSWI)[16] and the right ventricular failure risk score (RVFRS)[17] have been used to estimate the likelihood of RHF after LVAD implantation. Although the number of RVADs used in the HeartMate II DT trial was low for both continuous- and pulsatile-flow LVADs, the patients who received a continuous-flow LVAD had less RHF needing extended inotropes compared to patients randomized to pulsatile-flow LVADs (0.14 events per patient-years vs. 0.46 events per patient-years, $P < .001$).[11]

BLEEDING

Bleeding, defined as requiring surgery or requiring transfusions of packed red blood cells (pRBCs), is a common problem after LVAD insertion. The use of the HeartMate II continuous-flow LVADs has not decreased the rates of bleeding compared with the pulsatile-flow HeartMate XVE.[12] One reason suggested for this finding is that the recommended antithrombotic and antiplatelet regimen for the HeartMate II was warfarin therapy to a targeted international normalized ratio (INR) of 2.0 to 3.0 and aspirin therapy, whereas the HeartMate XVE-treated patients were treated with aspirin. Boyle et al.[18] found a low risk of thromboemolic events in 331 patients with a HeartMate II as BTT. Ten patients had thrombotic events (ischemic stroke or pump thrombosis), whereas 58 patients who had hemorrhagic events (hemorrhagic stroke, hemorrhage requiring surgery, or transfusion of pRBCs). The highest risk for bleeding occurred with an INR >3.0 and the highest risk for ischemic stroke occurred with an INR <1.5, arguing for a targeted INR of 1.5 to 2.5 to balance the risk of thromboemolism and hemorrhage. Crow et al.[19] evaluated gastrointestinal bleeding (GIB) rates and found much higher rates of GIB in patients with continuous-flow LVADs compared to pulsatile-flow LVADs (63 events per 100 patients-years vs. 6.8 events per 100 patient-years, $P = .0004$). A frequent cause of GIB in the continuous-flow LVAD patients was from arteriovenous malformations (AVMs). Heyde syndrome[20]—GIB from angiodysplasia seen in patients with severe aortic stenosis with a low pulse pressure—was posited as a similar mechanism to GIB seen in patients with continuous-flow, nonpulsatile LVADs.[19] It has been shown that patients with aortic stenosis develop acquired von Willebrand (vWB) syndrome owing to the high sheer stress associated with blood flow through a severely stenotic aortic valve causing proteolysis of the high-molecular-weight (HMW) vWB multimers.[21] After aortic valve replacement, HMW vWB levels rise and GIB resolves.[22] Recent work by Uriel et al.[23] examining 79 HeartMate II patients found 44.3% of patients had a bleeding event an average of 112 days after LVAD insertion. Thirty-one

of the HeartMate II LVAD patients had their levels of HMW vWB multimers measured, and levels were reduced to absent in all patients. Of these 31 patients, 18 of them (58%) had bleeding episodes. In six patients who underwent cardiac transplantation, the HMW vWB multimer levels normalized. In one patient who had HMW vWB levels checked prior to HeartMate II insertion, the levels decreased with LVAD support. Further work is needed to see if other kinds of continuous-flow LVADs in clinical trials cause decrease in HMW vWB multimers and bleeding as well as what the best antithrombotic and anticoagulant strategy is for patients with a HeartMate II LVAD.

AORTIC INSUFFICIENCY

Aortic insufficiency (AI) may be present in both systole and diastole with a continuous-flow LVAD. This results in significant volume overload as a part of the LVAD forward cardiac output returns into the pump through the incompetent aortic valve.[12] For patients with pulsatile-flow LVADs, AI has been addressed by oversewing the valve, repairing the valve, or valve replacement.[24] In patients who have their aortic valve oversewn, all cardiac output now exits the LV into the LVAD. AI has also been seen to develop after continuous-flow LVAD placement. Mudd et al.[25] noted eight of nine patients with a Heartmate II who were bridged to cardiac transplant had gross pathological evidence of commissural fusion of the aortic valve leaflets at the time of explant. Review of the patients' echocardiograms showed a decreased prevalence of aortic valve opening and an increase in the presence of AI with time. Pak et al.[26] compared the prevalence of de novo AI in patients undergoing HeartMate XVE and HeartMate II support. Overall, significant AI developed in 6.0% of patients with a HeartMate XVE and 14.3% of patients with a HeartMate II ($P = .14$). For Heartmate II patients who remained on LVAD support for 1 year, the prevalence of significant AI was 25%. Of 26 patients whose aortic valve did not open, AI occurred in 11 patients. For those whose aortic valve did open, AI developed in only 1 of 14 patients ($P = .03$). Aortic root diameter tended to be larger at baseline and during follow-up in patients who developed AI, indicating aortic root dilatation as another possible mechanism for AI in LVAD patients. Given the long-term use of continuous-flow LVADs in the DT population as well as the use in the BTT population that is having longer waits for cardiac transplantation, strategies to prevent the development of significant AI must be developed.

VENTRICULAR ARRHYTHMIA

For patients with ventricular tachycardia (VT) storm, LVAD therapy is an effective treatment modality to provide full hemodynamic support.[27] However, in a study of 100 patients who received a HeartMate XVE LVAD for advanced CHF, new-onset monomorphic VT was 4.5 times more likely than the elimination of previously present VT ($P = .001$).[28] Most of the patients who developed VT did so early after LVAD placement when serum electrolytes were in flux and arrhythmogenic inotropes were commonly used. Sustained ventricular arrhythmias were also common in patients on HeartMate II support. In a study by Andersen et al.[29] of 23 patients implanted with a Heartmate II, 5 of the patients had sustained VT or ventricular fibrillation (VF) prior to implantation. After implantation, 12 patients had VT or VF with 4 of them previously having ventricular arrhythmia and 8 having new onset VT or VF. Nine of the patients had the onset of the ventricular arrhythmia within 4 weeks of LVAD implantation. Several patients had suction-induced nonsustained VT during echocardiographic adjustment of the HeartMate II motor speed, but these events were not counted as VT or VF events in the study. Excessive ventricular unloading by continuous-flow LVADs and diminution of the LV cavity size can cause direct contact of the LVAD inflow cannula and the endocardium causing ventricular arrhythmias much like a catheter in the RV or LV inducing VT.[30] Vollkron et al.[30] showed that suction events caused by continuous flow LVADs caused a significant increase in VT compared with baseline arrhythmic activity, regardless of whether the patient had frequent or infrequent ventricular arrhythmias. These ventricular arrhythmias ceased after resolution of the suction event. Ventricular arrhythmias have also been correlated with failure to use a β-blocker after LVAD implantation (odds ratio 7.04, P = .001).[31] The period after LVAD implantation when inotropes are employed and before β-blockers are restarted would seem to be a particularly high-risk period for ventricular arrhythmias.

PATIENT AND DEVICE SELECTION

Figure 13.7 outlines a pathway for selection of patients for an appropriate LVAD therapy. Figure 13.8 outlines an algorithm of choosing an LVAD pathway.

The first step in deciding which patient should get an LVAD and what is the correct device for that patient should involve the recognition of a patient with advanced heart failure that is failing medical therapy, either acutely or chronically. Next, one must decide for what indication the patient will receive an LVAD (i.e., bridge to recovery, BTT, or DT). For a patient with postcardiotomy shock, cardiogenic shock after a myocardial infarction, or fulminant myocarditis, a short-term paracorporeal device (such as the CentriMag) should be implanted as there is a likelihood the patient could recover from their hemodynamic embarrassment quickly, allowing for device explantation. Should the patient not recover sufficient cardiac function, they could then be transitioned to a long-term LVAD as BTT or DT as appropriate. A short-term device can also be used in patients who have had a cardiac arrest and their neurologic status is unknown.[32] In this situation, a short-term device can provide hemodynamic support until appropriate neurologic assessment is made (bridge to decision). If the patient recovers neurologically from their cardiac arrest, they can be switched to a long-term device or have the device explanted if rapid cardiac recovery ensues. For patients with neurologic compromise, the short-term device can be explanted and palliative care measures pursued. BTT patients are actively listed for cardiac transplantation with the United Network of Organ Sharing. DT patients meet the inclusion criteria of the randomized studies proving the benefit of DT.[11] These include EF of <25%, a peak

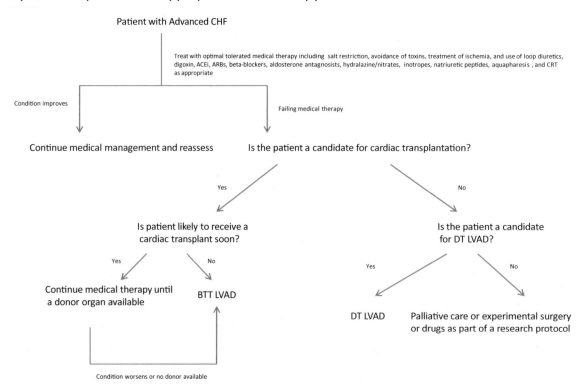

Pathway to select patients for appropriate LVAD therapy

ACEi = angiotensin converting enzyme inhibitor, ARB = angiotensin receptor blocker, BTT = bridge to transplantation, CHF = chronic heart failure, CRT = cardiac resynchronization therapy, DT = destination therapy, LVAD = left ventricular assist device

Figure 13.7. Outlines a pathway for selection of patients for an appropriate LVAD therapy.

Choosing an LVAD Pathway

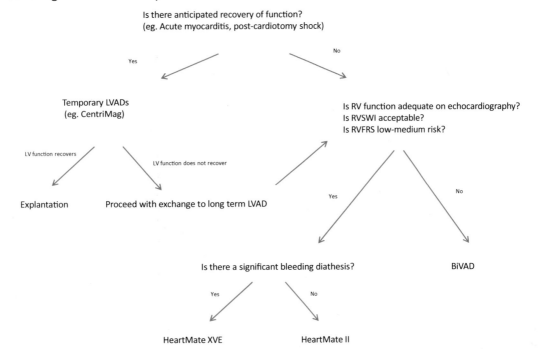

BiVAD = biventricular assisteddevice, LV = left ventricle, LVAD = left ventricular assist device, RV = right ventricle,
RVFRS = right ventricular failure risk score, RVSWI = right ventricular stroke work index

Figure 13.8. Outlines an algorithm of choosing an LVAD Pathway.

oxygen consumption of <14 ml/kg/minute, NYHA class IIIB or IV symptoms for at least 45 of the 60 days prior to placement or dependence on an intra-aortic balloon pump for 7 days or inotropes for ≥14 days in patients ineligible for cardiac transplantation. Patients with irreversible, severe pulmonary, renal, or hepatic dysfunction, or an active infection are not candidates for an LVAD.

In patients with advanced CHF, optimal medical and electrical therapies must be employed. If these therapies are insufficient, evaluation for mechanical circulatory support is appropriate. Risk scores have been developed to predict the outcomes of patients after LVAD implantation[33] and to estimate the risk of RV failure in LVAD candidates.[17] Lietz and colleagues[33] examined 280 patients who underwent HeartMate XVE placement for DT after the REMATCH trial and using multivariate analysis, devised a 9-variable weighted risk score for 90-day in-hospital mortality. The patient variables that afforded higher risk included: platelet count ≤148 ×10^3 per μl (7 points), serum albumin ≤3.3 g per dl (5 points), INR >1.1 (4 points), vasodilator therapy at the time of implant (4 points), mean PAP ≤25 mm Hg (3 points), AST >45 U per ml (2 points), hematocrit ≤34% (2 points), BUN >51 U per dl (2 points), and lack of intravenous inotropes (2 points). A cumulative risk was calculated with low-risk patients having a score of 0 to 8, medium-risk patients a score of 9 to 16, high-risk patients a score of 17 to 19, and very high-risk patients a score of >19. Low-risk patients had an in-hospital mortality within 90 days of 2%, medium risk of 12%, high risk of 44%, and very high risk of 81%. One-year survival was 81.2%, 62.4%, 27.8%, and 10.7% for the

low-, medium-, high-risk, and very high-risk patients, respectively (Figure 13.9). Sepsis, multiorgan failure, and RHF were the main causes of in-hospital mortality. Because DT is supposed to be an elective surgical therapy for patients with end-stage CHF, attending to correctable factors such as nutritional deficiencies, active infection, coagulation abnormalities, or lack of inotropes may make the patient a better DT LVAD candidate. This Lietz risk

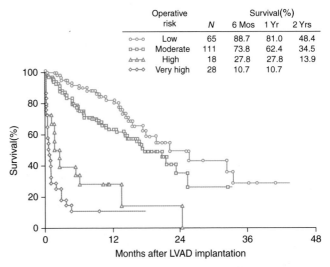

Operative risk	N	Survival(%)		
		6 Mos	1 Yr	2 Yrs
Low	65	88.7	81.0	48.4
Moderate	111	73.8	62.4	34.5
High	18	27.8	27.8	13.9
Very high	28	10.7	10.7	

Figure 13.9. Survival of HeartMate XVE DT patients according to operative risk.

score was derived from DT patients implanted with pulsatile-flow devices. How well this risk score stratifies patients who receive continuous-flow LVADs or are BTT candidates is unknown.

RHF IN LVAD RECIPIENTS

Twenty percent of patients develop RHF after LVAD implantation, and RHF is associated with diminished frequency of successful BTT, cardiac recovery, or continued LVAD support at 180 days. Because 77% of patients with RHF who received an RVAD within the first 24 hours survived at 180 days compared with 39% of patients who received an RVAD later than 24 hours,[15] accurate assessment of the risk of RV failure prior to LVAD placement is important. One of the initial hemodynamic predictors of RHF was the RVSWI.[16] The RVSWI is defined as the mean PAP minus the mean right atrial pressure multiplied by the stroke volume index, where stroke volume index was calculated as the cardiac index divided by the heart rate. A preoperative RVSWI of >400 mm Hg × ml per m^2 predicted the successful implantation of an LVAD without the need for an RVAD. Matthews and colleagues[17] developed an RVFRS based on a multivariable analysis of 197 patients who underwent LVAD implantation, 94% of which was as BTT. Vasopressor requirement (4 points), AST ≥80 IU per L (2 points), bilirubin ≥2 mg per dl (2.5 points), and creatinine ≥2.3 mg per dL (3 points) were found to be significant predictors of RHF, defined as need for IV inotropes >14 days after surgery, inhaled nitric oxide for ≥48 hours, right-sided circulatory support, or hospital discharge on an inotrope. The odds ratio for RV failure with an RVFRS <3 points was 0.49, 4.0 to 5.0 was 2.8, and ≥5.5 was 7.6. The survival rate for 180 days for these risk scores was 90%, 80%, and 66%, respectively. The RVFRS was derived from a mostly BTT cohort and the data set included seven different types of LVADs, with most of the cases of RHF occurring in the HeartMate VE and XVE devices, thus limiting the applicability to continuous-flow LVADs.

CHOICE OF LVAD TYPE

After calculation of the Lietz risk score and RVFRS and deciding that the patient has an acceptable risk profile, choosing a device is the next step. If there is anticipation of the need for biventricular support, the Thoratec PVAD or IVAD may be appropriate. Patients with a known significant bleeding diathesis may be considered for a HeartMate XVE, thus avoiding the acquired vWB deficiency universally seen with the HeartMate II. Because of the increased durability and smaller size of the HeartMate II, this would be the preferred device in most instances for BTT and DT.

Mechanical circulatory support with LVADs has made tremendous advances in the last 20 years. Technology has evolved from large, loud, pulsatile-flow LVADs with many moving parts and limited durability, to continuous-flow LVADs which are smaller, quieter, and with only one moving part, much more durable. In short, LVADs have become a viable option for many of the end-stage CHF patients as both BTT and for DT. Innovation will continue to occur to solve the current problems of bleeding, driveline infections, AI, and ventricular arrhythmias. Newer generations of LVADs hold significant promise in treating what has been considered the terminal phase of CHF.

REFERENCES

1. Ammar KA, Jacobsen SJ, Mahoney DW, et al. Prevalence and prognostic significance of heart failure stages: application of the American College of Cardiology/American Heart Association heart failure staging criteria in the community. *Circulation.* 2007;115:1563–1570.
2. Lloyd-Jones D, Adams RJ, Brown TM, et al. Heart disease and stroke statistics—2010 update: a report from the American Heart Association. *Circulation.* 2010;121:e46–e215.
3. Birks EJ, Tansley PD, Hardy J, et al. Left ventricular assist device and drug therapy for the reversal of heart failure. *N Engl J Med.* 2006;355:1873–1884.
4. Maybaum S, Mancini D, Xydas S, et al. Cardiac improvement during mechanical circulatory support: a prospective multicenter study of the LVAD Working Group. *Circulation.* 2007;115:2497–2505.
5. Rose EA, Gelijns AC, Moskowitz AJ, et al. Long-term mechanical left ventricular assistance for end-stage heart failure. *N Engl J Med.* 2001;345:1435–1443.
6. Frazier OH, Rose EA, Oz MC, et al. Multicenter clinical evaluation of the HeartMate vented electric left ventricular assist system in patients awaiting heart transplantation. *J Thorac Cardiovasc Surg.* 2001;122:1186–1195.
7. Rogers JG, Butler J, Lansman SL, et al. Chronic mechanical circulatory support for inotrope-dependent heart failure patients who are not transplant candidates: results of the INTrEPID Trial. *J Am Coll Cardiol.* 2007;50:741–747.
8. Lietz K, Long JW, Kfoury AG, et al. Impact of center volume on outcomes of left ventricular assist device implantation as destination therapy: analysis of the Thoratec HeartMate Registry, 1998 to 2005. *Circ Heart Fail.* 2009;2:3–10.
9. Pagani FD, Miller LW, Russell SD, et al. Extended mechanical circulatory support with a continuous-flow rotary left ventricular assist device. *J Am Coll Cardiol.* 2009;54:312–321.
10. Russell SD, Rogers JG, Milano CA, et al. Renal and hepatic function improve in advanced heart failure patients during continuous-flow support with the HeartMate II left ventricular assist device. *Circulation.* 2009;120:2352–2357.
11. Slaughter MS, Rogers JG, Milano CA, et al. Advanced heart failure treated with continuous-flow left ventricular assist device. *N Engl J Med.* 2009;361:2241–2251.
12. Slaughter MS, Pagani FD, Rogers JG, et al. Clinical management of continuous-flow left ventricular assist devices in advanced heart failure. *J Heart Lung Transplant.* 2010;29:S1–S39.
13. Chinn R, Dembitsky W, Eaton L, et al. Multicenter experience: prevention and management of left ventricular assist device infections. *ASAIO J.* 2005;51:461–470.
14. Farrar DJ, Compton PG, Hershon JJ, et al. Right heart interaction with the mechanically assisted left heart. *World J Surg.* 1985;9:89–102.
15. Kormos RL, Teuteberg JJ, Pagani FD, et al. Right ventricular failure in patients with the HeartMate II continuous-flow left ventricular assist device: incidence, risk factors, and effect on outcomes. *J Thorac Cardiovasc Surg.* 2010;139:1316–1324.
16. Ochiai Y, McCarthy PM, Smedira NG, et al. Predictors of severe right ventricular failure after implantable left ventricular assist device insertion: analysis of 245 patients. *Circulation.* 2002;106:I198–I202.
17. Matthews JC, Koelling TM, Pagani FD, et al. The right ventricular failure risk score a preoperative tool for assessing the risk of right ventricular failure in left ventricular assist device candidates. *J Am Coll Cardiol.* 2008;51:2163–2172.
18. Boyle AJ, Russell SD, Teuteberg JJ, et al. Low thromboembolism and pump thrombosis with the HeartMate II left ventricular assist device: analysis of outpatient anti-coagulation. *J Heart Lung Transplant.* 2009;28:881–887.
19. Crow S, John R, Boyle A, et al. Gastrointestinal bleeding rates in recipients of nonpulsatile and pulsatile left ventricular assist devices. *J Thorac Cardiovasc Surg.* 2009;137:208–215.
20. Heyde E. Gastrointestinal bleeding in aortic stenosis [letter]. *N Engl J Med.* 1958;259:196–200.
21. Warkentin TE, Moore JC, Anand SS, et al. Gastrointestinal bleeding, angiodysplasia, cardiovascular disease, and acquired von Willebrand syndrome. *Transfus Med Rev.* 2003;17:272–286.
22. Vincentelli A, Susen S, Le Tourneau T, et al. Acquired von Willebrand syndrome in aortic stenosis. *N Engl J Med.* 2003;349:343–349.
23. Uriel N, Pak SW, Jorde UP, et al. Acquired von Willebrand syndrome after continuous-flow mechanical device support contributes to a high prevalence of bleeding during long-term support and at the time of transplantation. *J Am Coll Cardiol.* 2010;56:1207–1213.
24. Rao V, Slater JP, Edwards NM, et al. Surgical management of valvular disease in patients requiring left ventricular assist device support. *Ann Thorac Surg.* 2001;71:1448–1453.
25. Mudd JO, Cuda JD, Halushka M, et al. Fusion of aortic valve commissures in patients supported by a continuous axial flow left ventricular assist device. *J Heart Lung Transplant.* 2008;27:1269–1274.
26. Pak SW, Uriel N, Takayama H, et al. Prevalence of de novo aortic insufficiency during long-term support with left ventricular assist devices. *J Heart Lung Transplant.* 2010;29:1172–1176.
27. Gehi AK, Mehta D, Gomes JA. Evaluation and management of patients after implantable cardioverter-defibrillator shock. *JAMA.* 2006;296:2839–2847.
28. Ziv O, Dizon J, Thosani A, et al. Effects of left ventricular assist device therapy on ventricular arrhythmias. *J Am Coll Cardiol.* 2005;45:1428–1434.
29. Andersen M, Videbaek R, Boesgaard S, et al. Incidence of ventricular arrhythmias in patients on long-term support with a continuous-flow assist device (HeartMate II). *J Heart Lung Transplant.* 2009;28:733–735.
30. Vollkron M, Voitl P, Ta J, et al. Suction events during left ventricular support and ventricular arrhythmias. *J Heart Lung Transplant.* 2007;26:819–825.
31. Refaat M, Chemaly E, Lebeche D, et al. Ventricular arrhythmias after left ventricular assist device implantation. *Pacing Clin Electrophysiol.* 2008;31:1246–1252.
32. John R, Liao K, Lietz K, et al. Experience with the Levitronix CentriMag circulatory support system as a bridge to decision in patients with refractory acute cardiogenic shock and multisystem organ failure. *J Thorac Cardiovasc Surg.* 2007;134:351–358.
33. Lietz K, Long JW, Kfoury AG, et al. Outcomes of left ventricular assist device implantation as destination therapy in the post-REMATCH era: implications for patient selection. *Circulation.* 2007;116:497–505.

PATIENT AND FAMILY INFORMATION FOR:
Mechanical Circulatory Support

CHF is a condition where the heart's main pumping chamber, the LV (Figure 13.10), is unable to pump enough blood forward to supply oxygen to the rest of the body. Blood can back up in the lungs causing shortness of breath and an inability to breathe while lying flat. Blood can also back up into the abdomen causing abdominal pain or fullness and into the legs causing edema (swelling). Fatigue is a common symptom of CHF as well. Medications such as diuretics, digoxin, ß-blockers and angiotensin converting enzyme inhibitors (ACE inhibitors) have significantly improved patients symptoms and the latter two medications have helped people live longer. Implantable cardioverter defibrillators (ICDs) and a special kind of pacemaker (biventricular pacemaker) that causes the LV and right ventricle (RV) to beat in synchrony have also extended lives of patients with CHF. Unfortunately, there are many patients where medications and ICDs and biventricular pacemakers are not enough, and patients die of progressive CHF. Heart transplantation is a highly effective treatment for some patients with advanced CHF, but a severe organ shortage exists in the United States and the waiting time for a heart transplant can be years. LVADs were developed to treat patients with end-stage CHF who would otherwise die while waiting for a heart transplant.

An LVAD is a heart assist pump. It handles most of the work of the failing LV. Long-term LVADs are implanted via a surgical procedure in the upper abdomen and chest. An LVAD consists of many parts (Figure 13.11). There is an inflow tube attached to the LV where blood exits the LV and enters the LVAD pump. From the LVAD pump, the blood exits into the outflow graft which then delivers the blood back into the aorta, the major artery from which blood is

circulated to the rest of the body. There is an insulated driveline with electric wiring that is tunneled from the implanted pump through the skin to an external controller. This electronic controller is worn outside the body and controls the function of the pump. The controller is connected to two batteries that the patient can wear in a holster. If the patient is stationary at home or in the hospital such as when the patient goes to sleep, the controller can also be plugged into a power base unit, and the pump can be powered by electricity from the wall socket.

There are different types of LVADs: internal and external LVADs. Internal devices, as described above, have the LVAD pump implanted inside the body. Only the wire connecting the LVAD pump on the inside of the body to the system controller on the outside of the body comes out through the skin. These internal, implanted devices are intended for long-term support of the heart. External LVADs are similar to internal LVADs except that the LVAD pump is not implanted in the body but is instead outside the body. For these devices, a tube delivers blood from the LV to the pump outside the body. The pump then sends the blood back through the skin and into the body through another tube and into the aorta. There are two kinds of external LVADs: long-term and temporary devices. Long-term external LVADs were used when patients' bodies were too small to allow implantation of the LVAD pump. With newer generation LVADs that are smaller, this does not happen much anymore. Another situation where long-term external LVADs are used is when a patient has a failing RV as well as a failing LV and requires an assist pump for both ventricles. In that situation, a BiVAD is used. Temporary external devices are used for patients where there is an

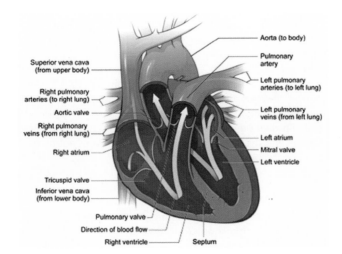

Figure 13.10. A healthy heart showing the direction of blood flow. Deoxygenated blood returns to the right heart from the superior and inferior vena cavae and then gets pumped to the lungs where it becomes oxygenated again. Oxygenated blood returns to the left heart from the pulmonary veins and then is pumped from the left ventricle (LV) into the aorta and to the rest of the body.

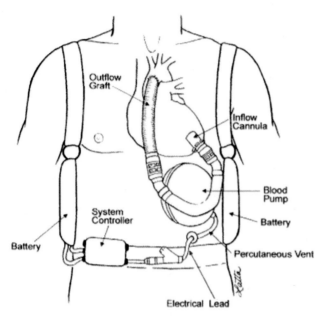

Figure 13.11. A left ventricular assist device (LVAD). Blood exits the left ventricle of the failing heart and enters the LVAD pump through the inflow cannula. The pump then pumps the blood through the outflow graft and into the aorta where it goes to the rest of the body. A controller located outside the body is connected to the internal pump through a percutaneous lead. The controller is attached to two batteries to provide electricity to the device.

expectation that the heart function will recover soon. An example of this is when a patient suffers a large heart attack causing the heart muscle to be stunned and unable to pump blood to the body. An LVAD would support the LV while the patient can have blood flow returned to their blocked artery by either a stent or by coronary artery bypass surgery. When the LV function recovers sufficiently, the LVAD can then be removed (explanted).

A major point in the treatment of CHF is deciding when a patient should receive an LVAD. There are three common scenarios when a patient receives an LVAD: bridge to recovery, Bridge To Transplantation (BTT) and Destination Therapy (DT).

Bridge to recovery refers to using an LVAD in a patient where there is an expectation that the heart function will recover and that a patient will eventually no longer need the LVAD. Examples of this are when a patient has a heart attack and the heart is stunned, or when a patient undergoes cardiac surgery and the heart is still weak from the surgery and not ready to function on its own without the heart–lung machine. Given enough time, the heart function usually recovers and the LVAD can be removed. Sometimes, a patient can get a virus that infects the heart and the heart function rapidly deteriorates (acute fulminant myocarditis). Supporting the weakened LV with an LVAD gives the patient time to recover from the infection and be treated with medications, with the hope of allowing LVAD removal. In all of these examples of bridge to recovery, the patient has an acute deterioration of LV function, and the purpose of the LVAD is to support the LV function until recovery occurs. There had been a great deal of enthusiasm for using long-term LVADs to support LV function and allow

patients with long-term LV dysfunction recover their LV function. Unfortunately, only small numbers of patients who have CHF and have a long-term LVAD have significant recovery of their LV function to allow the LVAD to be explanted and the patient to no longer have CHF.

BTT refers to using an LVAD in patient who has been listed for a heart transplant until a donor organ becomes available. This has become a very common occurrence given the huge donor shortage that could make the time on the heart transplant waiting list in the order of months and years. BTT patients have had progression of their CHF and often have more frequent hospitalizations, an inability to tolerate oral CHF medications because of low blood pressure, or more frequent ICD shocks. By receiving an LVAD, CHF symptoms and the function of other organs that depend on blood flow from the heart (e.g., kidneys) are improved in BTT LVAD patients. BTT patients are also able to improve their nutrition status and functional status by participating in physical therapy and cardiac rehabilitation. Adequate nutritional status and functional status are important components to successful heart transplantation when a donor organ becomes available.

DT involves the permanent, long-term placement of an LVAD in patients with end-stage CHF who are not candidates for a heart transplant. When treated with only the best medical therapy available, candidates for DT LVAD have a horrific 2-year survival of only 8%. However, when an LVAD is implanted for long-term therapy in such a patient, 2-year survival improves to 58%.

There has been a shift in the type of LVAD pumps used. Originally, LVADs used pulsatile pumps. Pulsatile pumps mimic the natural pulsatily of the heart. During systole, the LV works and ejects blood into the aorta, whereas during diastole the LV rests and fills with blood. The ejection of blood into the aorta during systole generates a person's pulse. With a pulsatile LVAD, the normal heart function is imitated when blood is pumped out of the LVAD pump and into the aorta during systole, and the LVAD pump fills with blood during diastole. Although these original pulsatile pumps worked to improve blood flow in patients with CHF, they had limited durability because of many moving parts that frequently wore out. Furthermore, pulsatile pumps were noisy and large, limiting their use in women and adolescents who have smaller body sizes. A newer type of pump, a continuous-flow LVAD, has been engineered with only one moving part, a rotor, which continuously spins and draws blood from the LV into the pump and continuously moves the blood into the aorta. These continuous-flow pumps are much smaller, and owing to their one moving part, are much more durable and operate quietly. An interesting point with continuous-flow LVADs, is that because blood is continuously being delivered to the aorta, patients often no longer have a palpable pulse to feel. Studies have proven the benefits of continuous-flow LVADs and the safety of having long-term continuous-flow rather than pulsatile-flow with a rhythmic pulse.

Not everyone is a good candidate for LVAD therapy. The LV cavity must be dilated enough to be able to supply blood into the LVAD pump. This makes LVADs inappropriate for most patients with hypertrophic and restrictive cardiomyopathies. Patients should not have an ongoing infection at the time of LVAD placement. Also, patients with irreversible, severe kidney, liver, or lung disease are not appropriate for LVADs. To receive an LVAD, patients must have a good social support network and someone who can help with dressing changes for where the electrical cable exits the skin. Most important, patients must have the desire to live with the assist pump for, potentially, a long period. For the patients where LVAD therapy is not possible, discussions should be had with the patients and their families regarding changing the focus of care from life prolonging to improvement in symptoms and other end-of-life issues.

As with other kinds of open heart surgery, after implantation of an LVAD, patients will require a stay in the intensive care unit where they will be treated with intravenous medications. During the initial phases of recovery, patients will need to work with physical and occupational therapy to regain strength and stamina as well as have an adequate diet to promote wound healing. During this process, patients and their support network are educated about the LVAD and prepared to live life outside of the hospital with an LVAD. Although the LVAD is designed to improve symptoms and quality of life, there are limitations. Patients must have extra batteries available to them at all times and depending on their LVAD, patients may not be able to take showers or baths because of the external electronic controller and wire. Serious complications can arise with LVAD treatment. Immediately after implantation, the patient can develop RV failure and require an RV assist device (RVAD). Serious infections leading to sepsis and multiorgan failure can occur. Strokes, abnormal heart rhythms, bleeding, and leaking of the aortic valve are complications being seen with increasing frequency as patients have an LVAD in place for longer durations. The main reason to implant a DT LVAD is to restore a full life not limited by weakness and shortness of breath and thus relieve the patient from the disabling symptoms of CHF. Although most patients will do well after the operation, it is critical to understand the patient's wishes in the event of a bad but not immediately fatal outcome (i.e., severe stroke or other chronically disabling outcomes) prior to going to the operating room.

LVADs are an important treatment option for patients with end-stage CHF. The technology has improved from large, loud pulsatile-flow devices to smaller, quieter, continuous-flow machines. Newer and smaller devices are currently being tested in clinical trials. Although serious complications can and do occur, LVADs are life-sustaining and life-restoring in the appropriate patient. With the continued scarcity of donor hearts and the aging of the population, LVADs will play an increasing role in treating patients with intractable CHF.

David S. Roffman

Medications Used in the Management of Heart Failure

The past 30 years have provided remarkable advances in the pharmacotherapeutic management of patients with acute and chronic heart failure. Major improvements in both survival and symptom management now provide practitioners with the ability to provide therapy that is well tolerated, decreases recurrent hospitalizations, and improves quality of life. As the incidence of heart failure continues to increase with the advancing age of the population, and improved postinfarction survival, maximizing the use of currently available agents, development of new class of drugs, and the continued development of implantable devices for treatment of mechanical and electrical complications of heart failure should further our ability to improve patient care.

INOTROPES

Intravenous inotropes are useful in patients with severe systolic dysfunction with relative hypotension and evidence of inadequate end-organ perfusion, who are not responsive to, or are intolerant of, vasodilators and diuretics. Inotropic agents relieve acute heart failure symptoms and may preserve end-organ function but have not been demonstrated to improve survival. On the contrary, several studies have demonstrated increased adverse outcomes, including increased mortality with chronic intravenous inotropic therapy.

DOBUTAMINE

Dobutamine, a synthetic catecholamine, is primarily a β-adrenergic stimulant with minimal α_1-cardiac sympathetic activity. Its β_1-sympathetic activity accounts for its inotropic activity through β-receptor mediated-activation of intracellular cyclic AMP. The resulting sarcoplasmic reticulum calcium release mediates myocardial contractility. Similar β_1 activity at the sinoatrial (SA) node accounts for its modest chronotropic activity. Patients taking β-blockers on admission may have an attenuated initial response to dobutamine, until the β-blocker has been metabolized or renally eliminated.[1] However, cardiac output response to increasing doses of dobutamine has been observed in patients on chronic carvedilol.[2] The dose-dependent β_2 effect produces mild peripheral arteriolar dilation. As with most intravenous sympathetic stimulants, dobutamine has a rapid onset of action (1 to 2 minutes) and has a peak effect within 10 minutes. The drug is rapidly methylated providing for a short duration of action (t 1 : 2 minutes), ideal for a drug requiring titration based on hemodynamic effects.

The hemodynamic effects of dobutamine in heart failure patients include increased cardiac output, arteriolar dilation, reduction of pulmonary artery occlusive pressure (PAOP or wedge pressure), and small but variable change in blood pressure (Table 14.1). In responsive patients, the hemodynamic benefits of the drug increase end-organ perfusion, manifest by improved renal function and urine output, decreased pulmonary vascular congestion, and improved skin perfusion and mentation.

Adverse effects that should be monitored in heart failure patients include dose-related tachycardia, most concerning in ischemic cardiomyopathy, and atrial (atrial fibrillation) or ventricular (ventricular tachycardia) arrhythmias.

Dobutamine dosing begins at 2.5 to 5 μg/kg/minute and is progressively increased based on clinical and hemodynamic response. Because it is not a vasoconstrictor (pressor), dobutamine does not need to be administered through a central line. Dosing may be increased to 15 μg/kg/minute, although maximum hemodynamic benefit may be achieved at lower doses, and ventricular ectopy risk increases as the dose is increased. Once hemodynamic stability has been accomplished, dobutamine infusions should be gradually tapered off. Although intermittent ambulatory dobutamine infusions have been used for quality of life enhancement in patients who are not candidates for transplantation or pump implantation, or as a pharmacologic bridge to cardiac transplantation, the practice has generally been replaced by implantation of ventricular assist devices.[3] In addition randomized trials have demonstrated increased mortality with the use of ambulatory dobutamine infusions.[4]

MILRINONE

Milrinone is a selective inhibitor of phospodiesterase III, an enzyme responsible for the intracellular breakdown of c-AMP. Cyclic-AMP accumulation increases intracellular calcium and thereby facilitates myocardial contractility. Although milrinone's hemodynamic effects are similar to those of dobutamine, milrinone produces more arterial and venous dilation, earning it the label "inodilator" (Table 14.1). Theoretical advantages of milrinone as compared with dobutamine include greater afterload reduction, augmenting the cardiac output produced by its inotropic effect, and its postreceptor mechanism of action, a potential benefit in patients receiving β-blockers for chronic heart failure. Hemodynamic improvement is usually observed within 15 minutes of initiation of therapy. The drug is renally eliminated with an elimination half-life of approximately

TABLE 14.1	Hemodynamic Effects of Intravenous Agents Used in the Treatment of Acute Decompensated Heart Failure					
Drug	*Dose*	*HR*	*MAP*	*PAOP*	*CO*	*SVR*
Dobutamine	2.5–15 µg/kg/min	0/+	0	–	+	–
Milrinone	0.375–0.75 µg/kg/min	0/+	0/–	–	+	–
Dopamine	0.5–3 µg/kg/min	0	0	0	0/+	–
Dopamine	3–10 µg/kg/min	+	+	0	+	0
Dopamine	>10 µg/kg/min	+	+	+	+	+
Nesiritide	Bolus: 2 µg/kg Infusion: 0.01 µg/kg/min	0	0/–	–	+	–
Nitroglycerin	5–200 µg/min	0/+	0/–	–	0/+	0/–
Nitroprusside	0.25–3.0 µg/kg/min	0/+	0/–	–	+	

CO, cardiac output; HR, heart rate; MAP, mean arterial pressure; PAOP, pulmonary artery occlusive pressure; SVR, systemic vascular resistance.
Adopted from DiPiro JT, Talbert RL, Yee GC, et al. *Pharmacotherapy: A Pathophysiologic Approach*. 7th ed. New York, NY: McGraw Hill; 1999.

3 hours in heart failure patients, and the maintenance infusion should be adjusted based on creatinine clearance (Table 14.2).

Although the package insert recommends a 50 µg per kg loading dose, many heart failure practitioners refrain from administering the loading dose to reduce the risk of hypotension. Typical maintenance doses of milrinone range from 0.375 to 0.75 µg/kg/minute (Table 14.1). At maintenance doses above 0.5 µg/kg/minute, once hemodynamic and clinical stability has been achieved, the infusion should be gradually tapered. However, because the drug has a longer elimination half-life than dobutamine, lower milrinone maintenance doses may be reduced more rapidly than dobutamine, provided hemodynamic stability has been achieved. In addition to hypotension, the most common side effects are tachyarrhythmias. Milrinone may produce less tachycardia than dobutamine, but it also has the potential to produce both atrial and ventricular arrhythmias.

Despite the potential adverse long-term impact on morbidity and mortality related to intravenous inotropic therapy, patients with acute decompensated heart failure benefit from the short-term hemodynamic improvement associated with the administration of these agents, pending the resolution of the underlying events that precipitate their hemodynamic deterioration.

DOPAMINE

Dopamine possesses dose-dependent hemodynamic effects, stimulating D_1 dopamine receptors, α_1-, β_1-, and β_2-receptors. Other than the diuretic effect of low-dose (renal dose) dopamine to enhance volume loss in patients with diuretic-resistant heart failure, dopamine use is typically reserved for use in markedly hypotensive patients including those with cardiogenic shock. Inotropic doses in the 2 to 5 µg/kg/minute range promote increase cardiac output; however, intermediate- and high-dose dopamine increase systemic vascular resistance, increase afterload and PAOP, and impede cardiac output (Table 14.1). In the setting of cardiogenic shock, dopamine may be required to maintain mean arterial pressure and coronary perfusion pressure until the underlying etiology can be treated or resolved.

DIGOXIN

Digoxin is a moderately potent inotrope with additional neurohormonal modulating effects producing increased parasympathetic nervous system activity and decreased central sympathetic nervous system drive. Its inotropic effect is related to inhibition of sarcolemmal sodium–potassium-ATPase, resulting in increased myocardial cell calcium, the final common pathway for all currently available inotropic agents. The benefit of digoxin in heart failure was debated for most of its first 200-year history. The drug has little use in the treatment of acute heart failure in patients with sinus rhythm. Perhaps the least controversial use of the drug in heart failure patients is to assist (in combination with β-blockers or amiodarone) in

TABLE 14.2	Renal Dosing of Milrinone
Creatinine Clearance (ml/min/1.73m²)	*Milrinone Infusion Rate (µg/kg/min)*
5	0.20
10	0.23
20	0.28
30	0.33
40	0.38
50	0.43

the management of rate control in patients with atrial fibrillation. The Digoxin Investigation Group (DIG) clarified the role for digoxin in the management of heart failure patients with normal sinus rhythm.[5] This study demonstrated that digoxin, in addition to background angiotensin converting enzyme inhibitor (ACEI) and diuretic therapy, improved exercise tolerance, and reduced heart failure related hospitalizations, but did not improve survival. Therefore, digoxin therapy for heart failure may be considered either in patients with atrial fibrillation, or in patients in sinus rhythm on target doses (if tolerated) of ACEI/ARB and β-blockers who exhibit continued exercise intolerance or recurrent heart failure related hospitalizations.

Digoxin is primarily renally eliminated with a serum elimination half-life of 1.6 days in patients with normal renal function. Recent trials have demonstrated that the efficacy of digoxin in heart failure can be achieved with doses that produce serum concentrations of 0.5 to 1.0 ng per ml, lower than those previously defined as "therapeutic."[6] Higher serum concentrations provide no added benefit and increase the risk of digoxin toxicity.

DIGOXIN TOXICITY

Digitalis intoxication is a clinical diagnosis based on the presence of signs and/or symptoms including anorexia, nausea, and vomiting, and atrial or ventricular arrhythmias. Given the establishment of lower effective serum concentration, the incidence of digoxin toxicity has likely diminished. It is important to understand that the diagnosis of digoxin toxicity is never based solely on the digoxin concentration. Elevated serum digoxin concentrations are only one etiology of drug toxicity, usually related to maintenance doses inappropriate for the level of renal function. Most patients with normal renal function require 0.125 mg digoxin daily. Patients with renal insufficiency typically require 0.125 mg every other day or less. Many

other factors that do not produce elevated serum digoxin concentrations are capable of causing digoxin toxicity including diuretic-induced hypokalemia or hypomagnesemia, hypoxemia, acidosis, hyperthyroidism, and others. Concurrent amiodarone therapy may double the serum digoxin concentration, and typical digoxin dosing in these patients should be reduced by 50% of the usual dose, considering renal function.

DIURETICS

Classical descriptions of acute decompensated heart failure characterize patients as volume overloaded but well perfused ("wet and warm"), or hypoperfused and not volume overloaded ("cool and dry"). The majority of hospitalized patients, however, will require acute diuretic therapy to relieve signs and symptoms associated with their acute presentation. Much of the efficacy data associated with diuretic therapy for acute heart failure are derived from experience prior to the era of randomized controlled trials. Despite their effectiveness for symptom relief, diuretics have not been demonstrated to improve survival in heart failure. Because of their potency, and rapid onset of action, loop diuretics (furosemide, torsemide, bumetanide) are considered the mainstay of treatment (Table 14.3). These agents inhibit sodium and chloride reabsorption in the ascending limb of the Loop of Henle. Their effect to reduce venous tone and therefore pulmonary capillary wedge pressure often begins to improve pulmonary symptoms prior to a significant increase in urinary output. It is important to recognize that patients with chronic heart failure may have increased pulmonary capillary pressures and progressive dyspnea in the absence of significant pulmonary crackles on physical examination. On the contrary, patients with new-onset heart failure are more likely to demonstrate pulmonary vascular congestion (crackles) on examination.

TABLE 14.3	Diuretics Used in the Treatment of Heart Failure		
Drug	Initial Daily Dose(s)	Maximum Total Daily Dose	Duration of Action
LOOP DIURETICS			
Bumetanide	0.5–1.0 mg once or twice	10 mg	4–6 h
Furosemide	20–40 mg once or twice	600 mg	6–8 h
Torsemide	10–20 mg once	200 mg	12–16 h
POTASSIUM SPARING DIURETICS			
Eplerenone	25 mg once	50 mg once	24 h
Spironolactone	12.5–25 mg once	50 mg	2–3 d
Triamterene	50–75mg	200 mg	7–9 h
SEQUENTIAL NEPHRON BLOCKADE			
Metolazone	2.5–10 mg once plus loop diuretic		
Chlorothiazide (IV)	500–1000 mg once plus loop diuretic		

Dosing of loop diuretics is empiric. In general, a 40-mg oral furosemide dose is equivalent to a 20-mg intravenous dose. In volume overloaded patients with normal renal function, an initial intravenous dose of furosemide should be one to two times the chronic oral dose. Response to an individual intravenous dose can be assessed in several hours. Patient response is based on relief of pulmonary vascular congestion, daily weight, hepatic congestion, and peripheral edema. Because Loop diuretics require a threshold serum concentration to affect their natriuretic response, patients with chronic heart failure, and those with moderate-to-severe renal insufficiency will usually require higher initial doses than patients with normal renal function or new-onset heart failure (diuretic naive patients). Alternative furosemide dosing strategies comparing bolus dosing to continuous infusions have been evaluated in a number of small uncontrolled trials. Earlier studies, in addition to a review of eight randomized trials, suggest that continuous intravenous infusions of furosemide ranging from 10 to 40 mg per hour, depending on renal function, produce a greater diuretic effect than similar total doses administered by intermittent bolus dosing, with fewer adverse effects.[7] The recent diuretic optimization strategies evaluation (DOSE) trial, a randomized, open-label comparison between twice daily furosemide and continuous infusion demonstrated no differences in outcomes in 41 hospitalized, volume-overloaded heart failure patients from admission to hospital day 3.[8] There was a trend towards less hypokalemia and hypotension in the continuous infusion group. Although no definitive data currently resolve the dosing route of administration controversy, it does not appear that continuous infusion offers a significant advantage over traditional bolus dosing of furosemide.

Monitoring for adverse effects of diuresis includes electrolytes, orthostatic hypotension, prerenal azotemia or increasing serum creatinine. Less commonly, patients with a history of chronic gout may experience an acute gout exacerbation. Excessive diuresis can enhance undesired neurohormonal activation, increasing the risk of excessive hypotensive effects from ACE inhibitors and β-blockers.

Diuretic resistance is not uncommon in patients with an acute exacerbation of chronic heart failure. A number of factors predispose to lack of diuretic response including worsening renal function, agents such as nonsteroidal anti-inflammatory drugs (NSAIDs) that antagonize the effects of diuretics, renal hypoperfusion secondary to heart failure, or overly aggressive diuresis or vasodilators. A number of strategies to produce an effective diuresis in nonresponsive patients have been employed. First, if appropriate diuretic response is not achieved within 4 hours, the intravenous dose can be successively doubled until an intravenous dose of furosemide 120 mg is reached. Higher single doses are unlikely to enhance diuresis and more likely to risk ototoxicity. Despite the lack of controlled data, anecdotal reports of successful diuresis with continuous furosemide infusions in diuretic-resistant patients may promote successful diuresis. Oral metolazone, unlike other oral thiazide diuretics, can be effective in patients with renal insufficiency. An oral dose of 5 to 10 mg should be administered 30 minutes prior to intravenous furosemide. Although other distal convoluted tubule diuretics such as oral hydrochlorothiazide, chlorthalidone, or intravenous chlorothiazide enhance the efficacy of loop diuretics, metolazone, perhaps related to its efficacy in patients with renal insufficiency and its longer elimination half-life, seems to be preferred by many clinicians.

Diuretics that act more distally, such as spironolactone or amiloride, are less likely to overcome diuretic resistance but may have a role in limiting hypokalemia and hypomagnesemia provoked by loop diuretics. These acute electrolyte disturbances in heart failure patients increase the risk of hemodynamically compromising or potentially life-threatening arrhythmias. Intravenous low-dose dopamine stimulates renal dopamine receptors and has been demonstrated to increase urine output; however, no controlled studies in diuretic-resistant heart failure patients have been undertaken. Interpatient variability in response to the β_1-adrenergic inotropic effects of dopamine may play a role in its ability to increase urinary output in heart failure. The UNLOAD trial demonstrated that ultrafiltration produced greater weight and fluid loss as well as fewer heart failure-related hospitalizations than intravenous diuretics in hospitalized heart failure patients.[9]

ALDOSTERONE ANTAGONISTS

The adverse effects of aldosterone in heart failure are related to its sodium and water retaining potential initiated by activation of the rennin–angiotensin–aldosterone system (RAAS) and from decreased hepatic aldosterone clearance. Important is the impact of aldosterone on myocardial and vascular remodeling producing increased collagen deposition and fibrosis. These effects produce ventricular systolic and diastolic dysfunction and contribute to the progressive nature of chronic heart failure. Although both ACEIs and angiotensin receptor blockers (ARBs) lower aldosterone production in the short term, long-term suppression may not be maintained. Aldosterone antagonists, spironolactone and eplerenone have both been demonstrated to improve symptoms, reduce heart failure-related hospitalizations, and improve survival in selected patients. The randomized aldactone evaluation study (RALES) trial evaluated the effect of spironolactone (maximum dose 25 mg daily) in patients with NYHA class IV symptoms, or class III symptoms in recently hospitalized patients.[10] The eplerenone post-acute myocardial infarction heart failure efficacy and survival study (EPHESUS) trial studied eplerenone (maximum dose 50 mg daily) in patients with heart failure or diabetes and LVEF <40% within 14 days of MI. Both drugs demonstrated an improvement in survival and reduction in heart failure-related hospitalization.[11]

The benefits associated with the use of aldosterone antagonists must be carefully weighed against the potential for life-threatening hyperkalemia. Because ACEI therapy has become a mainstay in the treatment of heart failure, and because some degree of renal insufficiency is common as the severity of heart failure increases, it is imperative that patients be chosen carefully, and that appropriate monitoring of serum potassium concentration takes place. The major trials excluded patients with serum creatinine >2.5 mg per dl; however, serum creatinine is a poor predictor of creatinine clearance, especially in elderly patients. Aldosterone antagonists should not be administered to patients with creatinine clearances <30 ml per minute, and the dose should be reduced at creatinine clearances <50 ml per minute. More frequent use of aldosterone antagonists in the general heart failure population, as opposed to patients enrolled in clinical trials, subsequent to the publication of the two major trials, has resulted in an incidence of hyperkalemia up to 24%.[12] Serum potassium concentrations should be monitored within 3 days after drug initiation and again at 1 week.

Serum potassium concentrations >5.5 mEq per L should promote discontinuation of the drug. The lack of routine monitoring has been well documented in the ambulatory care setting.[13] Although significantly more expensive, the advantage of eplerenone over spironolactone is a lower incidence of gynecomastia.

VASODILATORS

Nitroglycerin, nitroprusside, and nesiritide are all effective to improve hemodynamics and symptoms of pulmonary vascular congestions in patients who are not hypotensive. These agents are indicated in patients with ongoing pulmonary vascular congestion not responsive to diuretic therapy and standard oral therapy. Additional indications for intravenous vasodilator therapy include heart failure patients with ongoing ischemia, hypertension, or significant mitral regurgitation.

NITROGLYCERIN

Nitroglycerin is primarily a venodilator with dose-dependent arteriolar dilating properties. At higher doses, nitroglycerin is a potent coronary vasodilator, making it an ideal agent for patients with ischemic cardiomyopathy. Nitrate-induced preload reduction results in reduced PAOP, myocardial oxygen demand, and improvement in dyspnea. Because of its short onset and duration of action, the infusion rate can be quickly adjusted, allowing easy titration towards maximal beneficial hemodynamic effects, and rapid correction of adverse effects. The risk of hypotension with nitroglycerin as with the other intravenous vasodilators is critically dependent on intravascular volume. Hemodynamic monitoring may be useful to assess the beneficial effects and limit the risk of hemodynamic adverse effects with both nitroglycerin and nitroprusside as well as with intravenous inotropes. Tolerance to the hemodynamic effects of nitroglycerin can be seen in 12 to 72 hours in patients on continuous nitroglycerin infusions.[14]

NITROPRUSSIDE

Nitroprusside is a more balanced arteriolar and venous dilator than nitroglycerin. As a more potent arteriolar dilator, it has greater effect to increase cardiac output in patients with elevated systemic vascular resistance while retaining the preload lowering benefit of reducing PAOP and pulmonary congestion. Although nitroprusside has been associated with coronary steal in patients with obstructive coronary disease, in heart failure patients, the reduction in both preload and afterload generally decreases myocardial oxygen demand.[15] Obviously a significant reduction in aortic diastolic pressure has the potential to decrease coronary perfusion pressure and increase ischemia. As with nitroglycerin, nitroprusside is short acting, providing for easy titration. The most common side effect is hypotension. Two biochemical toxicities have potentially led to the underutilization of nitroprusside in acute decompensated heart failure—cyanide and thiocyanate toxicity. Malnourished patients or patients with liver disease are more prone to cyanide intoxication owing to their inability to combine cyanide produced in the serum from nitroprusside metabolism, with the hepatically produced sulfhydril group to form thiocyanate. The accumulated cyanide produces elevated lactate levels and

metabolic acidosis. Patients with decreased renal function are unable to eliminate the thiocyanate metabolite and develop neurotoxicity including headache, altered mental status, and seizures. Because thiocyanate has an elimination half-life of 4 days in patients with normal renal function, infusions of <3 μg/kg/minute administered for <3 days in patients with a serum creatinine <3.0 mg per dl are unlikely to result in toxicity. Serum thiocyanate concentrations can be measured in the hospital laboratory.

NESIRITIDE

Nesiritide is an intravenous form of recombinant human B-type natriuretic peptides (BNP). It produces a dose-dependent reduction in venous and arterial pressures, natriuresis, and diuresis. Its most consistent effect is decreased dyspnea and POAP, much like nitroglycerin. Questions remain as to the impact of nesiritide on hospitalization rates and mortality, especially in the face of its relatively high cost compared with nitroglycerin. In addition, in a review of a series of publications nesiritide significantly increased the risk of worsening renal function.[16] The acute study of clinical effectiveness of nesiritide in decompensated heart failure (ASCEND-HF) trial recently demonstrated that nesiritide had no beneficial effect on survival or rehospitalization in heart failure patients, and had a small, nonsignificant effect on dyspnea. Renal function was not adversely affected, but the rate of hypotension was increased.[17]

ANGIOTENSIN CONVERTING ENZYME INHIBITORS/ANGIOTENSIN RECEPTOR BLOCKING AGENTS

ACEIs have been demonstrated to improve survival in NYHA classes II–IV patients with systolic dysfunction and improve symptoms in many patients (Table 14.4). Their pharmacologic effects, inhibiting the conversion of angiotensin I to angiotensin II, result in a decreased production of angiotensin II and aldosterone. Limiting aldosterone production decreases the progression of left ventricular dysfunction and reduces ventricular remodeling, myocardial fibrosis, cardiac hypertrophy, and dilatation. The chronic hemodynamic effects of ACEIs to reduce afterload, and to a lesser extent, preload, improves exercise tolerance and quality of life. In addition to improving survival, ACEIs decrease the rate of heart failure-related hospitalizations and limit the need for increasing diuretic doses. For post-MI patients, ACEIs reduce the risk of developing heart failure, recurrent MI, and heart failure-related hospitalizations. Owing to the significant cumulative data demonstrating the benefit for ACEI in the treatment of chronic heart failure, these drugs, as opposed to ARBs are recommended as first line therapy for chronic heart failure. ARBs, which probably possess similar symptom and survival benefit, should be reserved for the 10% to 15% of patients who develop ACEI-induced cough.[18]

ACEI therapy for ischemic or nonischemic cardiomyopathy should be initiated at low doses but may be titrated to maximum doses within a few days to weeks, provided blood pressure and renal function remain stable. It is important to note that patients with more severe heart failure may have relatively low blood pressures (systolic pressures in the 100 mm Hg range), and as long as symptomatic hypotension is not present, ACEI therapy should be maintained. Dose reduction or transient

TABLE 14.4	Oral Agents FDA Approved for Treatment of Chronic Heart Failure		
Drug	*Initial Dose*	*Target Dose*	*Elimination*
ACE INHIBITORS			
Captopril	6.25 mg TID	50 mg TID	Renal
Enalapril	2.5–5 mg BID	10 mg BID	Renal
Lisinopril	2.5–5 mg daily	20–40 mg daily	Renal
Quinapril	10 mg BID	20–40 mg BID	Renal
ANGIOTENSIN RECEPTOR BLOCKERS			
Candesartan	4 mg daily	32 mg daily	Renal
Valsartan	40 mg BID	160 mg BID	Liver/some renal
β-BLOCKERS			
Carvedilol	3.125 mg BID	<85 kg: 25 mg BID >85 kg: 50 mg BID	Liver
Carvedilol extended release	10 mg daily	80 mg daily	Liver
Metoprolol extended release	12.5 mg daily	200 mg daily	Liver
HYDRALAZINE-ISOSORBIDE (Bidil)	Hydralazine 37.5 mg Isosorbide 20 mg TID	Hydralazine 75 mg Isosorbide 40 mg TID	Liver

withholding of ACEI administration should not be based only on the systolic blood pressure reading but also on the presence of symptomatic hypotension. In addition, new onset hypotension or an increase in serum creatinine, in the setting of ACEI therapy warrants an evaluation for cause, especially overly aggressive diuretic therapy, or hyponatremia in the setting of NYHA Class IV heart failure. Although survival enhancement can be achieved with low doses of ACEIs (5 mg lisinopril or its equivalent), maximum symptom improvement and limitation of heart failure-related hospitalizations are best achieved with higher doses (20 to 40 mg lisinopril).

For patients with acute decompensations of chronic heart failure, ACEI or ARBs have minimal acute hemodynamic benefit but should remain part of the therapeutic regimen as long as they are hemodynamically tolerated. There are two additional goals associated with ACEI and ARB administration in hospitalized heart failure patients: first, to prevent other hospital-related diagnostic or therapeutic interventions, such as the administration of intravenous contrast dye, from increasing the risk of ACEI/ARB toxicity; and second, to maximize the dose of ACEI/ARB to doses that have been shown to have the most benefit for symptom relief prior to hospital discharge.

The two most likely adverse effects associated with ACEI/ARB administration in hospitalized patients are hypotension and worsening renal function. The risks of both these outcomes are enhanced by overly aggressive diuresis. Small (10%) increases in serum creatinine are commonly associated with initiating ACEI/ARB therapy in heart failure patients and should not provoke dosage reduction or drug withdrawal. Progressive increases in serum creatinine, however, are a typical manifestation of decreased renal blood flow, commonly the result of aggressive diuretic therapy or worsening heart failure. Reducing the rate of diuresis rather than holding the dose of ACEI/ARB will usually allow renal function and/or blood pressure to return to its baseline level. It is not usually necessary to temporarily withhold administration of the ACEI/ARB, unless the rise in serum creatinine continues. Drug-induced

hypotension, even in the face of total body volume overload, will usually require holding the diuretic until intravascular volume equilibrates.

A second common cause of worsening renal function associated with the administration of ACEIs/ARBs is the concomitant use of other nephrotoxic agents, most notably, intravenous contrast administered for coronary artery imaging. Because of the risk of nephrotoxicity associated with iodinated contrast, especially in the diabetic patient, withholding ACEIs/ARBs for patients with suspected dye-induced nephrotoxicity is appropriate until renal function returns to baseline. Although volume repletion is an effective method of reducing the risk of dye-induced nephrotoxicity, this may be more difficult in heart failure patients than in patients with coronary artery disease without heart failure.[18] The presence of preexisting renal disease in heart failure patients should not be considered a contraindication to ACEI/ARB therapy in chronic heart failure. Several trials in various patient populations including post-MI patients with decreased left ventricular function have demonstrated that ACEIs are more effective in the subset of patients with mild-to-moderate renal insufficiency than in patients with normal renal function.[19] Judicious routine monitoring of renal function is required in hospitalized heart failure patients, irrespective of the addition of ACEIs/ARBs. Prevention of hyperkalemia is especially important in heart failure patients with CKD receiving ACEI/ARB therapy.

β-BLOCKERS

β-Blockers were originally considered contraindicated in heart failure patients owing to their negative inotropic effects (Table 14.4). Once the paradigm for the pathogenesis of heart failure shifted away from primary myocardial dysfunction to a syndrome resulting from the action of "compensatory" mechanisms related to the sympathetic nervous system and the renin–angiotensin–aldosterone axis, it became clear that agents that antagonize these mechanisms might be beneficial. Several large randomized trials in the 1990s demonstrated that β-blockers improve survival in patients with NYHA classes II–IV heart failure.[20–23] In addition, they decrease the risk of overt heart failure in patients with asymptomatic left ventricular dysfunction. The progression and degree of chronic heart failure severity are associated with the serum concentration of norepinephrine. Patients with the highest norepinephrine concentrations have the poorest prognosis. Hemodynamically, norepinephrine-induced tachycardia and inotropic effects increase myocardial oxygen demand. In addition, the peripheral vasoconstriction increases left ventricular afterload, further increasing oxygen demand and decreasing cardiac output. Chronically, sympathetic stimulation produces myocardial cell loss through apoptosis and cell necrosis as well as downregulation of myocardial β_1-receptors and loss of sensitivity to sympathetic stimulants. As had been previously discovered with the use of ACEIs—to interfere with the adverse effects of the RAAS on progressive ventricular dysfunction, survival, and symptoms—blocking the detrimental effects of catecholamines on the failing ventricle with β-blockers resulted in improved left ventricular function, attenuating ventricular remodeling, decreasing the risk of life-threatening arrhythmias, and decreasing myocardial oxygen demand.

A number of issues are relevant to the use of β-blockers in the hospitalized heart failure patient. These include timing of drug therapy initiation, methods for increasing doses towards chronic target dosing, strategies for dosing in patients on chronic β-blockers who are admitted for acute heart failure decompensation, and choosing between various β-blockers approved for use in chronic heart failure.

β-Blocker therapy should be initiated in patients with new-onset heart failure only after volume status has been optimized. Patients who remain volume overloaded are more likely to develop increasing heart failure symptoms, whereas patients who are intravascularly volume depleted are more likely to become hypotensive. Several studies have addressed the order in which ACEI/ARB or β-blockers should be administered, because initiation of both agents is recommended within 24 hours of the onset of MI.[24] These studies, however, have been performed in mild-to-moderate chronic heart failure patients, not hospitalized patients with new onset, or acutely decompensated heart failure. Although both β-blockers and ACEIs are effective for myocardial remodeling postMI, current guidelines recommend initiation of ACEI within 24 hours of the MI, and delaying the introduction of β-blockade until the signs and symptoms of heart failure have been resolved. It is not necessary to achieve the "target dose" of ACEI/ARB prior to initiating starting doses of β-blocker.

Unlike the initial dosing strategy with ACEIs/ARBs, β-blockers should be titrated towards their target doses more gradually, with a minimum of 2-week interval between dosage increases. It is well documented that many patients with chronic heart failure do not receive doses consistent with target doses determined by large controlled trials. As with ACEIs/ARBs, although small doses of β-blockers do positively affect survival, greater reduction in heart failure hospitalizations and improvement in LVEF are achieved with dosing strategies intended to achieve target doses. It is common for ambulatory care providers to maintain patients on the low-dose β-blockers that were initiated during an acute hospitalization, presumptively based on concerns for worsening heart failure as the dose is increased, or assuming that the patient has achieved his or her ultimate level of symptom control. Clearly, monitoring for adverse effects such as worsening heart failure, symptomatic

bradycardia, or hypotension are a requisite part of chronic monitoring during titration towards target doses of β-blocker therapy. Especially for new-onset heart failure patients, however, maintaining a starting dose, without an attempt to titrate to target doses, diminishes the potential benefit that the combination of ACEI/ARB and β-blockers can achieve for prevention of disease progression.

Recent data have addressed the question of withdrawing β-blockers in patients on chronic therapy who present with an acute decompensation of heart failure. Until recently, the approaches have generally been either to temporarily discontinue the β-blocker or to decrease the chronic dose to some degree. The appropriate strategy clearly depends on the level of severity of the acute decompensation. Patients who present with severe hemodynamic decompensation (hypotensive, or approaching cardiogenic shock) or those with severe pulmonary vascular congestion are obvious candidates for transient withdrawal of β-blockers. Data prospectively analyzed from the OPTIMIZE-HF Program demonstrated that patients withdrawn from β-blocker therapy had a higher risk for mortality, compared with those who continued on β-blockers.[25] Patients who were eligible for β-blocker therapy, but did not receive them had similar risk for mortality as those who had therapy withdrawn. During the 60- to 90-day follow-up period, 94% of patients remained on β-blockers after discharge. Only 57% of patients who had their β-blocker withdrawn received β-blocker treatment during the 60- to 90-day follow-up period. Of the patients maintained on therapy during hospitalization, only 12% had their maintenance dose reduced during follow-up. The remaining 88% were maintained on their preadmission dose or had their dose increased (12%). It appears therefore from limited registry data that patients with chronic heart failure admitted to the hospital on β-blocker therapy should not have this therapy withdrawn unless they are hemodynamically compromised. An additional risk associated with β-blocker withdrawal is failure to reinstate the drug after hospital discharge.

Two β-blockers are currently approved in the United States for the treatment of heart failure—metoprolol controlled release/extended release (CR/XL) and carvedilol. Bisoprolol has also been demonstrated to reduce the incidence of sudden death and of heart failure-related death, but is not approved by the FDA for this indication in the United States. Metoprolol is a cardioselective β-blocker, whereas carvedilol is a nonselective β-blocker with α-adrenergic blocking activity. Both agents have demonstrated similar reductions in morbidity and mortality in large randomized controlled studies of heart failure patients. Subtle pharmacodynamic features may influence the decision to use one drug or the other. The cardioselectivity of metoprolol may be beneficial in patients with reversible airway disease such as asthma; however, cardioselectivity diminishes with increasing dosage. The recommended target dose of metoprolol of 200 mg daily likely provides little cardioselectivity. The α-blocking property of carvedilol has a theoretical advantage in patients with a history of cocaine abuse in whom pure β-blocker pharmacology leaves unopposed coronary artery α-receptors susceptible to the vasospastic potential of cocaine. Both metoprolol XL and carvedilol are available as once daily dosing formulations to enhance patient compliance.

The commonest adverse effects of β-blockers in heart failure patients include worsening of heart failure symptoms, especially in volume-overloaded patients or in those whose dose titration has occurred too rapidly, symptomatic bradycardia, or hypotension.

HYDRALAZINE–ISOSORBIDE

The combination of the direct arteriolar dilator, hydralazine and isosorbide dinitrate (ISDN), a long-acting nitrate venodilator was the first vasodilator regimen to demonstrate improved survival in chronic heart failure (V-HeFT).[26] Within a few years, ACEIs had been shown to enhance survival to a greater degree than the original vasodilator combination and had become the standard of care for chronic heart failure. A post hoc analysis of the original hydralazine—nitrate trial suggested that the combination was particularly effective in African Americans. The A-HeFT trial compared a fixed combination of hydralazine and ISDN (maximum dose hydralazine 75 mg plus ISDN 40 mg three times a day) versus placebo in self-identified African American patients on background ACEI, β-blocker, and a diuretic with or without digoxin and spironolactone.[27] The hydralazine–ISDN group had a significant reduction in mortality, heart failure-related hospitalizations, and an improvement in quality of life.

Oral vasodilator therapy with ACEIs and the combination of hydralazine have primarily been studied in patients with chronic heart failure. However, in hospitalized patients with acute heart failure for whom ACEIs may be transiently withheld owing to acute elevations of serum creatinine, hydralazine–isosorbide has been substituted for its beneficial hemodynamic effect.[28] Once stable renal function has been reestablished, ACEIs are the preferred choice for chronic management. In addition to its use in African-American patients, chronic hydralazine–isosorbide therapy may be appropriate for patients who do not tolerate either ACEIs or ARBs owing to renal insufficiency or hyperkalemia.

The frequency of side effects such as headache and gastrointestinal complaints from the hydralazine–isosorbide combination in large trials is significant, and in both VA heart failure trials many patients did not tolerate target doses of these drugs. In addition, the necessity of three times daily dosing increases the risk of noncompliance.

REFERENCES

1. Dec GW. Management of acute decompensated heart failure. *Curr Probl Cardiol.* 2007;32:321–366.
2. Tsvetkova TFD, Abraham WT, Kelly P, et al. Comparative hemodynamic effects of milrinone and dobutamine in heart failure patients treated chronically with carvedilol [abstract]. *J Card Fail.* 1998;4(suppl 1):36.
3. Applefeld MM, Newman KA, Grove WR, et al. Intermittent, continuous outpatient dobutamine infusion in the management of congestive heart failure. *Am J Cardiol.* 1983;51:455–458.
4. Silver AM, Horton DP, Ghali JK, et al. Effect of nesiritide versus dobutamine on short-term outcomes in the treatment of patients with acutely decompensated heart failure. *J Am Coll Cardiol.* 2002;39:798–803.
5. The Digitalis Investigation Group. The effect of digoxin on mortality and morbidity in patients with heart failure. *N Engl J Med.* 1997;336:525–533.
6. Adams KF, Gheorghiade M, Uretsky BF, et al. Clinical benefits of low serum digoxin concentrations in heart failure. *J Am Coll Cardiol.* 2002;39:946–953.
7. Salvador DR, Rey NR, Ramos GC, et al. Continuous infusion versus bolus injection of loop diuretics in congestive heart failure. *Cochrane Database Syst Rev.* 2005;CD003178.
8. Allen LA, Turer AT, DeWald T, et al. Continuous versus bolus dosing of furosemide for patients hospitalized for heart failure. *Am J Cardiol.* 2010;105:1794–1797.
9. Costanzo MR, Guglin ME, Saltzberg MT, et al. Ultrafiltration versus intravenous diuretics for patients hospitalized for acute decompensated heart failure. *J Am Coll Cardiol.* 2007;49:675–683.
10. Pitt B, Zannad DF, Remme WJ, et al. The effect of spironolactone on morbidity and mortality in patients with severe heart failure. *N Engl J Med.* 1999;341:709–717.
11. Pitt B, Remme WJ, Zannad DF, et al. Eplerenone, a selective aldosterone blocker in patients with left ventricular dysfunction after myocardial infarction. *N Engl J Med.* 2003;348:1309–1321.
12. Juurlink DM, Mamdani M, Kopp A, et al. Drug–drug interactions among elderly patients hospitalized for drug toxicity. *JAMA.* 2003;289:1652–1658.
13. Shah KB, Rao K, Sawyer R, et al. The adequacy of laboratory monitoring in patients treated with spironolactone for congestive heart failure. *J Am Coll Cardiol.* 2005;46:845–849.
14. Elkayam U, Kulick D, McIntosh N, et al. Incidence of early tolerance to hemodynamic effects of continuous infusion of nitroglycerin in patients with coronary artery disease and heart failure. *Circulation.* 1987;76:577–584.
15. Robertson RM, Robertson D. Drugs used for the treatment of ischemia. In: Limbird LE, Hardman JG, eds. *Goodman and Gillman's the Pharmacological Basis of Therapeutics.* 10th ed. New York, NY: McGraw Hill; 2001:840–871.
16. Sackner-Bernstein JD, Skopicki HA, Aaronson KD. Risk of worsening renal function with nesiritide in patients with acutely decompensated heart failure. *Circulation.* 2005;111:1487–1491.
17. O'Connor CM, Starling RC, Hernandez AF, et al. Effect of nesiritide in patients with acute decompensated heart failure. *N Engl J Med.* 2011;365:32–43.
18. Maeder M, Klein M, Fehr T, et al. Contrast nephropathy: review focusing on prevention. *J Am Coll Cardiol.* 2004;44:1763–1771.
19. Solomon SD, Rice MM, Jablonski KA, et al. Renal function and effectiveness of angiotensin-converting enzyme inhibitor treatment in patients with chronic stable coronary disease in the prevention of events with ACE inhibition (PEACE) trial. *Circulation.* 2006;114:26–31.
20. Packer M, Bristow MR, Cohn JN, et al. The effect of carvedilol on morbidity and mortality in patients with chronic heart failure. U.S. Carvedilol Heart Failure Study group. *N Engl J Med.* 1996;334:1349–1355.
21. Effect of metoprolol CR/XL in chronic heart failure: Metoprolol CR/XL Randomized Intervention Trial in-Congestive Heart Failure (MERIT-HF). *Lancet.* 1999;353:2001–2007.
23. The Cardiac Insufficiency Bisoprolol Study II (CIBIS-II): a randomized trial. *Lancet.* 1999;353:9–13.
24. Willenheimer R, van Veldhuisen DJ, Silke B, et al. Effect on survival with hospitalization of initiating treatment for chronic heart failure with bisoprolol followed by enalapril, as compared with the opposite sequence: results of the randomized Cardiac Insufficiency Bisoprolol Study (CIBIS) III. *Circulation.* 2005;112:2426–2435.
25. Fonarow GC, Abraham WT, Albert NM, et al. Influence of beta blocker continuation or withdrawal on outcomes in patients hospitalized with heart failure. Findings from the OPTIMIZE-HF Program. *J Am Coll Cardiol.* 2008;52:190–199.
26. Cohn JN, Archibald DG, Zeische S, et al. Effect of vasodilator therapy on mortality in chronic congestive heart failure. Results of a Veterans Administration Cooperative Study. *N Engl J Med.* 1986;314:1547–1552.
27. Taylor AL, Ziesche S, Yancy C, et al. Combination of isosorbide dinitrate and hydralazine in blacks with heart failure. *N Engl J Med.* 2004;351:2049–2057.
28. Verma SP, Silke B, Reynolds GW, et al. Vasodilator therapy for acute heart failure: haemodynamic comparison of hydralazine/isosorbide, alpha-adrenergic blockade, and angiotensin-converting enzyme inhibition. *J Cardiovasc Pharmacol.* 1992;20:274–281.

PATIENT AND FAMILY INFORMATION FOR:

Medications in the Management of Heart Failure

DRUGS FOR HOSPITALIZED HEART FAILURE PATIENTS

Patients with heart failure symptoms often need hospitalization when their symptoms become severe. Several drugs are useful to relieve the symptoms of heart failure and to return them to the quality of life they experienced prior to the need for hospitalization. For most patients, relieving symptoms related to shortness of breath and swelling of their extremities are important goals. For patients who are more severely ill, improving their heart function will provide better blood flow to their organs and muscles. There are three drug categories that are frequently used for hospitalized heart failure patients: drugs that relieve swelling and shortness of breath: diuretics such as furosemide (Lasix); drugs that improve heart pumping function (dobutamine or milrinone); and drugs that relax blood vessels and make it easier for the heart to pump blood into the blood vessels (nitroglycerin or nitroprusside).

Diuretic drugs decrease the amount of volume that is in the bloodstream by increasing the amount of salt and water that is removed by the kidneys. Patients with heart failure are often short of breath because the amount of fluid in their lungs makes it difficult to breathe. In addition, many patients have fluid accumulation in their ankles, legs, and even in their abdomen. The primary goal in hospitalized heart failure patients is to eliminate fluid from the lungs, followed by a reduction of fluid in other parts of the body. It is important for heart failure patients to know their "dry weight," the target weight they should maintain as outpatients. Appropriate use of diuretic drugs in the hospital should bring patients close to their dry weight. It equally important for heart failure patients to weigh themselves daily at home because this is a practical method to determine fluid accumulation. Weight gain of more than 2 to 3 pounds within a few days is an indication that their heart failure may not be well controlled. Dietary salt intake has the greatest potential to promote fluid accumulation. Patients should be aware of the salt (sodium) content of the foods they eat, especially prepared foods such as canned vegetables and soups, prepared meats, and snack foods such as pretzels, potato chips, and similar snack foods. They should also avoid adding salt to their meals at the table. Excessive salt intake can easily overcome the effects of diuretic drugs and result in fluid accumulation. Some physicians have successfully educated patient to increase the dose of their diuretic drugs (furosemide or Lasix) when their weight increases by several pounds. If weight gain continues, or patients become increasingly short of breath with exertion or when lying down at night, they should contact their physician. The side effects of diuretics that are closely monitored are decreases in blood pressure, kidney function, and other body salts such as potassium and magnesium. A careful balance is maintained between too much volume in the circulation—producing symptoms of shortness of breath and swelling, and too little volume—resulting in diminished kidney function or low blood pressure.

In addition to diuretics such as furosemide, which are used in the hospital and chronically to manage fluid balance, two other diuretic drugs may be used in selected heart failure patients with moderate to severe forms of heart failure. Spironolactone (aldactone) and eplerenone (inspra) are diuretic drugs that work by a different mechanism than furosemide, and, unlike other diuretic agents, have been shown to improve survival in selected heart failure patients. Although they add to the ability of diuretic drugs to maintain appropriate fluid balance, their major impact is to add to the survival benefit of drugs such as ACE inhibitors and ß-blockers (see below). The most important side effect of these added diuretics is their ability to increase the level of potassium in the blood. As ACE inhibitors or ARBs also have the ability to cause the kidneys to hold on to potassium, serum potassium level should be closely monitored, especially in patients whose kidney function is impaired.

Intravenous drugs that increase the force of contraction in heart failure patients are sometimes required in hospitalized patients when more conservative therapy has failed to improve symptoms and blood flow. Dobutamine and milrinone are drugs that increase the force with which the heart contracts, and therefore increase the amount of blood to kidneys, muscles, and other vital organs. These drugs are intended for short-term use—several days, and are effective at improving blood flow, stabilizing blood pressure, and improving symptoms. Because these drugs have a short duration of action, doses can be easily adjusted to the heart pressures that are being closely monitored in severely ill patients. Most patients with heart failure have poorly contracting ventricles (lower heart chambers). Although it seems logical that drugs that improve the force of contraction of the heart should improve survival, the effect of these drugs is to improve symptoms and restore normal pressures in the circulation rather than to benefit survival. The major side effects of dobutamine and milrinone include increased heart rate and heart rhythm disturbances. These potential side effects are closely monitored in hospitalized patients in intensive care units. In rare cases, dobutamine may be used as an intermittent outpatient infusion to relieve symptoms in patients with severe heart failure who are not candidates for heart transplants or implantable heart pumps.

The only oral drug used in heart failure to increase the force of contraction is digoxin. The drug, used for more than 200 years in the treatment of heart failure, is much less powerful than agents such as dobutamine or milrinone. There are two circumstances in which digoxin may be used in heart failure. In hospitalized patients whose heart failure is complicated by the cardiac rhythm disturbance, atrial fibrillation, a rhythm disturbance of the upper chambers of the heart, digoxin may be used with other drugs to reduce pulse rate. In chronic heart failure patients, digoxin may be added to other chronic heart failure medications to improve symptoms of exercise intolerance and to decrease the rate of hospitalizations for heart failure symptoms. Digoxin must be administered at lower dose or less frequently (every other day) to patients whose heart failure is complicated by reduced kidney function. Loss of appetite, nausea, and changes in heart rhythm are side effects that should be monitored in patients receiving digoxin therapy.

Nitroglycerin and nitroprusside are intravenous drugs that dilate arteries and/or veins and may be used in patients with severe heart failure. By relaxing arteries, more blood can be ejected from the heart, increasing blood flow to vital organs. Because these drugs have the potential to lower blood pressure in patients whose heart function is already compromised, they must be administered under close supervision, making sure that blood flow is improved while blood pressure is maintained. Fortunately, both nitroprusside and nitroglycerin are very short-acting drugs, whose doses can be quickly altered if necessary. Because nitroprusside has some side effects that occur more commonly in patients whose kidneys are not functioning normally, some physicians prefer nitroglycerin in such patients. Because nitroprusside is better able to dilate arteries than nitroglycerin, it may be preferred in patients with normal kidney function. Nitroglycerin dilates veins, to a greater extent than arteries, and is especially useful in patients with significant shortness of breath owing to fluid accumulation in the lungs, and in patients with coronary artery disease, who may be experiencing chest pain associated with their heart failure symptoms.

DRUGS FOR CHRONIC HEART FAILURE

Most drugs used for the treatment of chronic heart failure will be continued when patients are hospitalized. At times during a patient's hospitalization, especially if their blood pressure decreases, or their kidney function worsens, these drugs may be withheld for short periods. However, once the patient's symptoms and vital organ function (especially kidneys) have improved, these agents will be restarted prior to discharge from the hospital.

ACE Inhibitors (lisinopril and others) are drugs that relax (dilate) blood vessels, making it easier for the heart to eject blood into the circulation. They thereby decrease the amount of work that the heart has to perform to provide adequate blood flow to vital organs and muscles. Most important, these drugs reduce the rate of deterioration of heart function responsible for the progression of heart failure and prolong survival. Heart failure patients and their caretakers should understand that although most patients experience some symptom improvement, continued compliance with the medication is critical, even in those whose symptoms do not improve, or improve only slightly, because the drugs prolong life. About 10% of patients experience a dry cough with ACE inhibitor therapy. The cough may occur at any time during therapy, and the patient's caretaker may notice the symptoms before the patient. Should the cough become bothersome, replacing the ACE inhibitor with an ARB will provide the same benefit without the associated cough. Many heart failure experts, however, prefer ACE inhibitors as first line therapy for heart failure. Seldom do patients experience swelling of the lips, tongue, or throat from ACE inhibitors. This reaction is a medical emergency and the patient should be taken to an emergency department for treatment to make sure that the airway is not blocked.

ARBs provide similar benefit for heart failure patients but are generally reserved for patients who do not tolerate ACE inhibitors. The incidence of swelling of the lips and throat is lower than with ACE inhibitors, but there are rare cases of such swelling in patients receiving ARBs who had previous reactions with ACE inhibitors. Patients receiving ACE inhibitors or ARBs will both require monitoring of blood pressure, kidney function, and potassium levels in the blood.

Similar to ACE inhibitors, ß-blocker drugs are an important part of the treatment of chronic heart failure. ß-Blockers work in heart failure by preventing chemicals produced by the nervous system from interacting with heart muscle. This interaction is partially responsible for the chronic decrease in pump function with progression of symptoms experienced by heart failure patients. ß-Blockers, like ACE inhibitors and ARBs may also be used to treat high blood pressure, but their use in heart failure is not primarily directed at blood pressure. Similar to ACE inhibitors, ß-blockers prevent the progression of pump function loss, improve survival, and for most patients, improve exercise tolerance and other symptoms of heart failure. Also similar to ACE inhibitor therapy, lack of symptom improvement should not cause patients to stop taking the drug because it also prolongs life. For patients with new-onset heart failure, ß-blockers will be started at a low dose, whether the patient is in the hospital or treated as an outpatient. However, ß-blocker therapy will not be started until the patient's heart failure symptoms, especially fluid overload, have been treated, and the patient is considered stable. The dose of ß-blocker will be gradually increased towards a maximum target dose no more frequently than every 2 weeks, provided no adverse effects are noticed. The most important ß-blocker side effects are excessive slowing of heart rate or reduction of blood pressure, producing symptoms of dizziness or lightheadedness. Other side effects may be observed in patients with other diseases such as asthma or diabetes. Patients with asthma may experience shortness of breath or wheezing. This side effect can be minimized with certain ß-blocker drugs such as metoprolol (Toprol) but may still occur and should be closely monitored. Diabetic patients, especially those receiving insulin should closely monitor their blood sugars at home because ß-blockers may either increase or decrease blood sugar. In addition, these drugs may interfere with a patient's ability to recognize the symptoms of low blood sugar. Sweating and change in mental status may still occur, but the patient may not experience tremor, rapid heart rate, or anxiety typically observed with low blood sugar in the absence of ß-blockers. ß-Blocks should not be discontinued abruptly without close medical supervision owing to the risk of heart attack or serious heart rhythm disturbances.

The combination of hydralazine and isosorbide, when added to standard ACE inhibitor, ß-blocker, and diuretic therapy in African American patients has been shown to improve survival, reduce hospitalizations, and improve quality of life in patients with moderate-to-severe heart failure. These drugs relax arteries (hydralazine) and veins (isosorbide), improving blood flow, decreasing the work of the heart, and possibly preventing changes in the structure of heart muscle associated with heart failure. This drug combination is available as a single fixed combination dosage form (Bidil) or as separate drug entities, which are less costly. A significant disadvantage of the combination is the necessity of administering the drugs three times a day. Because most drug therapies for heart failure are administered once or twice a day, the addition of this combination may challenge the likelihood of successful compliance. The incidence of side effects with this combination is also higher than with most other heart failure regimens. Headache, dizziness, and gastrointestinal distress increase with dose and are fairly common. Dosage should be gradually increased towards the target maximum dose (hydralazine 75 mg and isosorbide 40 mg three times daily) or to a dose that is tolerated by the patient.

There are many drugs that should be avoided in heart failure patients. Most of these drugs are available only by prescription and will be known by your physician. These include some drugs used for high blood pressure, diabetes, heart rhythm disturbances, and arthritis. Patients must be aware that some over-the-counter medications have the potential to worsen the symptoms of heart failure. Most important among these is NSAIDs such as ibuprofen (motrin), naproxen (aleve, naprosyn), and similar drugs for pain and inflammation. Acetaminophen (Tylenol) in appropriate doses is safer. NSAIDs may cause salt and water retention, leading to edema (swelling), worsening shortness of breath, and to a decrease in kidney function. In addition, many herbal products including ginseng, and licorice, and St. John's wart should be avoided in heart failure patients. It is best to consult with your pharmacist or physician before adding any new over-the-counter medication or herbal preparation to the prescribed regimen. Patients with heart failure are commonly prescribed complicated drug therapy regimens and have other medical conditions related to heart disease including diabetes, high cholesterol, high blood pressure, or others. Behaviors that improve drug therapy compliance can help reduce the need for hospitalizations. Patients should always keep a list of their current drug therapy regimen with them, especially when visiting health care providers or on admission to the hospital.

SECTION III

Arrhythmia in the Cardiac Care Unit

Seongwook Han
Mithilesh K. Das

CHAPTER

15

Bradyarrhythmia Including Heart Block

Bradycardia refers to a heart rate of <60 beats per minute (bpm). The term bradyarrhythmia should be reserved for any heart rhythm <60 bpm. Bradyarrhythmias may be associated with symptoms such as dizziness, near-syncope or syncope, congestive heart failure, exercise intolerance, fatigue, or a confusion that improves with resolution of the bradycardia. The mere presence of a slow heart rate of <60 bpm that is not associated with any symptoms almost never justifies aggressive interventions. However, it may be important to determine whether the bradyarrhythmia will not resolve spontaneously or with the alleviation of a condition that is the likely cause of the bradyarrhythmia. Management of bradycardia includes the management of reversible causes such as drugs. Nonreversible symptomatic bradycardia warrants pacemaker implant. However, if a hemodynamically stable patient can be observed safely while being treated for a metabolic or ischemic condition or an adverse drug reaction, then it is not justified to implant a permanent pacemaker, even though a temporary pacemaker may be necessary in the interim.

SINUS RHYTHM

Sinus rhythm is present when the dominant pacemaker controlling impulse generation is the sinus node. In this setting, activation of the atria is from right to downwards and left as well as from anterior to posterior. The normal P wave in sinus rhythm may appear slightly notched as the activation of the right atrium precedes that of the left atrium. The normal P wave is positive (upright) in leads 1 and 2, negative in aVR, and it may be positive, negative, or biphasic in lead 3. It is of variable polarity in lead aVL. In the precordial (chest) leads, V_1 and V_2, there is often a terminal negative component of the P wave, reflecting the posterior location (with respect to the right atrium) and later activation of the left atrium. The P wave is typically positive in the remaining precordial leads. In normal sinus rhythm with 1:1 atrioventricular conduction, a P wave with a uniform morphology precedes each QRS complex. The rate is between 60 and 100 bpm and the variation in the heart rates fairly uniform between sequential P waves and QRS complexes. In addition, the P wave morphology and PR intervals appear identical from beat to beat.

INFLUENCE OF THE AUTONOMIC NERVOUS SYSTEM ON SINUS RHYTHM

Although the sinus node has an intrinsic automaticity and always produces an impulse, the rate of impulse generation is controlled by other factors, particularly the autonomic nervous system. With augmented parasympathetic (vagal) influence or reduced sympathetic stimulation, the sinus rate slows, and the PR interval prolongs owing to a vagal-mediated slowing of conduction through the atrioventricular node. By comparison, increased sympathetic activity and decreased vagal effects increase the sinus nodal rate and enhance atrioventricular nodal conduction, resulting in a shortened PR interval.

SINUS ARRHYTHMIA

Sinus arrhythmia is present when there is a sinus rhythm with variability in the cycle lengths between successive P waves. The physiologic variability observed in sinus arrhythmia is the result of respiratory-related changes in autonomic tone that influence the heart rate. Inspiration and the stretching of lung tissue cause a reflex inhibition of vagal tone, which will increase the heart rate. The reverse occurs during expiration. A continuous electrocardiographic recording of sinus arrhythmia reveals a gradual increase and decrease in the heart rate because the cycle lengths between QRS complexes vary with the respiratory cycle. Although sinus arrhythmia is a normal finding, it may be confused with other arrhythmias if the respiratory changes in the RR intervals are prominent.

SICK SINUS SYNDROME OR SINUS NODE DYSFUNCTION

Sick sinus syndrome results from intrinsic disease of the sinus node. Some individuals with this syndrome also have underlying disease of other portions of the conduction system, particularly the AV node. Manifestations of the sick sinus syndrome are symptomatic sinus bradycardia, sinus pauses or arrest, chronotropic incompetence, and tachy–bradycardia syndrome.

SINUS BRADYCARDIA

Sinus bradycardia is defined as a sinus rhythm with a rate <60 bpm. Sinus bradycardia is most frequently caused by an increase in vagal tone or a reduction in sympathetic tone (and thus a physiologic change). Sinus bradycardia occurs in normal children and adults, particularly during sleep when rates of 30 bpm and pauses of up to 2 seconds are not uncommon. It may also be seen in the absence of heart disease in the following settings:

- At rest, in 25% to 35% of asymptomatic individuals under 25 years of age
- In well-conditioned athletes
- In some elderly patients.

As a result, sinus bradycardia is very common at night. When sinus bradycardia results from increased vagal tone, slowing of impulse conduction through the atrioventricular node also results in PR interval prolongation. There is no prognostic significance to sinus bradycardia in otherwise healthy subjects.

PATHOPHYSIOLOGIC SINUS BRADYCARDIA

Sinus bradycardia can be the result of pathophysiologic condition including intrinsic disease of the sinus node ("sick sinus") and several extrinsic causes, manifested as a decrease in spontaneous automaticity and the impulse generation rate (Table 15.1).

- *Exaggerated vagal activity*: Vasovagal responses may be associated with a profound bradycardia owing to heightened parasympathetic activity and sympathetic withdrawal on the sinus node. The combination of the slow heart rate and an associated decline in peripheral vascular resistance is often sufficient to produce presyncope or syncope. There are a variety of stimuli for vagal activation: Pressure on the carotid sinus, as may occur with a tight collar or with the impact of the stream of water in a shower, vomiting, or coughing, Valsalva maneuver when straining at stool, sudden exposure of the face to cold water, and prolonged standing through a Bezold–Jarisch reflex. Hypervagotonia can also result in chronic (i.e., nonepisodic) resting sinus bradycardia. This is the primary mechanism of resting bradycardia in well-trained athletes. Junctional bradycardia and Mobitz type I AV block can also be seen in this setting.
- *Increased intracranial pressure*: Increased intracranial pressure should be excluded when sinus bradycardia occurs in a patient with neurologic dysfunction.
- *Acute myocardial infarction (AMI)*: Sinus bradycardia occurs in 15% to 25% of patients with AMI, particularly those affecting the inferior wall as the right coronary artery supplies the sinus node in approximately 60% of people. Increased vagal activity is primarily responsible, and the bradycardia is typically transient.
- *Obstructive sleep apnea*: Individuals with obstructive sleep apnea frequently have sinus bradycardia and sinus pauses during apneic episodes. Therapies to improve the apnea frequently alleviate the bradycardia.
- *Drugs*: A number of drugs can depress the sinus node and slow the heart rate. These include parasympathomimetic agents, sympatholytic drugs (β-blockers, reserpine, guanethidine, methyldopa, and clonidine), cimetidine, digitalis, calcium channel blockers, amiodarone and other antiarrhythmic drugs, and lithium.
- *Others*: Other causes of sinus bradycardia include hypothyroidism, hypothermia, and severe prolonged hypoxia.

Infectious agents associated with relative sinus bradycardia include Chagas' disease, legionella, psittacosis, Q fever, typhoid fever, typhus, babesiosis, malaria, leptospirosis, yellow fever, dengue fever, viral hemorrhagic fevers, trichinosis, and Rocky Mountain Spotted fever.

SINUS PAUSE OR SINUS ARREST

Sinus pause or sinus arrest is the result of intermittent failure of sinus node impulse generation. Sinus pause or arrest may be owing to intrinsic sinus node disease and dysfunction or from drugs that directly or indirectly (through the autonomic nervous system) depress sinus node activity. On the surface ECG, a sinus pause or arrest is manifest as a long PP cycle length that is longer than the P-P interval of the underlying sinus rhythm but less than two P-P intervals. There is no relationship between the cycle length of the pause and that of the intrinsic sinus rhythm. This occurs in intrinsic sinus node disease or in the setting of vagal stimulation such as respiratory lavage in an intubated patient in intensive care unit.

SINOATRIAL EXIT BLOCK

Sinoatrial (SA) exit block most commonly arises from a change in the electrophysiologic characteristics of the tissue surrounding the sinus node resulting in an inability to respond to or

TABLE 15.1	Major cause of bradycardia
Intrinsic	*Extrinsic*
Idiopathic degeneration (aging)	Autonomically mediated syndromes
Infarction or ischemia	Neurocardiac syncope
Infiltrative diseases	Carotid-sinus hypersensitivity
Sarcoidosis	Situational disturbances
Amyloidosis	Coughing
Hemochromatosis	Micturition
Collagen vascular diseases	Defecation
Systemic lupus erythematosus	Vomiting
Rheumatoid arthritis	Drugs
Scleroderma	β-Adrenergic blockers
Myotonic muscular dystrophy	Calcium-channel blockers
Surgical trauma	Clonidine
Valve replacement	Digoxin
Correction of congenital heart disease	Antiarrhythmic agents
Heart transplantation	Hypothyroidism
Familial diseases	Hypothermia
Infectious diseases	Neurologic disorders
Chagas' disease	Electrolyte imbalances
Endocarditis	Hypokalemia
	Hyperkalemia

conduct an impulse from the sinus node into the atrium. This can be owing to drugs, disease, or increased vagal activity. SA nodal exit block is classified as the first degree, second degree, and third degree.

- First degree SA nodal exit block reflects a slowing of impulse exit but there is still 1:1 conduction. This abnormality cannot be recognized on the surface ECG.

- Second degree SA nodal exit block has two types. Type I (Wenckebach type) is characterized by progressively decreasing P-P intervals prior to a pause caused by a dropped P wave; the pause has a duration that is less than two P-P cycles. The mechanisms of progressive shortening of P-P interval is Wenckebach phenomenon between sinus node to atrium (Figure 15.1). In type II exit block, the P-P output is an arithmetic multiple of the presumed sinus pacemaker input (e.g., 2:1, 3:1, 4:1). Therefore the P-P cycle length surrounding the pause is a multiple of the normal P-P interval (Figure 15.2).

- Third degree SA nodal exit block prevents pacemaker impulses from reaching the right atrium, giving the appearance of sinus arrest (i.e., no P waves).

TACHYCARDIA–BRADYCARDIA SYNDROME

This form of the syndrome is most often characterized by bursts of an atrial tachyarrhythmia (usually atrial fibrillation) which terminate spontaneously and are followed by long offset pauses and symptoms (Figure 15.3). The pause is often long, and there may be no junctional escape rhythm because of associated AV nodal disease. The tachy–bradycardia syndrome is the result of overdrive suppression of the sinus node by the atrial arrhythmia. After arrhythmia termination, there is a variable delay before the sinus node recovers and again generates an impulse because of sinus node dysfunction. Catheter ablation of atrial arrhythmia sometimes cures the arrhythmia. Symptomatic patients, who are not a candidate for catheter ablation, receive permanent pacemakers for bradycardia, and tachycardia is treated by calcium or β-blockers.

CHRONOTROPIC INCOMPITENCE

Chronotropic incompetence is defined as inability to accelerate sinus rate appropriate to the level of exercise. This definition includes inability to reach 70th to 80th percentile of maximum predicted heart rate, delayed peak of heart rate (heart rate peaks during recovery period after the exercise), early peaking of heart rate (prior to the peak exercise), fluctuations of heart rate during exercise or inability to reach a heart rate of 100 to 120 bpm. The heart rate response to exercise also depends on several factors such as deconditioning, drug therapy, and comorbidities.

ATRIOVENTRICULAR BLOCK

AV block can be defined as a delay or interruption in the transmission of an impulse from the atria to the ventricles owing to an anatomical or functional impairment in the conduction system. The conduction disturbance can be transient or permanent, and it can have many causes (Table 15.2). The conduction can be delayed, intermittent, or absent. The commonly used terminology includes first degree (slowed conduction without missed beats), second degree (intermittent conduction, often in a regular pattern, for example, 2:1, 3:2, or higher degrees of block), and third degree or complete AV block.

PHYSIOLOGIC AND PATHOPHYSIOLOGIC AV BLOCK

- *Increased vagal tone.* Enhanced vagal tone owing to sleep, athletic training, pain, carotid sinus massage, or hypersensitive carotid sinus syndrome can result in slowing of the sinus rate and/or the development of AV block.

- *Idiopathic progressive cardiac conduction disease.* Fibrosis and sclerosis of the conduction system accounts for about one-half of cases of AV block and may be induced by several different conditions that often cannot be distinguished clinically. Progressive cardiac conduction defect, also called *Lenegre's*

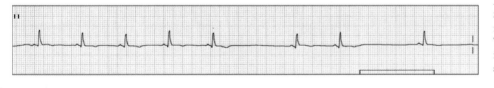

Figure 15.1. Type I second degree SA block. The rhythm strip shows sinus rhythm with normal AV conduction. There is progressive shortening of P-P interval followed by a dropped P wave suggestive of second degree type 1 (Wenckebach) SA block.

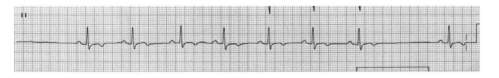

Figure 15.2. Type II second degree SA block. The rhythm strip shows a fixed P-P interval and dropped P waves similar to the rhythm strip of the upper panel.

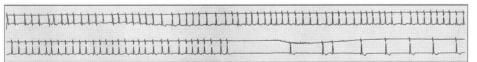

Figure 15.3. Tachy–bradycardia syndrome. The rhythm strip shows atrial fibrillation that terminates into a prolonged pause followed by a slow junctional rhythm.

TABLE 15.2	Major Causes of Atrioventricular Block

Physiologic and Pathophysiologic	Iatrogenic
Increased vagal tone	Drugs
Fibrosis and sclerosis of the conduction system	digitalis, calcium channel blockers,
Ischemic heart disease	β-blockers, amiodarone
Cardiomyopathy and myocarditis	Cardiac surgery
Congenital heart disease	Transcatheter closure of VSD
Familial AV block	Alcohol septal ablation for HCM
Other	
Hyperkalemia, infiltrative malignancies, neonatal lupus syndrome, severe hypo- or hyperthyroidism, trauma, degenerative neuromuscular diseases	

or *Lev's disease*, is characterized by progressive impairment of the conduction system: The term Lenegre's disease has been traditionally used to describe a progressive, fibrotic, sclero-degenerative affliction of the conduction system in younger individuals. It is frequently associated with slow progression to complete heart block and may be hereditary. Lev's disease has referred to "sclerosis of the left side of the cardiac skeleton" in older patients, such as that associated with calcific involvement of the aortic and mitral rings. It is caused by fibrosis or calcification extending from any of the fibrous structures adjacent to the conduction system into the conduction system. Fibrosis of the top of the muscular septum is a common cause of right bundle branch block (RBBB) with left anterior fascicular block in the elderly patient. Involvement of the mitral ring or the central fibrous body, for example, may be the commonest cause of complete heart block with a narrow QRS complex in the elderly. Aortic valve calcification, on the other hand, can invade the bundle of His, the right and/or left bundle branch as well as the left anterior fascicle. Thus, the QRS complex may be prolonged.

- *Ischemic heart disease*: Ischemic disease accounts for about 40% of cases of AV block. Conduction can be disturbed with either chronic ischemic disease or during an AMI. It is estimated that approximately 20% of patients with AMI develop AV block: 8% with first degree 5% with second degree, and 6% with third degree. Intraventricular conduction disturbances (IVCDs), including bundle and fascicular blocks, also occur in 10% to 20% of cases of acute MI. Left bundle branch block (LBBB) and RBBB with left anterior fascicle block are most common, each occurring in about one-third of patients with an IVCD. RBBB with or without left posterior fascicular block and alternating bundle branch block are less frequently seen, whereas isolated left anterior or posterior fascicle block is distinctly unusual.

- *Cardiomyopathy and myocarditis*: AV block can be seen in patients with cardiomyopathies, including hypertrophic obstructive cardiomyopathy and infiltrative processes such as amyloidosis

and sarcoidosis, and in patients with myocarditis owing to a variety of causes including rheumatic fever, Lyme disease, diphtheria, viruses, systemic lupus erythematosus, toxoplasmosis, bacterial endocarditis, and syphilis. The development of AV block in myocarditis is often a poor prognostic sign.

- *Congenital heart disease*: Congenital complete heart block may be an isolated lesion or may be associated with other types of congenital heart disease.

- *Familial disease*: Familial AV conduction block, characterized by a progression in the degree of block in association with a variable apparent site of block, may be transmitted as an autosomal dominant trait. Several sodium channel gene (*SCN5A*) mutations have been associated with sinus node and AV nodal disease. Some of these mutations produce AV block in childhood, whereas others present in middle-age and have been called hereditary Lenegre's disease. In some families with *SCN5A* mutations, AV block or other conduction abnormalities are present with or without associated dilated cardiomyopathy. Different *SCN5A* mutations are associated with other cardiac abnormalities including congenital long QT syndrome type 3, the Brugada syndrome, familial sick sinus syndrome, and familial dilated cardiomyopathy with conduction defects and susceptibility to atrial fibrillation.

- *Other*: AV block can also occur in a variety of other disorders:
  - Hyperkalemia, usually when the plasma potassium concentration is above 6.3 mEq per L.
  - Infiltrative malignancies, such as Hodgkin lymphoma and other lymphomas, and multiple myeloma.
  - Hereditary neuromuscular degenerative disease such as myotonic dystrophy, Kearns–Sayre syndrome, and Erb's dystrophy.
  - Rheumatologic disorders including dermatomyositis and Paget disease.
  - Hyperthyroidism, myxedema, and thyrotoxic periodic paralysis.
  - Neonatal lupus syndrome, which results from transplacental passage of anti-Ro/SSA or anti-La/SSB antibodies from the mother.

IATROGENIC AV BLOCK

- *Drugs*: A variety of drugs can impair conduction and cause AV block. Examples include digitalis, calcium channel blockers (especially verapamil and to a lesser extent diltiazem), amiodarone, adenosine, and β-blockers. In comparison, antiarrhythmic drugs that modulate the sodium channel, such as quinidine, procainamide, and disopyramide, can produce block in the more distal His–Purkinje system. Most patients with AV block who are taking drugs that can impair conduction probably have underlying conduction system disease.

- *Cardiac surgery*: AV block is not uncommonly associated with replacement of a calcified aortic or mitral valve, closure of a ventricular septal defect (VSD), or other surgical procedures.

- *Catheter ablation for arrhythmias*: AV block is a potential complication of catheter ablation of reentrant tachycardia when the reentrant pathway lies within or near the AV node.

- *Transcatheter closure of VSD*: A variety of devices (septal defect occluder) have been used to close muscular VSDs, both congenital and those that occur after myocardial infarction. The presumed mechanism is that the right ventricular retention disk overlaps the ventricular conduction system as it passes above or anterosuperiorly to the defect.

- *Alcohol (ethanol) septal ablation*: Percutaneous transluminal septal myocardial ablation, also called alcohol (ethanol) septal ablation is a nonsurgical treatment for obstructive hypertrophic cardiomyopathy. This intervention consists of infarction and thinning of the proximal interventricular septum through infusion of alcohol into the first septal perforating branch of the left anterior descending coronary artery through an angioplasty catheter. Complete heart block is seen in about half of patients after this procedure.

FIRST DEGREE AV BLOCK

The PR interval includes activation of the atrium, AV node, His bundle, bundle branches and fascicles, and terminal Purkinje fibers. The normal PR interval is between 120 and 200 milliseconds (0.12 to 0.20 second) and tends to shorten with increases in heart rate in part owing to rate-related shortening of action potentials. Children under age 14 tend to have a PR interval of about 140 milliseconds. Atrioventricular impulse transmission is delayed in first degree AV block, resulting in a PR interval >200 milliseconds (>210 milliseconds at slow heart rates). On occasion, the PR interval may be prolonged in the absence of apparent heart disease. For example, first degree AV block, with PR intervals as long as 280 milliseconds has been reported in 1.6% of healthy aviators. Using these criteria, first degree AV block is more common in African Americans than in Caucasians in most age groups. The conduction delay in this setting can occur in the atrium, the AV node, the bundle of His, and in the specialized infra-Hisian conduction system. Involvement of more than one of these sites has been reported

in 20% to 80% of cases. Generally, the first degree AV block does not need treatment.

SECOND DEGREE AV BLOCK

In second degree AV block, some atrial impulses fail to reach the ventricles. Wenckebach described progressive delay between the atrial and ventricular contractions and the eventual failure of an atrial beat to reach the ventricle. Mobitz divided second degree AV block as determined by the ECG into two types:

- Type I block where the phenomenon described by Wenckebach was now translated into ECG terms in which progressive PR interval prolongation preceded a nonconducted P wave (Figures 15.4 and 15.5).
- Type II block in which the PR interval remained unchanged prior to the P wave that suddenly failed to conduct to the ventricles (Figure 15.6).
- The term advanced second degree AV block refers to the block of two or more consecutive P waves, but some beats are conducted in contrast to third degree or complete heart block (Figure 15.7).

Types I and II AV block have different sites of involvement and different prognoses for progression to complete heart block. Type I block most often involves the AV node (70% to 75%) and is generally benign, whereas type II block is almost always below the AV node and can progress to complete heart block. The distinction between type I and type II AV block cannot be made from the ECG when 2:1 block is present. In this situation, every other beat is dropped, and there is no opportunity to observe the PR prolongation that is characteristic of type I block. To aid in the diagnosis, a long rhythm strip should be obtained or a previous ECG examined to try to find a 3:2 cycle.

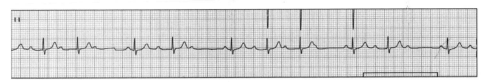

Figure 15.4. Classic type I second degree AV block. The rhythm strip shows progressive PR prolongation preceded a nonconducted P wave.

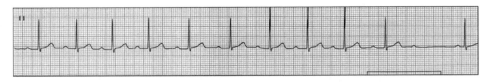

Figure 15.5. Atypical type I second degree AV block. With a long conduction ratio 6:5 or 7:6 or more progressive increment in PR interval becomes unpredictable and the PR interval remains prolonged but constant as shown in this rhythm strip.

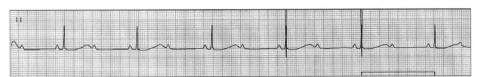

Figure 15.6. The rhythm strip shows sinus rhythm with 2:1 AV block. This can be a type I or type II second degree AV block.

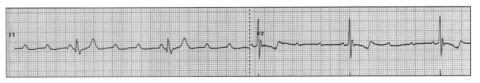

Figure 15.7. Advanced second degree AV block. The rhythm strip shows failure of conduction of two or more consecutive P waves when AV synchrony is otherwise maintained.

If necessary, atropine can be given in an attempt to induce 3:2 conduction.

Mobitz type I AV block (Wenckebach). Uncomplicated Mobitz type I block does not produce symptoms. If, however, the sinus rate is slow and the ratio small (2:1 or 3:2 block), there may be a significant reduction in cardiac output and symptoms of hypoperfusion (including angina or syncope) or heart failure. A Mobitz type I block can occur in normal subjects, athletes, older adults, and in patients who are taking drugs that block the AV node. Mobitz type I block can occur in patients with intrinsic AV nodal disease, myocarditis (including Chagas disease), acute inferior MI or ischemia, and cardiac surgery.

- *Classic:* Classic Mobitz type I block occurs most commonly in the AV node but may also reflect a delay in the transmission of an impulse from the sinus node to the atrium or in any part of the conduction system. It can also be observed in antegrade AV conduction, retrograde VA conduction across the AV node, or as part of exit block with ectopic and parasystolic pacemakers. Regardless of the site involved, what follows is a sequence in which there is a gradually increasing PR interval, usually a gradually falling R-R interval, and an eventual dropped beat. The classic Wenckebach pattern occurs usually with ratios of 3:2, 4:3 or 5:4. This gives rise to a clustering of beats with decreasing R-R intervals that tends to repeat (group beating). One other characteristic of the Wenckebach phenomenon is the cycle of the dropped beat is less than the summed cycles of any two previous cycles. This also results from the incremental conduction delay as the P wave that is not conducted is closer to the preceding QRS than any other in the cycle.

- *Atypical:* Once conduction ratios exceed 6:5 or 7:6, the progressive increment in PR interval becomes unpredictable and the PR interval remains prolonged but constant. The commonest explanation is that the sinus rate changes which, in turn, influences the PR interval through hemodynamic and autonomic effects. The PR interval is still longest in the beat before the dropped beat, shortest in the first beat of the cycle, and then increases in the second beat.

Mobitz type II AV block. The failure of one or more P waves to conduct to the ventricles can lead to dizziness, presyncope, or syncope (called Stokes–Adams attacks), as the lower spontaneous pacemakers are sluggish. An increase in heart rate owing to exercise, atropine, or atrial pacing can worsen the AV block. On the contrary, vagal maneuvers may slow the sinus rate, allow more time for excitability to recover in or below the bundle of His, and facilitate conduction. Type II block is permanent and frequently progresses to higher or even complete heart block. The incidence of requiring insertion of a pacemaker is uncertain, varying in part on the presence or absence of other conduction disturbances.

COMPLETE AV BLOCK

No atrial impulses reach the ventricle in third degree or complete heart block (Figure 15.8). The block can exist in the AV node or in the infranodal conduction system. Escape rhythms occur when a pacemaker other than the sinus node has sufficient time to depolarize, attain threshold, and produce a depolarization. In complete heart block, the escape rhythm that controls the ventricles can occur at any level below that of the conduction block, and the morphology of the QRS complex can help to determine the location at which this is occurring. If third degree block occurs in the AV node, about two-thirds of the escape rhythms have a narrow QRS complex, that is, a junctional or AV nodal rhythm. Block at the level of the bundle of His is also typically associated with a narrow QRS complex. If the escape rhythm has a normal QRS duration of <120 milliseconds, the block occurs with almost equal frequency in the AV node and the bundle of His. In comparison, involvement of these sites is infrequent with a prolonged QRS; the block in this setting is in the fascicles or bundle branches in >80% of cases. As a general rule, the more distal the block, the slower will be the escape pacemaker. Low pacemakers have a rate of 40 bpm or less and are often unreliable, resulting in a very slow rate or asystole. Syncope is most common in this group. The effects of autonomic tone, exercise, and atropine may all be helpful in determining the site of block. High junctional pacemakers may respond with an increase in heart rate to exercise, catecholamines, or atropine, and a decrease in heart rate after vagal maneuvers. In comparison, lower pacemakers are less responsive to autonomic manipulation. In addition to affecting the heart rate, these interventions also may improve AV conduction.

ATRIOVENTRICULAR DISSOCIATION

AV dissociation is characterized by independent atrial and ventricular rhythms, and the duration ranges from fleeting (greater than or equal to a single beat) to permanent. It is not a mechanism per se; rather, it is the result of a number of different electrophysiologic mechanisms, each occurring in relation to a clinicopathologic substrate:

1. *Isorhythmic AV dissociation:* The intrinsic atrial activation rate falls below that of a subsidiary pacemaker, allowing the latter to produce an escape complex. The escape complex cannot activate the atria retrograde. In cases in which rates of the independent atrial and ventricular pacemakers are close, dissociation may be termed, isorhythmic.

2. *AV block:* Both incomplete and complete AV block can result in AV dissociation.

3. *Interference AV dissociation:* The rate of subsidiary pacemaker becomes abnormally fast, exceeding that of the atrium, and its activity does not influence the atria retrograde. Examples include junctional and ventricular tachycardia.

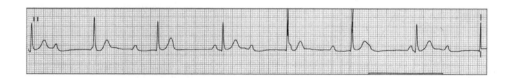

Figure 15.8. Complete AV block. The P-P interval and the R-R intervals are fixed but is no AV synchrony.

CLINICAL MANIFESTATION OF BRADYARRHYTHMIA

The symptoms related to the bradyarrhythmia include light-headedness, presyncope or syncope, and worsening of angina pectoris or heart failure. Symptoms may be subtle, with many patients noting only fatigue, which is frequently ascribed to aging rather than bradycardia. The sick sinus node often does not respond appropriately to exercise (chronotropic incompetence), and fatigue or dyspnea on exertion may be the presenting feature. A slow heart rate may also allow the appearance of supraventricular and ventricular extrasystoles or even arrhythmias that would normally be suppressed at a more rapid rate.

TREATMENT OF BRADYARRHYTHMIA

Bradycardia is defined conservatively as a heart rate <60 bpm. The advanced cardiac life support (ACLS) guidelines recommend that clinicians not intervene unless the patient exhibits evidence of inadequate tissue perfusion thought to result from the slow heart rate (Figure 15.9). Signs and symptoms of inadequate perfusion include hypotension, altered mental status, evidence of acute pulmonary edema, or ongoing ischemic chest pain. If any such symptoms are present in the setting of bradycardia, immediately prepare for transcutaneous pacing.

Preparations for pacing are not delayed to administer medications. Before using transcutaneous pacing, assess whether the patient can perceive the pain associated with this procedure, and if so provide appropriate sedation and analgesia. While preparing for transcutaneous pacing, it is reasonable to administer atropine (0.5 mg IV, which may be repeated every 5 minutes to a total dose of 3 mg), unless there is evidence of high degree (type II second degree or third degree) AV block. Atropine exerts its antibradycardic effects at the AV node and is unlikely to be effective if this block is at or below the bundle of His. If transcutaneous pacing fails to capture, prepare for transvenous pacing. While doing so, epinephrine (2 to 10 μg per minute) or dopamine (2 to 10 μg/kg/minute) infusions, titrated to the patient's response, may be started. Patients requiring transcutaneous or transvenous pacing also require immediate cardiology consultation, and admission for evaluation for permanent pacemaker placement. Glucagon may be given (3-mg IV followed by a 3-mg per hour drip as necessary) if symptomatic bradycardia is thought to result from supratherapeutic levels of β-blockers.

TEMPORARY CARDIAC PACING

Temporary cardiac pacing involves electrical cardiac stimulation to treat a bradyarrhythmia until it resolves or until long-term therapy can be initiated. The purpose of temporary

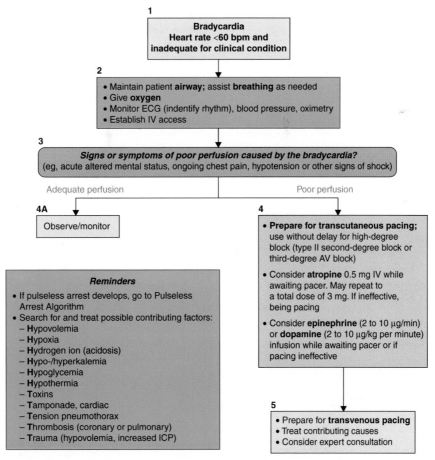

Figure 15.9. ACLS bradycardia algorithm. (Reproduced from 2005 American Heart Association Guidelines for Cardiopulmonary Resuscitation and Emergency Cardiovascular Care. Part 7.3: Management of Symptomatic Bradycardia and Tachycardia. *Circulation* 2005;112:IV-67-IV-77, with permission.)

pacing is the reestablishment of circulatory integrity and normal hemodynamics that are acutely compromised by a slow heart rate by maintaining an appropriate heart rate; in some situations, temporary pacing can be lifesaving.

TECHNICAL SKILLS

Prior to implantation, knowledge about normal anatomy and endocardial endocardial structures, and the ability to distinguish between normal ECG and artifact are important to guide proper lead positioning. An ACP/ACC/AHA task force, and others, have made recommendations about numbers of devices that a physician needs to place to be considered competent[1]:

- Invasive, hemodynamic skills must be demonstrated by performing a minimum of 25 procedures.
- A minimum of 10 ventricular temporary pacemaker implants is suggested.
- Technical skills, adhering to strict surgical sterile technique, including the ability to perform venous access from two or multiple sites using a percutaneous or cut down approach are necessary.
- The ability to perform and operate all instrumentation must be demonstrated. This includes use of pacing catheters, ability to correct technical problems with pacing instrumentation and pacing catheters, and ability to obtain sufficient and high-quality data.
- To maintain competence, hospitals should require continuous experience for physicians and at least one to two pacemaker implants per year are recommended.

MODES OF TEMPORARY CARDIAC PACING

A number of pacing modes are available for temporary use; pacing can be atrial (AAI, AOO), ventricular (VVI, VOO), or dual chamber (DDD, VDD, DDI, or DVI) (Tables 15.3 and 15.4). Pacing can be asynchronous or demand although with dual chamber pacing atrial sensing can trigger ventricular pacing. The most frequent use of temporary pacing is for therapy of symptomatic bradycardia because of sinus node dysfunction or AV nodal block. Once pacing is initiated for bradycardia, the patient can become rapidly dependent on the pacemaker. In this setting, dislodgement of the lead or failure of the pacer to capture can result in asystole, which may not have otherwise occurred.

Once a patient has a temporary pacemaker inserted, checking its threshold parameters and assuring proper functioning is the nurse's responsibility. To do this you need to understand the concepts and principles of cardiac pacing and how to adjust the settings on the pulse generator.

APPROACHES TO TEMPORARY PACING

Temporary pacing can be performed with the following:

- Internal or endocardial leads
- Atrial or ventricular epicardial leads placed at the time of surgery
- External or transthoracic.

TYPES OF ELECTRODE CATHETERS

Various types of electrode catheters are available. Endocardial pacing catheters are stiff but can be balloon-tipped for easier insertion. They come with various curves, including a preformed atrial "J" wire, and in 2, 5, 6, and 7 French sizes; they are generally bipolar or quadripolar. Stiff endocardial leads can maintain stability over a period, but careful positioning is recommended. Endocardial screw-in temporary leads can be used to help maintain stability. These leads, purposefully flimsy, are thin and deployed through a sheath that is then removed. Two such leads can be placed from one vein, if needed, and maintained with no indwelling intravenous access. These leads can maintain excellent pacing and sensing thresholds for many days. Epicardial wires have unipolar and bipolar design. Electrode catheters can be used to pace atria and/or ventricles. In general atrial leads are not inserted when bradycardia alone is the indication for pacing. However, an atrial lead is inserted for pace termination of atrial tachyarrhythmias, particularly atrial flutter, and to provide AV synchrony if a dual chamber pacing system is required. Atrial pacing may be crucial in a situation where junctional rhythm is present with hemodynamic compromise. Atrial pacing may provide hemodynamic advantage in patients with

TABLE 15.3	NBG Codes for Pacing Nomenclature			
Position	*I*	*II*	*III*	*IV*	*V*
	Chamber(s) paced	Chamber(s) sensed	Response to sensing	Rate modulation	Multisite pacing
	O	O	O	O	O
Category	A	A	T	R	A
	V	V	I		V
	D	D	D		D
	(A+V)	(A+V)	(T+I)		(A+V)

O, none; A, atrium; T, triggered; R, rate modulation; V, ventricle; I, inhibited; D, dual.
Adapted from Bernstein AD, Daubert JC, Fletcher RD, et al. The revised NASPE/BPEG generic code for antibradycardia, adaptive-rate, and multisite pacing. North American Society of Pacing and Electrophysiology/British Pacing and Electrophysiology Group. *Pacing Clin Electrophysiol.* 2002;25(2):260–264, with permission.

TABLE 15.4	Types of Cardiac Pacemakers and NBG Codes
Code	*Meaning*
A(V)OO	Asynchronous atrial (ventricular) pacemaker without sensing of patient's atrial (ventricular) rhythm
AA(VV)I	Nonphysiologic atrial (ventricular) demand pacemaker; sensing and pacing in atrium (ventricle) only
DDD	Multiprogrammable physiologic dual chamber pacemaker
DDI	Dual chamber pacing and sensing without atrial synchronous ventricular pacing
VDD	Ventricular pacing with dual chamber sensing with atrial synchronous ventricular pacing
DVI	Sequential dual chamber pacing; without atrial sensing and atrial synchronous ventricular pacing
XXX-R	Adaptive-rate pacemaker (AAIR, VVIR or DDDR)

Adapted from Bernstein AD, Daubert JC, Fletcher RD, et al. The revised NASPE/BPEG generic code for antibradycardia, adaptive-rate, and multisite pacing. North American Society of Pacing and Electrophysiology/British Pacing and Electrophysiology Group. *Pacing Clin Electrophysiol.* 2002;25(2):260–264, with permission.

diastolic dysfunction, such as those early after cardiac (especially valvular) surgery. The benefits of atrial pacing for conditions of sinus bradycardia or junctional rhythm are most prominent after cardiac surgery for patient with ischemia, ventricular hypertrophy, or heart failure. Transthoracic pacing patches are high impedance to cause better current density and less pain.

ACCESS SITE

The best access site for temporary pacing leads is through the left subclavian vein or the right internal jugular vein. Brachial and femoral approaches are not recommended because of the risk of cardiac puncture and instability using a brachial approach and the risk of deep vein thrombosis and infection using the femoral approach. Direct cardiac puncture is seldom needed. Although the right internal jugular approach is usually preferred, the best approach to minimize complications is the one with which the physician has the most experience. When a patient is pacemaker-dependent, it is crucial that the lead be placed in a stable position and fluoroscopy should be used.

The subclavian approach permits more freedom of patient motion and might be useful in a patient who requires a long-term temporary pacemaker. However, once the pacemaker is in place, a permanent pacemaker should not be implanted on that side owing to the risk of infection. After obtaining venous access, a modified Seldinger technique is usually used; a peel-away sheath is recommended if the lead is to be in place for >5 days. Another approach is to use a sheath with a sterile connector covering so that the lead can be repositioned at a later time. A temporary pacemaker placed in the subclavian or right internal jugular that has been inserted in a sheath (or without an indwelling introducer sheath) that does not allow for intravenous infusion can be maintained for as long as 7 to 10 days without major concern. However there is a need for careful care and proper bandaging of the site to prevent infection.

TABLE 15.5	Indications of Temporary Pacemaker

EMERGENCY/ACUTE

Acute myocardial infarction
- Asystole
- Symptomatic bradycardia (sinus bradycardia with hypotension and type I second degree AV block with hypotension not responsive to atropine)
- Bilateral bundle branch block (alternating BBB or RBBB with alternating LAHB/LPHB)
- New or indeterminate age bifascicular block with first degree AV block
- Mobitz type II second degree AV block

Bradycardia not associated with acute myocardial infarction
- Asystole
- Second or third degree AV block with hemodynamic compromise or syncope at rest
- Ventricular tachyarrhythmia secondary to bradycardia

ELECTIVE

Support for procedures that may promote bradycardia
General anesthesia with:
- Second or third degree AV block
- Intermittent AV block
- First degree AV block with bifascicular block
- First degree AV block with LBBB

Cardiac surgery
- Aortic surgery
- Tricuspid surgery
- Ventricular septal defect closure
- Ostium primum repair

Rarely considered for coronary angioplasty (usually to right coronary artery)
Overdrive suppression of tachyarrhythmias

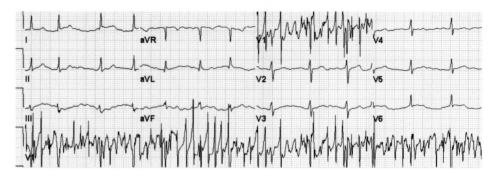

Figure 15.10. The temporary pacemaker wire (distal pole) is connected to the lead V1. When the temporary pacemaker lead touches the right atrium, the lead V1 recording shows rapid irregular electrograms due to atrial fibrillation.

LEAD PLACEMENT

The lead can be advanced under fluoroscope guidance. In absence of fluoroscopic guidance, the ECG guidance can be used. The distal pole of temporary lead connection can be connected to the ECG lead V1 (Figure 15.10). When the lead advances the right atrium, intracardiac recording of the atrial impulse (equivalent to the P wave) is recorded. When the lead is placed in the right ventricle the current of injury is recorded (Figure 15.11). The right ventricular apex can be confirmed by the 12-lead ECG polarities (LBBB and left axis deviation, Figure 15.12), whereas right ventricular outflow tract pacing will have LBBB left inferior axis, which may not be the stable lead position because of risk of lead migration to the pulmonary artery. There should be slight excess lead (pressure at the tip, with a bend at the tricuspid ring) to insure that the lead does not become dislodged. The lead should be tied down in at least two different sites, one where the lead exits from the vein and the other to a loop formed with the lead. The loop should be large enough to prevent tension on the lead, preventing it from becoming dislodged and the pacemaker losing capture. For the patient who has symptomatic bradycardia and requires transthoracic or external temporary pacing, if available, it should be used before a temporary wire is placed. External pacing functions only in a VVI mode and is used only for emergent pacing. It should not be relied upon if temporary pacing for a longer period is required.

PACEMAKER SYSTEM

Several types of pulse generators that permit single and dual chamber pacing are available. The connector cable linking the catheter lead to the pacemaker generator is a simple aspect of the system, but it is important for these connectors to be screwed tightly and securely fastened with a clamp. An improper connection or inadvertent disconnection can result in pacing malfunction or even asystole and possibly death in a patient who is pacemaker-dependent. Even if a patient is not initially pacemaker-dependent but is then paced, abrupt disconnection of the pacing or turning off of the pacemaker could lead to asystole owing to newly acquired pacemaker-dependence. To insure proper pacemaker sensing and capture, the pacemaker output should be set at least two to three times the pacing threshold (i.e., the minimum current in milliamps [mA] and, therefore, energy necessary for pacemaker capture) and two to three times the sensing threshold. The threshold, especially in the ventricle, should be ≤1 mA, especially for the patient who is pacemaker-dependent.

Epicardial pacing. This route is used following cardiac surgical procedures as it requires direct access to the external surface of the myocardium. Fine wire electrodes are placed within the myocardium of the atrium, ventricle, or both chambers from the epicardial surface and the connectors emerge through the skin. These electrodes can be removed with gentle traction when no longer required; however, their electrical performance (lead longevity) tends to deteriorate quite rapidly with rising threshold, and reliable sensing/pacing capability is often lost within 5 to 10 days, especially when used in the atrium.

External (transcutaneous) pacing. As part of advanced life support, current trend recommends this approach as pacing can be achieved rapidly with very little training and without the need to move the patient. Clinical studies have demonstrated the efficacy of external pacemaker for periods of up to

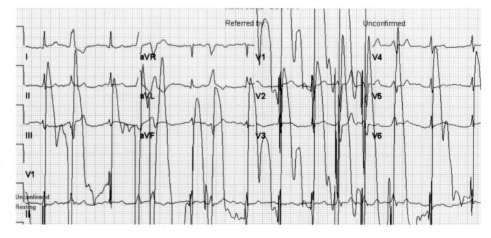

Figure 15.11. The temporary pacemaker wire (distal pole) is connected to the lead V1. When the temporary pacemaker lead touches the right ventricular, the lead V1 recording shows rapid irregular electrograms with ST elevation due to endocardial contact of the lead (current of injury pattern).

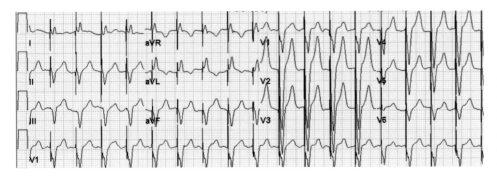

Figure 15.12. The 12-lead ECG shows ventricular pacing with QRS configuration showing left bundle branch block with left axis deviation suggests right ventricular apical position of the temporary ventricular apex.

14 hours of continuous pacing with success rates of 78% to 94%, although many patients require sedation if conscious. This approach certainly offers a "bridge" to transvenous approach for circumstances where the patient cannot be moved or staff with transvenous pacing experience are not immediately available. Large chest wall electrodes with a high impedance interface are required for external pacing. However, it causes significant discomfort and sedation or a state of unconsciousness is required to use this approach effectively for more than backup or emergency pacing. Reliability limits its use, and it is often difficult to determine whether there is adequate ventricular capture. Positioning of the transcutaneous pacing electrodes is usually in an anteroposterior configuration, but if this is unsuccessful, if external defibrillation is likely to be needed, or if electrodes are placed during a cardiac arrest situation, the anterolateral configuration should be considered (Figure 15.13). It is also recommended as a standby therapy for patients at high risk for developing a symptomatic bradycardia such as those with an asymptomatic bradycardia who require pharmacologic therapy that may worsen the bradycardia or for patients with an AMI who have a conduction abnormality that may result in a serious bradycardia (Table 15.6).

MANAGEMENT OF TEMPORARY PACEMAKER ELECTRODES

Continuous monitoring is mandatory during the entire period the patient has a temporary pacemaker, and a separate intravenous line or a heparin lock is recommended should there be a need for drug therapy. Patients with temporary pacemakers require a daily check of pacing thresholds to make certain that there is proper capture and sensing, and at least one 12-lead ECG recorded during pacing to determine the electrocardiographic appearance of the QRS complex to ensure the proper location of the leads. The endocardial ventricular lead should be at the apex and, when the pacemaker is in the proper position, the QRS should have a LBBB morphology and a superior axis (i.e., an upright QRS complex in lead 1 and aVL).

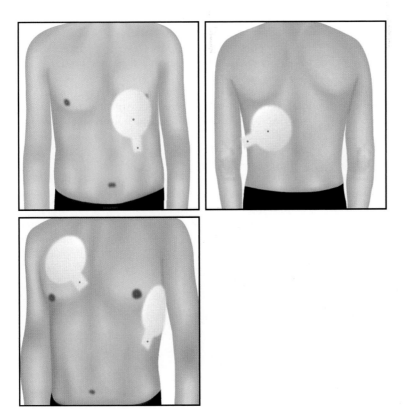

Figure 15.13. Typical anteroposterior and anterolateral (bottom panel) positioning of transcutaneous pacing electrodes.

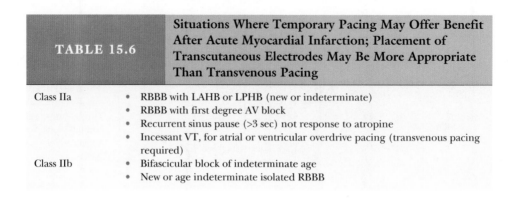

TABLE 15.6	Situations Where Temporary Pacing May Offer Benefit After Acute Myocardial Infarction; Placement of Transcutaneous Electrodes May Be More Appropriate Than Transvenous Pacing
Class IIa	• RBBB with LAHB or LPHB (new or indeterminate) • RBBB with first degree AV block • Recurrent sinus pause (>3 sec) not response to atropine • Incessant VT, for atrial or ventricular overdrive pacing (transvenous pacing required)
Class IIb	• Bifascicular block of indeterminate age • New or age indeterminate isolated RBBB

A chest X-ray should be obtained to determine the position of the endocardial leads. This test should be repeated if there is failure to capture or sense the leads or if a ventricular tachyarrhythmia occurs, which suggests electrode dislodgement.

A physical examination should be performed regularly to evaluate for a pericardial friction rub, which is indicative of a perforation; for the presence of asymmetrical or absent breaths sounds, indicating the presence of a pneumothorax; for hypotension and jugular venous distension suggesting tamponade or a pacing problem; or fever suggestive of an infection. In addition, the need for continuous pacing should be established. The dressing at the site of pacemaker insertion should be changed daily and antibiotic ointment applied to prevent infection. The stability of the wire and the loop should be checked to prevent inadvertent dislodgement of the lead. All connections and pacemaker programmed settings should be checked routinely.

Achieving capture. The ability of the myocardium to contract when stimulated by the pacemaker is called capture. It is determined by the amount of voltage delivered to the muscle measured in mA. The stimulation threshold is the lowest amount of mA needed for capture. Successful capture will show up on an EKG or telemetry as a spike—a perfectly vertical line—followed by a P wave if the atrium is paced, or by QRS complex if the ventricle is paced. Before determining the stimulation threshold, make sure the pacemaker is in the demand mode. Then, set the pacemaker rate 10 beats above the patient's own heart rate, or as high as needed to see 100% capture—a pacer spike with every beat. Next, slowly turn down the mA until 1:1 capture is lost (Figure 15.14). The EKG or telemetry strip will show spikes without complexes following them. Slowly turn up the mA until capture is regained. This is the stimulation threshold. The mA should be set two to three times higher than the stimulation threshold. Pacing thresholds will vary according to the underlying pathology for which the patient is paced, and these can be affected further by concomitant drug treatment. Initial

thresholds should be recorded and then checked and recorded at least once daily thereafter by competent staff. If pacing output needs to exceed 5.0 volts or 10.0 mA, repositioning of the lead should be considered. If pacing fails suddenly, always check connections to the external generator, generator batteries, and possible oversensing (go to VOO, fixed rate pacing). If pacing spikes can be seen but no capture occurs, increase output and consider repositioning or replacing the electrode.

Sensing. Sensing refers to the ability of the pacemaker to detect the heart's electrical activity and deliver paced beats only when needed. To determine whether the pacemaker is sensing properly, set the rate 10 beats below the patient's inherent rate. (Note: This step is contraindicated if a patient has no intrinsic rate or has symptomatic bradycardia.) Then, turn the sensitivity dial towards a higher numerical setting (the sensing light, which flashes when sensing, will stop). The pacemaker is now less sensitive to the patient's heartbeat. Now, turn the sensitivity dial towards a lower number until the sensing light starts flashing again. This is the sensitivity threshold. Set the sensitivity, measured in millivolts (mV), at half the sensitivity threshold value obtained. It is important to note that an atrioventricular (AV sequential) pulse generator may have dials for atrial settings on the left and ventricular settings on the right.

If you are not seeing pacer spikes it may mean the pacemaker is oversensing. A pacemaker will sense, or pick up and interpret, muscle movement and artifact as heart beats if the sensitivity threshold is set too high (too small number), or there are items in the vicinity of the pacemaker that interfere with its signals, or the lead wire is fractured.

If oversensing is the likely cause of the failure to pace, increase the number on the sensitivity dial as it lowers the sensitivity of the pacemaker, and remove items that could cause electromechanical interference such as electric razors, radios, or cautery devices. You will need a chest X-ray to rule out a fractured lead wire. However, not seeing pacer spikes can be normal, such as

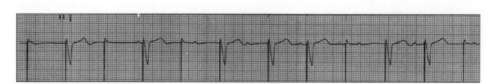

Figure 15.14. Noncapture in VVI pacemaker.

when the patient's heart is beating faster than the rate set on the pacemaker. Another problem can occur when the pacemaker fails to sense the patient's intrinsic beats. Undersensing can be dangerous: Pacer spikes that fire indiscriminately throughout the cardiac cycle can trigger a lethal ventricular arrhythmia if a spike falls on a T wave. In this case, higher the pacemaker's sensitivity to the heart by turning down the dial to a lower mV.

REFERENCES

1. Epstein AE, DiMarco JP, Ellenbogen KA, et al. ACC/AHA/HRS 2008 guidelines for device-based therapy of cardiac rhythm abnormalities: a report of the American College of Cardiology/American Heart Association Task Force on Practice Guidelines (Writing Committee to Revise the ACC/AHA/NASPE 2002 Guideline Update for Implantation of Cardiac Pacemakers and Antiarrhythmia Devices) developed in collaboration with the American Association for Thoracic Surgery and Society of Thoracic Surgeons. *J Am Coll Cardiol.* 2008;51(21):e1–e62.

PATIENT AND FAMILY INFORMATION FOR:
Bradyarrhythmia, including Heart Block

WHAT IS A BRADYCARDIA?

In most healthy people, the heart at rest beats approximately 60 to 100 times per minute. A small bunch of heart cells located in the right upper chamber of the heart is called the sinus node. Sinus node generates rhythmic electricity, which is responsible for the heart beat. Arrhythmia is a medical term that refers to a heart rate that is outside of this normal range. An arrhythmia that is too slow is called a bradyarrhythmia. When the heart is beating under 60 bpm, this is referred to as bradycardia. Although in some people this can be a sign of a serious condition, it is also important to note that some people with healthy hearts may have a heart rate <60 bpm. Many well-conditioned athletes have heart rates at rest <60 bpm. Some individuals may have heart rates that fall below 60 bpm while sleeping. If the slow heart rate is not associated with symptoms, it almost never justifies aggressive intervention. The two commonest causes of bradycardia are diseases of the sinus node (sick sinus syndrome), which is the heart's natural pacemaker or other problems with the heart's electrical conduction system (heart block). These diseases can cause the heart to beat too slowly all the time or occasionally.

WHAT CAUSES BRADYCARDIA?

Bradycardia can be caused by the following conditions:
- Changes in the heart that are the result of aging.
- Diseases that damage the heart's electrical system. These include coronary artery disease, heart attack, and infections such as endocarditis and myocarditis.
- Conditions that can slow electrical impulses through the heart. Examples include a low thyroid level (hypothyroidism) or an electrolyte imbalance, such as too much potassium in the blood.
- Some medicines for treating heart problems or high blood pressure, such as ß-blockers, calcium blockers, antiarrhythmic drugs, and digoxin.

WHAT ARE THE SYMPTOMS?

As the heart rate declines, the heart may not pump enough blood to meet the body's needs. A very slow heart rate may cause you to:

- Feel dizzy, lightheaded
- Feel short of breath and find it harder to exercise
- Feel tired
- Have chest pain or a feeling that your heart is pounding or fluttering (palpitations)
- Feel confused or have trouble in concentrating
- Faint, if a slow heart rate causes a drop in blood pressure.

Some people do not have symptoms, or their symptoms are so mild that they think they are just part of getting older. You can find out how fast your heart is beating by taking your pulse at your wrist. If your heartbeat is slow or uneven, talk to your doctor.

HOW IS BRADYCARDIA DIAGNOSED?

Your doctor may be able to diagnose bradycardia by doing a physical exam, asking questions about your past health, and doing an EKG. An EKG measures the electrical signals that control heart rhythm, so it is the best test for bradycardia. Bradycardia often comes and goes; therefore, a standard EKG done in the doctor's office may not detect it. An EKG can identify bradycardia only if you are actually having it during the test. You may need to use a portable (ambulatory) EKG. This lightweight device is also called a Holter monitor or a cardiac event monitor. You wear the monitor for a day or more, and it records your heart rhythm while you go about your daily routine. You may also have blood tests to find out if another problem is causing your slow heart rate.

HOW IS IT TREATED?

How bradycardia is treated depends on what is causing it. Treatment also depends on the symptoms. If bradycardia does not cause symptoms, it usually does not require treatment. If damage to the heart's electrical system causes your heart to beat too slowly, you will probably need to have a pacemaker. A pacemaker is a device placed under your skin that helps correct the slow heart rate. People older than 65 are most likely to have a type of bradycardia that requires a pacemaker. If another medical problem, such as hypothyroidism or an electrolyte imbalance, is causing a slow heart rate, treating that problem may cure the bradycardia. If a medicine is causing your heart to beat too slowly, your doctor may adjust the dose or prescribe a different medicine. If you cannot stop taking that medicine, you may need a pacemaker. The goal of treatment is to raise your heart rate so that your body gets the blood it needs. If severe bradycardia is not treated, it can lead to serious problems. These may include fainting and injuries from fainting as well as seizures or even death.

WHAT CAN YOU DO AT HOME FOR BRADYCARDIA?

Bradycardia is often the result of another heart condition; therefore taking steps to improve your cardiac health will usually improve your overall health. The following steps you can take are best to improve heart condition:

- Control your cholesterol and blood pressure.
- Eat a low-fat, low-salt diet.
- Get regular exercise. Your doctor can tell you what level of exercise is safe for you.
- Stop smoking.
- Limit alcohol.
- Take your medicines as prescribed.
- See your doctor for regular follow-up care.

People who get pacemakers need to be careful around strong magnetic or electrical fields, such as MRI machines or magnetic wands used at airports. If you get a pacemaker, your doctor will give you information about the type you have and what precautions to take.

Edgar Argulian
Dan G. Halpern
Emad F. Aziz
Eyal Herzog

CHAPTER

16

Supraventricular Arrhythmias and Atrial Fibrillation

Most common supraventricular arrhythmias encountered in the cardiac care unit (CCU) are sinus tachycardia and atrial fibrillation. The current chapter focuses on the general approach to narrow QRS complex tachycardias followed by the description of common forms of supraventricular tachycardias (SVTs) with a special emphasis of atrial fibrillation. The algorithms described in the chapter apply to the most common clinical scenarios and do not intend to be all-inclusive or highly specific.

SVTs usually present with a narrow QRS complex (<120 milliseconds) on ECG because of the normal sequence of ventricular activation using the His-Purkinje system. Occasionally, SVTs present with a wide QRS complex (≥120 milliseconds) because of the following reasons: preexisting conduction abnormalities (e.g., bundle branch block), rate-related aberrant conduction, or conduction using an accessory pathway. In those cases, differentiation from ventricular tachycardia can be challenging, and it is discussed in details in Chapter 17.

GENERAL APPROACH TO NARROW QRS COMPLEX TACHYCARDIAS

HEMODYNAMIC IMPACT

Patients presenting with narrow QRS complex tachycardias should be assessed for symptoms potentially attributable to the arrhythmia. These include hypotension, poor peripheral perfusion, altered mental status, shortness of breath, and chest pain.

Although commonly well tolerated by otherwise healthy individuals, SVTs can have a significant hemodynamic impact on patients with cardiac comorbidities such as coronary artery disease, valvular diseases, and congestive heart failure. Before attributing hemodynamic instability to the arrhythmia, the underlying precipitants should be thought. For example, sepsis or pulmonary embolism in a patient with atrial fibrillation can be the driver of the rapid ventricular response. If SVT is thought to be *the cause* of hemodynamic instability, immediate treatment such as electrical cardioversion is warranted. One should keep in mind that sinus tachycardia is almost always a compensatory response, and it should not be considered the cause of hemodynamic instability. The underlying cause of sinus tachycardia (such as myocardial ischemia, congestive heart failure, etc.) should be identified and addressed.

REGULARITY OF THE RHYTHM

After determination of the hemodynamic impact of the arrhythmia, the 12-lead ECG should be inspected for regularity of QRS complexes (Figure 16.1). This allows rapid differentiation into two major categories: irregular rhythms and regular rhythms.[1,2]

Irregular rhythms should be further inspected for the presence and morphology of P waves. Atrial fibrillation is the most common irregular tachycardia, and it has no identifiable P waves. One must remember that atrial fibrillation with a very fast heart rate may appear regular, and careful inspection and

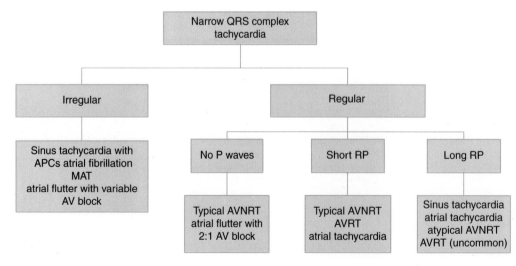

Figure 16.1. General approach to narrow QRS complex tachycardias. APC, atrial premature complex.

heart rate slowing maneuvers can help to disclose irregularity. Multifocal atrial tachycardia (MAT) has identifiable P waves indicative of atrial activity, but there is no single dominant focus (unlike sinus tachycardia with frequent atrial premature complexes). By definition, three different P-wave morphologies should be present on a single ECG with a heart rate exceeding 100 beats per minute (bpm) to diagnose MAT. Occasionally, atrial flutter presents as irregular tachycardia because of variable atrioventricular (AV) block.

Regular rhythms should be further analyzed for the presence of P waves as outlined below. Paroxysmal SVTs are a group of arrhythmias in this category that are intermittent in nature and commonly start and terminate abruptly. These include AV node reentrant tachycardia (AVNRT), AV reentrant tachycardia (AVRT), and unifocal atrial tachycardia.

ABSENCE OF P WAVES IN LIMB LEADS

Identification of P waves is essential in further characterization of regular narrow QRS complex tachycardias. It requires familiarity and experience in ECG interpretation since P waves can be subtle and superimposed on other waves.[1] Absence of identifiable P waves usually means that the atrial and ventricular activations are occurring almost simultaneously and P waves are completely buried within the QRS complex. The typical cause for such supraventricular arrhythmia is AVNRT with other causes (such as unifocal atrial tachycardia) being rare.

AVNRT develops in individuals with peculiar electrophysiologic (EP) properties of the AV node called dual AV node physiology. Within the AV node or in its proximity, there are two pathways having different conduction properties and refractoriness: fast pathway and slow pathway. As a result, an impulse can circulate between those pathways creating a regular arrhythmia at the rate of 130 to 250 bpm. Typically, the impulse travels down the slow pathway and up the fast pathway leading to simultaneous (no identifiable P waves) or almost simultaneous (P wave slightly after QRS complex) atrial and ventricular activation. Uncommonly, the impulse travels down the fast pathway and up the slow pathway (atypical AVNRT) leading to QRS complexes preceded by P waves.

Atrial flutter is an atrial macroreentrant rhythm, which is *usually* located in the right atrium with a counterclockwise circuit around the tricuspid valve (typical atrial flutter). The atrial rate is close to 300 bpm (240 to 340 bpm) typically conducting through the AV node with 2:1 block. Therefore, the ventricular rate is most commonly regular and close to 150 bpm. Any SVT with the ventricular rate close to 150 bpm should be specifically inspected for atrial flutter! On surface ECG, there are no P waves. Instead, "sawtooth" undulations of the baseline (F waves) are present in inferior leads (II, III, avF). In V1, small positive deflections are seen (two per each QRS complex). One should know that identification of F waves can be challenging because they are commonly obscured by other waves (Figure 16.2).

RP INTERVAL

If P waves are identified, the relationship between R wave and P wave should be determined. If the RP interval is less than one-half of the RR interval, the tachycardia is called a short RP tachycardia, otherwise it is a long RP tachycardia (Figure 16.1). Typical AVNRT is a common form of short RP tachycardia as described above. AVRT is another common form of short RP tachycardia.

AVRT develops in patients with an accessory pathway, an extranodal tissue that electrically connects the atrium with the ventricle bypassing the AV node. The pathway can manifest on baseline ECG as a Wolff–Parkinson–White (WPW) pattern if it conducts in both antegrade and retrograde directions. Some pathways conduct only retrograde (from the ventricle to the atrium). They are called concealed because they are not recognized on the baseline surface ECG. Typically, AVRT results from an impulse traveling down the AV node and up the accessory pathway (orthodromic AVRT). Therefore, orthodromic AVRT is a narrow QRS complex, short RP tachycardia resembling AVNRT. On average, the RP interval is slightly longer with AVRT compared with AVNRT (P wave is seen on top of ST segment as opposed to the end of QRS complex), but the difference is usually subtle. Uncommonly, AVRT results from an impulse traveling down the accessory pathway and up the AV node (antidromic AVRT). Antidromic AVRT is a *wide complex*, not a narrow complex tachycardia!

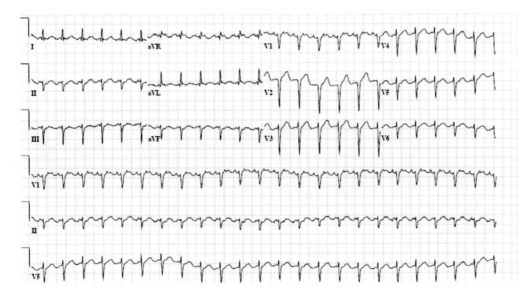

Figure 16.2. Atrial flutter with 2:1 AV block. Note F waves as undulations of the baseline in the inferior leads (II, III, avF) and small positive deflections in lead V1 (two per each QRS complex). The ventricular rate is regular at 142 bpm.

P-WAVE MORPHOLOGY

P-wave morphology assessment helps in further differential diagnosis of narrow QRS complex tachycardias. Sinus P waves are positive in lead II and negative in lead AVR. Retrograde P waves are always negative in inferior leads (II, III, avF) and commonly positive in V1. P waves originating from different foci in atria can have variable morphology including one closely mimicking sinus P waves (e.g., the rhythm originating from the crista terminalis). Therefore, comparison with the baseline ECG for P-wave morphology and documentation of the abrupt onset/termination is useful in differentiating long-RP tachycardias because of ectopic atrial activity from sinus tachycardia. AVNRT is always associated with retrograde P waves; any other morphology excludes AVNRT. AVRT can occasionally present with non-retrograde P-wave morphology depending on the location of the accessory pathway.

TRANSIENT SLOWING OF AV CONDUCTION

Transient slowing of AV conduction is essential in the differential diagnosis and acute treatment of SVTs.[3] It is accomplished by bedside vagal maneuvers (such as Valsalva and carotid sinus massage) or if those are ineffective with medications (most commonly adenosine, sometimes βblockers and calcium channel blockers). Before performing carotid sinus massage, check for contraindications such as history of cerebral vascular disease, recent myocardial infarction, or carotid bruits. Never perform bilateral carotid sinus massage. As adenosine has a very short half-life, it is given as a rapid intravenous push followed by saline infusion. The initial dose of adenosine is 6 mg (lower if using a central venous line), which can be followed by 12 mg if no response is seen. Adenosine can precipitate transient atrial fibrillation in up to 12% of patients that is potentially dangerous in patients with known WPW syndrome.[4] Ventricular fibrillation and transient asystole in response to adenosine administration are rare. Patients should be warned that side effects (such as flushing, chest tightness, and shortness of breath) are very common but short lasting. Table 16.1 outlines the common responses to the transient slowing of AV conduction that help in differential diagnosis. Arrhythmias that use the AV node in the reentry circuit (such as AVNRT and AVRT) commonly terminate with the slowing of the AV nodal conduction. Other arrhythmias can slow down helping identification of the abnormal rhythm.

LONG-TERM MANAGEMENT OF PAROXYSMAL SVTS

Patients with infrequent episodes of AVNRT that are well tolerated can be managed by AV node blocking medications (such as βblockers or nondihydropyridine calcium channel blockers). In patients with frequent episodes of AVNRT or poorly tolerated episodes, catheter ablation is usually safe and effective. Catheter ablation should be strongly considered in patients with AVRT and WPW syndrome.

MAT is most commonly seen in the setting of advanced lung disease. It is also associated with some structural heart diseases and congestive heart failure. It requires rate control and management of the underlying condition. The former is commonly achieved by calcium channel blockers or βblockers if there are no contraindications. Unifocal atrial tachycardias can be managed by rate control using AV node blocking medications. Occasionally, antiarrhythmic medications or catheter ablation is required.

ATRIAL FIBRILLATION

Atrial fibrillation is a common arrhythmia affecting 1% to 2% of general population. The prevalence increases dramatically with age affecting as many as 5% to 15% at the age of 80 years.[5,6] Therefore, it is commonly encountered in hospitalized patients, especially in the CCU. Atrial fibrillation is strongly associated with both the risk and severity of stroke. It is also associated with higher all-cause mortality and rates of hospitalizations compared with normal sinus rhythm.

RECOGNITION

Atrial fibrillation is characterized by disorganized atrial activity exceeding 300 bpm. This results in the loss of effective atrial contraction and typically a rapid ventricular response. Atrial fibrillation is recognized on the surface ECG as an irregularly irregular rhythm with no distinct P waves (Figure 16.3). Sometimes signs of regular atrial activity are seen in lead V1. Ventricular rates during atrial fibrillation are usually in the range of 90 to 160 bpm. A slow ventricular rate without AV node blocking medications may indicate conduction system disease. Regular and slow ventricular response is seen in patients with atrial fibrillation who are in complete heart block. Very fast rates (>200 bpm) are also unusual because of concealed conduction in the AV node. They can be seen in the

TABLE 16.1	Response of Narrow QRS Complex Tachycardias to the Transient Slowing of AV Nodal Conduction by Vagal Maneuvers or Mediations (e.g., Adenosine)
Response	*Interpretation*
No change	No diagnostic information gained; try adenosine or escalate adenosine dose
Gradual slowing of ventricular rate	Sinus tachycardia, atrial tachycardia
Some transient slowing of ventricular rate without termination	Almost always excludes AVRT and AVNRT
Transient slowing of ventricular rate with unmasking of F waves	Atrial flutter
Abrupt termination with a P wave after the last QRS complex	AVRT, AVNRT, very uncommonly atrial tachycardia
Abrupt termination with a QRS complex	AVRT, AVNRT, atrial tachycardia

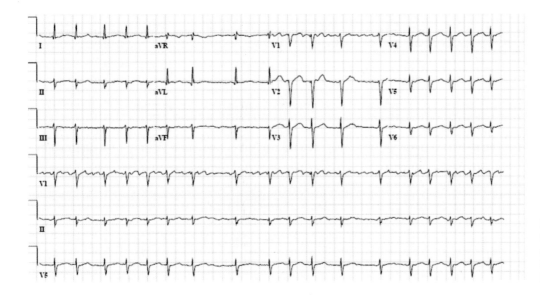

Figure 16.3. Atrial fibrillation. Note irregularly irregular and rapid ventricular response. Coarse fibrillatory waves can be best seen in lead V1.

states of significant catecholamine excess or in patients with an accessory pathway. One should recognize that atrial fibrillation is commonly an intermittent arrhythmia, at least early in the natural course of the disease. When clinically suspected, a long telemonitoring may be required for the correct diagnosis.

DISEASE ASSOCIATIONS AND DEFINITIONS

Atrial fibrillation is strongly associated with valvular pathologies such as mitral valve diseases and advanced aortic valve diseases as well as certain congenital heart diseases such as atrial septal defect. Those patients comprise a separate category with the risk profile and management different from nonvalvular atrial fibrillation patients. One should bear in mind that most studies in atrial fibrillation including rhythm versus rate control and stroke risk stratification were performed in patients with nonvalvular atrial fibrillation. Nonvalvular atrial fibrillation is commonly associated with hypertension, congestive heart failure, coronary artery disease, obesity, diabetes, obstructive sleep apnea, and primary cardiomyopathies such as hypertrophic cardiomyopathy. Atrial fibrillation can be a manifestation of sick sinus syndrome (tachycardia-bradycardia syndrome). Transient and reversible causes of atrial fibrillation include thyroid disease, acute pericarditis, pulmonary embolism, pulmonary diseases, heavy alcohol consumption, and cardiac surgery. In patients with no identified structural heart disease or predisposing condition, the term *lone atrial fibrillation* is sometimes used.

At our institution, a pathway for the management of atrial fibrillation has been developed and implemented.[7] The pathway contains abbreviated etiology of atrial fibrillation using the acronym of TRAPS for noncardiac etiology (to refer to Thyroid or Trauma, Recreational drug use, Alcohol, Pulmonary disease, Sepsis/infection) and CATCH WAVE for cardiac etiology (to refer to Congestive heart failure, Acute coronary syndrome, Tachycardia-bradycardia syndrome/sick sinus syndrome, Hypertension, WPW syndrome, After cardiac surgery, Valvular heart disease, medical noncompliance).[7]

It is important to understand that atrial fibrillation in most cases is a chronic and progressive disease.[6] It usually starts with short bursts of arrhythmia, which are either asymptomatic (silent atrial fibrillation) or difficult to document on routine examination because of very transient nature. More sustained episodes develop over time, which commonly last for <48 hours and terminate spontaneously (paroxysmal atrial fibrillation). With further progression, the episodes last even longer progressing into persistent and eventually permanent atrial fibrillation. The timeline of progression is highly variable, and 90% of atrial fibrillation episodes are asymptomatic.[8] That makes history very unreliable in determining the presence and timeline of atrial fibrillation. Atrial fibrillation can be diagnosed clinically at any point during the progression of the disease (from paroxysmal to permanent), and then, it is called "newly diagnosed atrial fibrillation." The common clinical terms used to describe types of atrial fibrillation are presented in Table 16.2.[6]

CONSEQUENCES AND COMPLICATIONS

Atrial fibrillation is more likely to develop in patients with dilated left atrium and, by itself, causes left atrial dilation and remodeling creating vicious circle. Effective left atrial contraction is lost, which predisposes to blood stasis. Clot formation can occur in the left atrium, typically in the left atrial appendage (LAA) and greatly increase the risk of embolic stroke. The risk of stroke is greatest after the restoration of atrial contractility (such as cardioversion to normal sinus rhythm) when the clot formed earlier is ejected from LAA to circulation. Therefore, careful assessment of thromboembolic risk is essential before any attempted

TABLE 16.2	Types of Atrial Fibrillation
Term	*Definition*
Paroxysmal	Self-terminating, up to 7 days, usually <48 h
Persistent	Lasts >7 days or requires electrical or pharmacological cardioversion
Long-standing persistent	Lasts ≥1 year, but rhythm control strategy is chosen
Permanent	Lasts ≥1 year, accepted by patient and clinician with no attempt of cardioversion contemplated

cardioversion. Transthoracic echocardiogram cannot reliably assess the thromboembolic risk in atrial fibrillation. In contrast, transesophageal echocardiogram (TEE) offers great resolution of left atrial structures. Spontaneous aggregation of red blood cells due to blood stasis can be visualized as "smoke" in the left atrium. Although it is associated with a greater risk of stroke, it is not an absolute contraindication to cardioversion. LAA is directly visualized and assessed for the presence of a clot that would preclude cardioversion. LAA emptying velocity measured by Doppler correlates with the risk of clot formation in LAA.

Loss of effective atrial contraction with atrial fibrillation as well as irregular and rapid ventricular response decreases cardiac output. In a subset of patients, persistently elevated ventricular rate (typically >110 bpm) causes progressive decline in the left ventricular systolic function, a condition called ventricular tachycardiomyopathy.

INITIAL ASSESSMENT

Patients with atrial fibrillation can present with a wide range of symptom severity. Atrial fibrillation can be diagnosed in minimally symptomatic patients on routine ECG or can manifest as an acute, severe condition because of complications such as stroke or acute decompensated heart failure. Initial evaluation should focus on the assessment of symptom burden and possible complications, presence and severity of structural heart disease and other predisposing conditions, and long-term thromboembolic risk assessment. An attempt should be made to establish the type of atrial fibrillation (Table 16.2). Transthoracic echocardiogram is obtained in all patients. Routine blood tests include basic metabolic profile, complete blood count, thyroid function tests, glycohemoglobin, and urinalysis for protein. Stress testing is recommended only in patients with concomitant symptoms suggestive of coronary artery disease.

INITIAL TREATMENT

Ventricular rate control usually brings symptomatic relief in patients with newly diagnosed atrial fibrillation. It is achieved by AV nodal blocking agents such as β-blockers, nondihydropyridine calcium channel blockers, and/or digoxin. Digoxin should not be used as a first-line agent in rate control of atrial fibrillation except in patients with acute decompensated heart failure and hypotension. In occasional patients intolerant of those medications or when those medications are ineffective, intravenous amiodarone can be used for acute, short-term rate control. Emergent cardioversion should be considered if the patient is hemodynamically unstable and atrial fibrillation is thought to be the cause of the instability. Those include patients with WPW syndrome and rapid ventricular rate since conduction through the accessory pathway can precipitate ventricular fibrillation. In symptomatic patients with newly diagnosed atrial fibrillation without advanced structural heart disease, many cardiologists perform elective cardioversion before deciding on the long-term strategy of rate control or rhythm control since some of those patients may stay in sinus rhythm for a long period of time.[5] Precipitating factors should be aggressively thought and corrected (e.g., thyroid dysfunction, fluid overload in patients with heart failure, and alcohol abuse).

After initial evaluation and treatment, two major questions should be answered for the long-term management plan: (1) what is the risk of thromboembolic complications? and (2) which strategy (rate control or rhythm control) should be used?

LONG-TERM THROMBOEMBOLIC RISK ASSESSMENT

Although atrial fibrillation itself predisposes to thromboembolic complications such as a stroke, the risk in each individual patient is greatly modified by age and comorbidities. *All patients* regardless of type and duration of atrial fibrillation should be risk stratified in terms of long-term thromboembolic complications using a validated risk stratification tool. The simplest and most commonly used tool is CHADS2 score, which uses major modifiers of stroke risk (Table 16.3).[9]

Patients with CHADS2 score of 2 or more require long-term anticoagulation unless contraindicated since their annual risk of stroke is at least 4%. In patients with CHADS2 score of 0 to 1, the necessity of anticoagulation should be individualized, commonly using nonmajor stroke risk modifiers (Figure 16.4).[6]

Anticoagulation has been consistently shown to decrease the risk of thromboembolic complications in atrial fibrillation compared with no therapy or in comparison with antiplatelet therapy such as aspirin or clopidogrel. The benefits of anticoagulation should be balanced against the risk of major bleeding including intracranial bleed, especially in patients requiring combined anticoagulation and antiplatelet therapy (e.g., patients with recent intracoronary stent). In general, the benefits outweigh the risks of therapy in most patients, especially with higher CHADS2 scores, but careful individual risk/benefit assessment may be necessary for some patients. Anticoagulation is commonly accomplished by warfarin targeting international normalized ratio (INR) 2.0 to 3.0. Newer oral therapies such as dabigatran, apixaban, and rivaroxaban appear to have good efficacy and safety profiles compared with warfarin, and they do not require INR checks and dose adjustments based on INR.[10]

RATE CONTROL VERSUS RHYTHM CONTROL

Long-term rhythm control in patients with atrial fibrillation can be achieved with antiarrhythmic medications, a catheter ablation procedure, or a surgical procedure. Despite appealing theoretical benefits of maintaining sinus rhythm in patients with atrial fibrillation, large studies showed that both strategies are associated with similar rates of mortality and serious morbidity.[11,12] Besides,

TABLE 16.3	CHADS2 Score Used to Assess the Long-Term Thromboembolic Risk in Patients with Atrial Fibrillation
Clinical Parameter	*Score*
Congestive heart failure/systolic LV dysfunction	1
Hypertension	1
Age ≥75 years	1
Diabetes mellitus	1
Stroke/transient ischemic attack/other thromboembolism	2

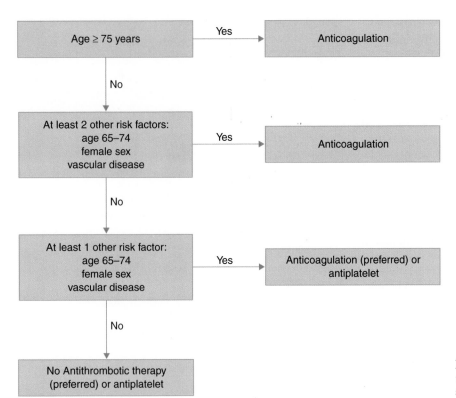

Figure 16.4. Further risk stratification in patients with CHADS2 <2 in choosing appropriate antithrombotic therapy.

quality of life measures also appear to be similar. Antiarrhythmic medications used for rhythm control add complexity and cost to the regimen, and they are associated with the risk of proarrhythmia and noncardiac complications. Their efficacy in maintaining sinus rhythm is limited, and they do not eliminate the need for anticoagulation. Therefore, most patients with atrial fibrillation especially those ≥65 years old, with many comorbidities and significant left atrial enlargement, can be successfully managed with rate control.[5,6] Current indications for rhythm control strategy include inability to achieve adequate rate control and persistent symptoms in patients who are adequately rate controlled, including patients with heart failure with worsening of symptoms and/or left ventricular systolic function while in atrial fibrillation.[5,6] Younger patients (<65 years old) with fewer comorbidities and recent onset of atrial fibrillation are usually more symptomatic, and they often opt for rhythm control.[5,6] Options for those patients include antiarrhythmic medications or radiofrequency ablation.

While choosing antiarrhythmic medications for patients with rhythm control strategy, the following should be kept in mind. β-Blockers are occasionally effective in maintaining sinus rhythm in patients with no structural heart disease and adrenergically medicated atrial fibrillation. Amiodarone is consistently better in maintaining sinus rhythm compared with other antiarrhythmic drugs including its derivative dronedarone, but amiodarone is associated with an array of extracardiac side effects. Therefore, in most situations, it is used as a second-line agent. Class IC agents (flecainide, propafenone) should be used after careful exclusion of coronary artery disease and structural heart disease because of significant proarrhythmic effect in those settings. Dronedarone is associated with adverse outcomes in certain patient populations such as advanced heart failure and permanent atrial fibrillation. Some antiarrhythmic medications such as dofetilide and sotalol should be initiated in the hospital with close ECG monitoring and patient follow-up.

Rate control is achieved with AV node blocking agents, typically β-blockers and nondihydropyridine calcium channel blockers. The goal of resting heart rate <110 bpm is acceptable in most patients.[13]

CARDIOVERSION

Restoration of sinus rhythm in patients with atrial fibrillation is achieved by electrical and pharmacologic cardioversion. Pharmacologic agents most commonly used for cardioversion include class IC agents (flecainide, propafenone) or class III agents (dofetilide, ibutilide, and amiodarone). In patients opting for the long-term rhythm control strategy, use of antiarrhythmic medications is often initiated before the electrical cardioversion to increase the change of maintaining sinus rhythm. The electrical cardioversion procedure is described in Chapter 21.

The indications for cardioversion in patients with atrial fibrillation include the following:

1. hemodynamic instability or worsening symptoms attributable to atrial fibrillation;

2. newly diagnosed atrial fibrillation in symptomatic patients without advanced structural heart disease before choosing long-term rate control or rhythm control strategy;

3. patients opting for long-term rhythm control strategy;

4. infrequent episodes of atrial fibrillation that can be managed by periodic cardioversions.

Before attempting cardioversion in nonurgent situation, the following issues should be addressed: (1) the probability of maintaining sinus rhythm after cardioversion and (2) the risk of thromboembolic complications. Certain patient populations are unlikely to maintain sinus rhythm after cardioversion. Those typically include patients with advanced structural heart disease and significant left atrial enlargement, advanced age, long-standing atrial fibrillation, previous failures to maintain sinus rhythm on antiarrhythmic medications, and serious comorbidities.

Thromboembolic complications associated with cardioversion of atrial fibrillation can be minimized by appropriate prevention strategies. As described above, blood clots can form in LAA during episodes of atrial fibrillation. Restoration of atrial contractility after cardioversion can dislodge those clots into the circulation causing thromboembolism. It is important to know that restoration of atrial contractility may not occur immediately after conversion to sinus rhythm because of atrial stunning, which can last up to 3 to 4 weeks. During that period, clots still can form in LAA and dislodge later once atrial contractility is fully restored. Therefore, appropriate pericardioversion thromboembolic prevention strategy must include the following components: (1) assure that there is no clot in LAA before attempted cardioversion, (2) assure that there is no clot formation postcardioversion during the atrial stunning period (up to 4 weeks), and (3) appropriate selection of long-term thromboembolic prevention strategy based on validated tools such as CHADS2 score.

Besides, before attempting cardioversion in patients with atrial fibrillation, one should look for contraindications for short-term and long-term anticoagulation such as active bleeding problems.

The following prevention strategies can be used before attempted cardioversion in patients with atrial fibrillation[5,6]:

1. In emergent situation, intravenous heparin should be administered before cardioversion if there are no contraindications. Anticoagulation should be continued for at least 4 weeks or longer depending on the long-term thromboembolic risk.

2. If atrial fibrillation is *documented* to exist <48 hours, cardioversion is usually safe. Intravenous heparin should be administered before cardioversion. Anticoagulation should be continued for at least 4 weeks or longer depending on the long-term thromboembolic risk. In patients with no stroke risk factors, anticoagulation can sometimes be omitted. While choosing this strategy, one should bear in mind that history can be unreliable in documenting the presence and duration of atrial fibrillation.

3. In patients with continuous 3 weeks of *documented* therapeutic anticoagulation, one can proceed with cardioversion followed by at least 4 weeks of anticoagulation or longer depending on the long-term thromboembolic risk.

4. In patients with no LAA clot visualized on TEE, one can proceed with cardioversion followed by at least 4 weeks of anticoagulation or longer depending on the long-term thromboembolic risk. If there is an LAA clot, cardioversion should not be attempted and repeat TEE should be done after at least 3 weeks of *documented* therapeutic anticoagulation to guide further management.

TEE-guided strategy is preferred at our institution.

ATRIAL FLUTTER

Atrial flutter is considered to have thromboembolic risk similar to atrial fibrillation. Therefore, the same long-term thromboembolic risk assessment tools can be used. In typical atrial flutter, radiofrequency catheter ablation is highly effective and

TABLE 16.4	Commonly Used Antiarrhythmic Medications for the Maintenance of Sinus Rhythm in Patients with Atrial Fibrillation based on Comorbidities
Patient Population	*Medications*
No structural heart disease	β-Blocker trial, class IC agents (flecainide, propafenone), dofetilide, sotalol, dronedarone, amiodarone
Coronary artery disease	Sotalol, dronedarone, amiodarone
Significant left ventricular hypertrophy (>1.4 cm)	Dronedarone, amiodarone
Hypertrophic cardiomyopathy	Amiodarone, disopyramide
Congestive heart failure	Amiodarone, dofetilide

relatively safe, whereas rate control is more difficult to achieve compared with atrial fibrillation.

SUMMARY

SVTs are commonly encountered in CCU. Narrow QRS complex tachycardias require a systematic approach to differential diagnosis and treatment. Sinus tachycardia is almost always a compensatory response that requires identification and treatment of the specific cause. Atrial fibrillation can lead to CCU admission or complicate the course of other heart diseases. Good understanding of specific issues related to atrial fibrillation management is necessary for health care providers in the CCU.

REFERENCES

1. Kalbfleisch SJ, el-Atassi R, Calkins H, et al. Differentiation of paroxysmal narrow QRS complex tachycardias using the 12-lead electrocardiogram. *J Am Coll Cardiol.* 1993;21:85–89.
2. Ganz LI, Friedman PL. Supraventricular tachycardia. *N Engl J Med.* 1995;332:162–173.
3. Ferguson JD, DiMarco JP. Contemporary management of paroxysmal supraventricular tachycardia. *Circulation.* 2003;107:1096–1099.
4. Strickberger SA, Man KC, Daoud EG, et al. Adenosine-induced atrial arrhythmia: a prospective analysis. *Ann Intern Med.* 1997;127:417–422.
5. Wann LS, Curtis AB, Ellenbogen KA, et al. 2011 ACCF/AHA/HRS focused update on the management of patients with atrial fibrillation (update on dabigatran): a report of the American College of Cardiology Foundation/American Heart Association Task Force on practice guidelines. *J Am Coll Cardiol.* 2011;57:1330–1337.
6. Camm AJ, Kirchhof P, Lip GY, et al. Guidelines for the management of atrial fibrillation: the Task Force for the Management of Atrial Fibrillation of the European Society of Cardiology (ESC). *Eur Heart J.* 2010;31:2369–2429.
7. Herzog E, Fischer A, Steinberg JS. The rate control, anticoagulation therapy, and electrophysiology/antiarrhythmic medication pathway for the management of atrial fibrillation and atrial flutter. *Crit Pathw Cardiol.* 2005;4:121–126.
8. Page RL, Wilkinson WE, Clair WK, et al. Asymptomatic arrhythmias in patients with symptomatic paroxysmal atrial fibrillation and paroxysmal supraventricular tachycardia. *Circulation.* 1994;89:224–227.
9. Gage BF, Waterman AD, Shannon W, et al. Validation of clinical classification schemes for predicting stroke: results from the National Registry of Atrial Fibrillation. *JAMA.* 2001;285:2864–2870.
10. del Zoppo GJ, Eliasziw M. New options in anticoagulation for atrial fibrillation. *N Engl J Med.* 2011;365:952–953.
11. Wyse DG, Waldo AL, DiMarco JP, et al. A comparison of rate control and rhythm control in patients with atrial fibrillation. *N Engl J Med.* 2002;347:1825–1833.
12. Van Gelder IC, Hagens VE, Bosker HA, et al. A comparison of rate control and rhythm control in patients with recurrent persistent atrial fibrillation. *N Engl J Med.* 2002;347:1834–1840.
13. Van Gelder IC, Groenveld HF, Crijns HJ, et al. Lenient versus strict rate control in patients with atrial fibrillation. *N Engl J Med.* 2010;362:1363–1373.

PATIENT AND FAMILY INFORMATION FOR:
Supraventricular Arrhythmias and Atrial Fibrillation

SVT is a general term that describes fast and abnormal heart rhythm (arrhythmia), which originates from the upper chambers of the heart (the atria) as opposed to the lower chambers of the heart (the ventricles). SVT is not a single disease but a wide range of arrhythmias that have different causes, pathophysiologic mechanisms, and management strategies.

HOW IS ARRHYTHMIA RECOGNIZED?

Symptoms experienced by the patient (such as fast heart beat, palpitations, syncope, etc.) are helpful in recognizing arrhythmias, but the specific type of the arrhythmia cannot be usually diagnosed by symptoms alone. Recognition of the specific type of arrhythmia requires careful analysis of ECG and/or telemonitoring strips. Owing to the transient nature of most arrhythmias, a prolonged monitoring is sometimes required that can be done in the hospital or in outpatient settings using external or internal (implantable) monitoring devices. On some occasions, an invasive study called EP study is performed. It uses multiple catheters/wires that help to map an abnormal electrical circuit in the heart and pinpoint the exact type of arrhythmia.

SINUS TACHYCARDIA

Sinus tachycardia refers to the fast heart rate that originates and propagates through the normal electrical circuits in the heart. It is a normal reaction of the heart to exercise and stress including anxiety, fever, and pain. It is also associated with various pathologic conditions affecting the heart itself (such as heart failure and heart attack) or other organs (such as pneumonia and blood clots in the lungs). Therefore, sinus tachycardia is usually a compensatory phenomenon, and it does not need to be specifically treated. Instead, the primary cause should be identified and treated.

PAROXYSMAL SVT

The term *paroxysmal SVT* refers to a group of arrhythmias that are caused by abnormal electrical circuits in the upper chambers of the heart. They are intermittent in nature and commonly start and terminate abruptly. Within the group, there are several types that differ in terms of pathophysiologic mechanisms. The patient typically feels a sudden onset of fast heart rate and palpitations occasionally accompanied by chest discomfort, lightheadedness, or shortness of breath. The episodes terminate spontaneously or in response to certain maneuvers such as holding a deep breath or straining. Doctors may instruct the patient to do those maneuvers or perform carotid sinus massage in attempt to stop the arrhythmia. Carotid sinus massage refers to applying pressure to a specific area in the neck to provoke slowing of the heart rate. As it carries certain rate of complications, it should not be performed by the patient. If those maneuvers do not work, certain medications are used to terminate SVT. The most commonly used medication is adenosine. It causes slowing of the heart rate and can break the abnormal electrical circuit in the heart resulting in termination of the arrhythmia. Adenosine is given as intravenous injection. Soon after injection, many patients feel skin flushing, chest tightness, and shortness of breath. Those sensations are uncomfortable but very transient since adenosine has a short half-life. If the episodes of SVT are infrequent and not highly symptomatic, medical follow-up and sometimes daily medications to prevent attacks are sufficient. In patients with severe symptoms and frequent episodes, EP study followed by ablation procedure can be performed. Ablation procedure refers to inducing tiny and very controlled burns of the abnormal electrical circuits in the heart. Certain uncommon types of SVT are potentially dangerous and also need the ablation procedure. In most patients with SVT, the arrhythmia is cured for good by the ablation procedure.

ATRIAL FIBRILLATION

WHAT IS ATRIAL FIBRILLATION?

Atrial fibrillation is a common arrhythmia caused by fast and disorganized electrical circuits in the upper chambers of the heart (atria) replacing the normal rhythm (sinus rhythm). It affects 1% to 2% of general population. The prevalence increases dramatically with age affecting as many as 5% to 15% at the age of 80 years. Usually, atrial fibrillation starts as intermittent arrhythmia that many patients feel like fast and irregular heart rate and palpitations occasionally accompanied by chest discomfort, lightheadedness, or shortness of breath. With time, in many patients, the episodes persist longer and eventually atrial fibrillation becomes a permanent condition. Many patients experience nonspecific symptoms like loss of energy or fatigue. Not every patient feels the abnormal rhythm, and most patients feel only some of the episodes. Actually, studies showed that patients do not feel up to 90% of atrial fibrillation episodes!

WHAT CAUSES ATRIAL FIBRILLATION?

Atrial fibrillation has been linked to an array of heart conditions such as valvular diseases (abnormal heart valves), congestive heart failure, and coronary artery disease. It is also strongly associated with high blood pressure, diabetes, and obesity. Heavy alcohol use can precipitate atrial fibrillation. Reversible causes of atrial fibrillation include lung diseases, thyroid diseases, infections, and cardiac surgery. In some patients, no apparent cause or precipitating factor can be identified.

WHY IS ATRIAL FIBRILLATION DANGEROUS?

Atrial fibrillation is strongly associated with the risk of stroke. Owing to atrial fibrillation, the flow inside the heart chambers becomes sluggish. This predisposes to formation of a blood clot inside the heart chamber structure called LAA. The clot can get dislodged and travel to different organs including the brain where it causes a stroke. Antithrombotic therapy (blood thinners) if taken regularly can greatly diminish the risk of stroke. The downside of antithrombotic therapy is the increased risk of bleeding.

The risk of stroke in patients with atrial fibrillation varies depending on age, gender, and other medical conditions. Certain heart valve diseases and prosthetic valves carry a very high risk of stroke. Otherwise, age ≥75 years and history of hypertension, diabetes, heart failure, and previous stroke are the major risk factors. Age 65 to 74 years, female sex, and vascular disease are the minor risk factors. On the basis of the presence of those risk factors, the physician calculates the risk of stroke, balances it against the risk of bleeding, and advises the patient in terms of antithrombotic therapy.

Warfarin (Coumadin) is a common antithrombotic therapy given to patients with atrial fibrillation. It requires frequent blood checks to establish appropriate antithrombotic level ("INR checks"), dosage adjustments, and dietary restrictions. There are newer blood thinners such as dabigatran (Pradaxa) and rivaroxaban (Xarelto) that do not require frequent blood checks. Appropriate indications for these medications are established by the treating physician. Occasionally, aspirin or clopidogrel is used as antithrombotic therapy although they are less effective in preventing stroke in patients with atrial fibrillation. In patients who do not have any risk factors for stroke antithrombotic therapy may not be indicated.

CAN ATRIAL FIBRILLATION BE CURED?

Most commonly, atrial fibrillation is a chronic and progressive disease. Long-term management of atrial fibrillation involves two strategies: rate control (slowing down the heart rate but accepting the presence of atrial fibrillation) and rhythm control (trying to convert the patient to normal sinus rhythm and keep him/her in the normal rhythm). Large studies showed that both approaches have similar clinical outcomes such as the risk of dying or getting serious medical complications. Besides, the quality of life also seems to be similar. Rate control is achieved by a relatively simple medical regimen and provides sufficient symptomatic relief to many patients. Rhythm control can be achieved by antiarrhythmic medications, by a catheter ablation procedure, or uncommonly by a surgical procedure. Antiarrhythmic medications used for rhythm control add complexity and cost to the medical regimen, and they are associated with a small risk of serious, sometimes life-threatening complications. Antiarrhythmic medications have limited efficacy, and they do not eliminate the need for antithrombotic therapy. At the same time, in experienced hands, they decrease the burden of atrial fibrillation and provide symptomatic relief by maintaining the normal sinus rhythm when rate control is not effective. Younger patients (<65 years old) with few comorbidities and symptomatic atrial fibrillation commonly opt for rhythm control. Catheter ablation of atrial fibrillation is a complex EP procedure that can dramatically decrease the burden of atrial fibrillation in carefully selected patients. The long-term management plan and the risks and benefits of each management strategy should be carefully discussed on individual basis.

WHAT IS CARDIOVERSION?

Atrial fibrillation episodes can resolve spontaneously or persist for a long period of time. Conversion to normal sinus rhythm called "cardioversion" can be done during those episodes by applying an electric current (electric shock) or less commonly by using antiarrhythmic medications. Compared with electric shock, antiarrhythmic medications are much less effective for cardioversion when the success rate exceeds 90%. Although it sounds scary, electrical cardioversion is usually a safe and well-tolerated same-day procedure. The appropriate indications and possible complications are explained in details by the treating physician. Sedation and analgesia are provided during electrical cardioversion.

As discussed above, atrial fibrillation carries the risk of clot formation inside LAA (a heart chamber structure). After cardioversion, normal contractility of the upper heart chambers is restored (which can take up to 4 weeks) and the clot formed in LAA can get dislodged into the circulation causing a stroke. Therefore, appropriate antithrombotic (blood thinning) medications should be taken before and after cardioversion. The importance of taking antithrombotic medications for stroke prevention as instructed by the physician cannot be overemphasized!

Commonly, an ultrasound procedure called TEE is performed before the attempted cardioversion. Unlike regular ultrasound of the heart (transthoracic echocardiogram), which is done by placing the probe on the chest, TEE is done through the mouth, esophagus, and stomach. After numbing the throat and giving some sedative medications, the physician asks the patient to swallow the ultrasound probe that is advanced from the mouth to the stomach. TEE allows good visualization of cardiac chambers from the back of the heart including assessment for a possible clot in LAA. If there is no clot in LAA, the risk of stroke after cardioversion procedure is low (provided the patient is taking antithrombotic medications as instructed by the physician). If the clot is seen in LAA, the cardioversion is typically deferred and appropriate antithrombotic medications are administered.

SUMMARY

Supraventricular arrhythmias are commonly seen in CCU. Sinus tachycardia is almost always a compensatory response that does not require specific treatment except for identification and treatment of its cause. Atrial fibrillation can lead to CCU admission or complicate the course of other heart diseases. Good understanding of specific issues related to atrial fibrillation management is important for patients and their families.

Prabhat Kumar
Jagmeet Singh

Ventricular Arrhythmias

Ventricular arrhythmias (VAs) are often encountered in intensive care settings. Patients presenting to the emergency room with VAs are often admitted to the cardiac care unit (CCU) for observation and evaluation. It is important to make a quick diagnosis of this arrhythmia and provide a prompt therapy to improve survival in this patient group. If not treated on time, VA may leads to deterioration of clinical status or a fatal outcome, depending on the hemodynamic compromise produced by the arrhythmia. Prevention, prompt detection, and early treatment of VA are important factors in favorable CCU survival.

CLASSIFICATION OF VENTRICULAR ARRHYTHMIA

The spectrum of VAs ranges from isolated ventricular premature complexes to ventricular tachycardia (VT) and ventricular fibrillation.[1] All these types may be a cause for concern or have clinical effects in a given clinical context.

1. *Premature ventricular complexes (PVCs)* are isolated complexes originating in the ventricle dissociated from the atrial activity. As the QRS complexes are of ventricular origin, ventricular depolarization does not occur through the His–Purkinje system leading to wide QRS complexes, with notable exceptions of origin in proximal His–Purkinje system. There may be a fusion of these complexes with conducted beat from the atrium.

2. *Couplets and nonsustained VT* may be more important as these may suggest higher chances of occurrence of sustained VT and/or ventricular fibrillation.

3. *Frequent PVCs* and *frequent nonsustained VT* may lead to clinical deterioration in the presence of compromised left ventricular function or ongoing ischemia.

4. *Accelerated idioventricular rhythm (AIVR)* is a specific kind of automatic slow ventricular rhythm at a rate of 60 to 100 beats per minute (bpm). This is incited by factors such as ischemia, cardiomyopathy, and some drugs.

5. *VT* is defined as three or more consecutive beats of ventricular origin at a rate >100 bpm (Figure 17.1).

    a. VT is called *sustained VT* if it continues for at least 30 seconds or causes hemodynamic compromise requiring termination within 30 seconds.

    b. VT lasting for <30 seconds and not causing hemodynamic compromise is classified as *nonsustained VT* (NSVT).

    c. VT is categorized as *monomorphic* if all the ventricular complexes are similar.

    d. *Polymorphic VT* has changing QRS morphology, as opposed to monomorphic VT with constant QRS morphology. *Torsades de pointes* is a type of polymorphic VT with QRS complexes of changing amplitude that appear to twist around the isoelectric line (Figure 17.2).

    e. *Bidirectional VT* is a specific type of VT seen in certain conditions (e.g., digoxin toxicity) and has alternating QRS axis in the consecutive beats.

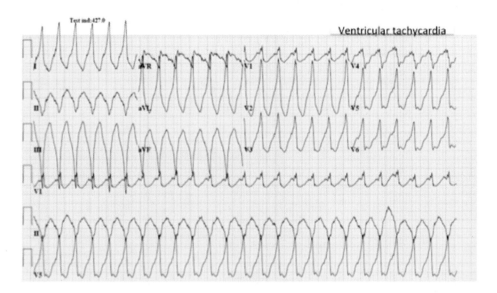

Figure 17.1. A 12-lead ECG of a patient recorded during ventricular tachycardia.

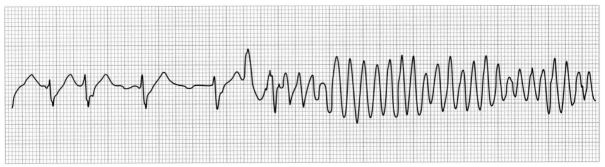

Figure 17.2. Rhythm strip recorded at the onset of torsades de pointes. Note the pause-dependent initiation of tachycardia and prolonged QT interval in the preceding beats.

6. *Ventricular fibrillation* is a ventricular rhythm with ill-formed irregular ventricular complexes owing to chaotic electrical activity of ventricles at a high rate (>300 per minute).

ETIOLOGY

VENTRICULAR TACHYCARDIA/FIBRILLATION

VT/fibrillation has multiple etiologies. They can be classified into three sections:

1. *Structural heart disease*: Patients with structural heart disease are at a risk of developing VAs. These can be broadly grouped as below:

   a. *Ischemic heart disease*: VA can be seen in patients with acute as well as chronic ischemic heart disease. Acute coronary syndrome with ongoing myocardial ischemia and acute myocardial infarction predispose the patients to VAs including PVCs, NSVT, and more malignant VT and ventricular fibrillation. Patients with chronic coronary artery disease (CAD) and with a history of myocardial infarction leading to myocardial scar are predisposed to scar-related VT, which is usually monomorphic. PVC and other forms of VA associated with acute ischemia are likely to be polymorphic.

   b. *Nonischemic cardiomyopathy*: Various forms of nonischemic cardiomyopathy have the propensity to develop VAs. These include idiopathic dilated, hypertrophic, and arrhythmogenic right ventricular cardiomyopathy (ARVC).

   c. *Infiltrative cardiac diseases and myocarditis*: Cardiac involvement with sarcoidosis is another cause of VA encountered in clinical practice. Various forms of myocarditis also have the potential of causing VAs, which at times may be clinically unstable.

2. *Ventricular arrhythmias without structural heart disease*: Many of these arrhythmias are considered to be owing to some defect in the handling of ions responsible for various phases of depolarization and repolarization of cardiac myocytes and conducting tissue of the heart. The exact molecular basis is not clear in some of these, which are categorized as idiopathic. Specific conditions in this group are as below:

   a. *Brugada syndrome*: This is a distinct syndrome seen frequently in south-east Asians, characterized by idiopathic ventricular fibrillation with presence of right bundle branch block (RBBB) pattern with ST-segment elevation in right precordial leads on baseline ECG (Figure 17.3).[2] Mutation in the Na⁺-channel gene has been seen in many of the families with Brugada syndrome.[3,4]

   b. *Catecholaminergic polymorphic ventricular tachycardia*: This is a rare form of inherited polymorphic VT caused by a mutation in the genes encoding ryanodine receptor and calsequestrin involved in handling calcium ion in the cells.[5,6]

   c. *Long QT syndromes*: These are a group of inherited syndromes caused by mutation in ion channels regulating the repolarization of myocytes, which lead to prolongation of the QT interval. These cause a specific form of VT, torsades de pointes, with characteristic ECG pattern (Figure 17.2).[7,8] The acquired form of long QT syndrome is caused by certain drugs (Table 17.1).

   d. *Idiopathic ventricular tachycardias*: These are focal monomorphic VTs originating in the outflow tracts or left ventricular septum. These can be subcategorized into outflow tract tachycardia (RV outflow tract being a commoner site of origin than LV outflow tract), fascicular (originating in the left ventricular side of the interventricular septum), and rare RV inflow tachycardia.[9] These probably have multiple mechanisms including reentry (fascicular VT) and triggered activity (outflow tract tachycardias and fascicular VT).[9]

3. *Reversible noncardiac etiologies*: VAs can be caused by certain factors leading to abnormal excitability of the myocardium.

   a. *Electrolyte abnormalities* such as hypokalemia and hypomagnesemia can precipitate VAs.

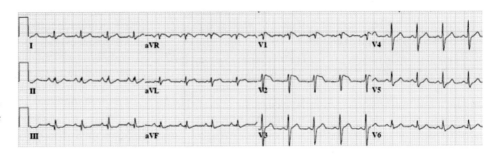

Figure 17.3. A 12-lead ECG of a patient with Brugada syndrome. Note the characteristic ST elevation in the right precordial leads.

TABLE 17.1	QT-Interval Prolonging Drugs Causing Torsades de Pointes

CARDIOVASCULAR	NEUROPSYCHIATRIC
Antiarrhythmic	*Antipsychotics*
Amiodarone	Chlorpromazine
Sotalol	Haloperidol
Ibutilide	Mesoridazine
Dofetilide	Pimozide
Procainamide	Thioridazine
Quinidine	*Opiates*
Disopyramide	Levomethadyl
Anti-anginal	Methadone
Bepridil	
ANTIMICROBIAL	GASTRO-INTESTINAL
Antibiotics	Cisapride[a]
Macrolides	Domperidone[b]
Clarithromycin	Droperidol
Erythromycin	ANTIHISTAMINES
Fluoroquinolones	Astemizole[c]
Sparfloxacin	Terfenadine[c]
Antiprotozoal	OTHERS
Pentamidine	Arsenic trioxide (anticancer)
Chloroquine	Probucol[c]
Halofantrine	

[a]Restricted availability; [b]Not available in the United States; [c]No longer available in the United States. Source: http://www.QTdrugs.org; look at the website for complete list of drugs with possible and conditional risk of torsades de pointes.

b. *Intracardiac leads* may occasionally cause irritation of the myocardium initiating VAs.
c. *Physiological stress* in general can lead to a hyperadrenergic state predisposing to VAs. This may be a causative factor in patients admitted to the intensive care unit. Hypoxia, hypotension, and other physiological stress factors may be causative.
d. *Drugs*: Other causes of VT are pro-arrhythmic medications. A high degree of suspicion should be exercised for this etiology in evaluating a patient's having VT, especially in patients admitted in the hospital on multiple medications. Certain drug interactions causing elevation of the serum level of pro-arrhythmic drugs should be kept in mind in these situations. Electrolyte abnormality can augment the pro-arrhythmic potential of a drug, for example, hypokalemia in patients on digoxin increases its arrhythmogenic potential.

These reversible factors can lead to VAs on its own, but they are even more likely to cause these arrhythmias in the presence of cardiac substrate abnormalities such as cardiomyopathy and ischemic heart disease. As can be seen, some of these have correctable factors and should be an important focus of management in these patients.

PREMATURE VENTRICULAR COMPLEXES AND NONSUSTAINED VT

Premature ventricular complexes and nonsustained VT also have similar etiologies as VT and ventricular fibrillation (VF). However, a large fraction of normal people can also have isolated infrequent PVCs, which have no significance in the absence of structural heart disease, if monomorphic.[10,11] Polymorphic PVCs suggest multifocal origin and may suggest myocardial ischemia and need more urgent attention.[12] The prognostic implication of NSVTs is dictated by the underlying myocardial substrate.[11,13]

ACCELERATED IDIOVENTRICULAR RHYTHM

As mentioned earlier, AIVR is seen in the setting of ischemic heart disease, cardiomyopathy, and drugs. In the setting of an acute coronary event, its occurrence has frequently been correlated with myocardial reperfusion, and this is considered to be a reperfusion arrhythmia.[14]

MANIFESTATIONS

1. *PVCs* may cause palpitations or a feeling of skipped beat in some patients, and it may remain asymptomatic in many. Hemodynamic deterioration may occur with PVCs if they are frequent. Frequent PVCs may lead to worsening of heart failure or worsening of myocardial ischemia and should be considered as a cause of worsening of heart failure or ischemia.
2. *AIVR* is usually a benign arrhythmia. However, in patients with compromised LV function, loss of LV synchrony may lead to hemodynamic deterioration leading to hypotension or heart failure. Patients with similar sinus rate may have rhythm switching between AIVR and sinus rhythm and may perceive the change in rhythm as palpitation.
3. *NSVT* such as PVCs have minimal symptoms of palpitations. However frequent NSVT such as frequent PVCs may exacerbate heart failure or myocardial ischemia.
4. *VT* may cause palpitations alone if hemodynamically stable. However, quite often VT is hemodynamically unstable and may cause heart failure, worsening of myocardial ischemia, syncope, or sudden cardiac death. Unstable VT if untreated usually degenerates into ventricular fibrillation.
5. *Ventricular fibrillation* always leads to cardiovascular collapse and loss of consciousness and unless promptly treated, leads to death.

DIAGNOSIS

1. Premature ventricular complex classically manifests a beat with QRS complex >120 milliseconds in duration, with a fully compensatory pause and absence of preceding P wave.
2. VT frequently manifests as wide complex tachycardia (QRS duration >120 milliseconds) on surface ECG. However, differentiation of such a wide QRS complex tachycardia from an SVT with aberrant intraventricular conduction is of paramount importance.
3. Various surface ECG criteria have been used to differentiate VT from SVT in the setting of wide complex tachycardia.

ECG CRITERIA FOR DIFFERENTIATION OF VT FROM SVT

Many EKG criteria had been developed for differentiation of VT from SVT.[15]

Fusion and capture beats and AV dissociation: These provide the strongest electrocardiographic evidence for differentiating VT from SVT with aberrant conduction. However in their absence, other clues from the ECG may be required to help with this differentiation.

Specific QRS contours can also be helpful in diagnosing VT:

1. Left-axis deviation.

2. QRS duration exceeding 140 milliseconds, with a QRS of normal duration during sinus rhythm.

3. In precordial leads with an RS pattern, the interval of the onset of R wave to the nadir of S wave exceeding 100 milliseconds suggests VT as the diagnosis.

4. Features supporting VT with an RBBB QRS morphology (predominantly positive QRS complex in V1):
   a. A QRS duration of >140 milliseconds
   b. The QRS complex is monophasic or biphasic in V1 with an initial deflection different from that of the sinus rhythm
   c. The amplitude of the first r wave in V1 exceeds r' and
   d. An rS or a QS pattern in V6.

5. Features supporting VT with a left bundle branch block (LBBB) type QRS morphology (predominantly negative QRS complex in V1):
   a. A QRS duration of >160 milliseconds
   b. The axis can be rightward, with negative deflections deeper in V1 than in V6
   c. A broad prolonged (> 40 milliseconds) R wave can be noted in V_1 and
   d. A qR or QS pattern in V6.

6. A QRS complex that is similar in V1 through V6, either all negative or all positive, favors a ventricular origin. However, this is not very specific as an upright QRS complex in V1 through V6 can also occur from conduction over a left-sided accessory pathway.

7. In the presence of a preexisting bundle branch block, a wide QRS tachycardia with a contour different from the contour during sinus rhythm is most likely a VT.

Features supporting supraventricular arrhythmia with aberrancy:

1. Onset of the tachycardia with a premature P wave

2. A very short RP interval (100 milliseconds)

3. A QRS configuration similar to recorded supraventricular rhythm at a similar heart rate

4. P wave and QRS rate and rhythm suggest that ventricular activation is associated with atrial activation (e.g., an AV Wenckebach block) and

5. Slowing or termination of the tachycardia by vagal maneuvers. Exceptions include the outflow tract VT and the fascicular VT.

Specific QRS contours supporting the diagnosis of SVT with aberrancy are a triphasic pattern in V1, an initial vector of the abnormal complex similar to that of the normally conducted beats.

A wide QRS complex that terminates a short cycle length following a long cycle (long–short cycle sequence) may support SVT.

Atrial fibrillation with conduction over an accessory pathway should be suspected with grossly irregular, wide QRS tachycardia with ventricular rates >200 beats per minute.

Several algorithms for distinguishing VT from SVT with aberrancy have been suggested based on the ECG features mentioned above. One such algorithm is shown in Figure 17.4. All the above features have some exceptions, especially in patients who have preexisting conduction disturbances or pre-excitation syndrome. Sound clinical judgment should always help in the decision based on ECGs in arriving at a diagnosis.

EVALUATION OF ETIOLOGY

REVERSIBLE FACTORS

1. Assessment should include serum electrolyte levels (particularly serum K^+ and serum Mg^{2+} levels).

2. Presence of ongoing myocardial ischemia should be kept as a possibility.

3. Pro-arrhythmic drugs are important in the causation of PVCs in such a setting. Drugs that prolong the QT interval should be carefully screened. QT interval should be measured on the ECG routinely.

4. Any factor that may be instrumental in autonomic stimulation such as hypoxia, heart failure, surgical stress, and anesthesia, should be considered the potential cause.

EVALUATION OF ARRHYTHMOGENIC SUBSTRATE

1. Baseline 12-lead surface ECG can give clues to etiology of VAs. Conditions such as long QT syndrome (QTc >0.46 millisecond in male and >0.47 in female) and Brugada syndrome (Figure 17.3) may have characteristic baseline ECG pattern.

2. Because cardiomyopathies form almost 90% of all patients with VAs with sudden cardiac arrest, echocardiography is of great help in evaluating the substrate of these arrhythmias.[16]

3. Because a significant fraction (up to 50% in various series) of VAs is caused by CAD, stress evaluation is an important part of diagnostic workup. Stress test may involve stress ECG or stress imaging (echocardiography or SPECT). Stress test is also helpful in evaluating catecholaminergic polymorphic VT, with characteristic onset of VA with exercise.[16]

4. Cardiac MRI is of diagnostic value in evaluating ARVC besides delineating myocardial scars and evaluation of myocardial ischemia.[16]

5. Procainamide challenge is helpful in the diagnosis of Brugada syndrome.[17]

TREATMENT

The treatment plan of VAs can be divided into two parts, (1) acute treatment for ongoing arrhythmia and (2) chronic therapy for prevention of recurrence of arrhythmia and sudden cardiac death.

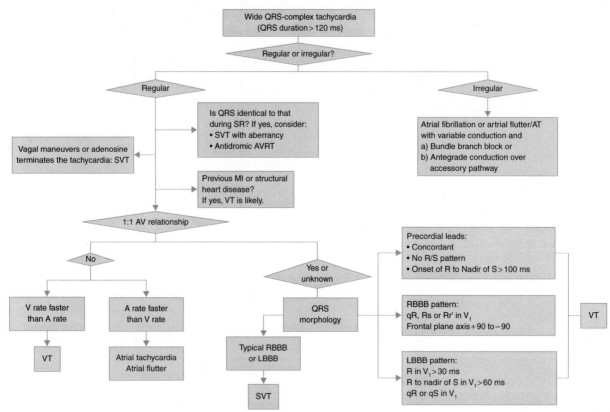

Figure 17.4. Algorithm for diagnosing a wide QRS tachycardia. AV, atrioventricular; AVRT, AV reentrant tachycardia; LBBB, left bundle branch block; RBBB, right bundle branch block; SVT, supraventricular tachycardia; VT, ventricular tachycardia. (Adapted from Blomstrom-Lundqvist C, Scheinman MM, Aliot EM, et al. ACC/AHA/ESC guidelines for the management of patients with supraventricular arrhythmias—executive summary: a report of the American College of Cardiology/American Heart Association Task Force on Practice Guidelines and the European Society of Cardiology Committee for Practice Guidelines (Writing Committee to Develop Guidelines for the Management of Patients with Supraventricular Arrhythmias). *Circulation.* 2003;108:1871.)

ACUTE THERAPY

Premature ventricular complexes and nonsustained ventricular tachycardia.

1. Any potential reversible factor should be corrected, for example, correction of electrolyte abnormality, withdrawal of causative drugs, treatment of myocardial ischemia with revascularization and repositioning of pacing leads.

2. Treating the basic condition, for example, correction of hypoxia and treatment of heart failure may control PVCs resulting from autonomic stimulation during various physiological stresses.

3. β-Blockers may be used to suppress frequent PVCs or episodes or NSVT causing exacerbation of heart failure or myocardial ischemia.[18] Other antiarrhythmic drugs should be used with caution owing to their pro-arrhythmic potential and lack of effect on mortality and actually increased mortality in some situations.[16]

Accelerated idioventricular rhythm.

1. This rhythm is usually benign and need not be treated unless it leads to hemodynamic compromise.

2. If need for treatment arises, it can be done by increasing the sinus rate by administering atropine or isoproterenol or by atrial pacing.

VENTRICULAR TACHYCARDIA

Treatment of VT depends on whether the tachycardia is associated with hemodynamic compromise or not. If there is associated hypotension, heart failure, angina, or cerebral hypoperfusion synchronized DC, cardioversion should be done emergently. In the absence of decompensation, pharmacotherapy can be attempted.

1. *Thumpversion:* Thumpversion is an effective way of cardioversion of VT, if the thump falls in the appropriate interval of cardiac cycle. However, it may also initiate more malignant arrhythmia such as ventricular fibrillation if the thump falls during the vulnerable period of the cardiac cycle.

2. *DC cardioversion:* Synchronized direct current cardioversion should be done immediately in patients with sustained VT associated with hypotension, angina, heart failure, or syncope.[19] Patients with continuing VT despite drug therapy should be taken for elective cardioversion. Conscious sedation is required during cardioversion unless the patient is unconscious owing to cerebral hypoperfusion. Biphasic defibrillators have been found to be more effective in converting the rhythm compared with older monophasic ones. Stable VT can be cardioverted with energy as low as 25 to 50 J. Patients with fast VT with hypotension should be converted with a biphasic energy delivery of 100 to 200 J (200 to 360 J

for monophasic cardioverter defibrillator).[20] Placement of defibrillating patches (or paddles) should be done in a manner that includes the maximum area of the heart in the current field and anteroposterior location of the patches may be more effective in cardioversion. Patients with digitalis toxicity are best treated with pharmacotherapy owing to the risk of precipitation of VF with DC cardioversion attempt.

3. *Overdrive pacing:* Some cases of VT such as scar-related reentrant VT can be reverted by pacing the right ventricle at a rate higher than the rate of VT through pacing lead or transcutaneously. This is particularly useful in patients with recurrent VT. However, overdrive pacing may also accelerate VT to ventricular flutter or fibrillation.

4. *Pharmacotherapy:* Acute treatment of sustained VT not causing hemodynamic decompensation can be done by medical therapy.[20] Intravenous bolus of lidocaine, amiodarone, or procainamide can be given followed by infusion of the effective drug. All three drugs raise the defibrillation threshold.

   a. *Amiodarone* is the most effective drug in cardioversion of VT. Intravenous loading with 150 mg over 10 minutes should be done followed by 1 mg per minute for 3 to 6 hours and 0.5 mg per minute thereafter. Repeat bolus of 150 mg over 10 minutes can be given in case of breakthrough VT/VF. Intravenous amiodarone administration prolongs QTc interval but seldom causes torsades de pointes.

   b. *Lidocaine* is a moderately effective drug for acute treatment of VT, especially in the setting of myocardial ischemia and after coronary revascularization. This can be given at a dose of 1 to 3 mg per kg bolus at the rate of 20 to 50 mg per minute followed by 0.5 mg per kg bolus after 10 minutes and can be continued as maintenance infusion at 1 to 4 mg per minute. Lidocaine administration can produce CNS toxicity such as dizziness, paresthesias, confusion, delirium, stupor, coma, and seizures.

   c. *Procainamide* is more effective in acutely reverting VT than lidocaine. However, its myocardial depressant action may lead to inability to use it in patients with LV dysfunction. Various dose regimens are used. Up to 17 mg per kg at a rate <50 mg per minute (usually 20 mg per minute) can be given as a bolus infusion. Infusion should be stopped once QRS duration increases by 50% of the baseline, or if arrhythmia is reverted or hypotension sets in. This can be followed by maintenance infusion at 1 to 4 mg per minute. Maintenance rate should be reduced in patients with renal failure, and serum levels should be monitored in such patients. Serum level should also be monitored if infusion is continued for more than 24 hours at a rate exceeding 3 mg per minute. Procainamide typically broadens QRS complex and slows VT before terminating it.

   d. Other antiarrhythmic medications as listed in Table 17.2 can be used to control and revert VT if the above drugs are not effective in controlling VT. Phenytoin is effective in treating VA associated with digoxin toxicity.

Ventricular flutter and fibrillation.
Pharmacotheraphy and electrical therapy are used to treat ventricular flatter and fribrillation.[19-21]

1. *Pharmacotherapy:*

   a. *Epinephrine:* Epinephrine remains the mainstay of therapy in ventricular fibrillation, which can be administered as 1 mg IV of 1:10,000 solution or 2 to 2.5 mg through endotracheal tube every 5 minutes during resuscitation. There is no evidence of efficacy of high-dose epinephrine therapy or intracardiac epinephrine injection.

TABLE 17.2	**Doses of Antiarrhythmic Drugs**			
	Intravenous		Oral	
Drug	Loading Dose	Maintenance	Loading Dose	Maintenance
Amiodarone	15 mg/min for 10 min mg IV bolus followed by 1 mg/min for 3 h followed by 0.5 mg/min. Total dose over 24 h not to exceed 2.2 g	0.5–1 mg/min	800–1,600 mg/d for 7–14 d	Oral maintenance of 200–600 mg/d
Lidocaine	1–3 mg/kg IV bolus at the rate of 20–50 mg min; repeat 0.5 mg/kg bolus after 10 min	1–4 mg/min		
Procainamide	Up to 17 mg/kg at a rate of 0.2–0.5 mg/kg/min (<50 mg/min)	2–6 mg/min	500–1,000 mg	250–1,000 mg Q4–6 h
Sotalol	10 mg over 1–2 min[a]			80–320 mg Q12 h
Quinidine	6–10 mg/kg at 0.3–0.5 mg/kg/min		800–1,000 mg	300–600 mg Q6 h
Mexiletine	500 mg[a]	0.5–1 g/24h	400–600 mg	150–300 mg Q8–12 h
Phenytoin	100 mg Q 5 min for ≤1 g		1,000 mg	100–400 mg Q12–24 h
Flecainide	2 mg/kg[a]	100–200 g Q12 h		50–200 mg Q12 h
Propafenone	1–2 mg/kg		600–900 mg	150–300 Q8–12 h
Moricizine			300 mg	100–400 mg Q8 h
Bretylium	5–10 mg/kg at 1–2 mg/kg/min	0.5–2 mg/min		4 mg/kg/d
Disopyramide	1–2mg/kg over 15–45 min[a]	1 mg/kg/h		100–300 mg Q6–8 h

[a]Intravenous use investigational.

b. *Vasopressin:* There are limited data suggesting the efficacy of single bolus of vasopressin (40 U IV) for the treatment of ventricular fibrillation.[22]

c. *Amiodarone:* Studies on out-of-hospital cardiac arrest have shown the efficacy of amiodarone (rapid IV infusion of 300 mg diluted in 20 to 30 ml of normal saline or 5% dextrose solution) in treating ventricular fibrillation.[23] Amiodarone has also been shown to increase the efficacy of electrical defibrillation in out-of-hospital cardiac arrest.[20]

d. There is no evidence of efficacy of lidocaine or any other antiarrhythmic medications in the management of ventricular fibrillation.

2. *Electrical therapy:*

a. *External defibrillation:* Prompt defibrillation is required for termination of ventricular flutter/fibrillation. An energy output of 360 J is used in succession if the previous shock does not terminate VF.[19] With biphasic defibrillator three shocks of 150 J each can be used in succession if previous shocks are unsuccessful.[19]

b. *Automated implantable cardioverter defibrillator:* If automated implantable cardioverter defibrillator (AICD) is in place, they can deliver shock to defibrillate acute VF.

LONG-TERM THERAPY

Long-term management of patients with VA depends on the risk of future event and potential of sudden cardiac death. The options of long-term therapy are (1) antiarrhythmic drugs, (2) catheter ablation, (3) AICD therapy, and more infrequently (4) procedures to modify cervical sympathetic outflow.

1. *Antiarrhythmic drugs* (see Table 17.2 for doses)

β-Blockers: These drugs are effective in suppressing ventricular ectopy and prevention of sudden cardiac death in patients with and without heart failure.[18,24] They can be used for suppression of symptomatic ventricular ectopics. They are also a mainstay of therapy in certain specific conditions (see section on management considerations in specific Types of ventricular Arrhythmias).

Amiodarone: Suppression of VA can be effectively achieved by amiodarone. However overall long-term survival benefit with amiodarone and its efficacy in preventing sudden cardiac death are controversial and definitely inferior to AICD.[25–27] There are considerable pulmonary, hepatic, thyroid, ocular, and skin toxicities associated with it.

Sotalol: Similar to amiodarone, sotalol is effective in suppressing VA.[28] However, it has a higher pro-arrhythmic potential.

Others: Other classes of antiarrhythmic drugs are seldom tried and most often in the setting of AICD implantation to reduce arrhythmia and shock burden.

Antiarrhythmic medications with the exception of β-blocker do not have an unequivocal efficacy in preventing sudden cardiac death. They can be best used to reduce the arrhythmia burden and frequency of device therapy needed in patients on AICD therapy.

2. *Catheter ablation:* Catheter ablation has emerged as an important modality of therapy in the treatment of arrhythmias in general and has been increasingly used for various forms of VT. Catheter ablation of a VT involves mapping of the arrhythmia by various methods to localize the origin of the arrhythmia and ablation of the focus with delivery of radiofrequency energy through ablation catheter. The efficacy of catheter ablation varies from <50% to >90% depending on the etiology of the arrhythmia.[29] This modality is highly effective in idiopathic outflow tract VTs and fascicular VTs. Efficacy in reentrant scar-related VT in chronic ischemic heart disease is lower, although it can be used to reduce arrhythmia burden.[29] Seldom is the procedure complicated by pericardial effusion or thromboembolism from the ablation site.

3. *AICD:* Implantable cardioverter defibrillator has become the mainstay of therapy in the long-term management of patients with various forms of VT and ventricular fibrillation. This therapy has been effectively used in preventing sudden cardiac death in patients with syncope or aborted sudden cardiac death owing to ventricular tachyarrhythmia. Besides its use in secondary prevention of sudden cardiac death[30–32] in these patients with history of ventricular tachyarrhythmia, they have been used increasingly for primary prevention purposes in patients with cardiomyopathy with high risk of developing ventricular tachyarrhythmia and sudden cardiac death (left ventricular ejection fraction or LVEF of <35%).[33,34]

4. *Modification cervical sympathetic outflow:* Sympathetically mediated triggering mechanisms are important in arrhythmogenesis of VT, and β-blocker therapy is one way of blocking these effects. Surgical cervical sympathectomy has been used in certain conditions to prevent ventricular tachyarrhythmia.[35,36] It has been effectively used in patients with long QT syndrome.[35]

MANAGEMENT CONSIDERATIONS IN SPECIFIC TYPES OF VENTRICULAR ARRHYTHMIAS

LONG QT SYNDROME AND TORSADES DE POINTES

1. Patients with long QT syndrome usually present with history of syncopal episodes and as survivors of sudden cardiac death owing to VT/VF. It is important to differentiate a polymorphic VT with associated long QT interval or U wave from those with normal QT interval as the pathogenesis and therapeutic implications of such a finding are different.

a. The term torsades de pointes is restricted to polymorphic VT associated with long QT syndrome. This may be seen in patients with congenital long QT syndrome, electrolyte abnormality such as hypokalemia, or drug-induced QT prolongation.

b. In acquired long QT syndrome, torsades de pointes is almost always precipitated by pause-dependent early afterdepolarizations.

2. In a large subgroup of patients with congenital long QT syndrome, torsades is largely adrenergic-dependent and precipitated by stress, which provides the rationale for β-blocker therapy in these patients.

3. *Treatment:*

a. Torsades de pointes in conjunction with prolonged QT interval is treated with IV magnesium ($MgSO_4$ at a dose of 1 to 2 g IV slow infusion over 1 to 2 minutes).

b. Temporary pacing can be used to prevent pause-dependent torsades de pointes.[37]

c. QT prolonging antiarrhythmic drugs (class IA, some class IC and class III) should not be administered in these patients. Polymorphic VT without QT prolongation at the baseline can, however, be treated with such medications.

d. Long-term therapy depends on risk of sudden cardiac death.

e. β-Blockers should be used for patients with long QT syndrome.[38] Patients with congenital long QT syndrome at high risk of sudden death (survivors of sudden cardiac death or history of syncope) should receive implantable cardioverter defibrillator (ICD) along with β-blocker therapy. Patients with prolonged QT interval without cardiac arrest or syncope with family history of sudden cardiac death should also be considered for ICD placement. In addition to cardioverting VT, ICD also prevents pause-dependent triggering of these arrhythmias in them.

f. Cervical sympathectomy may reduce arrhythmia burden in patients with congenital long QT syndrome on ICD with frequent episodes of torsades.[35]

ISCHEMIC HEART DISEASE

1. VT in the setting of chronic ischemic heart disease occurs typically by reentry. All patients with chronic CAD and history of VT/VF episode should have an implantation of AICD to prevent sudden cardiac death.

2. In the setting of old myocardial infarction, VT is typically monomorphic.

3. Polymorphic VT usually occurs in the setting of ongoing ischemia and acute myocardial infarction.

4. Patients with history of VF during the first 24 to 48 hours of myocardial infarction do not have increased risk of sudden death beyond the acute phase, and AICD is not recommended for secondary prevention.[39,40]

5. Patients with chronic CAD with ischemic cardiomyopathy, without history of VA should also receive AICD for primary prevention of sudden cardiac death owing to VA if they have a poor LV function with LVEF <35% and are in NYHA class II–III.[33,34]

6. Catheter ablation of focal reentrant tachycardia may be useful in reducing the burden of arrhythmia and shock in these patients.

DILATED CARDIOMYOPATHY

1. Management of VT/VF in dilated cardiomyopathy is similar to ischemic cardiomyopathy. In the presence of history of VT/VF, implantation of AICD is needed.

2. Implantation of AICD for primary prevention of sudden cardiac death is recommended in patients with dilated cardiomyopathy with severe LV dysfunction (LVEF <35%) and NYHA class II–III.[33,41]

3. Some patients with dilated cardiomyopathy may develop VT owing to bundle branch reentry. Patients with bundle branch reentry type of VT should be treated with ablation of the right bundle branch.

HYPERTROPHIC CARDIOMYOPATHY

1. VA is an important part of clinical manifestations in patients with hypertrophic cardiomyopathy.

2. Patients with presence of syncope, a family history of sudden death in first degree relatives, septal thickness of >3 cm and presence of nonsustained VT on 24-hour ECG recordings are at a high risk of sudden cardiac death.[42]

3. Asymptomatic or mildly symptomatic patients with infrequent episodes of NSVT are at low risk of sudden cardiac death.

4. Patients with high risk of sudden death by these considerations or those with history of sustained VT should be considered for AICD implantation.

ARRHYTHMOGENIC RIGHT VENTRICULAR CARDIOMYOPATHY

1. A type of cardiomyopathy with fatty or fibro-fatty infiltration of right ventricular myocardium mediated by patchy myocarditis.[43]

2. It is associated with reentrant VA and right ventricular failure in late stages.

3. In advanced cases, the left ventricle can also be involved in more than half of the patients.

4. ECG during sinus rhythm may exhibit complete or incomplete RBBB, terminal notch in the QRS complex (epsilon wave), and T inversion in V1–V3.[43]

5. Owing to the progressive nature of the disease and poor prognosis, AICD is preferred over drug therapy alone especially if the patient has had a poorly tolerated VT.

6. Radiofrequency ablation is not a good option because of multiple foci and progressive disease.

BRUGADA SYNDROME

a. Brugada syndrome should be a consideration in patients with idiopathic ventricular fibrillation presenting with aborted sudden cardiac death. The characteristic ECG pattern of RBBB and ST-segment elevation in V1—V3 may not be present in the baseline ECG of all the patients.

1. Sodium channel blocking drugs (e.g., procainamide) can unmask the ECG findings in patients without typical ECG finding at baseline and are used for provocative test for the diagnostic workup of idiopathic ventricular fibrillation.

2. AICD is the only effective therapy for this group of patients.

3. *Quinidine*, which blocks I_{to}–current, has been found to be effective in suppressing VA in these patients. *Cilostazol* is another drug that has been used with some success and acts by augmenting I_{CaL}. Newer drug (*tedisamil*) to block I_{to} specifically is under investigation.[44] Intravenous *isoproterenol*, which augments I_{CaL}, has been used to manage electrical storm owing to Brugada syndrome, usually in combination with general anesthesia and cardiopulmonary bypass.[44] Currently all these drugs should be used only in conjunction with AICD for long-term preventive therapy.

4. Role of risk stratification based on inducibility during electrophysiological study is controversial.

CATECHOLAMINERGIC POLYMORPHIC VENTRICULAR TACHYCARDIA

1. This is a rare form of inherited polymorphic VT seen in children and adolescents without any structural heart disease.

2. The manifestation is usually syncope or aborted sudden death usually precipitated by exercise.

3. Usual time course of rhythm disturbances during exercise is sinus tachycardia followed by premature ventricular complexes progressing to salvos of monomorphic and bidirectional VT preceding the development of polymorphic VT.

4. A family history of stress-induced syncope or sudden death is present in one-third of these patients, and many have a mutation in the ryanodine receptor gene.

5. These patients are treated with β-blockers[45] and AICD.

IDIOPATHIC VENTRICULAR TACHYCARDIAS

A. These are focal monomorphic VTs originating in the outflow tracts or left ventricular septum.[9]

B. The mechanism of these tachycardias is probably multiple, including reentrant as well as triggered activity.

C. These forms of tachycardia usually have good prognosis and can be managed with radiofrequency ablation in most cases, and antiarrhythmic medications can be effective in others.

   1. *Outflow tract tachycardia:*
     a. Tachycardias originating in the right ventricular outflow tract are the most common of these idiopathic forms of tachycardias. Other foci of origin can be LVOT and rarely RV inflow or RV apex.
     b. These tachycardias can be terminated by adenosine and can be suppressed by β-blockers and verapamil.

   2. *Left septal VT (fascicular VT):*
     a. This form of focal tachycardia originates in the left posterior septum and is preceded by fascicular potential. This is a heterogeneous group of tachycardia where multiple mechanisms may be operative.
     b. Demonstration of entrainment suggests reentry as the mechanism in some of the tachycardia. Verapamil, diltiazem, and rarely adenosine suppress the tachycardia.
     c. Suppression with verapamil suggests that delayed afterdepolarization and triggered activity may be a potential mechanism.

ELECTRICAL STORM (VT STORM)

The generally accepted definition of electrical storm or VT storm is three or more episodes of VT and/or ventricular fibrillation requiring therapy with device intervention (antitachycardia pacing or defibrillation shock delivery) or external cardioversion/defibrillation in a 24-hour period.[46]

In the era of AICD implantation recurrent malignant VA and electrical storm has become an important management problem. Besides causing discomfort, multiple shocks during an electrical storm also cause myocardial injury and inflammation and raise cardiac enzyme levels.

CLINICAL PRESENTATION

Clinical presentation of electrical storm may be quite variable. In patients with an AICD, it may be quite dramatic often with anxious patients getting repeated shocks. In the most severe form, the arrhythmia may become incessant despite all attempts to restore the baseline rhythm for any extended period by drugs and cardioversion.

MANAGEMENT

Basic principles of management are similar to management of a patient presenting with VT/VF. Precipitating factors such as acute ongoing ischemia, fulminant myocarditis, drug toxicity with QT prolonging drugs, and electrolyte abnormality should be assessed.

Suppression of ventricular arrhythmia. Anxiety associated with electrical storm and repeated AICD shocks usually augment sympathetic stimulation in these patients. Intravenous β-blockade combined with sedatives (benzodiazepines) should be a part of the initial management of these patients. In selected patients, intubation and anesthesia may be required to eliminate anxiety and sympathetic drive and may be effective in suppressing the arrhythmia acutely. Nonselective β-blockers such as propranolol and/or stellate ganglion blockade can be used if selective β-blockers are not effective.

Antiarrhythmic therapy should be used to suppress the arrhythmia. Amiodarone is effective in suppression of most VAs. With the exception of polymorphic VT with QT prolongation owing to drugs or electrolyte abnormality, amiodarone is the drug of choice. If IV β- blockade and amiodarone are not effective, addition of lidocaine or procainamide should be considered. These medications sometimes slow down the arrhythmia, so that they are tolerated hemodynamically.

Polymorphic VT with QT prolongation owing to drug toxicity or electrolyte abnormality (hypokalemia/hypomagnesemia) should be treated with intravenous magnesium and potassium.

Polymorphic VT with ongoing myocardial ischemia not immediately responding to antiarrhythmic therapy should be considered for coronary revascularization at the earliest. In the meantime, aggressive medical therapy of ongoing ischemia with drugs and possible intra-aortic balloon counterpulsation are usually necessary.

In Brugada syndrome, intravenous isoproterenol has been used in combination with general anesthesia and cardiopulmonary bypass.[44] Oral quinidine has also been used in this setting to suppress the arrhythmia.

Catheter ablation may be needed at times during the electrical storm, which is incessant or frequently recurrent despite other measures.

Long-term management. Future implications: Occurrence of electrical storm usually raises the likelihood of cardiac death several fold in the next few months compared with those on ICD without any arrhythmic event. The patients with electrical storm have threefold higher rate of cardiac death as compared with those having isolated VT/VF.[47] Most of these cardiac deaths are nonsudden.

Evaluation of cardiac substrate: The factors responsible for cardiac mortality after an electrical storm are essentially the same cardiac substrates that increase the likelihood of electrical storm and include worsening or new onset heart failure, recent ischemic event, or worsening of myocardial pathology.

Treatment of these patients should focus on comprehensive treatment of these basic conditions. Treatment of heart failure should be optimized. Evaluation of ischemia should be done and in case significantly ischemic segment is detected, treatment of ischemia should be maximized and myocardial revascularization, if feasible, should be done at the earliest. Close follow-up of these patients for the first few months after the event is warranted.

REFERENCES

1. Buxton AE, Calkins H, Callans DJ, et al. ACC/AHA/HRS 2006 key data elements and definitions for electrophysiological studies and procedures: a report of the American College of Cardiology/American Heart Association Task Force on Clinical Data Standards (ACC/AHA/HRS Writing Committee to Develop Data Standards on Electrophysiology). *J Am Coll Cardiol.* 2006;48:2360–2396.
2. Brugada P, Brugada J. Right bundle branch block, persistent ST segment elevation and sudden cardiac death: a distinct clinical and electrocardiographic syndrome. A multicenter report. *J Am Coll Cardiol.* 1992;20:1391–1396.
3. Chen Q, Kirsch GE, Zhang D, et al. Genetic basis and molecular mechanism for idiopathic ventricular fibrillation. *Nature.* 1998;392:293–296.
4. Vatta M, Dumaine R, Antzelevitch C, et al. Novel mutations in domain I of *SCN5A* cause Brugada syndrome. *Mol Genet Metab.* 2002;75:317–324.
5. Priori SG, Napolitano C, Tiso N, et al. Mutations in the cardiac ryanodine receptor gene (*hRyR2*) underlie catecholaminergic polymorphic ventricular tachycardia. *Circulation.* 2001;103:196–200.
6. Mohamed U, Napolitano C, Priori SG. Molecular and electrophysiological bases of catecholaminergic polymorphic ventricular tachycardia. *J Cardiovasc Electrophysiol.* 2007;18:791–797.
7. Antzelevitch C. Ionic, molecular, and cellular bases of QT-interval prolongation and torsade de pointes. *Europace.* 2007;9(suppl 4):iv4–iv15.
8. Antzelevitch C, Shimizu W. Cellular mechanisms underlying the long QT syndrome. *Curr Opin Cardiol.* 2002;17:43–51.
9. Badhwar N, Scheinman MM. Idiopathic ventricular tachycardia: diagnosis and management. *Curr Probl Cardiol.* 2007;32:7–43.
10. Hiss RG, Lamb LE. Electrocardiographic findings in 122,043 individuals. *Circulation.* 1962;25:947–961.
11. Engstrom G, Hedblad B, Janzon L, et al. Ventricular arrhythmias during 24-h ambulatory ECG recording: incidence, risk factors and prognosis in men with and without a history of cardiovascular disease. *J Intern Med.* 1999;246:363–372.
12. Viskin S, Belhassen B. Polymorphic ventricular tachyarrhythmias in the absence of organic heart disease: classification, differential diagnosis, and implications for therapy. *Prog Cardiovasc Dis.* 1998;41:17–34.
13. Kennedy HL, Whitlock JA, Sprague MK, et al. Long-term follow-up of asymptomatic healthy subjects with frequent and complex ventricular ectopy. *N Engl J Med.* 1985;312:193–197.
14. Solomon SD, Ridker PM, Antman EM. Ventricular arrhythmias in trials of thrombolytic therapy for acute myocardial infarction. A meta-analysis. *Circulation.* 1993;88:2575–2581.
15. Blomstrom-Lundqvist C, Scheinman MM, Aliot EM, et al. ACC/AHA/ESC guidelines for the management of patients with supraventricular arrhythmias—executive summary: a report of the American College of Cardiology/American Heart Association Task Force on Practice Guidelines and the European Society of Cardiology Committee for Practice Guidelines (Writing Committee to Develop Guidelines for the Management of Patients with Supraventricular Arrhythmias) developed in collaboration with NASPE-Heart Rhythm Society. *J Am Coll Cardiol.* 2003;42:1493–1531.
16. Zipes DP, Camm AJ, Borggrefe M, et al. ACC/AHA/ESC 2006 guidelines for management of patients with ventricular arrhythmias and the prevention of sudden cardiac death: a report of the American College of Cardiology/American Heart Association Task Force and the European Society of Cardiology Committee for Practice Guidelines (Writing Committee to Develop Guidelines for Management of Patients With Ventricular Arrhythmias and the Prevention of Sudden Cardiac Death): developed in collaboration with the European Heart Rhythm Association and the Heart Rhythm Society. *Circulation.* 2006;114:e385–e484.
17. Krahn AD, Gollob M, Yee R, et al. Diagnosis of unexplained cardiac arrest: role of adrenaline and procainamide infusion. *Circulation.* 2005;112:2228–2234.
18. Ellison KE, Hafley GE, Hickey K, et al. Effect of beta-blocking therapy on outcome in the Multicenter UnSustained Tachycardia Trial (MUSTT). *Circulation.* 2002;106:2694–2699.
19. Link MS, Atkins DL, Passman RS, et al. Part 6: electrical therapies: automated external defibrillators, defibrillation, cardioversion, and pacing: 2010 American Heart Association Guidelines for Cardiopulmonary Resuscitation and Emergency Cardiovascular Care. *Circulation.* 2010;122:S706–S719.
20. Neumar RW, Otto CW, Link MS, et al. Part 8: adult advanced cardiovascular life support: 2010 American Heart Association Guidelines for Cardiopulmonary Resuscitation and Emergency Cardiovascular Care. *Circulation.* 2010;122:S729–S767.
21. Berg RA, Hemphill R, Abella BS, et al. Part 5: adult basic life support: 2010 American Heart Association Guidelines for Cardiopulmonary Resuscitation and Emergency Cardiovascular Care. *Circulation.* 2010;122:S685–S705.
22. Aung K, Htay T. Vasopressin for cardiac arrest: a systematic review and meta-analysis. *Arch Intern Med.* 2005;165:17–24.
23. Kudenchuk PJ, Cobb LA, Copass MK, et al. Amiodarone for resuscitation after out-of-hospital cardiac arrest due to ventricular fibrillation. *N Engl J Med.* 1999;341:871–878.
24. Hallstrom AP, Cobb LA, Yu BH, et al. An antiarrhythmic drug experience in 941 patients resuscitated from an initial cardiac arrest between 1970 and 1985. *Am J Cardiol.* 1991;68:1025–1031.
25. Connolly SJ. Meta-analysis of antiarrhythmic drug trials. *Am J Cardiol.* 1999;84:90R–93R.
26. Steinberg JS, Martins J, Sadanandan S, et al. Antiarrhythmic drug use in the implantable defibrillator arm of the Antiarrhythmics Versus Implantable Defibrillators (AVID) Study. *Am Heart J.* 2001;142:520–529.
27. Packer DL, Prutkin JM, Hellkamp AS, et al. Impact of implantable cardioverter-defibrillator, amiodarone, and placebo on the mode of death in stable patients with heart failure: analysis from the sudden cardiac death in heart failure trial. *Circulation.* 2009;120:2170–2176.
28. Kuhlkamp V, Mewis C, Mermi J, et al. Suppression of sustained ventricular tachyarrhythmias: a comparison of d,l-sotalol with no antiarrhythmic drug treatment. *J Am Coll Cardiol.* 1999;33:46–52.
29. Stevenson WG, Soejima K. Catheter ablation for ventricular tachycardia. *Circulation.* 2007;115:2750–2760.
30. A comparison of antiarrhythmic-drug therapy with implantable defibrillators in patients resuscitated from near-fatal ventricular arrhythmias. The Antiarrhythmics Versus Implantable Defibrillators (AVID) Investigators. *N Engl J Med.* 1997;337:1576–1583.
31. Connolly SJ, Gent M, Roberts RS, et al. Canadian implantable defibrillator study (CIDS): a randomized trial of the implantable cardioverter defibrillator against amiodarone. *Circulation.* 2000;101:1297–1302.
32. Kuck KH, Cappato R, Siebels J, et al. Randomized comparison of antiarrhythmic drug therapy with implantable defibrillators in patients resuscitated from cardiac arrest: the Cardiac Arrest Study Hamburg (CASH). *Circulation.* 2000;102:748–754.
33. Bardy GH, Lee KL, Mark DB, et al. Amiodarone or an implantable cardioverter-defibrillator for congestive heart failure. *N Engl J Med.* 2005;352:225–237.
34. Moss AJ, Zareba W, Hall WJ, et al. Prophylactic implantation of a defibrillator in patients with myocardial infarction and reduced ejection fraction. *N Engl J Med.* 2002;346:877–883.
35. Schwartz PJ, Priori SG, Cerrone M, et al. Left cardiac sympathetic denervation in the management of high-risk patients affected by the long-QT syndrome. *Circulation.* 2004;109:1826–1833.
36. Atallah J, Fynn-Thompson F, Cecchin F, et al. Video-assisted thoracoscopic cardiac denervation: a potential novel therapeutic option for children with intractable ventricular arrhythmias. *Ann Thorac Surg.* 2008;86:1620–1625.
37. Viskin S, Glikson M, Fish R, et al. Rate smoothing with cardiac pacing for preventing torsade de pointes. *Am J Cardiol.* 2000;86:111K–115K.
38. Hobbs JB, Peterson DR, Moss AJ, et al. Risk of aborted cardiac arrest or sudden cardiac death during adolescence in the long-QT syndrome. *JAMA.* 2006;296:1249–1254.
39. Volpi A, Cavalli A, Franzosi MG, et al. One-year prognosis of primary ventricular fibrillation complicating acute myocardial infarction. The GISSI (Gruppo Italiano per lo Studio della Streptochinasi nell'Infarto miocardico) Investigators. *Am J Cardiol.* 1989;63:1174–1178.
40. Zipes DP, Camm AJ, Borggrefe M, et al. ACC/AHA/ESC 2006 guidelines for management of patients with ventricular arrhythmias and the prevention of sudden cardiac death: a report of the American College of Cardiology/American Heart Association Task Force and the European Society of Cardiology Committee for Practice Guidelines (Writing Committee to Develop Guidelines for Management of Patients with Ventricular Arrhythmias and the Prevention of Sudden Cardiac Death). *J Am Coll Cardiol.* 2006;48:e247–e346.
41. Kadish A, Dyer A, Daubert JP, et al. Prophylactic defibrillator implantation in patients with nonischemic dilated cardiomyopathy. *N Engl J Med.* 2004;350:2151–2158.
42. Maron BJ, McKenna WJ, Danielson GK, et al. American College of Cardiology/European Society of Cardiology clinical expert consensus document on hypertrophic cardiomyopathy. A report of the American College of Cardiology Foundation Task Force on Clinical Expert Consensus Documents and the European Society of Cardiology Committee for Practice Guidelines. *J Am Coll Cardiol.* 2003;42:1687–1713.
43. Gemayel C, Pelliccia A, Thompson PD. Arrhythmogenic right ventricular cardiomyopathy. *J Am Coll Cardiol.* 2001;38:1773–1781.
44. Riera AR, Zhang L, Uchida AH, et al. The management of Brugada syndrome patients. *Cardiol J.* 2007;14:97–106.
45. Leenhardt A, Lucet V, Denjoy I, et al. Catecholaminergic polymorphic ventricular tachycardia in children. A 7-year follow-up of 21 patients. *Circulation.* 1995;91:1512–1519.
46. Huang DT, Traub D. Recurrent ventricular arrhythmia storms in the age of implantable cardioverter defibrillator therapy: a comprehensive review. *Prog Cardiovasc Dis.* 2008;51:229–236.
47. Sesselberg HW, Moss AJ, McNitt S, et al. Ventricular arrhythmia storms in postinfarction patients with implantable defibrillators for primary prevention indications: a MADIT-II substudy. *Heart Rhythm.* 2007;4:1395–1402.

PATIENT AND FAMILY INFORMATION FOR:
Ventricular Arrhythmias

WHAT IS VENTRICULAR ARRHYTHMIA?

Pumping activity of the heart is accomplished by the contraction of the muscles of the heart, which form the walls of its four chambers (two upper chambers called right and left atria that receive blood and the two lower chambers called right and left ventricles that pump out blood). This is normally accomplished by a coordinated sequential electrical activation of these muscles. During normal rhythm this electrical activity arises in the right atrium leading to a coordinated contraction of the atria first followed by the ventricles. Ventricles are filled optimally with blood during contraction of the two atria preceding the contraction of the ventricles by a fraction of a second. This normal sequence of contraction is important in the effective contraction of the ventricles to generate an adequate blood pressure in the arteries (blood vessels in the body supplying blood pumped by the heart to various parts of the body). Ventricular Arrythmias (VA) are disturbances of the rhythm of the heart when they originate in the ventricles (lower pumping chambers).

TYPES OF VENTRICULAR ARRHYTHMIAS

VA can be classified into the following categories:

1. *Isolated Premature Ventricular Contraction (PVC):* These are isolated beats originating in the ventricles interspersed between trains of normal heartbeats originating in the right atrium.
2. *Ventricular Tachycardia (VT):* These premature ventricular complexes can come in as a train of two (couplets) or three (triplets) beats. VT is defined as a train of three or more premature ventricular complexes at a rate >100 bpm. VT is called *sustained* if it lasts for >30 seconds or requires termination by shock therapy within 30 seconds.
3. *Ventricular Fibrillation (VF):* When the ventricles start beating at a rate >300 bpm, the electrical activation and contraction of different parts of the ventricle become completely uncoordinated. This chaotic ventricular rhythm is called ventricular fibrillation or VF. Because there is a complete lack of coordinated contraction of the ventricular muscles, the pumping becomes ineffective. Lack of blood circulation to vital organs including the brain owing to the resulting cardiovascular collapse leads to loss of consciousness. If the rhythm is not reverted promptly, it ends in irreversible injury to the brain and other organs leading to death.

MANIFESTATIONS AND SIGNIFICANCE

1. *Isolated PVCs and Non Sustained VT (NSVT)* may cause palpitations or a feeling of skipped beat in some patients, and it may remain asymptomatic in many. Frequent PVCs and NSVT may lead to worsening of heart failure (inefficient pumping) or worsening of myocardial ischemia (lack of adequate blood supply to heart muscles). Frequent PVCs should be considered as a cause of worsening of heart failure or ischemia.
2. *VT* may manifest in different ways depending on the rate of the arrhythmia and the underlying condition of the heart. In the mildest form, especially when the arrhythmia is not too fast, it may cause palpitations alone. However, VT may often lead to loss of consciousness and collapse owing to reduced pumping of blood. It may worsen the manifestations of a previous heart disease. Unstable VT if untreated usually degenerates into VF.
3. *VF* always leads to collapse of the patient with loss of consciousness and unless promptly treated, leads to death.

CAUSES OF VENTRICULAR ARRHYTHMIA

VAs can occur owing to various abnormalities of the heart, which may be either structural or electrical. Sometimes, certain abnormalities unrelated to heart per se might be a causative factor; for example, electrolyte abnormality (abnormal levels of certain ions in the blood) or certain drug toxicity.

These can be categorized follows:
1. **Structural heart disease**
   a. *Coronary Artery Disease (CAD):* Almost 50% of these serious VAs occur in the setting of CAD (blockage of vessels supplying blood to the heart) with scar in the heart after a heart attack or during acute heart attack. It is important to note that heart attack is results from sudden blockage of one of the arteries supplying blood to the heart owing to formation of blood clot and should not be confused with these potentially fatal rhythm disturbances leading to sudden cardiac death. Heart attack itself may sometimes lead to such rhythm disturbances and result in sudden cardiac death.
   b. *Cardiomyopathies:* Various diseases of the heart muscles (cardiomyopathies) cause these VAs. Cardiomyopathy may lead to weakness or thickening and stiffness of the heart muscles. Weakness of the heart muscles is a frequent cause of these

arrhythmias and may due to a previous heart attack and scar formation or previous inflammation of heart because of viral infection. Quite often the cause of heart muscle weakness remains unknown.

c. *Infiltrative heart disease and myocarditis*: These conditions lead to some lesions in the muscle wall of the heart and inflammation, which in turn act as a focus of origin of rhythm disturbances.

2. *VA without structural heart disease* may be result from some hereditary abnormalities of the electrical activity of the heart, which put patients at a high risk of developing arrhythmias. Many of these abnormalities are now known to be due to alteration in the proteins involved in handling the ions (sodium, potassium, and calcium), which are key to the electrical activity of the heart muscles. Some forms of these arrhythmias are readily treatable by drugs and catheter ablation (see below).

3. *Reversible factors unrelated to any heart disease*: At times VAs may result from some electrolyte abnormality (abnormal level of certain ions such as potassium or magnesium ions in blood), without any abnormality of the heart. Seldom can a pacing wire or catheter inside the heart irritate the heart muscles and cause these arrhythmias. Stress in some patients who are very sick and have certain metabolic problems such as hypoxia (deficiency of oxygen in the tissue) can also sometimes cause these arrhythmias. Some medications may alter the electrical activity of the heart and be responsible for ventricular rhythm disturbances. These include some of the antibiotics and some other medications used to treat rhythm disorders. Interaction between two drugs can also sometimes lead to toxic level of one of them, which may cause arrhythmia.

TREATMENT OPTIONS

The treatment plan of VA can be divided into two parts. The first is acute treatment when the patient is having arrhythmia. The second part is planning for prevention of arrhythmia, its detection, and prompt treatment of potentially fatal recurrent arrhythmias in future. There are three modalities of treatment:

ANTIARRHYTHMIC MEDICATIONS

Antiarrhythmic medications decrease the propensity of arrhythmia. These drugs can be used for treating the acute rhythm disturbances as well as for prevention of recurrence of arrhythmia. However, these are also associated with development of new and more severe arrhythmia and worsening of the existing arrhythmia as well as other side effects such as depression of the pumping function of the heart. Amiodarone, the most commonly used drug over the long term, has many toxic side effects involving liver, lungs, thyroid, and eyes.

CATHETER ABLATION OF VENTRICULAR TACHYCARDIA

Another method of treating arrhythmia is to destroy or modify the pathway of abnormal electrical conduction or points generating an abnormal rhythm. This is done by delivery of heat energy by a catheter to the point of interest in the heart wall. Depending on the type of disease, success of catheter ablation in preventing the recurrence of VT may range from as low as 50% to as high as 95%. In patients with structural heart disease with multiple scars in the heart there may be multiple points of origin of arrhythmia, and ablation may not be sufficient to eliminate all the foci, although ablation may decrease the chances of arrhythmia by eliminating some of the foci. These procedures are quite safe and there is a very low chance of formation of clot at the burn site, which may rarely break away and go to vital organs (<1%). Another potential but infrequent complication is collection of blood around the heart, which may require drainage.

PACING AND ELECTRIC SHOCK

Another modality of treating these arrhythmias is by pacing the heart with a pacemaker at a rate higher than the arrhythmia (called overdrive pacing or antitachycardia pacing for VT) or by delivering an electric shock (for VT and VF). This therapy reverts the rhythm back to normal. However, unlike antiarrhythmic medication, this therapy does not have any preventive effect on recurrence of arrhythmia. This therapy can be administered by an external device by a health care provider in the hospital setting or by a bystander in a public place. An implanted device (AICD or ICD) has become commonplace for this kind of treatment now and does not need the presence of another person for delivering therapy. ICD is used in high-risk patients for prevention of sudden cardiac death. ICD placement is done similar to a pacemaker by placing one or two wires in the heart (called a lead) through major veins below the collarbone. These leads are connected to the device that delivers the therapy when needed by automatic detection and interpretation of the rhythm disturbances.

WHEN TO TREAT AND WHAT MODALITY TO USE?

As mentioned earlier, often these rhythm disturbances can result from certain conditions that are reversible and treatable (e.g., electrolyte abnormality, drugs). Treating these causative conditions may itself eliminate the arrhythmia altogether. No long-term plan may be required in such a situation. However, in the absence of any such condition, one or more of the above-mentioned modalities might be required to treat the ongoing arrhythmia and to prevent its recurrence.

ISOLATED PREMATURE VENTRICULAR COMPLEXES AND NONSUSTAINED VENTRICULAR TACHYCARDIA

1. Significance and need for treatment of isolated premature ventricular complexes and NSVTs depend on the underlying heart condition.

2. In the absence of any structural heart disease and any symptoms, isolated PVCs may not require any treatment. If they are frequent or produce significant symptoms, medication (usually a ß-blocker) may be tried to suppress it.

3. The risk of VT/VF in these patients is better predicted by functional capacity and pumping function of the heart. Patients at high risk of developing life-threatening VT/VF should receive ICD implantation to treat further episodes and prevent sudden death.

VENTRICULAR TACHYCARDIA AND VENTRICULAR FIBRILLATION

1. All patients with VT need some kind of treatment. In the acute setting with ongoing arrhythmia, drug therapy can be used in patients who are stable with normal blood pressure and do not have symptoms of compromised function of the heart. Otherwise, treatment with pacing or shock may be needed.

2. Long-term therapy for VT is guided by etiology of the arrhythmias and risk stratification by comprehensive evaluation of these patients.

3. Some forms of VT occurring in the patients with structurally normal heart do very well with catheter ablation with an efficacy rate exceeding 90%. ICD may be considered if drug therapy and catheter ablation are not effective.

4. In the absence of reversible condition, most of the patients who have had the VT or VF owing to conditions other than some forms of focal idiopathic VT should get an ICD implantation to treat future episodes. Drug therapy and catheter ablation can be used to supplement the therapy to reduce the episodes of VT/VF requiring shock.

5. Patients with cardiomyopathy with severely depressed pumping function of the heart (ejection fraction <35%) without any history of VAs are also at high risk of life-threatening VT and VF. They should be treated by placement of ICD for prevention of sudden cardiac death.

6. Certain groups of patients are at high risk of VA (e.g., Brugada syndrome, ARVD) and sudden cardiac death. These patients should always be treated with ICD in conjunction with drug therapy and catheter ablation as applicable. However, certain other groups (e.g., long QT syndrome, hypertrophic cardiomyopathy) need risk stratification by comprehensive evaluation to decide about the need for ICD implantation.

Emad F. Aziz
Eyal Herzog

The Approach to the Patient with Syncope

Syncope is a syndrome consisting of a relatively short period of temporary and self-limited loss of consciousness caused by transient diminution of blood flow to the brain.[1,2] The term derives from the Greek word *synkoptein*, which means "to cut short,"[3] and is used to classify a common clinical problem. The incidence of self-reported syncope is 6.2 per 1,000 person-years in the Framingham study with a cumulative incidence of 3% to 6% over 10 years.[4,5] In selected patient populations, the lifetime prevalence of syncope could reach almost 50%. In the United States, 1 to 2 million patients are evaluated for syncope annually accounting for 3% to 5% of emergency department visits and 1% to 6% of urgent hospital admissions.[6]

Several guidelines have been published for the diagnostic approach to patients with syncope; however, they do not apply to every clinical situation encountered.[7,8] The European Societies of Cardiology[9] and the American College of Cardiology[10] have published detailed documents specifying a classification of the principle causes of syncope (Table 18.1). However, given the vast differential diagnosis and the potential variation of required therapies for patients presenting with syncope and owing to the lack of consensus guidelines, there was a need for a structured approach for the management of these patients. To address this issue, we developed a standardized pathway that is comprehensive, yet simple, and provides guidelines for the management of all patients presenting with a complaint of syncope[11] (Figure 18.1).

INITIAL ASSESSMENT OF A PATIENT WITH SYNCOPE

The initial assessment of a patient with syncope (Table 18.2) includes a meticulous and comprehensive medical history, incorporating eyewitness accounts that can help determining the cause of syncope.[7] Important questions to be asked in assessing patients with syncope are listed in Table 18.3. Orthostatic hypotension and autonomic dysfunction are identified by measuring blood pressure and pulse rate in the upper and lower extremities in both the supine and the upright positions. A 12-lead ECG and basic laboratory tests including a basic metabolic panel and a complete blood cell count should be performed in all patients with syncope.

DEFINITION OF TRUE SYNCOPE

We use the acronym of **SELF-1**, which reflects the four criteria that should be met in order for an event to be considered true syncope.

These criteria include:

S—**S**hort period, **S**elf-limited, **S**pontaneous recovery

E—**E**arly rapid onset

L—**L**oss of consciousness—transient

F—**F**ull recovery, **F**all

Patients who do not lose consciousness are defined as "not true syncope."

CLASSIFICATION OF SYNCOPE WHEN THERE IS A CERTAIN OR SUSPECTED DIAGNOSIS

The following are certain disorders causing true syncope with a transient loss of consciousness:

1. *Reflex syncope:* Neurally mediated reflex syndrome[12] in absence of structural heart disease. It refers to a reflex that, when triggered, gives rise to vasodilatation and bradycardia. These triggers include fear, pain, instrumentation, blood phobias, prolonged standing, crowded warm places, nausea, vomiting, and abdominal pain.

2. *Orthostatic hypotension syncope:* In orthostatic hypotension syncope, syncope occurs with assumption of upright position. It can occur after starting a medication that can lead to hypotension, or it can be due to an autonomic neuropathy.[13] Volume depletion is an important cause of orthostatic hypotension.

3. *Cardiovascular disease:* Structural heart disease can cause syncope when circulatory demands overwhelm the impaired ability of the heart to increase its output. Cardiac arrhythmia can cause a decrease in cardiac output, which usually occurs irrespective of circulatory demands.

RISK STRATIFICATION FOR ADMISSION

One of the main dilemmas faced by emergency department physicians is whether to admit patients to the hospital or to refer them for an outpatient evaluation. Many risk assessment scores have been developed. These includes the San Francisco Syncope Rule,[14] the *Osservatorio Epidemiologico della Sincope nel Lazio,*[15] and the Evaluation of Guidelines in Syncope Study.[16] In all of these risk scores, there is a consensus to admit patients with abnormal ECG, hypotension, heart failure, and anemia. In our standardized SELF pathway,[11] we use the **SELF-2** criteria to evaluate the need for admission.

TABLE 18.1	Classification of the Principle Causes of Syncope

REFLEX (NEURALLY MEDIATED) SYNCOPE
- Vasovagal:
  - Mediated by emotional distress: fear, pain, instrumentation, blood phobia
  - Mediated by orthostatic stress
- Situational:
  - Cough, sneeze
  - Gastrointestinal stimulation (swallow, defecation, visceral pain)
  - Micturition (postmicturition)
  - Postexercise
  - Postprandial
- Carotid sinus syncope

SYNCOPE DUE TO ORTHOSTATIC HYPOTENSION
- Primary autonomic failure:
  - Pure autonomic failure, Parkinson disease with autonomic failure, dementia
- Secondary autonomic failure:
  - Diabetes, amyloidosis, uremia, spinal cord injuries
- Drug-induced orthostatic hypotension:
  - Alcohol, vasodilators, diuretics, phenothiazine, antidepressants
- Volume depletion:
  - Hemorrhage, diarrhea, vomiting

CARDIAC SYNCOPE (CARDIOVASCULAR)
- Arrhythmia as primary cause:
  - Bradycardia:
    - Sinus node dysfunction (including bradycardia/tachycardia syndrome)
    - AV conduction system disease
    - Implanted device malfunction
  - Tachycardia:
    - Supraventricular
    - Ventricular (idiopathic, secondary to structural heart disease or to channelopathies)
  - Drug-induced bradycardia and tachyarrhythmias
- Structural disease:
  - Cardiac: cardiac valvular disease, acute MI/ischemia
  - Hypertrophic cardiomyopathy, cardiac masses (atrial myxoma, tumors)
  - Pericardial disease/tamponade, congenital anomalies of coronary arteries, prosthetic valves dysfunction
- Others: pulmonary embolus, acute aortic dissection, pulmonary hypertension

Adapted from Brignole M, Alboni P, Benditt D, et al. Task force on syncope, European Society of Cardiology. Part 1. The initial evaluation of patients with syncope. *Europace.* 2001;3(4):253–260.

These criteria include:

S—**S**tructural heart disease
E—abnormal **E**CG
L—atrial f**L**utter
F—atrial **F**ibrillation

Admitted patients should be monitored for a minimum of 24 hours, which could potentially reveal bradyarrhythmias or tachyarrhythmias. The management of bradyarrhythmias may include an electrophysiologic testing with or without subsequent pacemaker implantation. Tachyarrhythmia includes ventricular tachycardia, supraventricular tachycardia, atrial fibrillation, and atrial flutter. The treatment for these patients may include radiofrequency ablation or a device therapy with a pacemaker or an implantable cardioverter-defibrillator (ICD). We recommend that all patients with a diagnosis of cardiac syncope will be evaluated by an electrophysiologist during their hospitalization.

MANAGEMENT OF CARDIAC SYNCOPE

The major goal of the evaluation of syncope in patients with heart disease is to identify a potentially life-threatening diagnosis, particularly arrhythmias. Workup and management of these patients can include medical therapy, stress testing with cardiac imaging, cardiac catheterization, and possible revascularization with a percutaneous coronary intervention or cardiac surgery.

DIAGNOSTIC TOOLS THAT AID IN THE MANAGEMENT OF CARDIAC SYNCOPE

ECG. ECG is essential in the workup of patients with unexplained syncope; however, it may only reveal a direct cause in 5% of patients. Abnormal ECGs include the following findings: sinus bradycardia resulting from sinus node dysfunction or atrioventricular (AV) block resulting from AV node or His-Purkinje system dysfunction, preexcitation patterns, a long/short QT-interval, Brugada syndrome, and characteristic ECG features of arrhythmogenic right ventricular dysplasia. Patients with unexplained bradycardia (heart rate of <50 beats per minute) should be evaluated for potential medical causes, explicitly hypovolemia, hypoxia, acidosis, hypoglycemia, and hypothermia. Mild hyperkalemia when combined with a low *glomerular filtration rate* can also be a recipe for cardiac syncope in the elderly.[17] Hypothyroidism should also be considered in this age group.

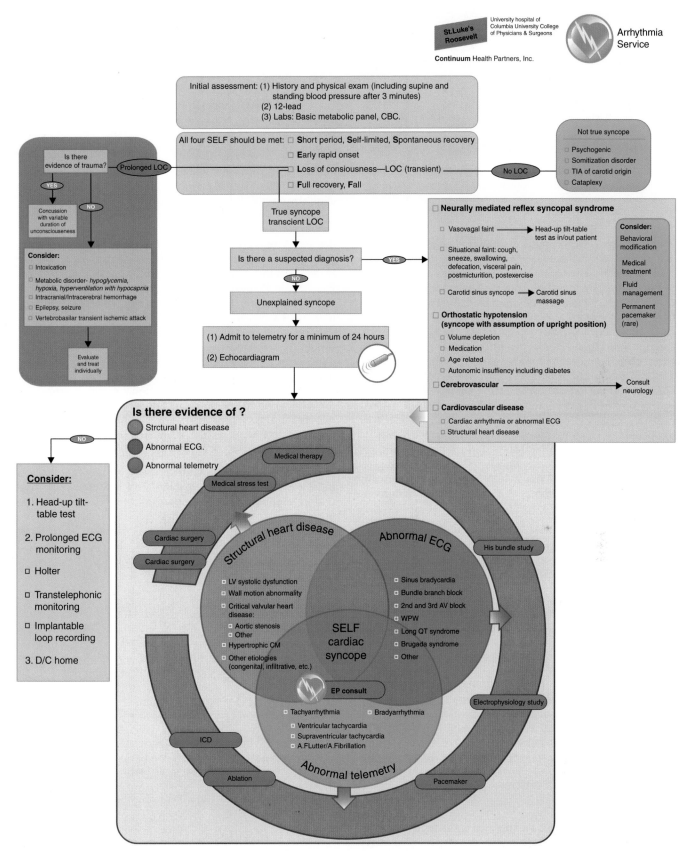

Figure 18.1. The SELF pathway for the management of syncope.

TABLE 18.2	Initial Assessment of a Patient with Syncope

FOR EVERY PATIENT PRESENTING WITH SYNCOPE
- Detailed history
- Comprehensive physical examination
- Standard 12-lead ECG
- Basic labs (including basic metabolic panel, complete blood cell count)

TO ALL ADMITTED PATIENTS (WHEN APPROPRIATE)
- Echocardiogram
- In-hospital 24-hr telemetry monitoring (out-of-hospital telemetry may be applicable where available)
- Neurologic evaluation

Marked bradycardia can be the results of many medications like β-blockers, calcium channel blockers, and digoxin, particularly in the presence of renal disease; this should be assessed and managed promptly. Lyme disease can be an unusual cause of heart block and needs to be considered in a traveling patient from an endemic area. Finally, heart block can be a manifestation of myocardial infarction (MI), and patients with acute anterior wall MI and Mobitz type II second-degree AV block have a class IIa indication for a temporary transvenous pacing. This is in contrast to patients with inferior wall MI where heart block can be a manifestation of the Bezold–Jarisch reflex. This is a cardiovascular decompressor reflex involving a marked increase in vagal efferent discharge to the heart, elicited by stimulation of chemoreceptors, primarily in the left ventricle. It causes a slowing of the heartbeat and dilatation of the peripheral blood vessels with resulting lowering of the blood pressure. In patients with inferior wall MI, the heart block usually has a narrow escape rhythm and it usually resolves within few days.

Echocardiography. Echocardiography should be performed in all patients with true syncope as it can identify patients with critical aortic stenosis, aortic dissection, severe pulmonary hypertension, acute pulmonary embolism, left atrial myxoma, and pericardial tamponade, situations that can lead to obstruction of flow in the heart and will cause syncope.[18] These patients tend to be seriously ill and may require a lengthy intensive care stay. Echocardiography is considered the gold standard diagnostic for the diagnosis of hypertrophic cardiomyopathy, segmental wall motion abnormalities suggestive of ischemic heart disease, and left ventricular systolic dysfunction.

Holter monitoring. Holter monitoring enables correlation of symptoms with episodes of bradycardia; diagnostic clues are obtained in 50% to 70% of patients with bradycardia suspected on clinical grounds. However, events can be missed if symptoms do not occur in the 24- to 48-hour monitoring period. Holter monitoring can reveal sinus pauses, sinus arrest, second- or third-degree AV block, or severe sinus bradycardia with symptoms. Nocturnal asymptomatic bradycardia and pauses are not uncommon in the normal heart and are probably nondiagnostic. First-degree AV block or Mobitz type I AV block may be noted while patients are asleep owing to a high vagal tone. A long-monitored strip should be obtained because a 2:1 AV block is unlikely to persist. The other forms of AV block (Mobitz I or II) should then become apparent. Monitoring while the patient does perform some form of exertion (e.g., arm exercise, standing, and walking) may also help to demonstrate the level of block. Block at the level of the AV node should improve with the adrenergic stimulation, but block below the AV node in the His-Purkinje system may worsen as AV nodal conduction improves and increases the frequency of inputs to the His-Purkinje system.

Cardiac event monitoring. Cardiac event monitors particularly those with auto-triggering capability are widely used in the diagnosis of symptomatic and asymptomatic bradycardia and can be worn for up to 30 days. These devices can detect sinus pauses, sinus arrest, second- or third-degree AV block, or severe sinus bradycardia with symptoms[19]; however, their diagnostic yield for syncope and presyncope is only 6% to 25%.[20,21]

TABLE 18.3	Important Questions That Can Be Asked in Assessing Patients with Syncope

QUESTIONS ABOUT SITUATIONS BEFORE SYNCOPE
- Position (supine, sitting, or standing)
- Activity (rest, change in posture, during or after exercise, during or immediately after urination, defecation, cough, or swallowing)
- Predisposing factors (crowded or warm places, prolonged standing, postprandial period) and precipitating events (fear, intense pain, neck movements)

QUESTIONS ABOUT ONSET OF SYNCOPE
- Nausea, vomiting, abdominal discomfort, feeling of cold, sweating, pain in neck or shoulders, blurred vision, dizziness
- Trauma

QUESTIONS FOR EYEWITNESS
- Way of falling (slumping forward, backward or kneeling over), skin color (pallor, cyanosis, flushing), duration of loss of consciousness, breathing pattern (snoring), movements (seizure-like) and their duration, onset of movement in relation to fall, tongue biting

QUESTIONS AFTER THE EPISODE
- Nausea, vomiting, sweating, feeling of cold, confusion, muscle aches, skin color, injury, chest pain, palpitations, urinary or fecal incontinence

QUESTIONS ABOUT PAST FAMILY AND MEDICAL HISTORY
- Family history of sudden death, congenital arrhythmogenic heart disease, or fainting
- Previous cardiac disease (coronary artery disease, heart failure)
- Neurologic history (epilepsy, narcolepsy)
- Metabolic disorders (diabetes, hypo- or hyperthyroidism)
- Medication (antihypertensive, antianginal, antiarrhythmic, diuretics, and QT prolonging agents)
- In instance of recurrent syncope, information on recurrences such as the time from the first syncopal episode and on the number of spells

Exercise testing. A subnormal increase in heart rate after exercise (*chronotropic incompetence*) can be useful in diagnosing sick sinus syndrome. However, sensitivity and specificity are unclear, and the results obtained may not be reproducible.[22] Exercise-induced AV block, even if asymptomatic, can be significant and suggests disease of the His-Purkinje system. Identifying symptoms owing to sinus bradycardia can be difficult; nonetheless, exercise testing can be useful to help determine the sinus node dysfunction as the cause of symptoms.

Electrophysiologic testing. Electrophysiologic testing is recommended when symptoms cannot be correlated clearly with a syncopal event and when significant bradyarrhythmias are suspected but cannot be diagnosed by noninvasive modalities. The sinus node dysfunction (*diagnosed as sinus node recovery time over 1,600 to 2,000 milliseconds and/or corrected sinus node recovery time over 525 milliseconds*) serves only as an adjunct to clinical and noninvasive parameters because these tests are based on assumptions that limit their validity and clinical utility. There is little utility for electrophysiologic testing in already documented second- and third-degree AV block. Testing can be useful in patients with AV block and no clear symptom association, in patients with symptoms of bradycardia in whom AV block is suspected but not documented, and when the site of the AV block cannot be determined reliably by surface tracings. His-ventricle interval of over *100 milliseconds* in a patient with bradycardia, even in the absence of symptoms, is a high-risk finding. Asymptomatic patients with Mobitz II AV block may benefit from this test to localize the site of block and to guide therapy. Overall, the role of electrophysiologic testing for bradycardia is limited because of low sensitivity and specificity. Positive findings may not be the reason for patient symptoms.[23]

MANAGEMENT OF PATIENTS WITH UNEXPLAINED SYNCOPE BUT WITH NO EVIDENCE OF CARDIAC ETIOLOGY

In the absence of underlying heart disease, syncope is not associated with excess mortality. Our recommendation for these patients is for early discharge, with consideration of head-up tilt-table testing and prolonged ECG monitoring (including Holter monitoring, transtelephonic monitoring, and implantable loop recording).

OUTPATIENT DIAGNOSTIC TOOLS

Tilt-table testing. Tilt-table testing is used to evaluate the adequacy of the autonomic system, especially when there is suspicion of neurocardiogenic syncope.[24] The test can be performed either by using head-upright tilting, which causes dependent venous pooling thereby provokes the autonomic response, or by using adenosine to facilitate the induction of vasovagal syncope. However, this test is limited by its poor sensitivity and the lack of uniformity.

Implantable loop monitor. Implantable loop recorders (ILRs) are subcutaneous monitoring devices that are typically implanted in the left parasternal or pectoral region and used for the detection of cardiac arrhythmias (Figure 18.2). The monitor has a loop memory and a battery life of 15 to 18 months. The current version stores an ECG that includes tracings recorded up to 40 minutes before and 2 minutes after activation by the patient. If the patient activates the device when his consciousness

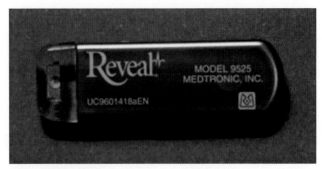

Figure 18.2. ILR; Reveal (Medtronic, USA).

returns, the probability of demonstrating a correlation between the ECG signals and the syncope is high. Krahn et al.[25] were among the first to describe a high diagnostic yield of the ILR in 16 patients with recurrent syncope. Extensive investigations including electrophysiology studies, treadmill testing, 48-hour ambulatory monitoring, and tilt-table testing failed to obtain a definite diagnosis in these patients. In 94% of the cases, recurrent syncope had occurred after implantation of the device revealing an arrhythmogenic cause in 60%. Consequently, no arrhythmias were detected in 40% of these patients. In all patients with an arrhythmogenic cause, successful therapy was implemented. The Place of Reveal in the Care Pathway and Treatment of Patients with Unexplained Recurrent Syncope (*PICTURE*) registry,[26] a prospective, multicenter, observational study that followed 570 patients with recurrent unexplained presyncope or syncope who received an ILR, showed that these patients were evaluated on average by three different specialists and underwent a median of 13 nondiagnostic tests (ranges between 9 and 20). Within the first year, syncope recurred in one-third of the patients; the ILR provided a diagnosis in 78% of the patients, most commonly a cardiac etiology.

In summary, having a standardized protocol for the management of patients with unexplained syncope should begin with a thorough medical history and a detailed physical examination including basic laboratory testing. High-risk patients (meeting SELF-2 criteria) should be admitted for at least 24-hour monitoring and echocardiography evaluation. Low-risk patients do not require hospital admission, and they can be evaluated as outpatients with tilt-table testing or with a prolonged monitoring including ILR.

REFERENCES

1. Brignole M, Alboni P, Benditt DG, et al. Guidelines on management (diagnosis and treatment) of syncope-update 2004. Executive Summary. *Eur Heart J.* 2004;25(22):2054–2072.
2. Brignole M, Alboni P, Benditt DG, et al. [Guidelines on management (diagnosis and treatment) of syncope. Update 2004. Executive summary]. *Rev Esp Cardiol.* 2005;58(2):175–193.
3. Soteriades ES, Evans JC, Larson MG, et al. Incidence and prognosis of syncope. *N Engl J Med.* 2002;347(12):878–885.
4. Savage DD, Corwin L, McGee DL, et al. Epidemiologic features of isolated syncope: the Framingham Study. *Stroke.* 1985;16(4):626–629.
5. Chen L, Chen MH, Larson MG, et al. Risk factors for syncope in a community-based sample (the Framingham Heart Study). *Am J Cardiol.* 2000;85(10):1189–1193.
6. Shen WK, Decker WW, Smars PA, et al. Syncope Evaluation in the Emergency Department Study (SEEDS): a multidisciplinary approach to syncope management. *Circulation.* 2004;110(24):3636–3645.
7. Linzer M, Yang EH, Estes NA III, et al. Diagnosing syncope. Part 1: Value of history, physical examination, and electrocardiography. Clinical Efficacy Assessment Project of the American College of Physicians. *Ann Intern Med.* 1997;126(12):989–996.
8. Linzer M, Yang EH, Estes NA III, et al. Diagnosing syncope. Part 2: Unexplained syncope. Clinical Efficacy Assessment Project of the American College of Physicians. *Ann Intern Med.* 1997;127(1):76–86.

9. Brignole M, Alboni P, Benditt D, et al. Task force on syncope, European Society of Cardiology. Part 1. The initial evaluation of patients with syncope. *Europace.* 2001;3(4):253–260.

10. Strickberger SA, Benson DW, Biaggioni I, et al. AHA/ACCF scientific statement on the evaluation of syncope: from the American Heart Association Councils on Clinical Cardiology, Cardiovascular Nursing, Cardiovascular Disease in the Young, and Stroke, and the Quality of Care and Outcomes Research Interdisciplinary Working Group; and the American College of Cardiology Foundation In Collaboration With the Heart Rhythm Society. *J Am Coll Cardiol.* 2006;47(2):473–484.

11. Herzog E, Frankenberger O, Pierce W, et al. The SELF pathway for the management of syncope. *Crit Pathw Cardiol.* 2006;5(3):173–178.

12. Sheldon R, Rose S, Connolly S, et al. Diagnostic criteria for vasovagal syncope based on a quantitative history. *Eur Heart J.* 2006;27(3):344–350.

13. Pont M, Froment R. [Essential orthostatic hypotension persisting for 25 years; syncope during defecation and post-syncopal obnubilation]. *Lyon Med.* 1950;183(50):389–390.

14. Quinn JV, Stiell IG, McDermott DA, et al. Derivation of the San Francisco Syncope Rule to predict patients with short-term serious outcomes. *Ann Emerg Med.* 2004;43(2):224–232.

15. Ammirati F, Colivicchi F, Minardi G, et al. [The management of syncope in the hospital: the OESIL Study (Osservatorio Epidemiologico della Sincope nel Lazio)]. *G Ital Cardiol.* 1999;29(5):533–539.

16. Del Rosso A, Ungar A, Maggi R, et al. Clinical predictors of cardiac syncope at initial evaluation in patients referred urgently to a general hospital: the EGSYS score. *Heart.* 2008;94(12):1620–1626.

17. Aziz EF, Javed F, Korniyenko A, et al. Mild hyperkalemia and low eGFR a tedious recipe for cardiac disaster in the elderly: an unusual reversible cause of syncope and heart block. *Heart Int.* 2011;6(2):e12.

18. Recchia D, Barzilai B. Echocardiography in the evaluation of patients with syncope. *J Gen Intern Med.* 1995;10(12):649–655.

19. Sivakumaran S, Krahn AD, Klein GJ, et al. A prospective randomized comparison of loop recorders versus Holter monitors in patients with syncope or presyncope. *Am J Med.* 2003;115(1):1–5.

20. Fogel RI, Evans JJ, Prystowsky EN. Utility and cost of event recorders in the diagnosis of palpitations, presyncope, and syncope. *Am J Cardiol.* 1997;79(2):207–208.

21. Zimetbaum P, Kim KY, Ho KK, et al. Utility of patient-activated cardiac event recorders in general clinical practice. *Am J Cardiol.* 1997;79(3):371–372.

22. Kosinski D, Grubb BP, Karas BJ, et al. Exercise-induced neurocardiogenic syncope: clinical data, pathophysiological aspects, and potential role of tilt table testing. *Europace.* 2000;2(1):77–82.

23. DiMarco JP. Value and limitations of electrophysical testing for syncope. *Cardiol Clin.* 1997;15(2):219–232.

24. Benditt DG, Ferguson DW, Grubb BP, et al. Tilt table testing for assessing syncope. American College of Cardiology. *J Am Coll Cardiol.* 1996;28(1):263–275.

25. Krahn AD, Klein GJ, Yee R, et al. Use of an extended monitoring strategy in patients with problematic syncope. Reveal Investigators. *Circulation.* 1999;99(3):406–410.

26. Edvardsson N, Frykman V, van Mechelen R, et al. Use of an implantable loop recorder to increase the diagnostic yield in unexplained syncope: results from the PICTURE registry. *Europace.* 2011;13(2):262–269.

PATIENT AND FAMILY INFORMATION FOR:
Syncope

Syncope (*sin-co-pee*) is a medical term used to describe a temporary loss of consciousness that is caused by a sudden lack of blood flow to the brain. Syncope is commonly called fainting or "passing out." If an individual is about to faint, he or she will feel dizzy, lightheaded, or nauseated and his/her field of vision may "white out" or "black out." The skin may be cold and clammy. After fainting, an individual may be unconscious for a short period of time but will eventually return to his/her baseline. Syncope can occur in otherwise healthy people and affects all age groups, but it is more common among the elderly. It can occur in many situations like standing up fast, working or playing hard especially in hot weather, breathing too fast (called hyperventilating), being upset, during long standing, during coughing, urinating, or all other situations that get in the way of the flow of oxygen to the brain.

There are several types of syncope. Vasovagal syncope usually has an easily identified triggering event such as emotional stress, trauma, pain, the sight of blood, or prolonged standing. Carotid sinus syncope is a medical term used for a situation in which there is pressure on the carotid artery in the neck, and this may occur after turning the head, while shaving, or even when wearing a tight collar. Situational syncope is the term used when syncope occurs with urination, defecation, coughing, or as a result of gastrointestinal stimulation. Syncope is not usually a primary sign of a neurologic disorder, but it may indicate an increased risk for some neurologic disorders such as Parkinson disease, diabetic neuropathy, and other types of neuropathy. Certain medicines can cause fainting, including diuretics, calcium channel blockers, angiotensin-converting enzyme inhibitors, nitrates, antipsychotic medications, antihistamines, levodopa, and narcotics. Alcohol, cocaine, and marijuana can also cause fainting.

INITIAL EVALUATION OF A PATIENT WITH SYNCOPE

Your doctor will like to know what exactly happened when you fainted and all the details about how you felt. Symptoms vary from patient to patient; however, the most common symptoms are light headedness, dizziness, and nausea. Some people will feel very hot and clammy, will feel sweaty, and will complain of visual and hearing disturbances. Information about current medications and preexisting medical conditions such as diabetes, heart disease, or psychiatric illness can help pinpoint the cause of syncope. There are certain tests and procedure that might be ordered to help guide your management. These tests might lead your physician to a definitive diagnosis and would guide your treatment.

PHYSICAL EXAMINATION AND LABORATORY TESTING

Your doctor will compare your heart rate and blood pressure while lying down with your heart rate and blood pressure in a standing position. The doctor will listen to your heartbeats for abnormal sounds that can be present in conditions such as narrowing of your aortic valve. Your doctor will listen for *bruit* in the sides of your neck to rule out narrowing of the neck arteries (called carotid arteries). The doctor may firmly massage your carotid artery while your heart rate is closely monitored with an EKG. The heart's response to this maneuver can give clues to the cause of your syncope.

Laboratory tests may identify low red blood cell count (*anemia*) or other abnormalities including thyroid abnormalities, and electrolyte imbalances (sodium, potassium, glucose, and magnesium).

ADDITIONAL DIAGNOSTIC TESTS

EKG. An EKG will be performed on your arrival. Sticky pads will be placed on your chest, arms, and legs and will be connected to a recording device with long, thin cables. This is not a painful procedure, and there is no risk with an EKG. The EKG provides a picture of the electrical activity throughout the heart muscle. A normal EKG does not necessarily mean that syncope is not caused by a heart rhythm problem. Heart rhythm problems are often brief and intermittent and may not be present at the moment when the EKG is performed.

Tilt-table testing. Tilt-table testing is a noninvasive test that is performed to diagnose recurrent or unexplained light-headedness or fainting spells. The test can define if a patient has a condition called vasovagal syncope in which there is malfunction of nerves that causes the heart to slow down and the blood pressure to drop with a change in position. The test takes about an hour to complete, and in preparation for it, you would be asked not to eat or drink for 5 hours before the test including holding your medications. You will be asked to lie down on a special flat table. A nurse will insert an intravenous line in a vein in your arm. EKG electrodes will be attached to your chest to monitor your heart rate and your rhythm during the procedure. A blood pressure cuff will be placed on your arm. Safety straps will secure you to the table. After obtaining your blood pressure and EKG while lying on the table, the table will be tilted to a 60° angle. You will be standing on a footboard at the bottom of the table. Your blood pressure and EKG will be monitored as you remain tilted up for 20 to 30 minutes. You will be instructed to tell your nurse if you experience any symptoms, such as feeling sweaty, nauseous, lightheaded, or cold and clammy. If your blood pressure starts to fall, you will be returned to a flat position. A doctor will be in the room during the entire procedure. If you experience no symptoms, the table will be lowered to a flat position and the test will be terminated. On occasion, a short-acting medication may be given intravenously to assist in the test. You may need to rest for several minutes after the test before going home. A nurse will stay with you until you meet the conditions for discharge.

Electrophysiology study. An electrophysiology study is an invasive procedure, which is performed in the hospital setting. You will be given sedative medications before the procedure, but you may stay awake during the procedure. The physician uses a local anesthetic to numb a small area over your blood vessels (veins), usually in the groin, and then threads small catheters (thin electrical wires) through the blood vessels into your heart using x-ray (fluoroscopic) guidance. Once in the heart, precise measurements of the heart's electrical function can be obtained. This procedure typically lasts 60 to 90 minutes.

Implantable loop recorder. With implantable loop recorder (ILR), your heart rate and rhythm can be monitored for a long period of time. The device has a memory and a battery that can last between 18 and 24 months. The ILR is implanted under the skin usually in the upper left chest area. It stores events automatically according to programmed criteria, or it can be activated by the patient. The ILR may be useful if your symptoms are sporadic and an arrhythmia is suspected, and other forms of testing were negative or inconclusive.

THERAPIES

Permanent pacemaker. A pacemaker is a small device, the size of a silver dollar, which is implanted under the skin just below the collarbone. The device is connected to wires that are threaded into the heart muscle where they emit impulses that help regulate the heartbeat. Pacemakers are occasionally recommended if your syncope is caused by a very slow heartbeat, carotid sinus hypersensitivity, or heart block. Pacemaker battery typically lasts 7 to 11 years and would require replacement after that with a simple procedure.

Implantable cardioverter-defibrillator. Certain dangerous conditions arise when irregular heartbeat originates from the lower chamber of the heart (ventricles), particularly in patients with a very weak heart. These patients may benefit from an implantable cardioverter-defibrillator (ICD). Like a pacemaker, the ICD is typically implanted under the skin just below the collarbone. The device is connected to wires that are threaded into the heart muscle. However, in addition to its pacemaker capability, the ICD has the ability to detect fatal arrhythmias and deliver a high-energy electrical shock to the heart that in turn will terminate the arrhythmia and return the heart to normal rhythm.

Emad F. Aziz
Fahad Javed
Eyal Herzog

CHAPTER

19

Strategies for the Prevention of Sudden Cardiac Death

Sudden cardiac death (SCD) also known as sudden cardiac arrest, is a major health problem worldwide.[1] Estimates for the United States range from <200,000 to >450,000 SCDs annually, with the most widely used estimates in the range of 300,000 to 350,000 SCDs annually.[2,3] It is usually defined as an unexpected death from a cardiac cause occurring within a short duration of time in a person with or without preexisting heart disease owing to the abrupt loss of heart function (cardiac arrest). A dynamic triggering factor usually interacts with an underlying heart disease either genetically determined or acquired, and the final outcome is the development of lethal tachyarrhythmias or less frequently, bradycardia.[4]

There is no comprehensible consensus on the definition of SCD, which is witnessed in only two-thirds of cases. As the duration of symptoms preceding the terminal event usually defines the sudden nature of death, the World Health Organization defines SCD as unexpected death within 1 hour of symptom onset if witnessed or within 24 hours of the person having been observed alive and symptom-free if unwitnessed.[5] Exclusion of noncardiac causes such as pulmonary embolus or drug overdose is also critical because sudden cardiac arrhythmias may be the final decisive pathology in these disease conditions.

According to the Framingham Heart Study, during a 20-year follow-up 13% of deaths were due to SCD.[6] In >80% of cases, sudden death is caused by coronary disease.[7] The mechanism of SCD is ventricular fibrillation (VF) in 65% to 85% cases, ventricular tachycardia (VT) in 7% to 10% cases, and electromechanical dissociation in 20% to 30% cases. Pathoanatomical findings can be observed on myocardium as fibrosis, edema, necrosis, cell infiltration, but rarely myocardium can be unchanged.

RISK FACTORS

Approximately 80% of individuals who suffer from SCD have coronary artery disease (CAD); the epidemiology of SCD to a great extent parallels that of CAD. Based on recent published data, the following variables have been associated with patients at higher risk of SCD: (1) syncope at the time of the first documented episode of arrhythmia, (2) NYHA class III or IV, (3) VT/VF occurring early after MI (3 days to 2 months), and (4) history of previous MI.[8] Other factors such as age, hypertension, left ventricular (LV) hypertrophy, intraventricular conduction block, elevated serum cholesterol, glucose intolerance, decreased vital capacity, smoking, relative weight, and heart rate also are as contributory in identifying individuals at risk for SCD.[9–11] Family history of MI has been reported to be associated with the risk of primary cardiac arrest.[12] Another entity of patients at highest risk for early SCD are those with hereditary ion channel or myocardial defects such as a long or short QT syndrome (LQTS or SQTS), hypertrophic cardiomyopathy (HCM), and arrhythmogenic right ventricular dysplasia (ARVD).

PATHOPHYSIOLOGY OF ARRHYTHMIAS

The most common electric sequence of events in SCD is degeneration of VT into VF during which disorganized contractions of the ventricles fail to eject blood effectively, often followed by asystole or pulseless electrical activity. Polymorphic VT or torsade de pointes may be the initial arrhythmia in patients with genetic or acquired forms of structural heart disease.[13] Bradyarrhythmias or electromechanical dissociation may be the primary electrical event in advanced heart failure or in the elderly patients.[14,15] Among patients with implantable cardioverter defibrillators (ICDs), arrhythmic death accounts for 20% to 35% of deaths, and electromechanical dissociation after shock is a frequent cause of death. Asystole may be the first rhythm observed in the field, but this may be a marker of the duration of arrest because coarse VF ultimately degenerates into asystole.

MANAGEMENT

RISK STRATIFICATION

Current parameters for risk stratification of patients with (CAD for SCD include medical history (presence of nonsustained VT or syncope), Ejection fraction (EF), electrocardiogram (QRS duration, QT interval, and QT dispersion), signal-averaged electrocardiogram, heart rate variability, and baroreflex sensitivity. However, the sensitivity and specificity of these parameters has not been studied yet in detail in large patient populations. The single major parameter associated with higher incidence and studied in many clinical trials is left ventricular ejection fraction (LVEF). At present, only LV dysfunction with reduced EF reliably defines "high risk" for SCD in patients with ischemic and nonischemic cardiomyopathy. The heart failure functional class and history of prior MI or CAD are also important prognostic risk factors along with sudden specific definitive indications.[16]

PREVENTION

Prevention of SCD is rendered as detection of high-risk patients and application of medical treatment to postpone it. The high risk of development of SCD is attributed principally to fatal ventricular arrhythmias. Electrophysiologic anomalies in cells lead to development of ventricular ectopic activity or ventricular arrhythmias, which comes to the end with fibrillation and eventually death if not terminated in time. As survival rates for out-of-hospital cardiac arrests are extremely low, ranging from 2% to 25% in the United States,[17] secondary prevention strategies address only a small portion of patient population at risk of SCD. The accumulated data has allowed guidelines to be formulated, which allows us to predict with more certainty about patients at risk for SCD and address the challenge to identify patients at risk before the first event as primary prevention. However, applying those guidelines in practice requires systems to structure the environment in which care is delivered so that "doing the right thing" becomes automatic.[18] This requires tools that simplify and provide focus by embedding the recommendations for evidence-based care into the care itself.

PHARMACOLOGIC THERAPY

β-BLOCKERS

Of the different drugs that have been evaluated, only β-blockers have reduced SCD in the MI survivors.[19] The β-blocker heart attack trial (BHAT) study showed that β-blockade with propranolol reduced all-cause mortality by 25% especially in patients with diminished LV function and/or ventricular arrhythmias.[20] A randomized trial of approximately 46,000 patients showed that in the acute MI setting, early administration of high-dose β-blocker drugs orally has been shown to prevent VF.[21] In the metoprolol CR/XL randomized intervention trial in congestive heart failure trial (MERIT-HF), 3,991 patients with NYHA class II–IV heart failure and EF = 40% were randomized to long-acting metoprolol with a dose escalation protocol.[22] At 1-year follow-up, overall mortality was lower in the treated group compared with placebo (7.2% vs. 11% per patient-years of follow-up). There was also a 41% relative risk reduction in SCD with long-acting metoprolol. These data provide unequivocal benefit of β-blockade in acute MI, post-MI, and congestive heart failure for prevention of mortality and SCD.

ANTIARRHYTHMIC DRUGS

The sine qua non for efficacy of common antiarrhythmic drugs in prevention against SCD based on well-designed, placebo-controlled clinical trials have shown no added benefit.[19–23] Class I drugs (mexiletine, encainide, flecainide), calcium antagonists, and class III drugs (d-sotalol, dofetilide) all failed to reduce the incidence, rather even increased the incidence of SCD after an MI.[24] Amiodarone also has been shown to have no definitive effect on mortality in patients after MI in preventing SCD, as manifested in the sudden cardiac death in heart failure trial (SCD-HeFT).[25]

STATINS

The role of statins has been well studied in the patients with CAD and has been shown to be extremely beneficial in reducing mortality but whether they play any significant role in preventing SCD remains controversial. A multicenter automatic defibrillator implantation trial (MADIT-II) substudy[26] demonstrated that among patients treated with ICDs, those with background statin therapy had a lower rate of ventricular tachyarrhythmias. This finding was intriguing because it was unclear whether this observation was due to reduction in coronary events, decreased inflammation, unique antiarrhythmic properties, or unidentified confounders. Recently, the Cholesterol Lowering and Arrhythmia Recurrences After Internal Defibrillator Implantation study demonstrated that intensive lipid-lowering therapy using 80 mg of atorvastatin led to a 40% relative risk reduction (from 38% to 21%) in VT/VF recurrence in ICD patients during a 12-month follow-up. Yet there are no definite guidelines supporting addition of statins as adjuvant therapy for prevention of SCD beyond conventional indications.

THE ROLE OF IMPLANTABLE CARDIOVERTER DEFIBRILLATOR DEVICES IN PRIMARY AND SECONDARY PREVENTION AGAINST SUDDEN CARDIAC DEATH

Multiple prospective randomized multicenter clinical trials have documented improved survival with ICD therapy in high-risk patients with LV dysfunction owing to either prior MI or nonischemic cardiomyopathy. On a background of optimal medical therapy (with or without antiarrhythmic drug therapy), ICD therapy has been associated with a 23% to 55% mortality reduction, almost exclusively owing to a reduction in SCD.

IMPLANTABLE CARDIOVERTER DEFIBRILLATOR TRIALS

AVID TRIAL

Superiority of an ICD over antiarrhythmic drug therapy for secondary prevention against SCD (predominantly amiodarone) was primarily noticed in the antiarrhythmic versus implantable defibrillator (AVID) trial.[27] The AVID trial enrolled 1,016 patients resuscitated from an episode of VT (if associated with hemodynamic collapse, cardiac symptoms, or occurring in the setting of an EF = 40%) or VF. Patients were randomized to receive either medical therapy alone or in conjunction with an antiarrhythmic drug, which was most commonly amiodarone. The trial was stopped prematurely when a survival benefit was noted in patients receiving ICDs compared with those treated with sotalol or amiodarone. The unadjusted survival rates for the ICD versus drug groups were 89% versus 82% at 1-year, 82% versus 75% at 2-years, and 75% versus 65% at 3-years. The major effect of the ICD was to prevent arrhythmic death (4.7% vs. 10.8% in patients treated with an antiarrhythmic drug). Results consistent with the AVID study were also reported from the Canadian Implantable Defibrillator Study (CIDS)[28] and the Cardiac Arrest Study Hamburg (CASH).[29]

MADIT TRIAL

To test the efficacy of ICDs in prevention of SCD, the MADIT trial randomized 196 patients with ischemic cardiomyopathy,[30] EF ≤35%, a documented episode of nonsustained VT (NSVT), and inducible VT on electrophysiology study to ICD (*n* = 95) versus conventional medical therapy(*n* = 101). After a mean follow-up of 27 months, the relative risk reduction for all-cause mortality in the patients receiving ICDs was 54% (*P* = .009) thus showing the benefit of prophylactic ICD placement in a high-risk population.

MADIT II TRIAL

However, to make an impact on the overall population at risk for SCD, high-risk patients need to be identified before an episode of VT or VF (primary prevention). The MADIT II study highlighted the possibility of preventing sudden death in patients with CAD. According to this trial, patients with a previous MI and low LVEF (=30%) on optimal medical therapy were randomized to receive either an ICD or no ICD.[26] Patients implanted with an ICD had mortality rate of 14.2% versus 19.8% in the conventional therapy group (*P* = .016); a 31% relative risk reduction in mortality during a follow-up period of 20 months. The survival benefit was entirely owing to a reduction in the incidence of SCD and became apparent at 9 months after device implantation. This trial was novel because there was no requirement for invasive electrophysiological testing of prior ventricular arrhythmias. This trial expanded on the findings of MADIT I, which showed the superiority of ICD therapy in patients with CAD with EF ≤35%.

SCD-HEFT TRIAL

The significant role of ICD therapy in primary prevention against SCD in both ischemic and nonischemic cardiomyopathy patients was further clarified by the SCD-HeFT.[31] This trial enrolled 2,521 patients with New York Heart Association (NHYA) class II or III CHF and an EF of ≤35%. Patients were randomized to receive optimal medical therapy alone (847 patients), optimal medical therapy along with amiodarone (845 patients), or optimal medical therapy along with a conservatively programmed, shock-only, single-lead ICD (829 patients). Placebo and amiodarone were administered in a double-blind fashion. The primary endpoint of the study was all-cause mortality with mean follow-up of 3.8 years. A 23% reduction in mortality (*P* = .007) was observed with the ICD; the benefit of ICD was similar in both ischemic (hazard ratio, 0.79; *P* = .05) and nonischemic cardiomyopathy (hazard ratio, 0.73; *P* = .06). In contrast, mortality was similar in patients on either medical therapy alone or when combined with amiodarone. The benefit of ICD therapy was comparable for ischemic and nonischemic cardiomyopathy.

DEFINITE TRIAL

The defibrillators in nonischemic cardiomyopathy treatment evaluation (DEFINITE) trial was the MADIT II counterpart. This trial included 458 patients with nonischemic dilated cardiomyopathy, EF ≤35%, NSVT or premature ventricular contractions, and NYHA class I, II, or III who were randomly divided to standard medical therapy or ICD.[33] At a 2-year follow-up, there was a trend in mortality reduction with ICD (7.9% vs. 14.1%; hazard ratio = 0.65, *P* = .08). The largest benefit was seen in NYHA class III patients (hazard ratio = 0.37). In part based on the results of this trial, the Centers for Medicare & Medicaid Services expanded coverage for ICD implementation to patients with nonischemic cardiomyopathy for more than 9 months in duration who have NYHA class III or IV heart failure and EF ≤35%.

TIMING OF CARDIOVERTER DEFIBRILLATOR IMPLANTATION

CABG PATCH TRIAL

In the CABG Patch study, 900 patients with LVEF of <36% and abnormal signal-averaged ECG who were undergoing elective coronary bypass surgery were randomized to ICD or antiarrhythmic therapy.[34] This trail showed no difference in survival between the two groups at an average of 32-month follow-up. Of note, 88 patients enrolled were not randomized because they were deemed too unstable at time of surgery for ICD placement. In addition, EFs of these patients were not assessed postoperatively. Nevertheless, results suggest that revascularization should be performed when feasible and SCD risk stratification should be performed after revascularization.

DEFIBRILLATOR IN ACUTE MYOCARDIAL INFARCTION TRIAL

In this randomized, open-label trial comparing ICD therapy to optimal medical therapy, 674 high-risk patients (defined by an EF <35%) were enrolled 6 to 40 days after MI.[35,36] The primary endpoint was death from any cause; death from arrhythmia was a secondary endpoint. During a mean follow-up of 30 months, there was no difference in overall mortality between two treatment groups. A reduction in arrhythmia was balanced by an increase in overall mortality (cardiac but nonarrhythmogenic) in ICD group. The reason for this surprising finding is unclear but may be related to impaired cardiac autonomic function early after MI. The benefits of ICD therapy for prevention of SCD may not become evident until years after MI and may not have been captured in the mean 30-month follow-up of defibrillator in acute myocardial infarction trial (DINAMIT). Current guidelines therefore recommend deferring ICD placement for at least 40 days following MI.

Aggressive treatment of myocardial ischemia, including revascularization is the main treatment in these patients, and early placement of ICD does not reduce overall mortality after early MI (the DINAMIT study). Placement of ICD should be deferred in these cases as is currently recommended, with reassessment of LV function after "40 days" to determine whether ICD is still required for primary prevention of SCD (if the LVEF <35%), although in some individuals circumstances it may be considered (e.g., in patients with recurrent, sustained arrhythmias).

CARDIAC RESYNCHRONIZATION THERAPY

Cardiac resynchronization therapy (CRT) or biventricular pacing can improve cardiac pump function in advanced heart failure by simultaneous activation of the left and right ventricles, especially in patients with underlying or pacing-induced bundle branch block. CRT[37] is approved in the United States for EF ≤35%, evidence of dyssynchrony, and class III–IV heart failure despite optimal medical therapy. A brief review of the clinical data supporting their current use is as below.

COMPANION TRIAL

Cardiac-resynchronization therapy with either a pacemaker or a pacemaker-defibrillator has been shown to be very beneficial in the COMPANION trial[38] This trial randomized patients with class III or IV heart failure, normal sinus rhythm, LVEF <35%, LV end diastolic volume >60 mm, and QRS interval >120 milliseconds. In this trial cardiac-resynchronization therapy with a pacemaker decreased the risk of the primary endpoint (hazard ratio, 0.81; P = .014), as did cardiac-resynchronization therapy with a pacemaker-defibrillator (hazard ratio, 0.80; P < .01). The risk of the combined endpoint of death or hospitalization for heart failure was reduced by 34% in the pacemaker group (P < .002) and by 40% in the pacemaker-defibrillator group (P < .001). A pacemaker reduced the risk of the secondary endpoint of death from any cause by 24% (P = .059), and a pacemaker-defibrillator reduced the risk by 36% (P = .003).

CARDIAC RESYNCHRONIZATION VALIDATED IN HEART FAILURE TRIAL

The Cardiac Resynchronization in Heart Failure (CARE-HF) study trial was a nonblinded European study, which enrolled patients with class III or IV heart failure LVEF <35%, LV end diastolic volume >30 mm, QRS interval >150 milliseconds, or QRS >120 milliseconds with echocardiographic parameters of dyssynchrony.[39] This trial earlier trials that the benefits of CRT are in addition to those achieved with standard pharmacologic

therapy in patients with moderate-to-severe heart failure owing to LV systolic dysfunction with evidence of cardiac dyssynchrony. CARE-HF is the first study to demonstrate both survival benefit as well as progressive clinical improvement for a period > 2 years in patients with CRT.

MADIT–CARDIAC RESYNCHRONIZATION THERAPY

In this large randomized study of NYHA class I and II patients, the primary endpoint showed that CRT-D were associated with 34% relative reduction in the risk of all-cause mortality or first heart failure event; in addition there were 41% relative reduction of heart failure events compared with ICD patients. One-year follow-up confirmed an improvement of 11% in LVEF compared with 3% improvement for ICD patients.[40]

THE ESCAPE PATHWAY FOR PREVENTION OF SUDDEN CARDIAC DEATH

Multiple pathways have been developed in recent past to address these complex issues faced in the management of SCD; however most of them lack simplicity and practicality of implementation, which in turn affect their overall outcome and patient care. We have developed a novel pathway for SCD prevention named ESCAPE pathway,[41] which is a simple pathway for primary and secondary prevention of sudden cardiac death aiming to increase physician awareness and incorporate a tool for appropriate referral for ICD evaluation (Figure 19.1).

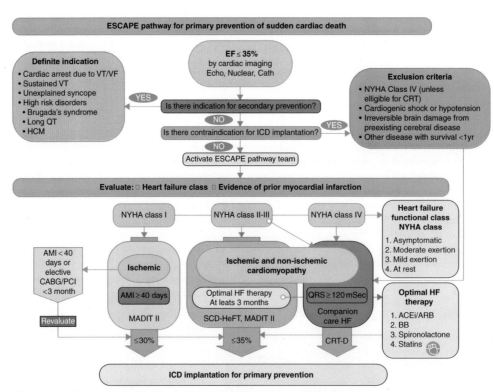

Figure 19.1. The ESCAPE pathway for primary prevention of sudden cardiac death. ACE; AMI, acute myocardial infarction; CABG, coronary artery bypass grafting; EF, ejection fraction; SCD, sudden cardiac death; VF, ventricular fibrillation; VT, ventricular tachycardia.

We recommend the following steps in managing patients.

Step A: Initial evaluation of patients.

The initial and foremost thing to observe while assessing for the prevention against SCD; is the EF. According to the ACC/AHA/ESC 2006 guidelines for management of patients with ventricular arrhythmias and the prevention of SCD new criteria includes patients with either ischemic or nonischemic cardiomyopathy with EF ≤35%, and NYHA class II or III heart failure, removing the controversial criteria from 2003 that restricted ICDs to patients with ischemic cardiomyopathy, EF ≤30%, and QRS >120 milliseconds, respectively.

Based on the initial evaluation of the patients with EF ≤35%, they can be divided into three subgroups: (A) Patients with a clear indication for secondary cardiac arrest prevention; (B) patients who have a contraindication to ICD or have no proven benefit from ICDs for SCD prevention as per clinical data available to date; and (C) patients who neither have any indication for ICD placement at this time as a part of secondary prevention of SCD nor have any contraindication.

Group A involves following patients (Figure 19.2):

- Survivors of sudden cardiac arrest owing to VT/VF.
- With a previous documented episode of hemodynamically destabilizing sustained VT.
- Unexplained syncope in the setting of underlying structural heart disease.
- Patients with high-risk SQTS or LQTS.
- Patients with high-risk Brugada syndrome.
- Patients with high-risk HCM.
- Patients with ARVD.

This group of patient population on presentation should be referred directly for ICD placement for secondary prevention against SCD.

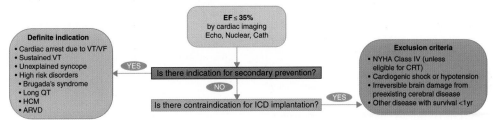

Figure 19.2. Indications and contraindications of implantable cardioverter defibrillator (ICD) for secondary prevention. ARVD, arrhythmogenic right ventricular dysplasia; CRT, cardiac resynchronization therapy; EF, ejection fraction; HCM, hypertrophic cardiomyopathy; VF, ventricular fibrillation; VT, ventricular tachycardia.

Group B involves patients with a contraindication for ICD placement and includes the following (Figure 19.2):

- NYHA class IV patients (unless QRS ≥120 milliseconds who are eligible for CRT).
- Cardiogenic shock or hypotension.
- Irreversible brain damage from preexisting cerebral disease.
- Other disease (e.g., cancer, uremia, liver failure) associated with a likelihood of survival <1 year.

Group C patients need further workup to decide whether and when they should get ICDs and should enter into step B.

Step B: Evaluation of heart failure class (Figure 19.3).

To determine the best course of therapy, these patients require assessment of the stage of heart failure according to the NYHA classification.[42,43]

Class I: No limitation of physical activity. Ordinary physical activity does not cause undue fatigue, palpitation, or dyspnea (shortness of breath).

Class II: Slight limitation of physical activity. Comfortable at rest, but ordinary physical activity results in fatigue, palpitation, or dyspnea.

Class III: Marked limitation of physical activity. Comfortable at rest, but less than ordinary activity causes fatigue, palpitation, or dyspnea.

Class IV: Unable to carry out any physical activity without discomfort. Symptoms of cardiac insufficiency at rest. If any physical activity is undertaken, discomfort is increased.

Step C: Evaluation of CAD or prior MI in NYHA class I patient (Figure 19.4).

Evaluation for any evidence of prior MI or CAD requiring intervention is further necessary.

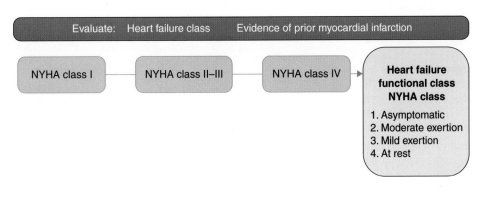

Figure 19.3. Assessment of the heart failure patients as per NYHA class category.

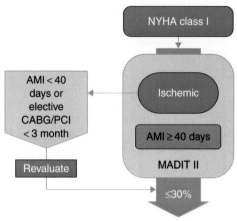

Figure 19.4. Primary prevention of sudden cardiac death in NYHA class I patients with low ejection fraction. AMI, acute myocardial infarction; CABG, coronary artery bypass grafting; PCI, percutaneous coronary intervention.

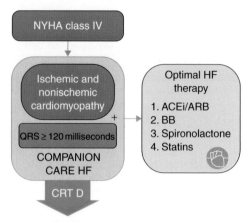

Figure 19.5. Primary prevention of SCD in NYHA classes III and IV heart failure patients with widened QRS complexes.

- Patients with NYHA class I heart failure whose EF is ≤30%, and who are at least 40 days post-MI should be referred for a placement of ICD according to MADIT-II trial.

- Patients with low EF and are ≤40 days post-MI, should be managed medically for their heart failure at present.[44] If repeat imaging at 40 days confirms EF ≤30% (or ≤35% in patients with class II or III NYHA class CHF), these patients should be referred for an ICD placement.

- Patients with low EF who underwent elective revascularization either by percutaneous intervention or coronary bypass surgery in ≤3 month should be managed medically with optimal therapy for heart failure and if repeated imaging at 3 months confirms EF ≤30% (or ≤35% in patients with class II or III NYHA class CHF), these patients should be referred for an ICD placement.

Step D: Primary prevention of SCD in NYHA class II–III patients with low EF.

According to the ACC/AHA published Update Guidelines for the Diagnosis and Management of Chronic Heart Failure in the Adult[43] this treatment includes the following:

- Angiotensin converting enzyme (ACE) inhibitors are recommended for routine administration to symptomatic and asymptomatic patients with LVEF ≤40% (strength of evidence = A).

- β-Blockers shown to be effective in clinical trials of patients with HF and are recommended for patients with an LVEF ≤40% (strength of evidence = A).

- Angiotensin receptor blockers (ARBs) are recommended for routine administration to symptomatic and asymptomatic patients with an LVEF ≤40% who are intolerant to ACE inhibitors for reasons other than hyperkalemia or renal insufficiency (strength of evidence = A).

- Administration of an aldosterone antagonist should be considered in patients following an acute MI, with clinical HF signs and symptoms and an LVEF ≤40%. Patients should be on standard therapy, including an ACE inhibitor (or ARB) and a β-blocker (strength of evidence = A).

If repeated imaging at 3 months confirms EF ≤35% and still in NYHA class II–III, these patients will be referred for an ICD placement.

Step E: Primary prevention of SCD is NYHA class III and IV heart failure patients with prolonged QRS (>120 milliseconds) (Figure 19.5).

Patients with QRS ≥120 milliseconds and in NYHA class (III or IV) according to COMPANION and CARE-HF trial will be referred for CRT with an ICD (CRT-D).[38]

CONCLUSION

Over the last three decades, revolutionary advancements in the understanding and treatment of SCD have been accomplished. Structural and electrical mechanisms of terminal arrhythmias have been elucidated. Over two dozen genetic mutations and polymorphisms have been identified, which in turn have increased our understanding of ion channel structure and function. At the same time, randomized trials that demonstrated harm from antiarrhythmic drugs have curtailed the use of such drugs alone in the prevention of SCD. The ICD was developed and has proven to be a highly effective therapy in the prevention of SCD to date. However, most cases of SCD occur in patients without these high-risk features, the biggest challenge still remains: to accurately identify patients at risk for SCD for primary prevention.

REFERENCES

1. Seidl K, Senges J. Worldwide utilization of implantable cardioverter/defibrillators now and in the future. *Card Electrophysiol Rev.* 2003;7:5–13.
2. Myerburg RJ, Kessler KM, Castellanos A. Sudden cardiac death: epidemiology, transient risk, and intervention assessment. *Ann Intern Med.* 1993;119:1187–1197.
3. Zheng ZJ, Croft JB, Giles WH, et al. Sudden cardiac death in the United States, 1989 to 1998. *Circulation.* 2001;104:2158–2163.
4. Stevenson WG, Stevenson LW, Middlekauff HR, et al. Sudden death prevention in patients with advanced ventricular dysfunction. *Circulation.* 1993;88:2953–2961.
5. Chugh SS, Jui J, Gunson K, et al. Current burden of sudden cardiac death: multiple source surveillance versus retrospective death certificate-based review in a large U.S. community. *J Am Coll Cardiol.* 2004;44:1268–1275.
6. Topalov V, Radisic B, Kovacevic D. [Sudden cardiac death]. *Med Pregl.* 1999;52:179–183.
7. Zipes DP, Wellens HJ. Sudden cardiac death. *Circulation.* 1998;98:2334–2351.
8. Brugada P, Talajic M, Smeets J, et al. The value of the clinical history to assess prognosis of patients with ventricular tachycardia or ventricular fibrillation after myocardial infarction. *Eur Heart J.* 1989;10:747–752.
9. Burke AP, Farb A, Malcom GT, et al. Coronary risk factors and plaque morphology in men with coronary disease who died suddenly. *N Engl J Med.* 1997;336:1276–1282.
10. Albert CM, McGovern BA, Newell JB, et al. Sex differences in cardiac arrest survivors. *Circulation.* 1996;93:1170–1176.
11. Escobedo LG, Zack MM. Comparison of sudden and nonsudden coronary deaths in the United States. *Circulation.* 1996;93:2033–2036.

12. Friedlander Y, Siscovick DS, Weinmann S, et al. Family history as a risk factor for primary cardiac arrest. *Circulation*. 1998;97:155–160.

13. Huikuri H. Abnormal dynamics of ventricular repolarization—a new insight into the mechanisms of life-threatening ventricular arrhythmias. *Eur Heart J*. 1997;18:893–895.

14. Luu M, Stevenson WG, Stevenson LW, et al. Diverse mechanisms of unexpected cardiac arrest in advanced heart failure. *Circulation*. 1989;80:1675–1680.

15. Pratt CM, Greenway PS, Schoenfeld MH, et al. Exploration of the precision of classifying sudden cardiac death. Implications for the interpretation of clinical trials. *Circulation*. 1996;93:519–524.

16. Choudhury L, Mahrholdt H, Wagner A, et al. Myocardial scarring in asymptomatic or mildly symptomatic patients with hypertrophic cardiomyopathy. *J Am Coll Cardiol*. 2002;40:2156–2164.

17. Eisenberg MS, Horwood BT, Cummins RO, et al. Cardiac arrest and resuscitation: a tale of 29 cities. *Ann Emerg Med*. 1990;19:179–186.

18. Cannon CP, Hand MH, Bahr R, et al. Critical pathways for management of patients with acute coronary syndromes: an assessment by the National Heart Attack Alert Program. *Am Heart J*. 2002;143:777–789.

19. The cardiac arrhythmia suppression trial. *N Engl J Med*. 1989;321:1754–1756.

20. Lampert R, Ickovics JR, Viscoli CJ, et al. Effects of propranolol on recovery of heart rate variability following acute myocardial infarction and relation to outcome in the Beta-Blocker Heart Attack Trial. *Am J Cardiol*. 2003;91:137–142.

21. Chen ZM, Pan HC, Chen YP, et al. Early intravenous then oral metoprolol in 45,852 patients with acute myocardial infarction: randomised placebo-controlled trial. *Lancet*. 2005;366:1622–1632.

22. Effect of metoprolol CR/XL in chronic heart failure: Metoprolol CR/XL Randomised Intervention Trial in Congestive Heart Failure (MERIT-HF). *Lancet*. 1999;353:2001–2007.

23. Effect of the antiarrhythmic agent moricizine on survival after myocardial infarction. The Cardiac Arrhythmia Suppression Trial II Investigators. *N Engl J Med*. 1992;327:227–233.

24. Waldo AL, Camm AJ, deRuyter H, et al. Effect of d-sotalol on mortality in patients with left ventricular dysfunction after recent and remote myocardial infarction. The SWORD Investigators. Survival With Oral d-Sotalol. *Lancet*. 1996;348:7–12.

25. Julian DG, Camm AJ, Frangin G, et al. Randomised trial of effect of amiodarone on mortality in patients with left-ventricular dysfunction after recent myocardial infarction: EMIAT. European Myocardial Infarct Amiodarone Trial Investigators. *Lancet*. 1997;349:667–674.

26. Moss AJ, Zareba W, Hall WJ, et al. Prophylactic implantation of a defibrillator in patients with myocardial infarction and reduced ejection fraction. *N Engl J Med*. 2002;346:877–883.

27. A comparison of antiarrhythmic-drug therapy with implantable defibrillators in patients resuscitated from near-fatal ventricular arrhythmias. The Antiarrhythmics versus Implantable Defibrillators (AVID) Investigators. *N Engl J Med*. 1997;337:1576–1583.

28. Connolly SJ, Gent M, Roberts RS, et al. Canadian Implantable Defibrillator Study (CIDS): study design and organization. CIDS Co-Investigators. *Am J Cardiol*. 1993;72:103F–108F.

29. Kuck KH, Cappato R, Siebels J, et al. Randomized comparison of antiarrhythmic drug therapy with implantable defibrillators in patients resuscitated from cardiac arrest: the Cardiac Arrest Study Hamburg (CASH). *Circulation*. 2000;102:748–754.

30. Farre J. [Implantable automatic defibrillator after MADIT and EMIAT]. *Rev Esp Cardiol*. 1996;49:709–713.

31. Bardy GH, Lee KL, Mark DB, et al. Amiodarone or an implantable cardioverter-defibrillator for congestive heart failure. *N Engl J Med*. 2005;352:225–237.

32. Barshop BA, Nyhan WL, Naviaux RK, et al. Kearns-Sayre syndrome presenting as 2-oxoadipic aciduria. *Mol Genet Metab*. 2000;69:64–68.

33. Ellenbogen KA, Levine JH, Berger RD, et al. Are implantable cardioverter defibrillator shocks a surrogate for sudden cardiac death in patients with nonischemic cardiomyopathy? *Circulation*. 2006;113:776–782.

34. Bigger JT Jr. Prophylactic use of implanted cardiac defibrillators in patients at high risk for ventricular arrhythmias after coronary-artery bypass graft surgery. Coronary Artery Bypass Graft (CABG) Patch Trial Investigators. *N Engl J Med*. 1997;337:1569–1575.

35. Hohnloser SH, Kuck KH, Dorian P, et al. Prophylactic use of an implantable cardioverter-defibrillator after acute myocardial infarction. *N Engl J Med*. 2004;351:2481–2488.

36. Hohnloser SH, Crijns HJ, van Eickels M, et al. Effect of dronedarone on cardiovascular events in atrial fibrillation. *N Engl J Med*. 2009;360:668–678.

37. New CRT technology boosts care for heart failure patients. Cardiac resynchronization therapy can provide better rhythm control and better communication with the doctor to help lower your risks. *Heart Advis*. 2008;11:10.

38. Bristow MR, Saxon LA, Boehmer J, et al. Cardiac-resynchronization therapy with or without an implantable defibrillator in advanced chronic heart failure. *N Engl J Med*. 2004;350:2140–2150.

39. Cleland JG, Daubert JC, Erdmann E, et al. The CARE-HF study (Cardiac REsynchronisation in Heart Failure study): rationale, design and end-points. *Eur J Heart Fail*. 2001;3:481–489.

40. Moss AJ, Hall WJ, Cannom DS, et al. Cardiac-resynchronization therapy for the prevention of heart-failure events. *N Engl J Med*. 2009;361:1329–1338.

41. Herzog E, Aziz EF, Kukin M, et al. Novel pathway for sudden cardiac death prevention. *Crit Pathw Cardiol*. 2009;8:1–6.

42. Hunt SA, Baker DW, Chin MH, et al. ACC/AHA guidelines for the evaluation and management of chronic heart failure in the adult: executive summary: a report of the American College of Cardiology/American Heart Association Task Force on Practice Guidelines (Committee to Revise the 1995 Guidelines for the Evaluation and Management of Heart Failure): Developed in Collaboration with the International Society for Heart and Lung Transplantation; Endorsed by the Heart Failure Society of America. *Circulation*. 2001;104:2996–3007.

43. Hunt SA, Abraham WT, Chin MH, et al. 2009 Focused update incorporated into the ACC/AHA 2005 Guidelines for the Diagnosis and Management of Heart Failure in Adults: a report of the American College of Cardiology Foundation/American Heart Association Task Force on Practice Guidelines Developed in Collaboration with the International Society for Heart and Lung Transplantation. *J Am Coll Cardiol*. 2009;53:e1–e90.

44. Herzog E, Varley C, Kukin M. Pathway for the management of acute heart failure. *Crit Pathw Cardiol*. 2005;4:37–42.

PATIENT AND FAMILY INFORMATION FOR:

The Prevention of Sudden Cardiac Death

Sudden Cardiac Death (SCD), also known as sudden cardiac arrest, is an escalating public health hazard. It is estimated that 300,000 to 350,000 SCDs occurs annually in the United States. It is generally defined as an unpredicted, rapid death from a cardiac cause occurring within a short duration time in a person with or without prior heart disease owing to abrupt loss of heart function (*cardiac arrest*). This chapter will provide you with an overview of this fatal condition and also equip you with the various preventive and treatment modalities available in current era by means of a simple yet comprehensive algorithmic approach called as an ESCAPE pathway for SCD prevention.

There is no clear agreement on any single definition of SCD among different disciplines of medicine, which is witnessed in only two-thirds of cases. As the name indicates, this condition is "unexpected" in nature without any prior indication or alarm in most of the patients. World Health Organization defines SCD as unexpected death in someone who suddenly started complaining of any distress and eventually died within 1 hour in front of another person (witnessed death), or death of a person who was seen completely normal without any distress but later found dead within 24 hours (unwitnessed death). The commonest cause of the SCD is Coronary Artery Disease (CAD) of the heart, but it is very important to understand that there are certain other causes of the SCD such as large blood clots in the arteries of the lungs known as pulmonary embolism or certain drug overdoses that can cause abnormal pattern of heart rhythm (cardiac arrhythmias) and can also result in SCD. SCD is not the same as a heart attack. The mechanism of death in SCD is mainly due to ventricular fibrillation (VF) (*fast irregular and lethal rhythm of the lower chambers of the heart called ventricles in which the contractions of the ventricles are very rapid and uncoordinated*). These arrhythmias result in quivering of ventricles, which then cannot pump blood to the vital organs of the body including the brain. Loss of consciousness, pulse, and breathing follow within seconds. VF almost never returns to a normal rhythm on its own, so if the victim does not receive immediate help, the brain dies.

EMERGENCY SIGNS OF SUDDEN CARDIAC DEATH

Although there is no standard list of SCD symptoms and SCD typically occurs without warning, following signs are mostly pathognomic of SCD.

- Sudden loss of consciousness
- No breathing
- No pulse.

RISK FACTORS

SCD can strike people of any age, gender, race, and even those who seem to be in good health, as witnessed in world-class professional athletes at the peak of fitness. About 80% of victims who suffer SCD have coronary heart disease. In some cases, a heart attack may lead to a SCD event. Most SCD victims are on average 60 years of age, and many victims are relatively healthy and lead active lives right up to the moment when SCD strikes. Based on recent medical data, following conditions have been found to be related to higher risk of SCD: (1) History of unexplained fainting or near fainting with palpitations (medically known as syncope or near syncope), (2) weak heart muscle with or advanced heart failure, (3) prior history of VT/VF occurring early (3 days to 2 months) after a heart attack, and (4) history of early heart disease, heart attack, or cardiac death in the family. Other cardiac risk factors such as advancing age, elevated blood pressure, enlarged heart chambers called dilated cardiomyopathy, elevated cholesterol levels, elevated blood glucose levels, smoking, obesity, and high heart rates are also attributed to the individuals at high risk for SCD. Principally, people who have had a previous heart attack (MI) have a four to six times higher risk of SCD than the general population. In people diagnosed with chronic heart failure, SCD occurs at six to nine times the rate of the general population.

SEQUENCE OF ARRHYTHMIAL EVENTS LEADING TO SUDDEN CARDIAC DEATH

SCD is an electrical problem and the commonest order of abnormal electric events in SCD is the deterioration of ventricular fibrillation (VF) (*abnormal speeding up of ventricular rate*) into VF, during which baffled contractions of the ventricles fail to pump blood effectively, often followed by a complete cessation of the heart muscle pumping. This results in termination of blood supply to brain. Breathing is one function of the brain that stops during SCD, which compounds the problem even further. Unless oxygenated blood returns to the brain in <4 to 6 minutes, potential reversible cardiac death leads to permanent brain death. It is therefore critical to recognize and respond to SCD because if caught early, it is possible to avoid brain death, which means, SCD is potentially reversible. Sometimes, bradyarrhythmias (slow heart beats) or in-coordination between the electrical and muscular function of the heart may be the principal electrical event triggering SCD especially in patients with advanced heart failure or in the elderly.

MANAGEMENT OF ARRYTHMIAS LEADING TO SCD

A life-threatening arrhythmia leading to SCD typically can be reversed but only if treated within minutes by an electric shock to the heart to restore a normal rhythm—an intervention called as defibrillation. Rhythms such as VF causing catastrophic consequences in the form of SCD are so abrupt that there is no time to begin medications. Fortunately, alternative forms of treatments are available for these conditions called as defibrillation and cardioversion (conversion of abnormal cardiac rhythm to normal). Defibrillation and cardioversion work by momentarily stopping the heart and the chaotic rhythm. This often allows the normal heart rhythm to take over again. ICDs are devices that provide protection against SCD. ICDs are battery-driven devices implanted in the body. ICDs have been found greatly effective in averting abnormal rhythms. Similar to pacemaker, wire electrodes attach the ICD's pulse generator to the heart. The ICD monitors the heart rhythm at all times. It can pace like a pacemaker for slow heart rates, rapidly pace for the tachyarrhythmias, and give smaller cardioversion or large defibrillation shocks. It is similar to the conventional external defibrillator, but the internal device has an advantage because it is always ready to deliver a lower-energy shock when needed. In short, ICD is always on hand, ready to deliver a life-saving shock.

THE "ESCAPE" PATHWAY FOR PREVENTION AND MANAGEMENT OF SCD

Prevention is better than cure. Considering the fact that key to successful prevention and management of SCD is early risk stratification of patients, prompt recognition of impending complications and achievement of certain measures to prevent or treat these risk factors, we utilized published guidelines to define the strategy and resolve differences in the literature in the form of a clinical pathway to effectively safeguard patients against SCD. This pathway called ESCAPE pathway is based on the principles of primary and secondary prevention (Figure 19.1). Primary prevention is treating or correcting risk factors to prevent a diseased condition from occurring, whereas secondary prevention is an attempt to reduce risk factors to prevent recurrence of that condition. You can think of this pathway as a preventive maintenance, taking steps to reduce your risk factors before SCD occurs. ESCAPE pathway is devised on the hypothesis that the best way to save lives is to prevent SCD by eliminating or reducing risk factors.

IDENTIFICATION OF PATIENTS AT RISK OF SCD

Certain parameters are used to identify patients at risk of SCD including medical history (*presence of nonsustained VT or unexplained fainting spells*), EF (*portion of blood that is pumped out of a filled left ventricle on each beat, normal value ranges between 55% and 65%*), ECGs (*transthoracic interpretation of the electrical activity of the heart over time captured and externally recorded by skin electrodes*), signal-averaged ECG (*a more advanced form of ECG*), and heart rate variability (*changes in heart rate*).

The initial and foremost thing to observe while assessing for the prevention against SCD is the EF. The EF is a good indicator of the overall function of one's heart. The left ventricle is by far the most important chamber of the heart. This chamber must generate enough pressure to drive blood to every region of one's body. When this chamber becomes weak, mostly owing to CAD the EF decreases. It is this reduction in EF that gives rise to various disastrous situations including but not limited to SCD.

Patients with a reduced EF of ≤35% are considered at high risk of SCD and need to be further evaluated for various interventions including placement of lifesaving ICD. This number of EF of ≤35% is derived from the results of various large clinical trials and consensus of various experts in the field. As shown in the Figure 19.2, patients with an EF of ≤35%, are divided into three subgroups: (A) Patients with a clear indication for secondary cardiac arrest prevention requiring an ICD, (B) patients who have a contraindication to ICD or have no proven benefit from ICDs for SCD prevention as per clinical data available to date, and (C) patients who neither have any indication for ICD placement at this time as a part of secondary prevention of SCD nor any contraindication.

Group A: Patients with a definite indication for secondary prevention. These are the patients who have EF of ≤35% with a clear indication for the placement of an ICD device for secondary prevention against SCD. These clear indications include patients with the following conditions:

- History of cardiac arrest in past owing to VT/VF.
- Any prior episode of prolonged VT that did not revert to normal rhythm spontaneously (medically referred to as sustained VT).
- Unexplained syncope as one loses consciousness when one's brain does not get enough blood and oxygen. Abnormal heart rhythm such as VT or VF can reduce heart's ability to pump enough blood to brain causing loss of consciousness.
- High-risk cardiac disorders including but not limited to
  - *Brugada syndrome.* A genetic disease with resultant abnormal ECG findings and increased risk of SCD.
  - *SQTS or LQTS.* The QT interval is the area on the ECG that represents the time it takes for the heart muscle to contract and then recover, or for the electrical impulse to fire impulses and then recharge. When the QT interval is shorter or longer than normal, it increases the risk of life-threatening forms of VT. LQTS sometimes is an inherited condition that can cause SCD in young people.

– *Hypertrophic Cardiomyopathy (HCM)*. HCM is the overgrowth of the heart muscle resulting from abnormal thickening of the heart walls for unknown reasons. The thickening can occur in several places throughout the ventricles, sometimes it impends the blood flow both into and out of the heart. Patients with HCM are prone to heart rhythm abnormalities and suffer frequently from syncope or SCD.

As evident from our pathway (Figure 19.1), these patients should get an ICD for secondary prevention against SCD for indefinite time.

Group B: Patients who are not an ideal candidate for ICDs. This group includes patients with a contraindication or no proven benefit from ICD implantation and comprises of the following:

- NYHA class IV patients who are those with severe heart failure and are prone to various irregular heart rhythms. These patients are mostly bedbound. The only exception is if the QRS interval on the ECG of these patients is ≥120 milliseconds making them eligible for CRT. CRT is a form of therapy for congestive heart failure caused by dilated cardiomyopathy and uses a specialized pacemaker to recoordinate the action of the right and left ventricles in patients with heart failure. CRT can also defibrillate, if needed.

- Cardiogenic shock that results when the heart muscle is too weak to contract with enough force to maintain blood pressure at a level that provides a sufficient amount of blood to body and the heart muscle itself. This circle is fatal in most cases.

- Irreversible brain damage from preexisting diseases that diminish brain blood supply.

- Other disease (e.g., cancer, kidney failure, liver failure), associated with a likelihood of survival of <1 year.

Group C: Patients requiring further evaluation. This group represents patients who need further workup to decide whether and when they should get ICDs. For patients in this group, a specialized cardiology team needs to be activated for further evaluation (Figure 19.1).This group consists of patients who either suffer from heart attack (MI) because of CAD with resultant weakening of heart owing to damaged heart muscle tissue leading to heart failure or patients who have diseases affecting directly the entire heart muscle medically referred to as cardiomyopathy (cardio means "heart," myo means "muscle," pathy means "disease"). This group undergoes stepwise segregation to determine what should be done on individual basis.

EVALUATION OF HEART FAILURE CLASS CATEGORY

To determine the best course of therapy, these patients require assessment to establish the class of heart failure they belong to, according to the NYHA classification system (Figure 19.3). This system relates symptoms to everyday activities and the patient's quality of life.

Class I: No limitation of physical activity. Ordinary physical activity does not cause unnecessary fatigue, palpitation, or dyspnea (shortness of breath).

Class II: Slight limitation of physical activity. Comfortable at rest, but ordinary physical activity results in fatigue, palpitation, or dyspnea.

Class III: Marked limitation of physical activity. Comfortable at rest, but less than ordinary activity causes fatigue, palpitation, or dyspnea.

Class IV: Unable to carry out any physical activity without discomfort. Symptoms of heart weakness at rest. If any physical activity is undertaken, discomfort is increased and mostly keeps them bed bound.

PRIMARY PREVENTION OF SUDDEN CARDIAC DEATH IN NYHA CLASS I PATIENTS WITH LOW EJECTION FRACTION

The patients who are identified as belonging to NYHA class 1 are further assessed to determine whether their weakened heart is owing to lack of reception of enough blood and oxygen through the coronary arteries—called as ischemia. Once it is established that patients has NYHA class 1 heart failure owing to ischemia, further management varies according to the number of days since the episode of heart attack (Figure 19.4).

- Patients with NYHA class I heart failure whose EF is ≤30%, and who are at least 40 days post-heart attack (post-MI) should be referred for an ICD placement.

- Patients with low EF but within 40-day period post-MI, should be managed medically for their heart failure. They should be reassessed after 40 days and if found to have an EF of ≤30%, they should be referred for an ICD placement.

- Patients with low EF who underwent elective revascularization either by percutaneous intervention or coronary artery bypass surgery (please see Chapters 4 and 8 for details of these procedures) in ≤3 months should be managed medically with optimal drug therapy for heart failure. These patients should be reassessed after 3 months and if found to have persistent lower EF of ≤30%, should be referred for an ICD placement.

PRIMARY PREVENTION OF SUDDEN CARDIAC DEATH IN NYHA CLASS II–III PATIENTS WITH LOW EJECTION FRACTION

The patients belonging to NYHA classes II and III may be suffering from either ischemic or nonischemic heart failure. Various nonischemic causes of heart failure include a mechanical problem (congenital or valvular), prolonged high blood pressure (which increases the workload on the heart), and various other forms of cardiomyopathies. All of these patients should receive optimal heart failure medical therapy for at least 3 months as these agents have been shown to be effective in improving the heart's pumping efficiency, reducing symptoms, and increasing survival. These treatment modalities include the following:

- ACE inhibitors are recommended for routine administration to symptomatic and asymptomatic patients with EF of ≤40%.

- ß-Blockers have been shown to be effective in clinical trials of patients with heart failure and are recommended for patients with an EF of ≤40%.

- ARBs are recommended for routine administration to symptomatic and asymptomatic patients with an EF of ≤40% who are intolerant to ACE inhibitors.

- Administration of an aldosterone antagonist (a diuretic used to promote urine production by kidneys and reduce fluid accumulation, a common problem in heart failure patients) should be considered in patients following an acute heart attack, with clinical heart failure signs or symptoms and an EF of ≤40%.

- Statins (*Cholesterol lowering drugs*) have been well studied in patients with CAD and have been shown to be extremely beneficial in reducing mortality but whether they play any significant role in preventing SCD remains controversial. However, we do advocate the use of statins in these patients.

After 3 months of continued optimal medical therapy consisting of ACE inhibitors/ARBs, ß-blockers, an aldosterone antagonist, and statins, these patients are reassessed to determine whether their EF has improved. If repeated evaluation after 3 months confirms that their EF is still ≤35%, these patients should be referred for an ICD implantation.

PRIMARY PREVENTION OF SCD IN NYHA CLASSES III AND IV HEART FAILURE PATIENTS WITH WIDENED QRS COMPLEXES

QRS complex is the element of an electrocardiogram that precedes the ST segment and indicates electrical activation of the ventricles. The normal duration ranges between 60 and 100 milliseconds. The widening of the QRS duration is an abnormality that can occur in certain conditions such as intraventricular conduction delay (disease of the electric conduction system of heart resulting in delayed conduction within ventricles) or right and left bundle branch blocks (Figure 19.5). This causes the two ventricles to beat in an asynchronous fashion. That is, instead of beating simultaneously, the two ventricles beat slightly out of phase. This asynchrony greatly reduces the efficiency of the ventricles in patients with heart failure, whose hearts are already damaged.

THE ROLE OF IMPLANTABLE CARDIOVERTER-DEFIBRILLATOR DEVICES IN PRIMARY AND SECONDARY PREVENTION AGAINST SCD

Multiple large multicenter clinical trials have documented improved survival with ICD therapy in high-risk patients with LV dysfunction because of prior heart attack or cardiomyopathy. On a background of optimal medical therapy with or without antiarrhythmic drug therapy (medical therapy to restore normal rhythm of heart), ICD therapy has been associated with a 23% to 55% mortality reduction, almost exclusively because of a reduction in SCD.

Over the last three decades, innovative advances in the understanding and treatment of SCD have been accomplished. The ICD was developed and has proven to be a highly effective therapy in the prevention of SCD to the date. However, most cases of SCD occur in patients without these high-risk features, and the death toll attributed to SCD remains higher.

Eyal Herzog
Eitan Klein
Emad F. Aziz
Janet M. Shapiro

CHAPTER 20

Pathway for the Management of Survivors of Out-of-Hospital Cardiac Arrest, Including Therapeutic Hypothermia

Cardiovascular disease (CVD) is the leading cause of death in the United States. Mortality data show that CVD as the underlying cause of death accounts for 35.3% of all deaths in the United States.[1] There is a wide variation in the reported incidence and outcome of out-of-hospital cardiac arrest (OHCA). Cardiac arrest is defined as cessation of cardiac mechanical activity with absence of signs of circulation. The estimated number of OHCA cases is approximately 300,000 per year in the United States.[1] The median reported survival to hospital discharge after OHCA with any first reported rhythm is 7.9%.[1]

Two landmark studies published together in 2002 demonstrated that the use of therapeutic hypothermia after cardiac arrest decreased mortality and improved neurological outcome.[2,3] Based on these studies, the International Liaison Committee on Resuscitation and the American Heart Association recommended the use of therapeutic hypothermia after cardiac arrest.[4,5]

Therapeutic hypothermia is defined as a controlled lowering of core body temperature to 32°C or up to 34°C. This temperature goal represents the optimal balance between clinical effect and cardiovascular toxicity.[6] Therapeutic hypothermia requires resources to implement—including device, close nursing care, and monitoring. It is important to select patients who have potential for benefit from this technique, which is a limited resource and carries potential complications. A collaborative team approach involving physicians and nurses is critical for successful development and implementation of this kind of protocol.[7]

In this chapter we describe our pathway for the comprehensive management of OHCA survivors.[8,9]

This pathway is limited to OHCA and does not include in-hospital arrest.

PATHWAY DESCRIPTION

The pathway is divided into three steps as shown in Figure 20.1.

Step I. From the field through the emergency department (ED) into the cardiac catheterization laboratory and to the critical care unit.

Step II. Induced invasive hypothermia protocol in the critical care unit.

Step III. The management following the rewarming phase including the recommendation for out-of-hospital therapy and the ethical decision to define goals of care.

STEP I

Presentation to the emergency department, proceeding to the cardiac catheterization laboratory and to the critical care unit. Upon arrival of a survivor of OHCA to the ED, the initial assessment (Figure 20.2) includes vital signs, physical examination, and neurologic examination with Glasgow coma score. Immediate 12-lead EKG is obtained and laboratory testing performed.

Initial laboratory testing includes complete blood count (CBC) with differential, basic metabolic panel, cardiac marker (troponin, CPK, CPK-MB), B-type natriuretic peptide (BNP), prothrombin time (PT), partial thromboplastin time (PTT), international normalized ratio (INR), lipid profile, phosphorus, calcium, magnesium, lactate, β-HCG (for women), TSH, and toxicology screening. We recommend a head CT without contrast only if it is clinically indicated and will not delay transfer to the cardiac catheterization laboratory.

The patient is stabilized in the ED where antiarrhythmic and vasopressor therapy may be administered, in addition to ventilator support.

The ED physician receives the emergency medical services (EMS) report of the primary rhythm and duration of cardiopulmonary resuscitation (CPR). This reported arrhythmia is the key decision point in our pathway.

The prognostically important distinction is between patients with documented ventricular fibrillation (VF) or sustained ventricular tachycardia (VT) who had a restoration of spontaneous circulation (ROSC) in <30 minutes and patients with reported asystole or pulseless electrical activity (PEA) (Figure 20.3).

1. If the initial rhythm was VF or VT with an ROSC of ≤30 minutes the cardiac arrest team is activated, and the patient will proceed to the cardiac catheterization laboratory (Figure 20.4).

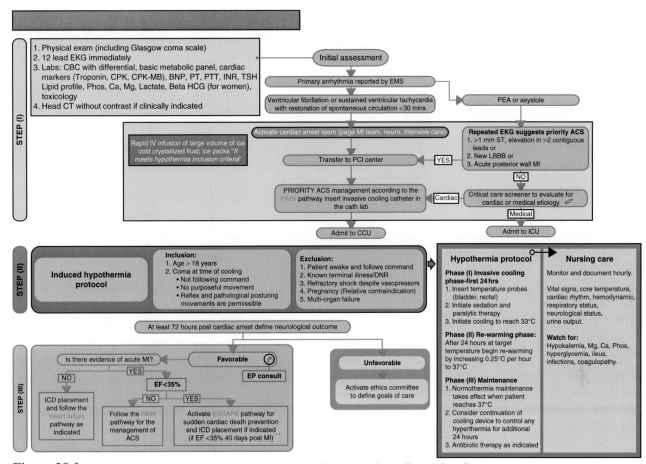

Figure 20.1. The comprehensive pathway for the management of survivors of out-of-hospital cardiac arrest.

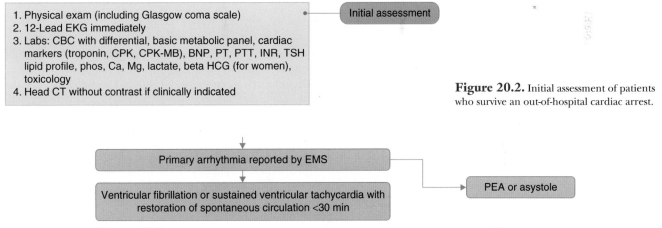

Figure 20.2. Initial assessment of patients who survive an out-of-hospital cardiac arrest.

Figure 20.3. Identification of the primary arrhythmia that led to the cardiac arrest. PEA pulseless electrical activity.

2. If the initial reported arrhythmia was PEA or asystole, the next step will depend on the EKG performed in the ED (Figure 20.4). If the EKG performed in ED is suggestive of priority ACS (including ST elevation MI, left bundle branch block, or acute posterior wall MI), the MI team should be activated, and the care is similar to those patients with reported VF or VT arrest.

3. If priority EKG findings are not seen but the etiology of the arrest is most likely owing to primary cardiac disease, the cardiology fellow will admit the patient to the cardiac care unit. We recommend an emergency echocardiogram.

4. If the etiology is likely noncardiac, the patient will be admitted to the medical intensive care unit.

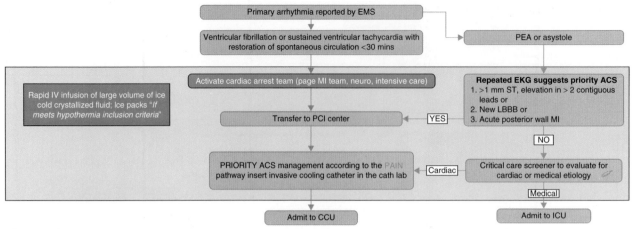

Figure 20.4. Activation of the cardiac arrest team, transfer to percutaneous coronary intervention (PCI) center, and transfer to the critical care unit. CCU, cardiac care unit; PAIN, *P*riority risk, *A*dvanced risk, *I*ntermediate risk, and *N*egative/low risk.

The *cardiac arrest team* includes the following 10 people.

The traditional (acute coronary syndrome) ACS-MI team comprises the following members[10]:

1. Interventional cardiologist on-call-the team leader
2. CCU director
3. Cardiology fellow on-call
4. Interventional cardiology fellow on-call
5. Cath lab nurse on-call
6. Cath lab technician on-call
7. CCU nurse manager on-call

In addition the following personnel form the team:

8. The neurologist on-call
9. The critical care attending on-call and
10. The medical resident screener

The MI team is activated by a single page to the central call center by the ED physician.

Steps in the emergency department.

1. Decision to initiate induced hypothermia is made jointly by the ED physician and the cardiology or critical care physician. It is very important to review the hospital center's inclusion and exclusion criteria and decide whether the patient is a candidate for the therapeutic hypothermia protocol (Figure 20.5).

2. The physician places an order to initiate hypothermia protocol.

3. Noninvasive hypothermia is initiated by the administration of iced saline in ED.

Our goal is to transfer the patient to the PCI center as soon as possible with a target door-to-balloon time of <90 minutes.

The management of the patient at this point is according to our *P*riority risk, *A*dvanced risk, *I*ntermediate risk, and

*N*egative/low risk (PAIN) pathway following the priority ACS algorithm.[10]

A detailed description of this pathway appears in Chapter 1 of this book.

Following cardiac catheterization, several steps occur while the patient is still in the catheterization laboratory:

1. The femoral arterial sheath is maintained as an arterial catheter, which is necessary to obtain blood pressure readings and arterial blood gas analyses.

2. The intravascular hypothermia catheter is inserted under strict aseptic technique.

All patients are then transferred from the catheterization laboratory to the CCU where invasive hypothermia is initiated.

STEP II

Induced invasive therapeutic hypothermia protocol in the critical care unit. The invasive hypothermia protocol begins in the critical care unit. The clinicians review the case and confirm the appropriateness of induced hypothermia (Figure 20.5).

In summary, we recommend induced hypothermia for patients >18 years of age, who sustained a cardiac arrest and remain in coma. Patient must be comatose, not following commands or demonstrating purposeful movements. Patients excluded from the hypothermia protocol include patients who: are awake, suffered prolonged ischemic times, experience refractory shock, demonstrate multiorgan failure, or have severe underlying illnesses, including terminal illnesses and do-not-resuscitate (DNR) status.

The hypothermia protocol is divided into three phases as seen in Figure 20.6:

Phase 1: Invasive cooling phase for the first 24 hours

Phase 2: Rewarming phase

Phase 3: Maintenance phase

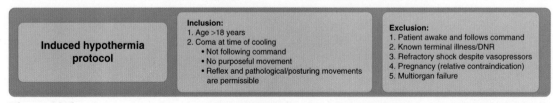

Figure 20.5. Inclusions and exclusions criteria for patients who are candidate for the therapeutic hypothermia protocol.

Hypothermia protocol

Phase (I) Invasive cooling phase-first 24 hours
1. Insert temperature probes (bladder, rectal)
2. Initiate sedation and paralytic therapy
3. Initiate cooling to reach 33°C

Phase (II) Rewarming phase:
After 24 hours at target temperature begin re-warming by increasing 0.25°C per hour to 37°C

Phase (III) Maintenance phase:
1. Normothermia maintenance takes affect when patient reach 37°C
2. Consider continuation of cooling device to control any hyperthermia for additional 24 hours
3. Antibiotic therapy as indicated.

Nursing care

Monitor and document hourly

Vital signs, core temperature, cardiac rhythm, hemodynamic, respiratory status, neurological status, urine output.

Watch for:
Hypokalemia, Mg, Ca, phos, hyperglycemia, ileus, infection, coagulopathy.

Figure 20.6. Induced invasive therapeutic hypothermia protocol.

Phase 1: Invasive cooling phase for the first 24 hours. In the two landmark studies published in 2002, Bernard et al.[2] cooled patients to 33°C for 12 hours, and the HACA trial[3] cooled patients to 32°C and up to 34°C for 24 hours.

We recommend 24 hours of the cooling therapy at a temperature goal of 33°C.

Endovascular catheters are an effective method of inducing therapeutic hypothermia.[11,12] The catheters are usually inserted into the inferior vena cava through the femoral vein.

Continuous core temperature monitoring is required and generally accomplished using a temperature probe in the bladder (urinary catheter) or the rectum.

Monitoring of clinical condition and potential complications during the invasive cooling phase.

As there are many physiologic effects of hypothermia, we recommend continuous monitoring and hourly documentation of vital signs; core temperature; cardiac rhythm; hemodynamic, respiratory, neurology status; and urine output. Common hemodynamic changes observed with cooling include hypertension, decreased cardiac output, and increased systemic vascular resistance. The hypertension and the increased systemic vascular resistance are believed to result from the cold-induced vasoconstriction.

Serum electrolyte imbalance is common during the cooling phase and results from the cooling-induced intracellular shifts of potassium, magnesium, calcium, and phosphate resulting in low levels of all these electrolytes. During the rewarming phase these electrolytes shift back to the extracellular space.

Our protocol therefore recommends measurements of the basic metabolic panel every 4 hours for a total of 48 hours, measuring electrolytes (calcium, magnesium, and phosphate) PT, PTT, and INR, and a CBC every 12 hours up to 48 hours.

Additional possible side effects of cooling to be monitored include the following:

1. *Coagulopathy.* Coagulopathy is generally not significant with careful temperature monitoring and avoiding temperature of <33°C. If active bleeding occurs during the cooling phase, evaluation of coagulation factors and platelets should be performed and deficiencies corrected.

2. *Hyperglycemia.* Hypothermia suppresses insulin release and causes insulin resistance. Our insulin infusion protocol for the management of hyperglycemia in critical care unit is used.[13]

3. *Infection.* Infection is usually multifactorial including emergency intubation and intravenous catheter insertion and aspiration pneumonia at the time of arrest.

    Furthermore, the hypothermia itself can suppress white blood cell production and impairs neutrophil and macrophage function. All measures to reduce ventilator associated pneumonia are employed including elevating the head of the bed.

4. *Shivering.* Our protocol aims to prevent shivering by administration of sedation and neuromuscular blocking agents on induction of hypothermia.

Phase 2: Rewarming phase. After 24 hours of the target temperature, the rewarming phase starts.

Controlled rewarming is a very important phase of this protocol.

Rewarming should be slow; we recommend a rate of 0.25°C per hour; therefore it typically requires 16 hours to rewarm to 37°C.

Potential complications during the rewarming phase include the following:

1. Hypotension—owing to peripheral vasodilatation during the rewarming phase.

2. Electrolyte imbalance—increased levels of potassium, magnesium, calcium, and phosphate owing to intracellular shifting of these ions back to the serum during the rewarming phase.

Phase 3: Maintenance of normothermia phase. The maintenance phase is the last phase of the therapeutic hypothermia protocol.

Normothermia maintenance takes effect when the patient's temperature reaches 37°C.

We recommend continuation of the cooling device to maintain a temperature of 37°C and avoid fever that can potentially worsen a cerebral injury.

STEP III

The management following hypothermia and rewarming depends on the neurologic prognosis (Figure 20.7).

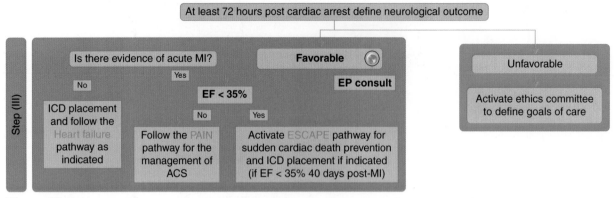

Figure 20.7. The management post the rewarming phase including the recommendation for out of hospital therapy and the ethical decision to define goal of care.

At least 72 hours postcardiac arrest, the neurologic examination is performed by the neurology team. The neurologic examination may be affected by the hypothermia protocol, including requirements for sedation and therapeutic paralysis, so that the formulation of a neurologic prognosis may be delayed.[14] The pathway for the patients will be divided based on whether the patient has a favorable neurologic prognosis or an unfavorable neurologic prognosis. An unfavorable neurologic prognosis would be defined as expectation for a persistent coma or vegetative state, or severe disability.

If the prognosis appears unfavorable, we recommend activating the ethics committee to meet with the family and clinicians to define the goals of care. From our experience, in most instances, life support is limited or withdrawn in such patients.

If the neurological prognosis appears favorable, then the key question regarding further therapy is based on whether the cardiac arrest was because of MI.

If there is no evidence of acute MI (negative cardiac markers) then we recommend electrophysiology service consultation for consideration of implantable cardioverter defibrillator (ICD) placement and treatment of heart failure based on our heart failure pathway.[15]

If acute MI is confirmed by positive cardiac markers we advise care based on the LV ejection fraction (LVEF) as it is defined by echocardiography or other imaging modalities. If LVEF ≤35% we recommend activation of the ESCAPE pathway for sudden cardiac death prevention[9] and to consider ICD placement if EF ≤35% at 40 days post-MI. Also, we recommend managing heart failure according to our heart failure pathway.[15]

If EF >35% we recommend following our PAIN pathway for the management of ACS[10] including the following:

– Lifestyle modification
– Cardiac rehabilitation
– Secondary prevention medication (aspirin, clopidogrel or prasugrel, β-blocker, high dose statin, ACE inhibitor/ARB)

REFERENCES

1. Lloyd-Jones D, Adams R, Carnethon M, et al. Heart disease and stroke statistics—2009 update: a report from the American Heart Association Statistics Committee and Stroke Statistics Subcommittee. *Circulation.* 2009;119:e21–e181.
2. Bernard SA, Morley PT, Hoek TL, et al. Treatment of comatose survivors from out-of-hospital cardiac arrest with induced hypothermia. *N Engl J Med.* 2002;346:557–563.
3. The Hypothermia after Cardiac Arrest Study Group. Mild hypothermia to improve the neurological outcome after cardiac arrest. *N Engl J Med.* 2002;346:549–556.
4. Nolan JP, Morley PT, Hoek TL, et al. Advancement Life Support Task Force of the International Liaison Committee on Resuscitation: therapeutic hypothermia after cardiac arrest: an advisory statement by the Advancement Life Support Task Force of the International Liaison Committee on Resuscitation. *Resuscitation.* 2003;57:231–235.
5. American Heart Association. Part 7.5: postresuscitation care. *Circulation.* 2005;112(suppl I):IV84–IV88.
6. Bernard SA. Therapeutic hypothermia after cardiac arrest. *Neurol Clin.* 2006;24:61–71.
7. Kupchik LK. Development and implementation of a therapeutic hypothermia protocol. *Crit Care Med.* 2009;37(7):S279–S284.
8. Herzog E, Shapiro J, Aziz EF, et al. Pathway for the management of survivors of out-of-hospital cardiac arrest. *Crit Pathw Cardiol.* 2010;9(2):49–54.
9. Herzog E, Aziz EF, Kukin M, et al. Novel pathway for sudden cardiac death prevention. *Crit Pathw Cardiol.* 2009;8:1–6.
10. Herzog E, Aziz E, Hong M. The PAIN pathway for the management of acute coronary syndrome. In: Herzog E, Hong M, eds. *Acute Coronary Syndrome: Multidisciplinary and Pathway-Based Approached.* New York, NY: Springer-Verlag London Limited; 2008:9–19.
11. Holzer M, Mullner M, Sterz F, et al. Efficacy and safety of endovascular cooling after cardiac arrest: cohort study and Bayesian approach. *Stroke.* 2006;37:1792–1797.
12. Feuchtl A, Lawrenz T, Bartelsmeier M, et al. Endovascular cooling improves neurological short-term outcome after prehospital cardiac arrest. *Intensive Care Med.* 2007;44:37–42.
13. Herzog E, Aziz E, Croiter S, et al. Pathway for the management of hyperglycemia in critical care units. *Crit Pathw Cardiol.* 2006;5:114–120.
14. Thenayan EA, Savard M, Sharpe M, et al. Predictors of poor neurologic outcome after induced mild hypothermia following cardiac arrest. *Neurology.* 2008;71:1535–1537.
15. Herzog E, Varley C, Kukin M. Pathway for the management of acute heart failure. *Crit Pathw Cardiol.* 2005;4:37–42.

PATIENT AND FAMILY INFORMATION FOR:

Survivors of Out-of-Hospital Cardiac Arrest, Including Therapeutic Hypothermia

Heart disease is the leading cause of death in the United States accounting for one-third of all deaths in the United States. Cardiac arrest is sudden loss of heart function in a person who may or may not have been previously diagnosed with heart disease. When cardiac arrest occurs outside the hospital it is referred to as Out of Hospital Cardiac Arrest (OHCA). The estimated number of OHCA cases is approximately 300,000 per year in the United States. Cardiac arrest occurs when the electrical system of the heart malfunctions leading to abnormal heart rhythms called *arrhythmias*. The two commonest arrhythmias that cause cardiac arrest are ventricular fibrillation (VF) and ventricular tachycardia (VT). In both VF and VT the lower chambers of the heart beat chaotically and cannot effectively pump blood to the organs including, and most important, the brain. Without blood flow to the brain, death will occur within minutes after the heart stops pumping. Cardiac arrest may be reversed if CPR is initiated immediately, and a device called a defibrillator is used to electrically shock the heart back to a normal rhythm. Even when cardiac arrest is reversed, and a normal heart rhythm is restored, many individuals who suffer cardiac arrest are left with irreversible brain damage. Less than 1 in 10 patients who suffer OHCA survives to be discharged from the hospital, and those who survive are often left with considerable brain damage and permanent disability. Effective CPR by either a bystander or a trained medical professional and early treatment with a defibrillator can minimize the amount of brain damage and increase the chance of survival.

Two important trials, published together in 2002, demonstrated that the use of a technique called "therapeutic hypothermia" after cardiac arrest can minimize brain damage and increase the likelihood of survival without significant disability. Based on these studies the International Liason Committee on Resuscitation and the American Heart Association recommend the use of therapeutic hypothermia after cardiac arrest.

Therapeutic hypothermia involves cooling the patient's body temperature from normal temperature (approximately 37°C, or 98.6°F) to a temperature between 32°C and 34°C (89.6°F and 93.2°F). This technique minimizes damage to brain cells by limiting a complicated inflammatory process that occurs in the brain after cardiac arrest. Because there are risks involved with therapeutic hypothermia, patients must be carefully selected to include only those in whom the benefit outweighs the risk. A collaborative team approach involving physicians and nurses is critical for successful implementation of this technique.

In this chapter we describe our pathway for the comprehensive management of survivors of OHCA. This pathway is limited to OHCA and does not include in-hospital cardiac arrest.

PATHWAY DESCRIPTION

The Pathway is divided into three steps.

Step I. Initial assessment and stabilization of the patient in the Emergency Department (ED). A plan of care is decided upon by a designated team of physicians, including whether to perform cardiac catheterization and whether to initiate therapeutic hypothermia.

Step II. Management of the patient in the critical care unit including implementation of the hypothermia protocol.

Step III. Management of the patient following completion of the hypothermia protocol. This begins with an evaluation of brain function and the likelihood of recovery, followed by recommendations for further therapy and, if necessary, evaluation by the ethics committee to assist in defining goals of care.

STEP I

Initial evaluation and treatment of a survivor of out of hospital cardiac arrest. The initial evaluation of a survivor of OHCA upon arrival to the ED includes vital signs, physical examination, and a standard assessment of brain function called the Glasgow coma score. An EKG is obtained immediately and laboratory testing is performed. Initial laboratory testing includes basic tests of kidney, liver, and thyroid function as well as blood count and chemical markers of heart muscle damage called cardiac biomarkers. If there is a suspicion of a stroke or bleeding in the brain a special type of X-ray of the head called a CT scan may be performed.

Although the initial evaluation is ongoing, steps are taken to stabilize the patient's condition. Virtually all patients who suffer a cardiac arrest are temporarily unable to breathe on their own and require support with a mechanical ventilator.

Many will require medications to maintain a normal blood pressure and to prevent any further abnormal heart rhythms.

Once the patient's condition is stable, a decision is made regarding therapeutic hypothermia. If the patient meets criteria for entry in our hypothermia protocol, then therapeutic hypothermia is initiated in the ED by infusion of cold saline through an IV catheter. The criteria for entry into the hypothermia protocol will be discussed in detail in the next section. These criteria are designed to ensure that only patients in whom the benefits of the therapy outweigh the risks are included in the protocol. The decision whether to initiate therapeutic hypothermia is made jointly by the ED physician and the cardiology or critical care physician.

Cardiac arrest may occur as a primary abnormality of the heart's electrical system but more often occurs in the setting of a heart attack. A heart attack is caused by a severe narrowing or complete blockage of one or more of the major coronary arteries—the blood vessels that deliver blood to the heart. In the case of a cardiac arrest that is caused by a heart attack, the patient must undergo an emergent procedure called a cardiac catheterization and possible angioplasty to open the blocked vessel.

Therefore, if the initial cardiac arrest was caused by VF or VT, or the EKG is suggestive of a heart attack, the patient is transferred immediately to the cardiac catheterization laboratory, where a cardiac catheterization is performed. Explanations of the catheterization procedure, angioplasty, and the management of a heart attack are provided in detail in Chapters 1 to 4. After completion of the cardiac catheterization the patient is transferred to the cardiac care unit (CCU).

If neither of above criteria is met, the patient is transferred directly to the CCU where an emergency echocardiogram is performed. An echocardiogram is an ultrasound of the heart that provides the physician with essential information regarding the structure and function of the heart muscle and heart valves. This is described in more detail in Chapter 5.

If the cardiac arrest is deemed not to be a primary malfunction of the heart but a consequence of serious medical illness, the patient is transferred to the medical intensive care unit for further care.

In the critical care unit therapeutic hypothermia is continued with initiation of the invasive hypothermia protocol.

STEP II

Induced invasive therapeutic hypothermia protocol in the critical care unit. The induced invasive hypothermia protocol begins when the patient arrives in the cardiac or medical critical care unit. The term invasive simply refers to the method of cooling that involves placement of a specialized catheter in a large vein in the leg called the femoral vein. This technique will be discussed in more detail later in this chapter. The physicians review the case and confirm that therapeutic hypothermia is appropriate. We recommend therapeutic hypothermia for patients older than 18 years of age who have suffered a cardiac arrest and remain in a coma. A coma is a deep state of unconsciousness. Patients who are in a coma cannot be awakened, do not respond normally to stimulation such as light, sound, and pain,

and do not make any voluntary movements. Patients excluded from the hypothermia protocol include those who are awake, have a severe or a terminal medical illness, or who suffered a prolonged period from the onset of cardiac arrest until the heart could be shocked back to a normal rhythm.

The hypothermia protocol is divided into three phases.

Phase 1: Invasive cooling phase for the first 24 hours
Phase 2: Rewarming phase and
Phase 3: Maintenance phase

Phase 1: Invasive cooling phase for the first 24 hours. Controlled cooling of the core body temperature is achieved by means of a catheter that is placed in the femoral vein. The catheter is attached to a specialized cooling system that is designed to continuously measure core body temperature and adjust the rate of cooling accordingly. This controlled method of cooling has proven to be safe and effective. Based on the available evidence from the two trials mentioned earlier we recommend cooling the patient to 33°C (91.4°F). At this temperature the patient receives the protective benefit of hypothermia with minimal side effects.

Patient monitoring and potential side effects of the hypothermia protocol.

Although major side effects are rare, there are a number of potential complications that can occur in patients being treated with therapeutic hypothermia. The most common effects of hypothermia include the following:

1. *Elevated blood pressure.* Cooling can cause increased blood pressure and decreased heart function. For this reason we recommend continuous monitoring and hourly documentation of many important clinical markers including, but not limited to, temperature, heart rhythm, blood pressure, and heart rate.

2. *Infection.* Cooling can weaken immune system function by interfering with normal white blood cell production and function. This can lead to an increased risk of infection. The risk of infection is further increased by the many emergent procedures that must be performed in any patient who suffers a cardiac arrest. Therefore, as part of our protocol, blood cultures and white blood cell counts are checked to help identify early signs of infection. Preventive measures are taken to minimize the risk of infection and antibiotics are administered when necessary.

3. *Blood electrolytes abnormalities.* Cooling can cause abnormalities of blood electrolytes especially potassium and magnesium. During the hypothermia protocol electrolyte levels are monitored every 4 hours and imbalances are corrected appropriately.

4. *Elevated blood sugar.* Cooling can cause abnormally elevated blood sugars. We control blood sugar levels using an insulin infusion protocol that we have developed for the management of elevated blood sugar in the critical care unit. Our protocol is described in detail in Chapter 32.

5. *Shivering.* Shivering can increase body temperature and interfere with cooling. Our protocol aims to prevent shivering by administration of medications that temporarily

paralyze muscle function. The patient is well sedated with medications and will not experience any discomfort from the muscle paralysis.

Phase 2: Rewarming phase. After keeping the patient at a body temperature of 33°C (91.4°F) for 24 hours we begin rewarming. To ensure patient safety we rewarm the patient in a controlled fashion at a slow rate of 0.25°C per hour. It should take 16 hours to raise the patient's body temperature back to normal (37°C or 98.6°F). The commonest side effects of rewarming include a drop in blood pressure and imbalances of blood electrolytes. The patient is carefully monitored during the rewarming phase to avoid these complications.

Phase 3: Maintenance of normal body temperature. The maintenance phase is the last stage of our hypothermia protocol. It is common for patients to develop fever after suffering a cardiac arrest. This can be owing to infection, medications, or damage to the part of the brain that regulates body temperature. Increased body temperature during the recovery period after a cardiac arrest can be particularly dangerous as it may worsen brain damage. We recommend using the cooling device to maintain a normal body temperature for at least an additional 24 hours after the rewarming stage is complete.

STEP III

Neurologic evaluation to determine long-term prognosis after completion of the hypothermia protocol. Once the hypothermia protocol is complete, it is important to perform a thorough neurologic evaluation—an evaluation of the patient's brain function to determine the likelihood of recovery. This evaluation is performed by a neurologist, a physician who specializes in brain function, and is generally performed approximately 72 hours after the cardiac arrest. Because some of the medications administered during the hypothermia protocol may interfere with the neurologic evaluation, it is often necessary to repeat the evaluation at a later time before making a final decision regarding prognosis.

If the brain damage is severe and it is likely that the patient will either remain in a coma or be left with permanent, severe disability we recommend involving the hospital's ethics committee. The Ethics Committee will meet with the physicians caring for the patient and the patient's family members to help decide on a plan of care. In this situation life support is often withdrawn, and aggressive measures are often limited, to maximize patient comfort.

If the prognosis is favorable and the patient is likely to recover without significant disability the next step is to determine whether the patient qualifies for an implantable cardioverter-defibrillator (ICD). An ICD is a small device similar in size to a pacemaker that is implanted under the skin during a minor surgical procedure. The ICD is programmed to recognize abnormal heart rhythms that can lead to cardiac arrest and restore the heart rhythm to normal by delivering a small electric shock. ICDs have been proven to save lives in patients who are at risk for cardiac arrest.

The decision whether to implant an ICD is complicated and will be made in agreement with an electrophysiologist, a cardiologist who specializes in pacemakers and abnormal heart rhythms. The decision depends largely on whether the patient is considered to be at risk for another cardiac arrest. The electophysiologist will consider the cause of the initial cardiac arrest as well as the heart muscle function as measured by echocardiogram in assessing the patient's risk of another cardiac arrest.

It is common for patients who recover from a cardiac arrest, especially when the cardiac arrest was caused by a heart attack, to be left with a weak heart that can no longer pump blood at full capacity. A weak heart can lead to congestive heart failure. There are many effective medications and therapies for the treatment of congestive heart failure. We recommend treatment according to our heart failure pathway outlined in Chapter 9.

CONCLUSION

Until recently, victims of OHCA seldom survived and most of those who did survive were left with severe, permanent disability. Only a small percentage of cardiac arrest survivors were able to recover normal brain function and return to live a normal life. Advances in the management of cardiac arrest, particularly the use of therapeutic hypothermia, have greatly improved the likelihood of survival without significant disability. We have described our protocol for the comprehensive management of OHCA. Implementation of protocols such as ours, and familiarity with the use of therapeutic hypothermia, provides victims of cardiac arrest with a much improved chance of a meaningful survival.

Eric M. Bader
Edgar Argulian
Eyal Herzog
Emad F. Aziz

CHAPTER 21

Procedures to Treat Arrhythmias in the Cardiac Care Unit

Cardiac arrhythmias are among the most common conditions encountered in the cardiac care unit (CCU). The confluence of technology, personnel, and expertise that the CCU provides makes it the ideal location to address these challenging states. Essential to the care of the critically ill cardiac patient is the constant monitoring of the patient's rhythm and vital signs, including blood pressure, respiration, and oxygenation. Symptomatic cardiac arrhythmias can be divided into bradycardias, where the native heart rate is insufficient to maintain an adequate cardiac output, and tachycardias, where the heart rate is accelerated or disorganized to the degree that the heart no longer functions as an effective pump. Either of these conditions can manifest clinically as heart failure, chest pain, dyspnea, dizziness or altered state of consciousness, hypotension, and pulmonary or peripheral edema.

The bradyarrhythmias include sinus bradycardia when, due to extrinsic or intrinsic reasons, the sinus node is chronotropically impaired. In other instances, the sinus node is intact, but there is a clinically significant interruption in the intracardiac conduction pathways. These include high-grade second-degree heart block (Mobitz type II) as well as third-degree (complete) heart block. Lower grade heart blocks, such as second-degree Mobitz type I (Wenckebach) and bundle branch blocks typically do not require acute intervention. Tachyarrhythmias can be divided into supraventricular and ventricular tachycardias (SVTs and VTs). SVTs are described in Chapter 16 and include atrial tachycardia, atrial fibrillation, and atrial flutter. VTs range from premature ventricular complexes, which typically do not require intervention, to ventricular fibrillation (VF), which is a medical emergency.

Many of the procedures to treat arrhythmias in the CCU require sedation that ensures patient comfort and can impact the success of the procedure. The desired degree of sedation, known as procedural or conscious sedation, should be provided by a health care practitioner who is certified in conscious sedation. Choice of medication should include careful consideration of the medication's side effects, time of onset, and half-life.

MANAGEMENT OF BRADYCARDIA WITH TEMPORARY PACING

Bradycardia in the critically ill patient becomes clinically significant when the cardiac output, as determined by the heart rate and the stroke volume, falls below that required to meet the body's metabolic demand. Once this occurs, temporary pacing may be required to increase the heart rate and correspondingly the patient's cardiac output. Temporary pacing is considered a temporizing measure until the patient recovers from the acute insult or is able to have a permanent pacemaker implanted. Temporary pacing can be carried out through a transcutaneous pacing or by means of temporary pacing wires.

TRANSCUTANEOUS PACING

Transcutaneous pacing[1] utilizes large cutaneous pads that pace the heart in a noninvasive manner. These pads are composed of an adhesive backing and a metallic plate, which is faced with a saline-based conductive gel. This method of pacing has the advantage of its ease of application and availability as a backup.

The noninvasive nature of this modality reduces the risk of complications associated with the more invasive pacing methods.[2] This is achieved, however, at the expense of patient comfort and a lower rate of capture. When properly applied, capture rates of up to 90% can be expected in the range of output typically provided by today's external defibrillator/pacing units. This electrical current, however, can also lead to painful stimulation of chest wall skeletal muscle requiring significant levels of analgesia and sedation for prolonged pacing durations.

Preprocedure preparation: The following are required:

- External defibrillator/pacer unit
- Pacer pads
- Adequate sedation and analgesia.

Procedure: The pads should be placed according to the individual manufacturer's instructions. Successful capture of external pacing impulses is dependent on proper placement of the pacing pads.[3] The choice of electrical output, typically between 10 and 200 mA, depends on the energy required for myocardial electrical capture. Unlike transvenous pacing, the EKG is not helpful in determining capture in transcutaneously paced patients, as the artifact from the long-duration pacing impulse can obscure the EKG. Instead, capture is determined by manual palpation of the pulse and other hemodynamic measurement.

Postprocedure: Continuous monitoring is essential to confirm continued capture, as well as to assess the patient's respiratory rate, level of sedation, and pain. At this time, serious consideration should be given to the next step in the treatment plan, including temporary and permanent transvenous pacing.

TEMPORARY TRANSVENOUS PACING

Transvenous pacing is an effective method for augmenting heart rate.[4,5] This method of pacing is more reliable than transcutaneous pacing but is not immune from problems like catheter migration, bleeding, infection, and perforation of the right ventricular (RV) free wall, which can lead to hemopericardium and tamponade.[6]

Table 21.1 outlines the class I indications for transvenous pacing.[7]

TABLE 21.1	Class I Indications for the Placement of Emergent Transvenous Pacemaker

BRADYARRHYTHMIAS
- Sinus node dysfunction
  - Sinus bradycardia
  - Sinus arrest
- High-degree atrioventricular (AV) block
  - Second-degree AV block, Mobitz type II
  - Third-degree AV block
  - Drug overdose
    - Intentional
    - Unintentional

TACHYARRHYTHMIAS
- Prevention by means of overdrive pacing

Preprocedure preparation: The following are required:

- 12-lead EKG machine
- Portable ultrasound
- Introducer sheath and central line kit (Figure 21.1)
- Sedation: As the level of discomfort experienced during this procedure is not comparable with transcutaneous pacing, sedation is rarely required. It may, however, be helpful at times to administer low doses of anxiolytics to ensure patient comfort.
- Pacing wire kit
- Generator box (Figure 21.2)
- Choice of access site: The right internal jugular (IJ) vein when accessed under direct ultrasound visualization is the preferred method of access. This location allows for the greatest combination of safety and long-term stability of the access point, with acceptably low rates of infection and catheter dislodgement. In addition, the use of the right IJ leaves the left subclavian vein available for the placement of a permanent pacing device should that be needed. The right IJ is followed in order of preference by the left subclavian vein, which is a relatively stable location but carries a higher rate of complications like pneumothorax. The right femoral vein is considered the safest access site. It is easily controlled in the event of a problem with the introducer sheath, but it carries the disadvantage of the highest rate of site infection and catheter dislodgment. It is advised to obtain an access in advance as temporary pacing may be required emergently. It is prudent in patients in whom you suspect that an emergency condition may require pacing support to place the introducer sheath in advance. Care should be exercised to ensure that the hub of the sheath remains sterile.

Procedure: Once the access site is chosen, the patient is prepped in a sterile fashion. A large drape should be used to provide an adequate sterile field.

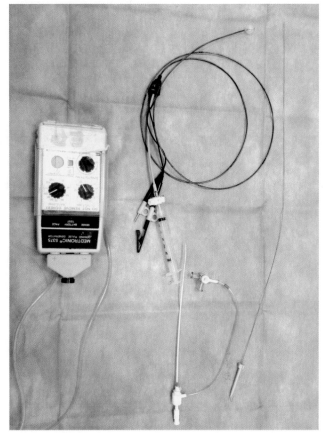

Figure 21.1. Four French introducer and transvenous pacing wire kit. (Note distal balloon inflated with provided syringe.)

1. IJ VENOUS CANNULATION[8] is guided by three anatomic landmarks: the two heads of the sternocleidomastoid muscle (SCM), the upper margin of the clavicle, and the midclavicular notch. After infiltrating the area with a small gauge needle, the IJ artery is palpated as it runs between the heads of the SCM. The artery is retracted medially, and if a sterile "site-finder" is available, the vein is accessed with an 18G needle at a 30° angle with the needle pointed toward the ipsilateral nipple. If no ultra-

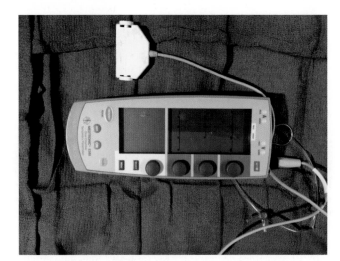

Figure 21.2. Typical external pacing generator box (dual chamber).

sound guidance is available, venous access is first achieved with a small finder needle and then repeated with a larger needle through which a J-tipped guidewire is advanced. The guidewire should then be advanced to about 20 cm with careful attention given to the cardiac monitor for ventricular ectopy. Should ventricular ectopic beats occur, the guidewire should be promptly withdrawn until the ectopy ceases. The dilator and sheath are then advanced over the wire. After placement of the sheath, the dilator and the guidewire are removed, blood is drawn out of the side port, and the sheath is flushed and sutured in place.

2. SUBCLAVIAN ACCESS[9] is obtained at the junction of the medial and mid–one-third of the clavicle. After preparing and sterilizing the area, a narrow gauge needle is used to infiltrate the area with local anesthetic. The 18G needle is then introduced immediately below the clavicle at a 35° angle pointing toward the midclavicular notch with the needle bevel facing caudally. Once behind the clavicle, the shaft of the needle should be positioned horizontal, parallel to the patient's body, as the needle advanced further toward the midclavicular notch. When venous return is obtained, a J-tipped guidewire is advanced to 25 cm with careful attention to the cardiac monitor for ventricular ectopy as discussed earlier. The needle is then removed, a small nick is made over the guidewire, and a dilator is advanced over the wire until blood appears in the hub of the dilator. The dilator is then removed and inserted into the introducer sheath, and the dilator and sheath are advanced over the wire. After placement of the sheath, the dilator and guidewire are removed, blood is drawn out of the side port, and the sheath is flushed and sutured in place.

3. FEMORAL VENOUS ACCESS[10] is obtained by directing an 18G needle 2 cm medial to the palpated femoral pulse at a point 4 cm below an imaginary line connecting the anterior superior iliac crest and the pubic symphysis. The needle should point toward the umbilicus and be at a 45° angle to the surface of the groin. After accessing the vein, a J-tipped guidewire is advanced to 25 cm. The sheath is placed in the same technique as described earlier. Of note, when femoral vein access is used, the pacing catheter must be advanced under fluoroscopic guidance.

POSITIONING OF TEMPORARY TRANSVENOUS PACING

When available, direct visualization using fluoroscopy provides an added level of security when placing balloon tipped pacing catheters. While maintaining sterile conditions, a pacing catheter is introduced through the sheath. The catheter should be oriented to take advantage of its natural curvature in transitioning from the right atrium to the RV. Once clear of the sheath, the balloon is inflated with the supplied syringe. The distal (negative) lead is attached by means of an alligator clip to lead V_1 on the 12-lead EKG; this provides a unipolar intracardiac electrogram that can be used to monitor the advancement of the pacer wire through the vena cava, right atrium, and RV.[11] The rest of the EKG leads should be applied to the chest in the usual fashion. The catheter is carefully advanced, monitoring its progress with the EKG and fluoroscopy (if available). When the EKG indicates that the catheter

has transitioned from the right atrium to the RV, the balloon should be deflated and the catheter should be advanced until the intracardiac EKG shows a current of injury, ST-segment elevation, which implies that the catheter is in contact with the ventricular myocardium.[12] Once in position, the collar around the introducer sheath is tightened to secure the catheter in place. Most kits provide a sterile sleeve to keep the pacing catheter sterile. The catheter is then disconnected from the EKG machine, and both poles are attached to the pacing generator, which is then set to maximum output with a rate of 60 beats per minute in an asynchronous pacing mode. If appropriately positioned, each pacing spike should result in a corresponding ventricular depolarization with left bundle branch block morphology.

Postprocedure: Postprocedure verification of appropriate wire placement is accomplished by means of chest x-ray as well as EKG verification of capture. A portable anteroposterior chest x-ray will confirm the catheter tip position aspect of the cardiac silhouette slightly to the left of the spine. Appropriate placement will manifest on the EKG as a left bundle branch block, with negative QRS complexes across the precordium. It is very important to look for pneumothorax and hemopericardium on chest x-ray.

Once capture has been demonstrated, the pacing threshold, or minimum current required to cause cardiac depolarization, measured in milliamperes, is evaluated.[13] This is done by setting the pacemaker at least 10 beats per minute faster than the intrinsic heart rate with the generator output set at the maximum amperage. The output is then incrementally decreased while monitoring the EKG until loss of ventricular capture occurs. The pacing threshold is the last setting at which all pacing impulses are captured. The generator output is then set at three times the threshold. A sudden increase in threshold or failure to capture could be the result of insufficient energy delivered by a pacer; low pacemaker battery; dislodged, loose, or fractured electrode; and electrolyte abnormalities (acidosis, hypoxemia, hypokalemia), which requires immediate evaluation.

The sensing threshold, measured in millivolts, is the pacemaker's ability to detect the native heart rate and is evaluated when the pacemaker is being used for synchronous pacing or as a backup. This is tested by setting the rate below that of the intrinsic rhythm and adjusting the sensitivity to the highest setting. The highest sensitivity setting has the lowest number value as it is sensing the smallest impulses. The sensitivity is then decreased until the pacemaker begins to fire irrespective of the intrinsic rhythm. The last value at which the pacemaker is completely inhibited is known as the sensing threshold. The pacemaker should then be set at sensitivity slightly greater than the threshold. Setting the threshold to high will result in oversensing of T-waves and inappropriate inhibition of the pacemaker function. Typically, a temporary single-chamber pacemaker will be set to pace the ventricle, sense the ventricle, and inhibit when a native beat is sensed. This mode is commonly referred to as VVI.

Table 21.2 outlines the nomenclature for the classification of pacemaker function as established by the North American Society of Pacing and Electrophysiology and British Pacing and Electrophysiology Group.

Complication rates that are encountered during temporary pacer placement are thought to be relatively high and range

TABLE 21.2	Classification of Pacemaker Function			
Position I—Chamber Paced	*Position II—Chamber Sensed*	*Position III—Response to Sensing*	*Position IV—Rate Modulation, Programmability*	*Position V—Antitachycardia*
A = Atrium	A = Atrium	T = Triggered	P = Simple	P = Pacing
V = Ventricle	V = Ventricle	I = Inhibited	M = Multi programmable	S = Shock
D = Dual	D = Dual	D = Dual	R = Rate adaptive	D = Dual
O = None	O = None	O = None	C = Communicating	
			O = None	

Adapted from Bernstein AD, Daubert JC, Fletcher RD, et al. The revised NASPE/BPEG generic code for antibradycardia, adaptive-rate, and multisite pacing. North American Society of Pacing and Electrophysiology/British Pacing and Electrophysiology Group. *Pacing Clin Electrophysiol.* 2002;25(2):260.

between 23% and 32%.[6,14-16] Among these complications are failure to secure venous access; failure to place the lead correctly; sepsis; puncture of arteries, lungs, or myocardium; and life-threatening arrhythmias (VT, VF).

MANAGEMENT OF TACHYARRHYTHMIA WITH CARDIOVERSION

SUPRAVENTRICULAR TACHYARRHYTHMIA

Supraventricular tachyarrhythmias (SVTs) include paroxysmal SVTs (atrioventricular node reentrant tachycardia, atrioventricular reentrant tachycardia, and atrial tachycardia), atrial fibrillation, and atrial flutter. Although the treatment for these conditions often involves advanced therapies such as radiofrequency ablation, the presence of a sustained arrhythmia and a hemodynamically unstable patient may require urgent cardioversion in the acute setting.

There are certain conditions in which cardioversion is less successful. These include thyroid storm and pulmonary embolism where the underlying condition creates an arrhythmogenic milieu. Patients with these conditions who are cardioverted may revert back to their unstable rhythm unless the underlying disease state is addressed.

Direct current cardioversion. The most important aspect of direct current (DC) cardioversion[17,18] of the hemodynamically unstable patient is the concept of synchrony. Synchronization ensures that the shock is delivered at the optimal point in the cardiac cycle corresponding to the R wave on the surface EKG. A shock delivered at the wrong time, during the T-wave, when the ventricle is refractory, can cause the patient to develop VF.

Early defibrillators delivered a monophasic DC impulse to simultaneously repolarize the entire myocardium. Although effective, these monophasic defibrillators required higher energy to achieve cardioversion. This could potentially cause myocardial stunning, conduction block, and surface damage to the patient. Newer rectilinear biphasic defibrillators that use DC and reverse polarity in mid discharge are more efficacious and require less energy with fewer adverse effects.[19,20]

Preprocedure: The following are required:

- Defibrillator
- Pads
- 12-lead ECG
- Sedation medications
- Code cart

If time and the patient's hemodynamic condition permit, adequate sedation and analgesia[21] should be administered before cardioversion.

In nonemergent atrial fibrillation or flutter, a transesophageal echocardiogram (TEE) should be obtained to exclude the possibility of an intracardiac thrombus, particularly in the left atrial appendage. A thrombus dislodged during cardioversion can lead to stroke, ischemic bowel, or a peripheral embolism.[22,23]

Adequate staff and a code cart should be available during the procedure.

Procedure: When possible, the patient should be appropriately sedated, while maintaining an adequate airway. Owing to the expectation that convulsion will accompany the delivery of shock, care must be taken to ensure that the patient has adequate space for possible uncontrolled limb movement. The defibrillator is set to its defibrillation function

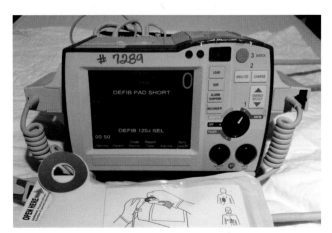

Figure 21.3. Typical external monitor/defibrillator.

and is placed in synchronized mode (Figure 21.3). The display should indicate that it is recognizing the presence of the QRS complex. The quality of the contact between the defibrillator pads and the chest wall is critical for successful defibrillation with minimizing trauma to the patient. In male patients, the chest should ideally be shaved to improve contact with the pads. When choosing the defibrillator output, consideration is given to the underlying rhythm. Atrial flutter/tachycardia typically requires 50 J, whereas atrial fibrillation requires 150 J. Many CCU physicians choose to start at the maximum output of 200 J to ensure success while minimizing the number of shocks. After ensuring that no one is in contact with the bed and confirming that the defibrillator is in synchronous mode, the Shock button is pressed. As the defibrillator requires several cycles to synchronize with the rhythm, the button should be held until the shock is delivered.

Postprocedure: Postcardioversion close monitoring is required to assess the cardiac rhythm for the possibilities of sinus arrest, recurrence of the original arrhythmia as well as prolongation of the Q-T interval.[24] The patient's skin should be inspected for burns and infection.[25] Cardioversion is not considered complete until the patient recovers from the sedation and his or her heart rate, respiration, blood pressure and pulse oximetry returns to baseline.

VENTRICULAR TACHYARRHYTHMIA

Ventricular tachyarrhythmias include VT and VF. Within the sustained hemodynamically significant VTs, one must differentiate between pulseless VT, which is treated with defibrillation, and VT with retained pulse for which the treatment is synchronized DC cardioversion.

The procedure for cardioversion of VT with a pulse is identical to that of a SVT, outlined earlier with the exception that output of the defibrillator is set at 200 J.

DEFIBRILLATION FOR PULSELESS VT/VF

Preprocedure: The following are required:

- Defibrillator
- Pads
- 12-lead EKG machine

Per Advanced Cardiac Life Support (ACLS) guidelines, the main goal of therapy in pulseless VT/VF is early defibrillation. To this end, cardiopulmonary resuscitation should be initiated as per ACLS protocol.[26]

Procedure: The procedure for defibrillation for pulseless VT/VF is identical to that of VT with a pulse, which outlined earlier, except that the defibrillator is not set to a synchronization mode.

Postprocedure: After restoration of organized cardiac electrical activity and a pulse, the patient requires close rhythm and hemodynamic monitoring.

REFERENCES

1. Syverud SA, Dalsey WC, Hedges JR. Transcutaneous and transvenous cardiac pacing for early bradyasystolic cardiac arrest. *Ann Emerg Med.* 1986;15(2):121–124. Epub 1986 Feb 01.
2. Peters RW. Temporary transcutaneous pacing. New indications for an old technique. *AORN J.* 1986;44(2):245–246, 8–9. Epub 1986 Aug 01.
3. Craig K. How to provide transcutaneous pacing. *Nursing.* 2006;36(suppl Cardiac):22–3. Epub 2006 Apr 28.
4. Lang R, David D, Klein HO, et al. The use of the balloon-tipped floating catheter in temporary transvenous cardiac pacing. *Pacing Clin Electrophysiol.* 1981;4(5):491–496. Epub 1981 Sept 01.
5. Jowett NI, Thompson DR, Pohl JE. Temporary transvenous cardiac pacing: 6 years experience in one coronary care unit. *Postgrad Med J.* 1989;65(762):211–215. Epub 1989 Apr 01.
6. Chin K, Singham KT, Anuar M. Complications of temporary transvenous pacing. *Med J Malaysia.* 1985;40(1):28–30. Epub 1985 Mar 01.
7. Chin K, Singham KT, Masduki A. Indications of temporary transvenous pacing. *Med J Malaysia.* 1984;39(2):139–1342. Epub 1984 Jun 01.
8. Widmann WD, Mangiola S, Thomas L, et al. Percutaneous cannulation of the internal jugular vein for temporary endocardial pacing. *Cathet Cardiovasc Diagn.* 1975;1(2):233–245. Epub 1975 Jan 01.
9. Evans DW, Clarke M. Temporary cardiac pacing using the subclavian vein. *BMJ.* 1970;4(5736):680. Epub 1970 Dec 12.
10. Weinstein J, Gnoj J, Mazzara JT, et al. Temporary transvenous pacing via the percutaneous femoral vein approach. A prospective study of 100 cases. *Am Heart J.* 1973;85(5):695–705. Epub 1973 May 01.
11. Goldberger J, Kruse J, Ehlert FA, et al. Temporary transvenous pacemaker placement: what criteria constitute an adequate pacing site? *Am Heart J.* 1993;126(2):488–493. Epub 1993 Aug 01.
12. Gulotta SJ. Transvenous cardiac pacing. Technics for optimal electrode positioning and prevention of coronary sinus placement. *Circulation.* 1970;42(4):701–718. Epub 1970 Oct 01.
13. Furman S, Hurzeler P, Mehra R. Cardiac pacing and pacemakers IV. Threshold of cardiac stimulation. *Am Heart J.* 1977;94(1):115–124. Epub 1977 Jul 01.
14. Aliyev F, Celiker C, Turkoglu C, et al. Perforations of right heart chambers associated with electrophysiology catheters and temporary transvenous pacing leads. *Turk Kardiyol Dern Ars.* 2011;39(1):16–22. Epub 2011 Mar 02.
15. Murphy JJ. Problems with temporary cardiac pacing. Expecting trainees in medicine to perform transvenous pacing is no longer acceptable. *BMJ.* 2001;323(7312):527. Epub 2001 Sept 08.
16. Sharma S, Sandler B, Cristopoulos C, et al. Temporary transvenous pacing: endangered skill. *Emerg Med J.* 2011. Epub 2011 ahead of print Sept 08.
17. O'Bryan EC Jr, Howard LW Jr, Gazes PC. DC-cardioversion in the treatment of arrhythmias, with a special note on the use of the platinum electrode for diagnostic purposes. *J S C Med Assoc.* 1966;62(9):341–346. Epub 1966 Sept 01.
18. Das JP, Lakshmikanthan C, Munsi SC, et al. DC electrical cardioversion (a preliminary report). *Indian Heart J.* 1968;20(4):383–392. Epub 1968 Oct 01.
19. Watson JN, Addison PS, Uchaipichat N, et al. Wavelet transform analysis predicts outcome of DC cardioversion for atrial fibrillation patients. *Computers Biol Med.* 2007;37(4):517–523. Epub 2006 Oct 03.
20. Page RL, Kerber RE, Russell JK, et al. Biphasic versus monophasic shock waveform for conversion of atrial fibrillation: the results of an international randomized, double-blind multicenter trial. *J Am Coll Cardiol.* 2002;39(12):1956–1963. Epub 2002 Jun 27.
21. Mitchell AR, Chalil S, Boodhoo L, et al. Diazepam or midazolam for external DC cardioversion (the DORM Study). *Europace.* 2003;5(4):391–395. Epub 2004 Feb 03.
22. Caution urged in the use of DC cardioversion. *Br J Hosp Med.* 1991;46(6):366. Epub 1991 Dec 01.
23. Missault L, Jordaens L, Gheeraert P, et al. Embolic stroke after unanticoagulated cardioversion despite prior exclusion of atrial thrombi by transoesophageal echocardiography. *Eur Heart J.* 1994;15(9):1279–1280. Epub 1994 Sept 01.
24. Caldwell JC, Woolfson P, Clarke B, et al. Ventricular fibrillation following successful DC cardioversion for atrial fibrillation. *Pacing Clin Electrophysiol.* 2011. Epub 2011 ahead of print Jan 22.
25. Ambler JJ, Sado DM, Zideman DA, et al. The incidence and severity of cutaneous burns following external DC cardioversion. *Resuscitation.* 2004;61(3):281–288. Epub 2004 Jun 03.
26. Field JM, Hazinski MF, Sayre MR, et al. Part 1: executive summary: 2010 American Heart Association Guidelines for Cardiopulmonary Resuscitation and Emergency Cardiovascular Care. *Circulation.* 2010;122:S640–S656.

PATIENT AND FAMILY INFORMATION FOR:
Arrhythmias in the CCU

CARDIOVERSION

An electrical cardioversion is a procedure used to treat an abnormal heartbeat. The abnormal heartbeat is caused by a disturbance in the electrical activity within the heart. Electrical cardioversion involves placing electrically conductive pads that adhere to the patient's chest. These patches are attached to a machine called a defibrillator, which delivers a small current of electricity to the heart converting it to the normal rhythm. Before having the procedure, the patient is given medications for sedation. This sedation lasts for the duration of the procedure. Before the procedure, the physician examines the overall heart function as well as the function of other vital organs (liver, lungs, kidneys, etc.). Important lab work is checked, and any medications that interfere with the procedure are stopped.

The patient should neither eat nor drink for the 6 to 8 hours ("nothing per mouth") preceding the procedure to prevent nausea and vomiting.

In most cases, cardioversion is an elective or nonurgent procedure. At these times, everything is done to ensure patient safety and comfort. This includes the complete explanation of the procedure to the patient and family as well as the presence of an anesthesiologist to assist with sedation. At times, a TEE may be obtained to exclude the possibility of a clot within the heart, which if present may detach and lodge elsewhere in the body and may lead to devastating complications like stroke.

When the patient is very sick, it might be necessary to perform these procedures urgently. An anesthesiologist may not be available, and there may be no time for a TEE. The patient or family should understand the urgent nature of the procedure and the risk of withholding it.

DEFIBRILLATION

In cases of unstable blood pressure, and in an extreme situation, when the patient no longer has a pulse, cardioversion/defibrillation is a medical emergency and must be done with the minimum of possible delay. The loss of circulation frequently requires chest compressions to maintain blood flow until restoration of a normal heart rhythm.

The main side effects of cardioversion/defibrillation are local burns and irritation of the skin in the area on which the pads were placed. This can be minimized for male patients if time allows, by shaving the chest and treated with the application of topical lotions. It may be necessary to monitor the patient for a period of time after the shock, and in the case of atrial fibrillation, the use of blood thinners should be addressed.

TEMPORARY PACING

If the heart rate becomes too slow to meet the body's requirements, it may be necessary to increase the heart rate by means of temporary pacing. Temporary pacemakers are intended for short-term use during hospitalization. They come in two forms, noninvasive or external pacing and the more invasive transvenous pacing. Noninvasive pacing is accomplished by means of large adhesive electrical pads, which once attached to the patient's skin are used to stimulate the heart externally. Although this is effective, it is less reliable and more painful and is usually used as an emergency backup. Transvenous pacing, by means of a pacing wire that is placed through a large vein into the heart, is more reliable but involves the procedure of placing a wire into the heart. There are risks involved with this procedure, mainly bleeding, infection, a small tear in the heart muscle, and abnormal heart rhythms. These risks are minimized by placing the wire under sterile conditions and whenever possible using x-ray guidance. In this procedure, a large intravenous line or "sheath" is inserted into a large vein, commonly in the neck. Through this sheath, a flexible wire is passed to the right side of the heart. This wire is connected to an external pacemaker box. Usually, this procedure is fairly brief and is well tolerated. Once the pacing catheter is in place, the pacemaker must remain close to the patient at all times, and for this reason, the patient is advised not to leave their bed.

CHAPTER

22

Dan Halpern Balaji Pratap

Harikrishna Makani Emad Aziz

Edgar Argulian Eyal Herzog

Commonly Used Medications for the Treatment of Arrhythmias

The management of cardiac arrhythmias requires familiarity with both the arrhythmia mechanism and the available pharmacologic and device approaches. Rhythm disturbances are related to abnormalities in the electrical impulse generation or conduction at the ion channel level of the cardiac pacemaker cells (native or ectopic). The Advanced Cardiac Life Support (ACLS) protocols provide a basic approach to the management of life-threatening rhythm disturbances, but broader understanding is required for providing day-to-day patient care.[1,2] The aim of this chapter is to overview the main pharmacologic options that are available in the management of rhythm disturbances.

In general, arrhythmias are divided into two broad categories: tachyarrhythmias (heart rate >100 beats per minute [bpm]) and bradyarrhythmias (heart rate <60 bpm). Tachyarrhythmias are broadly categorized as either supraventricular or ventricular tachycardias. The three main pathophysiologic mechanisms that explain tachyarrhythmias are reentry, increased automaticity, and triggered activity. Bradyarrhythmias are classified according to the anatomic level of abnormality in the conduction system (sinus node, atrioventricular [AV] node, or His-Purkinje system). Knowledge of the mechanism of action and the target tissue specificity (sinus node, atrial, AV node, ventricular) for each medication is pivotal in the management of the specific arrhythmia.

The Vaughan Williams classification[3] of antiarrhythmic drugs designates four groups of drugs according to the predominant electrophysiologic mechanism of action:

Class I Sodium channel blockage and slowing of conduction velocity

    Ia—Quinidine, procainamide, and disopyramide

    Ib—Mexiletine, phenytoin, and lidocaine

    Ic—Flecainide and propafenone

Class II β-Adrenergic receptor blocking medications that decrease catecholaminergic effect (e.g., propranolol, metoprolol)

Class III Potassium channel blockage with prolongation of repolarization (e.g., sotalol, amiodarone, bretylium)

Class IV Calcium channel blockage with prolongation of conduction and refractory time (e.g., verapamil, diltiazem)

Of note, the classification does not account for the fact that some medications exhibit more than one mechanism of action (e.g., amiodarone blocks potassium, calcium, α- and β-adrenergic receptors). The classification also does not include several commonly used drugs such as atropine (muscarinic receptor blocker), adenosine (A1-receptor blocker), or digoxin (neurally mediated effects).

Treatment strategies in the management of rhythm disturbances depend on the patient's presentation including history and the ECG tracing of the arrhythmia (preferably compared with a previous tracing) as well as his/her hemodynamic status. An aggressive approach is mandated if the patient is hemodynamically unstable including ventricular pacing for bradyarrhythmias and direct current (DC) cardioversion for tachyarrhythmias in conjunction with pharmacologic therapy.

MEDICATIONS FOR THE TREATMENT OF BRADYARRHYTHMIAS

Bradyarrhythmias may arise from dysfunction in the initiation or conduction of an electrical impulse as well as an increase in parasympathetic tone. The dysfunction may originate at the level of the sinus node, AV node, or His-Purkinje system. Cardiac Care Unit (CCU)admissions for symptomatic bradycardia commonly include high-degree AV blocks requiring ventricular pacing as a result of inherent conduction system disease (commonly degenerative), ischemia, or drug effect (overdose or decreased elimination). Other etiologies that may lead to bradycardia include increased vagal tone (vasovagal, increased intracranial pressure), infective endocarditis involving the aortic valve, Lyme disease, and infiltrative diseases. The most common medications used for the treatment of bradyarrhythmias are outlined in Table 22.1. According to ACLS guidelines, atropine is the first-line agent used for symptomatic

TABLE 22.1	Medications for the Treatment of Bradyarrhythmias				
Medication	*Initial Dose*	*Maintenance Dose*	*Onset of Action*	*Half-Life*	*Acute Adverse Effects*
Atropine	0.5 mg every 3–5 min; maximum 3 mg	—	2–4 min	2–3 hr	Blurry vision, palpitations, arrhythmias
Isoproterenol	0.02–0.06 mg bolus	2–10 μg/min	1–2 min	Few minutes	Angina, palpitations, dyspnea

bradycardia with certain exceptions (e.g., infranodal AV block) when it may be ineffective or even harmful. In those situations, chronotropic agents or temporary pacing is advised.[4]

ATROPINE

Electrophysiologic actions: Atropine sulfate is an anticholinergic and parasympatholytic alkaloid agent that competitively antagonizes the muscarinic receptors. It is derived from the deadly nightshade plant (*Atropa belladonna*).

Pharmacokinetics: The onset of action after intravenous (IV) administration begins after 2 to 4 minutes and has a half-life of 2 to 3 hours. It is metabolized mainly in the liver and excreted in the urine.

Dosage: According to the ACLS guidelines,[1,2] doses are 0.5 mg every 3 to 5 minutes, up to a total of 3 mg or 0.04 mg per kg. Dosages of <0.5 mg may be associated with paradoxical bradycardia.

Indications: Atropine is indicated for the treatment of acute symptomatic bradycardia (class IIa, level of evidence B) when the dysfunction is suspected to arise from the sinus node or the AV node. Atropine use in the setting of infranodal block, manifested with a wide QRS complex (e.g., Mobitz II AV block), may paradoxically increase the degree of block. The increase of the firing rate in the AV node "strains" the conduction system distally and prevents transmission of impulses. Atropine was frequently used during cardiac resuscitation but had been removed from the ACLS 2010 guidelines because of the lack of evidence.[1,2] Heart transplant patients may not have any effect of the drug because of the lack of parasympathetic innervation.

Adverse effects: Anticholinergic side effects of atropine include flushing, dry mouth, decreased sweating, blurred vision, delirium, hallucination, as well as tachyarrhythmias.

Contraindication: Patients with glaucoma may develop acute angle closure glaucoma, and those with benign prostatic hypertrophy may develop urinary retention.

ISOPROTERENOL

Electrophysiologic actions: Isoproterenol is not a commonly used drug nowadays as it is mainly used as a chronotropic agent in the electrophysiology lab and the CCU setting. It acts on the β_1- and β_2-receptors, conveying chronotropic and inotropic effect. It may also cause peripheral vasodilatation because of β_2 effect.

Pharmacokinetics: The onset of action after IV administration begins after 1 to 2 minutes, has a half-life of 2.5 to 5 minutes, and is mainly metabolized by conjugation in the liver and lungs and excreted through the urine.

Dosage: Initial bolus of 0.02 to 0.06 mg, followed by continuous IV infusion, dose range: 2 to 10 μg per minute; titrate until response is achieved.

Indications: The drug is indicated for the treatment of bradyarrhythmias and refractory torsade de point VT storm (by decreasing the QT interval). The use of isoproterenol during cardiac resuscitation was replaced by epinephrine and dopamine.

Dopamine, epinephrine, and dobutamine are chronotropic agents that may be used to treat the bradyarrhythmias—they are discussed in length in Chapter 14.

MEDICATIONS FOR THE TREATMENT OF TACHYARRHYTHMIAS

SUPRAVENTRICULAR ARRHYTHMIAS

Supraventricular arrhythmias are discussed in detail in Chapter 16, and their main pharmacologic therapy is outlined in Table 22.2.

Atrial fibrillation and atrial flutter are managed with rhythm control or rate control, depending on the patient's hemodynamics.[5,6] Emergent synchronized cardioversion is required in hemodynamically unstable patients. Otherwise, pharmacologic or electrical cardioversions should be carried out after ruling out a left atrial appendage thrombus on transesophageal echocardiogram or after verifying that the patient had been on anticoagulation for at least 4 weeks or the symptoms lasted <48 hours. Medications that are commonly used for rate control are β-adrenergic receptor blocker, calcium channel blockers, and digoxin. Amiodarone may slow the heart rate but may also convert the rhythm to sinus. Digoxin does not have the negative inotropic properties seen in other medications and can be used in conges-

TABLE 22.2	Medications for the Treatment of Supraventricular Tachyarrhthmias

Medication	Bolus Dose	Maintenance Dose	Onset of Action	Half-Life	Acute Adverse Effects
Adenosine	6 mg followed by 12 mg if needed	–	seconds	10 s	Dyspnea, flushing, chest pressure
Digoxin	0.5 mg followed by 0.25 mg × 2 every 6 hr	0.125–0.25 mg/d	5–30 min	34–44 hr	Conduction abnormalities, dizziness, nausea
Diltiazem	15–20 mg over 2 min, second dose of 25 mg in 15 min if needed	5–15 mg/hr	2–3 min	2–11 hr	Hypotension, bradycardia, AV block
Verapamil	2.5–5 mg over 2 min, second dose of 5–10 mg in 15 min if needed	–	2 min	2–8 hr	Hypotension, bradycardia, dizziness
Esmolol	500 μ/kg bolus over 1 min, up to three boluses	50–200 μ/kg/min	1–2 min	5–23 min	Hypotension, diaphoresis
Metoprolol	2.5–5 mg every 2–5 min (maximum of 15 mg over 10–15 minutes)	–	20 min	3–8 hr	Hypotension, bradycardia, worsening of heart failure
Amiodarone	150 mg bolus over 10 min	1 mg/min for 6 hr, then 0.5 mg/min for 18 hr	3–7 hr	9–47 days	Hypotension, bradycardia, heart block

tive heart failure cases. Anticoagulation is warranted according to the CHADS2 stratification score or if the patient has been cardioverted. Pharmacologic cardioversions are mostly performed with amiodarone and ibutilide—both may be used in patients with systolic dysfunction. For patients with no structural heart disease, flecainide and propafenone can be used for chemical cardioversion.

Adenosine. Adenosine is the first-line drug to terminate reentry circuits involving the AV node and helps to diagnose supraventricular arrhythmias. The drug is an endogenous nucleoside with a very short half-life of 10 seconds that can transiently block the AV node and slow down the sinus node by activating potassium channels. It is given in incremental dosages starting from 6 mg and followed by 12 mg and a repeated dose of 12 mg if needed. It is prudent to flush the injection port immediately after administration as slow rate of delivery may abate the drug's effects. Decreased doses (3 mg) are required if the administration is through central venous access, in patients taking dipyridamole or in heart transplant patients. Failure of adenosine to terminate a tachycardia means that the circuit does not involve the AV node but may indicate inconsistencies with the IV line or that the drug was given at too slow a rate. Following the administration of the drug, patients tend to feel a transient uncomfortable sensation that includes flushing, shortness of breath, and chest discomfort that quickly wears off. Notifying the patient in advance of the expected sensation helps reduce the fear during administration. The drug is contraindicated in patients with a history of asthma and bronchospasm. βBlockers or calcium channel blockers can be used in these situations.

β-Adrenergic receptor blockers. Electrophysiologic actions: βReceptor blockers are class II drugs that competitively inhibit catecholamine binding at β-receptors and decrease the adrenergic tone. They slow automaticity and firing rate in the sinus node and slow conduction over the AV node. ECG changes include decreased heart rate and PR prolongation. Commonly used drugs in this category include metoprolol, carvedilol, atenolol, propranolol, and esmolol. The medications that would be elaborated here are the ones most commonly used in the CCU setting such as metoprolol and esmolol.

Pharmacokinetics and dosages: **Metoprolol**: Commonly used as a short-acting β-blocker (half-life of 3 to 8 hours), metabolized primarily in the liver. Initial bolus of 2.5 to 5 mg every 2 to 5 minutes up to a maximum of 15 mg. Peak effect in 20 minutes. Additional IV dosages can be given every 6 to 12 hours, but transition to oral should be done when possible. The oral form metoprolol tartate should be started from 25 to 50 mg two to three times a day, and its peak effect is in 1.5 to 4 hours.

Esmolol: Commonly used as a continuous infusion β-blocking agent (half-life of 9 minutes, onset of action in 2 to 10 minutes); initially, 500 μg per kg bolus infusion over 1 minute, followed by 50 μg/kg/minute Infusion may be titrated up to a maximum of 200 μg/kg/minute. Increments of 50 μg/kg/minute can be made every 4 minutes with a 500 μg per kg bolus over 1 minute before each increment.

Indications: βBlockers can be used effectively to treat ventricular and supraventricular arrhythmias. βBlockers are first-line medications for tachyarrhythmias associated with excessive cardiac adrenergic stimulation, such as exercise and emotion, thyrotoxicosis, pheochromocytoma, and anesthesia-related tachycardia from inhaled gases such as halothane or cyclopropane.

Adverse effects: Acute cessation of β-blockade may cause reflex tachycardia that could worsen existing heart disease. This class of drugs can cause bradycardia and hypotension, worsening of asthma and chronic obstructive pulmonary disease, Raynaud phenomenon, increased risk of hypoglycemia in diabetic patients, depression, and impaired sexual function.

Calcium channel blockers. Electrophysiologic actions: Calcium channel blockers are class IV antiarrhythmic drugs. The cardioselective calcium blockers verapamil and diltiazem prolong conduction time through the AV node, the Purkinje system, and prolong refractory time (more apparent at faster rates). The sinus rate and rhythm do not change significantly because of peripheral vasodilation and reflex sympathetic stimulation. However, during non sinus tachyarrhythmias, the bradycardic effect of the calcium blocker is more pronounced. Dihydropyridine type calcium blockers do not exert significant electrophysiologic effects.

Pharmacokinetics: The onset of action time is 1 to 2 minutes with IV verapamil, whereas it is 30 minutes with oral doses, with duration of action lasting 6 hours in both. Elimination half-life of verapamil is 3 to 7 hours mostly being excreted by the kidneys. Diltiazem onset of action is 15 minutes, and half-life is 6 hours.

Dosage: Infusion of 5 to 10 mg of verapamil over 1 to 2 minutes. A repeat of an equal dose may be given in 30 minutes. Maintenance infusion is at a rate of 0.005 mg/kg/minute. Diltiazem is given IV at 0.25 mg per kg over 2 minutes with a repeat in 15 minutes if necessary and is also preferred over verapamil in patients with hypotension. Rate of infusion for diltiazem is 5 mg per hour. Oral dosing for verapamil ranges from 240 to 480 mg per day and for diltiazem from 120 to 360 mg per day in three to four divided doses. Long-acting formulations are available for both verapamil and diltiazem.

Indications: The drugs are useful in the treatment of sustained supraventricular arrhythmias. Verapamil and diltiazem terminate close to 90% of paroxysmal supraventricular tachycardias (SVTs) within minutes. It must be noted that in patients with preexcited ventricular complexes (accessory pathways) during atrial fibrillation associated with Wolff–Parkinson–White (WPW), IV verapamil may accelerate the ventricular response.

Adverse effects: Calcium blockers are negative inotropic agents and should be used cautiously in those with depressed cardiac function and sinus node dysfunction as they may cause significant bradycardia and hypotension. The drugs are contraindicated in advanced heart failure, advanced AV block without a pacemaker, atrial fibrillation in the setting of WPW, cardiogenic shock, most types of ventricular tachycardia (VT). These drugs interfere with digoxin excretion.

Digoxin. Electrophysiologic actions: The digitalis alkaloid primarily augments parasympathetic vagal tone, slowing down both the sinus node and AV node. The drug does not affect the His-Purkinje system or the ventricle in therapeutic concentration. Exercise decreases the effect of digoxin because of decrease in vagal tone.

Pharmacokinetics: Time to onset of action IV is within minutes whereas orally is up to 3 hours. Digoxin half-life is 36 to 48 hours and it is excreted in the urine.

Dosage: IV or oral loading dose up to 1 mg per day in separate dosages followed by 0.125 to 0.25 mg per day. The loading dose is not influenced by creatinine clearance, but the maintenance dose thereafter requires dose adjustment. Digoxin levels may be used to monitor toxicity and compliance.

Indication: At present, digoxin is a second-line drug for rate control of chronic atrial fibrillation or flutter. Digoxin has little effect in chemically cardioverting rapid atrial fibrillation and has probably less effect than other drug for rate control.

Adverse effects: Digoxin has narrow therapeutic window. Toxicity symptoms include gastrointestinal complaints, headaches, altered color vision, and halo vision. Commonly seen arrhythmias include sinus bradycardia/arrest, atrial or junctional tachycardia with variable block, and VT. Digoxin toxicity increases with age, renal failure, chronic lung disease, hypothyroidism, and hypokalemia. Diagnosis of digoxin toxicity is confirmed with serum levels of digoxin. Treatment includes cessation of digoxin use, digoxin-specific antibodies fragments when arrhythmias occur, phenytoin for atrial tachyarrhythmias, and lidocaine for infranodal tachyarrhythmias. Pharmacologic therapy is favored over DC cardioversion during tachyarrhythmias in digoxin toxicity.

VENTRICULAR TACHYARRHYTHMIAS

Ventricular arrhythmias are discussed in Chapter 17, and their main pharmacologic therapy is outline in Table 22.3.

Treatment of ventricular tachyarrhythmias relies primarily on the hemodynamic status of the patient. In the acute setting, decompensated patient should be immediately treated with DC cardioversion. Concomitantly, electrolyte imbalances should be corrected, revascularization should be sought if the patient is actively ischemic, and proarrhythmic agents should be discontinued. Amiodarone, procainamide, and lidocaine are the mainstay pharmacologic options for the stable patient with VT. β-Blockers are used for the prevention of recurrent ventricular arrhythmias, especially in the setting of ischemia. There are situations like digitalis toxicity when pharmacologic treatment is preferred to DC cardioversion. In Belhassen VT (idiopathic fascicular VT) that is manifested with an RBBB-right bundle branch block, and a relatively narrow QRS (0.12 to 0.14 seconds) verapamil is the treatment of choice.

Amiodarone. Electrophysiologic actions: Amiodarone is a class III antiarrhythmic agent that acts by primarily blocking the rapid component of the delayed potassium rectifier channels with moderate blockade of calcium channel, α- and β-adrenergic receptors, and some sodium channel inhibition. The drug prolongs the action potential and refractory period, decreases sinus firing, and slows AV conduction.[7]

Pharmacokinetics: Amiodarone is slowly absorbed orally, primarily metabolized in the liver by CYP2C8 and 3A4 to *N*-desethylamiodarone, the active form. Onset of action after IV administration is within 1 to 2 hours. Oral administration takes 2 to 3 days to reach a steady state but may take up to 2 to 3 weeks. The drug is lipophilic and thus has a prolonged half-life of around 53 days with a large variability between patients. The drug is excreted through the urine and feces.

Dose: In the CCU or in emergent settings, amiodarone is given as a 150 mg bolus over 10 minutes, followed by 1 mg per kg for 6 hours and then 0.5 mg per minute for 18 hours IV. During breakthrough ventricular arrhythmias, it can be given in additional boluses—usually at 150 mg over 10 minute. Caution should be used in patients with systolic dysfunction because of the threat of hypotension, and QT interval should be measured in all patients (although the incidence of torsades de points from amiodarone is low). Oral dosages of amiodarone are titrated down from an initial dose of 800 to 1,200 mg per day to 200 mg per day over a period of 2 months. Concomitant use of other drugs should be considered when dosing—for example, digoxin and warfarin increase the amiodarone levels and thus lower amiodarone doses are required.

Indications: Amiodarone is indicated for both ventricular and supraventricular arrhythmias. Amiodarone is probably the most commonly used drug for ventricular arrhythmias. The Amiodarone in Out-of-Hospital Resuscitation of Refractory Sustained Ventricular Tachycardia (ARREST)[8] trial and the Amiodarone versus Lidocaine in Pre-Hospital Refractory Ventricular Fibrillation Evaluation (ALIVE)[9] trials were two relatively large randomized controlled trials that have demonstrated higher survival to admission when IV amiodarone was given during cardiac resuscitation for pulseless VT or ventricular fibrillation (VF) as compared with placebo or lidocaine. Amiodarone is currently considered the drug of choice for the treatment of ventricular arrhythmias during resuscitation.[1,2] Amiodarone may suppress between 40% and 60% of the ventricular arrhythmias, decrease intracardiac defibrillator (ICD) firings, and suppress asymptomatic ventricular arrhythmias. In the Sudden Cardiac Death in the Heart Failure Trial,[10] (SCD-HeFT) it was proven that ICD treatment provided higher survival rate than amiodarone in patients with systolic heart failure (EF-ejection fraction <35% with NYHA class II and III symptoms). Amiodarone is also efficacious with supraventricular arrhythmias with a suppression rate ranging between 60% and 80%. It is used for atrial fibrillation cardioversion and maintenance and atrial fibrillation prophylaxis after heart surgery.

TABLE 22.3	**Medications for the Treatment of Ventricular Tachyrhythmias**				
Medication	*Initial Dose*	*Maintenance Dose*	*Onset of Action*	*Half-Life*	*Acute Adverse Effects*
Amiodarone	Pulseless VT or VF 300 mg bolus, stable VT 150 mg bolus over 10 min	1 mg/min for 6 hr, then 0.5 mg/min for 18 hr	3–7 hr	9–47 d	Hypotension, bradycardia, heart block
Lidocaine	1–1.5 mg/kg bolus followed by 0.5–0.75 mg/kg every 10 min (up to 3 boluses)	1–4 mg/min (reduce dose in patients with CHF-Congestive heart failure, shock, or hepatic disease)	45–90 s	7–30 min	Confusion, bradycardia, arrhythmia
Procainamide	15–18 mg/kg over 30 min or 100 mg every 5 min (maximum 1 g dose)	1–4 mg/min	10–30 min	3–5 hr	Hypotension, conduction abnormalities

Adverse effects: There are multiple side effects that are both dose and duration dependent. Among them are lung toxicity (interstitial lung disease), thyroid disorders (hyperthyroidism requires cessation of the drug), liver cirrhosis, photosensitivity, peripheral neuropathy, corneal deposits, bradycardia, worsening systolic heart failure, and torsades de pointes (related to the long QT interval; therefore, amiodarone should be used with caution with other QT prolonging drugs such as class Ia antiarrhythmics).

Lidocaine. Electrophysiologic actions: Lidocaine is a class Ib antiarrhythmic agent that exerts its effect by blocking the sodium channels. The drug acts primarily on ventricular tissue and the His-Purkinje system by increasing the electrical stimulation threshold, suppressing automaticity, and shortening the refractory period and action potential. The drug is more effective at fast heart rates (use dependent) and on damaged tissue (lower pH, hyperkalemia, and reduced membrane potential). The drug has no effect on atrial tissue including the sinus or the AV node and therefore not effective in supraventricular arrhythmias.

Pharmacokinetics: Lidocaine is used IV only with a rapid onset of action (45 to 90 seconds), effect duration of 10 to 20 minutes, and a half-life of 7 to 30 minutes. Metabolism is primarily hepatic with a significant first-pass metabolism (its metabolites may cause central nervous system toxicity). Decreased hepatic flow, shock, and decreased cardiac output may cause toxicity.

Dose: Initial bolus is 1 to 1.5 mg per kg followed by 1 to 4 mg per minute. Careful up-titration is needed because of its narrow therapeutic range. A second bolus of 0.5 mg per kg is usually given 20 to 40 minutes after the initial dose because of redistribution of the drug in the body. Repeated boluses (usually up to three) may be given for breakthrough arrhythmias at 10-minute intervals to achieve desired effect.

Indications: Lidocaine is used for the treatment of ventricular arrhythmias and pulseless VT/VF after failed defibrillation attempts.[1] It has no effect on the atrial tissues and thus is not effective in SVTs. The drug was commonly used in the 1980s for the prevention of arrhythmias after MIs but was shown to be associated with increased mortality in the Cardiac Arrhythmia Suppression Trial[11] (CAST) and is thus currently used as a second-line agent for ischemic VT. In the resuscitation setting, amiodarone was shown to be superior to lidocaine in the ALIVE trial.[9]

Adverse effects: Side effects and toxicity are dose dependent and include neurologic manifestations such as dizziness, mental status changes, paresthesias, and seizures.

Mexiletine. The drug is a class Ib antiarrhythmic agent that can be used as the oral alternative to lidocaine. It has a longer half-life than lidocaine and may be used for refractory VTs, especially when combined with amiodarone or a class I drugs (not effective for supraventricular arrhythmias). The drug has similar metabolic profile to lidocaine with dose adjustments in patients with liver disease or congestive heart failure. A dose of 400 mg orally once followed by 200 mg in 8 hours is used in the acute setting, whereas 200 mg orally every 8 hours is suggested in the postacute setting. Side effects include gastrointestinal complaints (the drug is usually taken with food), bradycardia, hypotension, and neurologic symptoms such as confusion, tremor, dysarthria, and mental status changes. The drug shows promise in the treatment of long QT syndrome type 3.

Procainamide. Electrophysiologic actions. Procainamide is a class Ia antiarrhythmic agent that exerts its effect by blocking the "fast response" sodium channels. It acts both at the atrial and ventricular levels. The drug suppresses myocardial excitability and contractility, decreases conduction velocity, and increases refractoriness. Procainamide is useful for both supraventricular (including bypass tracts) and ventricular arrhythmias. It is very useful in terminating sustained monomorphic VT and was shown to be superior to lidocaine.

Dose: Procainamide is available in both oral and IV forms. For the acute setting, initial infusion of 15-18 mg/Kg over 30 minutes or 100 mg every 5 minutes until one of the following occurs: the arrhythmia is terminated, hypotension ensues, QRS complex widens by 50% of its original width, QT prolongs, or a total of 17 mg per kg is given. Continuous infusion at a rate of 1 to 4 mg per minute may be given after the initial bolus.

Adverse effects: Procainamide may cause lupus-like syndrome (antihistone positive), agranulocytosis, and gastrointestinal symptoms.

CONCLUSION

Many antiarrhythmic drugs are available nowadays, but familiarity with their action, indications, and side effects will assist the health care provider in selecting the preferred drug.

REFERENCES

1. Field JM, Hazinski MF, Sayre MS, et al. Part 1: executive summary: 2010 American Heart Association Guidelines for Cardiopulmonary Resuscitation and Emergency Cardiovascular Care. *Circulation.* 2010;122(18)(suppl 3):S640–S656.
2. Neumar RW, Otto CW, Link MS, et al. Part 8: adult advanced cardiovascular life support: 2010 American Heart Association Guidelines for Cardiopulmonary Resuscitation and Emergency Cardiovascular Care. *Circulation.* 2010;122(18)(suppl 3):S729–S767.
3. Vaughan Williams EM. Classification of antidysrhythmic drugs. *Pharmacol Ther B.* 1975;1(1):115–138.
4. Kusumoto FM, Goldschlager N. Cardiac pacing. *N Engl J Med.* 1996;334(2): 89–97.
5. Fuster V, Rydén LE, Cannom DS, et al. ACC/AHA/ESC 2006 Guidelines for the Management of Patients with Atrial Fibrillation: a report of the American College of Cardiology/American Heart Association Task Force on Practice Guidelines and the European Society of Cardiology Committee for Practice Guidelines (Writing Committee to Revise the 2001 Guidelines for the Management of Patients With Atrial Fibrillation): developed in collaboration with the European Heart Rhythm Association and the Heart Rhythm Society. *Circulation.* 2006;114(7): e257–e354.
6. Fuster V, Rydén LE, Cannom DS, et al. 2011 ACCF/AHA/HRS focused updates incorporated into the ACC/AHA/ESC 2006 guidelines for the management of patients with atrial fibrillation: a report of the American College of Cardiology Foundation/American Heart Association Task Force on practice guidelines. *Circulation.* 2011;123(10):e269–e367.
7. Goldschlager N, Epstein AE, Nacarrelli GV, et al. A practical guide for clinicians who treat patients with amiodarone: 2007. *Heart Rhythm.* 2007;4(9):1250–1259.
8. Kudenchuk PJ, Cobb LA, Copass MK, et al. Amiodarone for resuscitation after out-of-hospital cardiac arrest due to ventricular fibrillation. *N Engl J Med.* 1999;341(12):871–878.
9. Dorian P, Cass D, Schwartz B, et al. Amiodarone as compared with lidocaine for shock-resistant ventricular fibrillation. *N Engl J Med.* 2002;346(12):884–890.
10. Bardy GH, Lee KL, Poole JE, et al. Amiodarone or an implantable cardioverter-defibrillator for congestive heart failure. *N Engl J Med.* 2005;352(3):225–237.
11. Preliminary report: effect of encainide and flecainide on mortality in a randomized trial of arrhythmia suppression after myocardial infarction. The Cardiac Arrhythmia Supression Trial (CAST) Investigators. *N Engl J Med.* 1989;321(6):406–412.

PATIENT AND FAMILY INFORMATION FOR:
Commonly Used Medications for the Treatment of Arrhythmias

Rhythm disorder or arrhythmias are disorders that involve the heart's electrical system. The heart has multiple cells that act as pacemakers to create an electrical impulse that is further transmitted through the heart to activate the contraction mechanism. Although most cells in the heart have pacemaker capabilities, only the fastest ones win to determine the heart rhythm. The fastest group is located in the right atrium (upper chamber) of the heart in an area that is called the sinus node; this explains why a normal rhythm is called normal sinus rhythm. Another group of specialized pacemaker cells sit at the junction between the atria and the ventricles (the two large squeezing chambers)—that area is called the AV node. The electrical impulse thus is generated in the sinus node, travels down to the AV node, and from there through a specialized web of conduction cells called the His-Purkinje system down to the ventricles. The heart rate mainly responds to signals dictated by the nervous system in addition to changes in blood flow and pressures from within the heart. The nervous system that is involved with the heart rate could be divided into two opposing powers—the sympathetic and parasympathetic systems. The sympathetic system is the activating branch, the driving force, exerting speed and increased heart rate. However, the parasympathetic system is the opposite—reducing speed and heart rate, "calming down" the system. The dialogue between the two systems where the heart rate goes up and down is the essence of life. Arrhythmias result from rhythms going too fast (tachyarrhythmias) or too slow (bradyarrhythmias). Both the fast and slow disorders generally originate from a problem in the creation of the signal or its conduction.

THE BRADYARRHYTHMIAS—WHEN THE HEART GOES TOO SLOW …

The bradyarrhythmias are more intuitive to understand; if a defect occurs throughout the conduction system and a signal is not created or transmitted, then the heart rate goes down and an artificial method (e.g., medication or pacemaker) is needed to restore the rate again. The most common reason for bradycardia (slow heart rate) is a predicated aging process that damages the cells ability to conduct an electrical impulse. Other important reasons are heart attacks that prevent blood flow to parts of the conduction system, infections (e.g., Lyme disease or valve infection), exaggerated effect of medications that slows down the heart rate, underactivity of the thyroid gland, diseases that have build up of clogging material inside the heart (e.g., sarcoidosis,

amyloidosis), and conditions where the parasympathetic system is in overdrive mode like during strokes and bleeding in the brain. The most important decision that a physician has to make with a patient who has bradycardia is to determine whether the slow rate can hold a blood pressure. Professional athletes, for example, usually have slower heart rate and that is considered normal, whereas an elderly patient with episodes of dizziness and falls with a heart rate of 30 bpm may need treatment. The most common ECG finding for bradycardia is called sinus bradycardia (the normal sinus node is active but too slow), and the most common ECG finding that would get the patient to the CCU is called heart block. The following medications are most commonly used during bradycardia with symptoms:

ATROPINE

This is perhaps the most commonly used medication in patients with bradycardia. Atropine negates the effect of the parasympathetic system, the "calming" system, and thus making the sympathetic system more pronounced that in turn gets the heart rate up. Side effects include reduced sweating, increase in pupil size, warm feeling, palpitations, and urinary retention.

Isoproterenol, dopamine, and epinephrine. This group of medications acts similarly to the sympathetic system, activating special receptors on the heart cell membrane that command the pacemaker cells to increase the heart rate. All of these medications are given IV and may increase the blood pressure and actually cause fast arrhythmias.

THE TACHYARRHYTHMIAS—WHEN THE HEART GOES TOO FAST …

The tachyarrhythmias are classified as supraventricular (above the large pumping chambers) or ventricular (main pumping chambers).

SUPRAVENTRICULAR TACHYARRHYTHMIAS

Supraventricular tachyarrhythmias are less dangerous than the ventricular ones and may be treated with medications, unless the patient's blood pressure decreases or the patient exhibits distressing symptoms (chest pain, shortness of breath, or confusion) that would warrant an electrical shock.

There are many types of supraventricular tachyarrhythmia that are discussed in Chapter 16. Atrial fibrillation is the most common arrhythmia and occurs when the upper chambers of the heart start fibrillating or "quivering" causing rapid, irregular heart rate. Other supraventricular arrhythmias include atrial flutter, atrial tachycardia, and different kinds of SVT. Typical symptoms to all of these kinds of arrhythmias include palpitations, fatigue, lightheadedness, and decreased exercise capacity. Patients may need to be admitted to CCU if they have a very fast heart rate with low blood pressure or if they have associated conditions such as heart failure, heart attack, or stroke. The following drugs are commonly used to treat supraventricular tachyarrhythmias:

Metoprolol. This drug is the most commonly used medication to slow down the heart rate. It acts by blocking specific receptors called β-receptors. It can be given IV for immediate action or can be given orally for slower and more prolonged action. The most common side effects are dizziness and lightheadedness resulting from low blood pressure and slow heart rate. Other side effects may include wheezing, low blood sugar, and depression.

Esmolol. This is another medication that blocks β-receptors and lowers heart rate. Its action is immediate and short lasting, thus it is given in continuous IV infusion. Most common side effects that may be observed are the same as metoprolol, low blood pressure and slow heart rate.

Diltiazem and verapamil. These medications slow heart rate by blocking the calcium channels of the heart cells. They act within 2 to 3 minutes if given IV. Most common side effects are low blood pressure and slow heart rate.

Adenosine. This medication transiently blocks the AV node when given IV. Its effect lasts only for few seconds but is able to terminate fast rhythms that circle through the AV node. Patient may feel symptoms like dyspnea or flushing transiently, usually lasting less than a minute.

Digoxin. This medication creates a parasympathetic surge (the "calming" nervous system arm) and thus slows down the heart without lowering the blood pressure. It is mainly used to slow down the heart rate in atrial fibrillation and atrial flutter that also have symptoms of heart failure and low blood pressure. The most common side effects of the drug are dizziness, nausea, and conduction abnormalities like bradycardia and AV block.

VENTRICULAR TACHYARRHYTHMIAS

The ventricular tachyarrhythmias (VT) are the most dangerous rhythm disorders and should be treated promptly—by medications or electrical shock. Structural heart diseases (e.g., prior heart attack or heart failure) are the most common causes of ventricular tachyarrhythmias. They usually originate from the muscles of the lower chambers of the heart outside the electrical system. Medications can be used to treat VT if patients have a stable blood pressure. However, if the patient has a low blood pressure an immediate electrical shock is needed. The following drugs are typically used in ventricular tachyarrhythmias:

Amiodarone. This drug acts on multiple ion channels (primarily the potassium channel of the heart cells). The drug is slowly absorbed when taken by mouth, but when injected IV, its effect is observed in 1 to 2 hours. Amiodarone is considered the drug of choice during cardiac resuscitation to terminate ventricular arrhythmias. Its effect lasts for days and weeks after stopping the drug. Low blood pressure is the most common adverse effect when used IV, along with slow heart rate and heart block. Caution needs to be advised while taking this drug since it interacts with several other drugs. When used on long-term basis, it has several side effects including liver, lung, and thyroid toxicity.

Lidocaine. This medication acts by suppressing both the initiation and conduction of the impulses in the ventricular tissue. Typically used as a second-line agent for the treatment of ventricular arrhythmias after amiodarone. It acts within seconds, and the effect lasts for around 30 minutes after stopping the drug. Side effects are dose dependent and include confusion and dizziness.

Procainamide. This medication exerts its effect by decreasing the excitability and contractility of both atrial and ventricular tissue. It acts within 10 to 30 minutes, and the effect lasts for 3 to 5 hours after stopping the drug. Most common adverse effect is low blood pressure when given IV and lupus-like symptoms (joint inflammation and rashes) when given orally on long-term basis.

In summary, there are many drugs for the treatment of arrhythmias, but familiarity with their action, indication, and side effects will assist the health care provider and the patients and their family in selecting the preferred drug.

SECTION IV

Management of Valvular, Aortic, and Pericardial Disease in the Cardiac Care Unit

Gila Perk
Itzhak Kronzon

CHAPTER

23

Acute Aortic Syndromes

ACUTE AORTIC SYNDROMES

The term "acute aortic syndrome" (AAS) has been used to describe a mixed group of thoracic aortic disorders that characteristically present with a typical combination of signs and symptoms.[1–4] The most distinctive presenting symptom is aortic pain, which is often described as sharp, tearing, or ripping. Although there are several pathophysiologic entities that can present as AAS (Table 23.1) occasionally one process can precede another or occasionally they may coexist. Importantly though, all can be life-threatening and require immediate medical attention (often including a surgical intervention). Given the similarity in the clinical presentation and the need for urgent assessment, diagnosis, and treatment, it is useful to classify these syndromes into one group of disorders, similar to "acute coronary syndromes" or an "acute abdomen."

AAS include the following:

1. Aortic dissection
2. Intramural hematoma, and
3. Penetrating aortic ulcer

Typically, patients with AAS present with an acute onset of chest pain with a long-standing history of hypertension or a known elastic tissue disorder (e.g., Marfan syndrome). The pain is classically described as abrupt in onset, intense, sharp, tearing, or ripping. Diseases that involve the ascending aorta typically produce pain that radiates to the neck or the jaw. Disease in the descending thoracic aorta often causes pain that radiates to the back or abdomen.[5]

A related process that will be discussed in this chapter as well is traumatic aortic rupture. Although aortic rupture is obviously a medical emergency that can present with symptoms of aortic pain similar to other AAS, patients present with a completely different scenario of onset of this process. For this reason, traumatic rupture is often not considered part of the classical AAS.

TABLE 23.1	Acute Aortic Syndromes
Aortic dissection	
Intramural hematoma	
Penetrating aortic ulcer	

Three conditions are considered in the classic clinical entity of acute aortic syndrome; classic aortic dissection, intramural hematoma and penetrating aortic ulcer.

AORTIC DISSECTION

Aortic dissection is characterized by an intimal tear and separation of the intima or media from the surrounding adventitia. Typically, the separation occurs within the media such that the outer layer of the media forms the outside wall of the false lumen and the inner part of the media, along with the intima, forms the intimomedial flap. The thickness of the media that forms the external layer of the false lumen determines the stability of the false lumen wall and is an important determinant of the risk of free wall rupture. The dissection can propagate through the aortic wall both distally and proximally to the initial tear. This propagation can be the cause for many of the complications of aortic dissection (e.g., myocardial ischemia, renal failure). In many patients a reentrance tear can be found or multiple communications between the true and false lumens can be identified.

There are two widely accepted anatomic classifications of aortic dissection; the DeBakey and the Stanford classification (Figure 23.1). The DeBakey system divides aortic dissection to three subtypes: types I, II, and III. Type I DeBakey is a dissection that starts at the ascending aorta and continues at least up to or beyond the arch. Type II starts at the ascending aorta and is confined to the ascending aorta. Type III is a dissection that starts at the descending thoracic aorta and propagates either distally or less commonly proximally. The Stanford classification differentiates aortic dissection according to presence or absence of ascending aorta involvement, regardless of the initial site of origin; type A is a dissection involving the ascending aorta, and type B is a dissection that does not involve the ascending aorta. The Stanford classification is the one clinically used for treatment purposes; urgent surgical intervention versus medical stabilization. Because Stanford classification is the more commonly used system, we will use it throughout this chapter.

EPIDEMIOLOGY

The incidence of aortic dissection is estimated to be 2.9 per 100,000 patient-years. The mean age of presentation is 65 years with approximately 60% predominance of men.[5–7] Women with acute aortic dissection present at an older age than men and tend to present later in the course of the disease than men.[8] Type A aortic dissection is more common than type B and accounts for 60% of cases of acute aortic dissection. Up to 30% of patients with acute type A dissection show involvement of the aortic arch as well.

Similar to acute ischemic syndromes, a circadian as well as seasonal variation in the frequency of acute aortic dissection

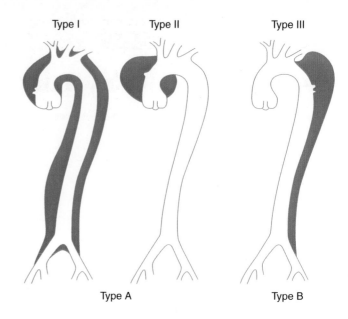

Figure 23.1. Classification systems for aortic dissection. There are two classification systems for aortic dissection. The De Bakey system divides dissection into three types: type I—starts at the ascending aorta and continues beyond it; type II—limited to the ascending aorta; and type III—starts beyond the aortic arch. The Stanford system divides aortic dissection to two types: type A—involving the ascending aorta (regardless of how far it extends) and type B—no involvement of the ascending aorta.

has been found.[9] Acute aortic dissection is significantly more prevalent between 6 a.m. and 12 noon, and in particular between 8 a.m. and 9 a.m. A seasonal variation in acute aortic dissection presentation has also been found, with more frequent occurrence in the winter as compared to summer, with a peak incidence in January.

Acute aortic dissection presents slightly different in North American and European adults.[10] North American patients tend to be older, demonstrate more ECG changes (significantly more nonspecific ST changes and a trend towards more ST elevations and acute myocardial infarcts), and have more atypical symptoms and less classic chest X-ray findings compared with European patients. Despite the differences in clinical presentation, there is no difference in the early outcome between North American patients and European patients.

ETIOLOGY

The underlying pathology in many cases of aortic dissection is cystic medial necrosis causing degeneration of the aortic media. Of note, this is in fact a misnomer as pathology specimens do not demonstrate either cysts or necrotic material. However, it is a commonly used term that describes the generative process of the aortic media that involves degeneration of the elastic tissue. There are several predisposing factors that have been identified as risk factors for aortic dissection. The commonest risk factor that has been recognized is systemic hypertension. Up to 72% of patients who present with acute aortic dissection have a history of systemic hypertension.[7] History of atherosclerosis is also common; it is found in up to 32% of patients presenting with acute aortic dissection. These risk factors are particularly noteworthy in patients above 40 years of age who present with acute aortic dissection.

Acute aortic dissection has also been found to be associated with collagen/elastic tissue diseases such as Marfan syndrome and Ehlers Danlos syndrome. Of all patients with acute aortic dissection, 4.9% have a history of Marfan syndrome.[5,7,11] However, among patients younger than 40 years of age who present with acute aortic dissection, 50% have Marfan syndrome.[11]

Several other predisposing risk factors have been identified in patients presenting with acute aortic dissection[5,7,11]:

- Prior aortic dilatation and aneurysm: Up to 16% of all patients (and 19% of patients younger than 40 years) presenting with acute aortic dissection have a prior history of aortic aneurysm.
- Bicuspid aortic valve: Among young patients (<40 years old) who present with acute aortic dissection, 9% have a bicuspid aortic valve. Bicuspid aortic valve is frequently associated with progressive dilatation of the ascending aorta, irrespective of the valvular function. This is likely due to significant loss of elastic fibers in the aortic media.[12] In patients with bicuspid valve-associate dissection, the ascending aorta is always involved (type A dissection).
- Prior history of aortic dissection is found in 4% to 7% of patients with acute aortic dissection, and up to 11% of patients presenting with type B dissection.
- Prior cardiac surgery is seen in up to 18% of patients presenting with acute aortic dissection. These include prior aortic surgeries (aneurysm or dissection repair) and other cardiac surgeries in which the aorta is surgically manipulated (such as coronary artery bypass grafting). Cardiac catheterization and percutaneous coronary interventions have been seen to precede in about 2% of cases of acute aortic dissection.
- Somewhat conflicting evidence exists regarding the casual relationship between cocaine use and acute aortic dissection.[13] In a multicenter, large international registry, cocaine use has been found seldom among patients presenting with acute aortic dissection (<1%). However, in an inner-city-based series, recent (minutes to hours before presentation) cocaine use has been reported in 37% of patients presenting with acute aortic dissection.[14] The difference is most likely related to the different patient populations represented in these studies. Cocaine has been suggested to cause weakening of the aortic elastic media, premature atherosclerosis, and sudden onset of severe sheer forces (from the significant hypertension and tachycardia associated especially with crack cocaine use). The combination of these chronic and acute effects of cocaine use could be related to the risk of acute aortic dissection.

- Inflammatory diseases involving the great vessels such as syphilitic aortitis, and vasculitis of the aorta (e.g., Takayasu vasculitis or giant cell arteritis) have been associated with aortic dissection in rare instances.
- Pregnancy: There have been several reports of acute aortic dissection complicating pregnancy. Most have been associated with Marfan syndrome as well, and it remains unclear whether pregnancy represents an additive risk or whether it is merely a common enough condition that these associations may not represent a causative relationship.

CLINICAL MANIFESTATIONS

The hallmark of the clinical presentation of acute aortic dissection is "aortic pain." This is frequently described as an abrupt onset of severe, sharp, tearing, or ripping chest pain. Radiation to the jaw or the neck is more common with type A dissection, whereas radiation to the back is seen more commonly with type B or abdominal aortic dissection. However, painless dissection has also been described, in up to 6.4% of patients presenting acute aortic dissection.[15] Patients who present with painless dissection are older than those with painful dissection, have a higher prevalence of type A dissection, and present more commonly with syncope, congestive heart failure, and stroke. The mortality rate in this group is also higher as compared to those who present with acute aortic pain, in particular in the group with painless type B dissection (who have a significantly elevated risk of aortic rupture).

Patients with acute aortic dissection can also present with syncope; this has been described as the presenting manifestation in 13% of patients and was found to be associated with significantly increased in-hospital mortality.[16] In multivariate analysis, syncope has been found to be associated with presence of cardiac tamponade, stroke, and proximal aorta involvement. The increased mortality risk associated with syncope persisted after controlling for patients' demographic characteristics but not after adjusting for the comorbid conditions (stroke, tamponade, and proximal dissection).

Pulse deficit (absence of carotid, brachial, or femoral pulse owing to intimal flap involving major branch vessels or compressing hematoma) has been described in up to 15% of patients, more commonly in type A dissection versus type B (19% vs. 9%, respectively). Pulse deficit has been associated with increased in-hospital complications (such as renal failure, coma, hypotension, and limb ischemia) as well as an independent predictor of 5-day in-hospital mortality.[17]

Patients with acute dissection can present with hypertension, normotension, hypotension, or shock.[5] Overall, 50% of patients present with hypertension. It is significantly more common for type B dissection to present with hypertension (70% of patients) as compared with type A dissection (36%). Hypotension or shock on presentation is significantly more common in type A dissection as compared with type B (25% and 5%, respectively).

Proximal dissection, involving the ascending aorta can result in one or more of the following clinical characteristics (Table 23.2):

- Pericardial tamponade was found in 18.7% of patients with acute aortic dissection.[18] It likely results from rupture of the aorta into the pericardial space. Tamponade has been found to correlate with presence of altered mental status

TABLE 23.2	Complications of Type A Aortic Dissection
Complication	*Incidence (%)*
Tamponade	18.7
Acute aortic insufficiency	44
Myocardial ischemia	5
Neurologic manifestations	15

Various clinical complications can occur with type A aortic dissection. These, and their incidence among patients who present with acute type A aortic dissection are shown in the table.

and hypotension. Using logistic regression models, it was also found to be an independent predictor of outcome, even when controlling for baseline clinical findings.
- Acute aortic insufficiency can be seen in up to 44% of patients presenting with type A dissection.[5,19] There are several possible mechanisms of acute aortic insufficiency in the setting of acute dissection: (1) Incomplete coaptation of otherwise normal aortic valve owing to dilatation of the sinotubular junction, (2) abnormal leaflet coaptation owing to prolapse of the dissection flap into the valve, (3) extension of the dissection flap below the sinotubular junction resulting in prolapse of one or more of the aortic valve leaflets, (4) aortic leaflet prolapse related to a bicuspid aortic valve, and (5) degenerative aortic valve disease with leaflet thickening and abnormal coaptation.
- Myocardial ischemia can complicate acute type A dissection by extension of the dissection flap into the coronary ostia. This can be seen in up to 5% of patients with type A dissection.[5] The right coronary artery is most frequently involved.
- Vocal cord paralysis from compression of the left recurrent laryngeal nerve has been reported.[20]
- Neurologic manifestations, including altered mental status and focal neurological deficits or frank stroke, can complicate acute aortic dissection in up to 15% of patients.[5,8] Neurologic complications can result from hypoperfusion secondary to shock or from direct extension of the dissection into the carotid vessels.

Descending thoracic aorta involvement can give rise to several distinct clinical characteristics including sudden onset of chest and back pain (86% of patients), abdominal pain, spinal cord ischemia (3% of patients), ischemic peripheral neuropathy (2% of patients), renal failure, shock, and lower extremity ischemia.[5,21]

Age and gender play a role in the clinical presentation of acute aortic dissection.[8,22] Atherosclerosis, hypertension, and iatrogenic dissection are significantly more common in the older patient population, whereas Marfan syndrome-associated dissection is seen solely in the younger age group. Typical symptoms and signs of acute dissection (e.g., sudden onset of "aortic pain," presence of aortic regurgitation murmur) are less common in the older (≥70 years) as compared with the younger (<70 years) patient population. Outcome and treatment of acute aortic dissection also differ between the age groups.

Women with acute aortic dissection are generally older and present later in the course of the disease.[8] Pericardial or pleural effusion, tamponade, periaortic hematoma, altered mental status or coma, and hypotension are more frequent in women

TABLE 23.3	ECG Abnormalities in Aortic Dissection
Nonspecific ST-T changes	41%
Left ventricular hypertrophy	26%
Ischemia or prior infarct	23%
Acute ischemic injury	3%

Based on International Registry of Aortic Dissection data.

and result in higher prevalence of in-hospital complications and mortality rate.

DIAGNOSIS

The diagnosis of acute aortic dissection remains challenging despite significant improvements in imaging and diagnostic modalities. The overall occurrence of the disease is relatively rare; it is estimated that out of 1,000 patients who present to the emergency department with chest or back pain, only 3 patients are diagnosed with acute dissection.[7] This is in contrast, for example, with acute coronary syndrome, which is probably 100 to 200 times more common. In one series,[6] acute aortic dissection was the initial diagnosis in only 15% of patients who were ultimately diagnosed with acute dissection, demonstrating how challenging this diagnosis remains. Given the low incidence of aortic dissection and the overlap of presenting symptoms with other, more common disease processes, the diagnosis requires high level of suspicion and appropriate utilization of imaging studies in a timely manner.

Of the clinical characteristics, presence of aortic pain (abrupt onset of tearing or ripping pain), mediastinal widening on chest X-ray, and presence of pulse deficit or blood pressure differential were found to be very important for the diagnosis of acute dissection.[23] In the absence of all three signs, the likelihood of dissection was low (7%). In the presence of aortic pain or mediastinal widening the probability of dissection was intermediate (31% or 39%). In the presence of pulse deficit or blood pressure differential or any combination of the three characteristics, the probability of dissection was high, >83%.

Electrocardiographic (ECG) abnormalities can be seen in acute aortic dissection; however up to 30% of patients present with normal electrocardiogram.[5] The ECG abnormalities that can be seen in acute dissection are summarized in Table 23.3.

Imaging studies are the key for the correct and timely diagnosis of acute aortic dissection (Figure 23.2). Currently available techniques include echocardiography (both transthoracic [TTE] and transesophageal [TEE]) contrast-enhanced computed tomography (CT), magnetic resonance imaging (MRI), and aortography.[7,22,24-45]

Often, several imaging studies are used to make and confirm the diagnosis of acute aortic dissection. CT, TEE, and MRI have a high sensitivity and specificity for the diagnosis of acute aortic dissection. A systematic review of the data available regarding the accuracy of these imaging modalities has shown that for a patient with a high (>50%) pretest probability of acute dissection, positive diagnosis on any one of these imaging modalities resulted in 93% to 96% posttest probability. For patients with low pretest probability (<5%), negative result on either imaging modality conferred a very low (0.1% to 0.3%) posttest probability of acute dissection.

Although both echocardiography (TTE and TEE) and CT scanning are overall utilized in >70% of patients with aortic dissection, CT is the commonest initial test used for the diagnosis (initial imaging modality in 61% of aortic dissection patients).

All the noninvasive imaging modalities have the advantage of providing information regarding the type and extent of the aortic dissection as well as evidence regarding presence and extent of complications. Involvement of the ascending aorta, branch vessels, coronary arteries, aortic valve with acute aortic insufficiency, and presence of pericardial effusion can be delineated using noninvasive assessment (Figure 23.3).

Because the accuracy of the various noninvasive tests for the diagnosis of acute aortic dissection are essentially very similar, other considerations ultimately determine the test that will be utilized. These can include accessibility, portability, patient's hemodynamic condition (which may require an urgent bedside test), and clinical characteristics (e.g., presence of renal failure limiting the use of intravenous contrast).

Aortography is seldom utilized these days. It is reported to be performed in <5% of patients presenting with aortic dissection. The main advantage of aortography is the ability to evaluate the coronaries at the time of the procedure (as well as assess for presence of aortic insufficiency).

Over the recent years, several biomarkers for acute aortic dissection have been recognized and studied.[27] For a biomarker to be clinically useful it must fulfill a set of or several prerequisites:

- It must be easy to use with a fast result.
- It must have a high sensitivity (to identify all cases of acute dissection) as well as high specificity (effectively rule out all cases that are not acute dissection).
- The appearance of the biomarker in the blood should be temporally related to the onset of the disease process.
- It should be widely available for use.
- Cost should be acceptable.

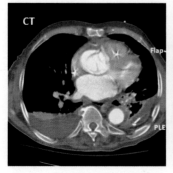
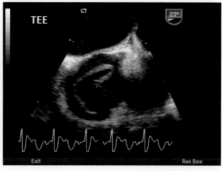

Figure 23.2. Type A aortic dissection. Left panel shows a CT image at the level of the ascending aorta with a dissection flap in it. Note the dilatation of the aorta and the dissection flap as well as the presence of pleural effusion (PLE). The right panel presents a short axis view of TEE image showing type A aortic dissection and demonstrating a circumferential dissection flap at the level of the aortic root.

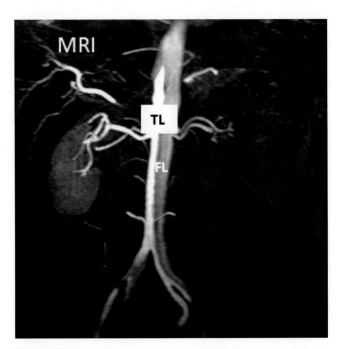

Figure 23.3. Type B aortic dissection. MRI image of a type B aortic dissection extending to the abdominal aorta. The true lumen and false lumen are easily differentiated. Also, differentiation between true lumen branches and false lumen branches is clear. On this image, the right renal artery is seen coming off the true lumen and the left renal artery is coming off the false lumen. FL, false lumen; TL, true lumen. (Courtesy of Pierre Maldjain, MD UMDNJ, Newark, NJ and Muhamed Saric MD, NYU School of Medicine, New York, NY.)

There is still no one biomarker that fits all the above criteria and can reliably identify or rule out acute aortic dissection. Marker combinations have not yet been studied. There are no biomarkers in routine clinical use; however, developments and advancements are ongoing. Several potential biomarkers that have been studied include the following:

1. *Smooth muscle myosin heavy chain*: This is a major component of smooth muscle, also present in uterine and intestinal smooth muscle (thus could potentially be elevated in diseases involving these systems). It appears to rapidly increase in the first few hours of acute aortic dissection (more in type A dissection than type B) but the levels rapidly drop within the first 24 hours. It does not seem to be increased in acute myocardial infarction. However, the rapid decrease in levels limits its use only to the first few hours after symptom onset.
2. *Calponin*: This is thin filament-associated protein that is related to modulation of smooth muscle contraction. Three isoforms have been isolated: acidic, neutral, and basic. Both the acidic and basic isoforms have been found to be elevated early in the course of acute dissection (more significantly in proximal dissection). Although the negative predictive value of calponin seems to be acceptable, the positive predictive value is poor. The acidic isoform seems to be highly specific in the early hours after symptoms onset but still requires further investigation and modification to be clinically useful.
3. *Elastin degradation products (sELAF)*: In acute aortic dissection, the pathological hallmark is degradation of the aortic media with elastin lamellar disruption, and sELAF levels have been found to increase in the setting of acute aortic

dissection. The levels of sELAF remain elevated up to 72 hours after the onset of aortic dissection, making it an attractive option as a dissection biomarker. However, in case of thrombosed, or even partially thrombosed false lumen, the sELAF levels may be falsely low.

4. *D dimer*: This is a fibrin degradation product that can be found in the circulation after fibrinolysis of a thrombus. Several studies have documented that D-dimer levels increase significantly with acute aortic dissection, making its sensitivity very high.[28] However, many other disease processes can give rise to elevated D-dimer levels, some of which are on the differential diagnosis of acute chest pain (e.g., pulmonary embolism). There are also subgroups of patients that have a lower level of D dimer despite the presence of acute dissection; these include younger patients, dissections of shorter length, and thrombosed false lumen thus lowering the negative predictive value of a negative or equivocal result.

MANAGEMENT AND PROGNOSIS

Despite advancements in the medical and surgical care of acute aortic dissection, the overall morbidity and mortality associated with it is still very high. The in-hospital mortality of all comers and all types of acute aortic dissection remains close to 30%.[5,7]

The in-hospital mortality of patients with type A dissection who are medically treated is reported to be as high as 60%. Even with prompt diagnosis and early surgical intervention, the in-hospital mortality remains high, at 26%. Among patients with type B aortic dissection, medically treated have the lowest mortality rate—11%; however those with type B surgically treated have mortality rate up to 31%.

Several clinical and anatomical characteristics affect the survival from acute aortic dissection.[5,7,8,22,29–35] Older age, female gender, hypotension, shock, tamponade, pulse deficit, or neurological symptoms on presentation correlate with increased mortality.[8,17]

For patients with type A aortic dissection, several factors have been identified as associated with increased mortality risk[22,29]: age (≥70 years), sudden onset of pain, pulse deficit on presentation, ECG changes, and in-hospital complications (hypotension, shock, and tamponade).

As mentioned above, age is a significant risk factor for mortality from acute aortic dissection. Surgical correction of type A aortic dissection also decreased with increasing age.[30] However, for every age group (up to 80 years of age), mortality rate in the surgically corrected group is lower than in the medically treated group. Even for the group of patients who are 80- to 90-year-old, surgical intervention appears to correlate with improved survival (although this has not reached statistical significance owing to the small number of patients at this age group that were studied).

Several risk models have been created to predict surgical outcome of acute type A dissection.[31] One model includes clinical characteristics on presentation (age, prior cardiac surgery, hypotension or shock on presentation, migrating pain, pulse deficit, ECG evidence of acute ischemia, and pericardial tamponade). The second model includes intraoperative characteristics (hypotension during surgery, need for coronary revascularization, and right ventricular dysfunction identified at surgery).

The overall 3-year survival after acute type A dissection treated surgically is 91%, and for those treated medically it is 69%.[32] The independent predictors of long-term mortality after type A dissection are history of atherosclerosis and history of prior cardiac surgery. It is interesting to note that the long-term survival is influenced by preexisting conditions and not by in-hospital complications of the acute dissection event (which of course affects the in-hospital mortality).

For patients with type B aortic dissection, painless dissection as well as refractory pain was found to be associated with increased mortality rate.[15,33] Factors identified as associated with increased surgical mortality include the short period between symptoms onset and surgical intervention, altered mental status or coma preoperatively, severely dilated descending aorta (diameter >6 cm), partially thrombosed false lumen, and peri-aortic hematoma. Factors associated with favorable operative outcome include radiating pain on presentation and shorter circulatory arrest time during surgery.[34]

The overall 3-year survival after acute type B dissection (medically or surgically treated) is 76% to 82%.[35] Several independent predictors of long-term mortality after type B dissection have been identified and include prior history of aortic aneurysm and history of atherosclerosis, female gender, and in-hospital complications (renal failure, pleural effusion, hypotension, and shock).

The commonest reported causes of death for patients with type A dissection include pericardial tamponade, visceral ischemia, and aortic rupture. For type B dissection, the commonest reported causes of death include aortic rupture and visceral ischemia. Reducing blood pressure and heart rate are critical and urgent for therapy of aortic dissection. Chapter 33 of this book outlines our recommended therapy.

INTRAMURAL HEMATOMA

Intramural hematoma (IMH) can be viewed as a variant of classic aortic dissection and has been described as "dissection without an intimal tear."[2,3] It is essentially a noncommunicating aortic dissection. The mechanism of its formation is still debated. It is likely the result of rupture of aortic vasa vasorum, with bleeding into the media and creation of a hematoma that disrupts the aortic wall. Most commonly the bleeding is intramedial although cases of subadventitial bleeding have been described. Expansion of the hematoma can result in encroaching on the aortic lumen. Yet surgical analysis as well as in-autopsy series shows that a small intimomedial tear can often be identified. Furthermore, cases of classic dissection and IMH in different parts of the aorta have been described. These findings raise the question about the pathogenesis of IMH and its relation to classics aortic dissection. It is possible to consider the development of classic dissection or IMH as the result of interplay between two governing factors; the source (intimal tear or vasa vasorum bleed) and the resistance to flow in the aortic media. Large source of blood combined with low resistance to flow will result in classic dissection, whereas if the combination of forces creates restricted flow, an IMH will result.

Similar to classic aortic dissection, IMH is divided into type A IMH involving the ascending aorta, and type B IMH that spares the ascending aorta. In accordance with classic dissection, this distinction is important for management, and prognosis purposes.

EPIDEMIOLOGY

Assessing the prevalence of IMH is difficult owing to significant geographical differences. Reported incidence varies between 6% of AAS in western registries[36] and 22% to 28% in eastern registries.[37,38] In the International Registry of Aortic Dissection (IRAD),[36] distal aorta involvement with IMH was more common than proximal aorta involvement (60% vs. 35%), which is different than what was found for classic aortic dissection. Patients who present with IMH are older than those with classic dissection (69 vs. 62 years). Gender distribution is similar for IMH patients and classic dissection patients with approximately 60% of patients being men.

ETIOLOGY

IMH and classic aortic dissection share some risk factors. Hypertension is very prevalent in patients with IMH, even more than in patients with classic dissection.[36] Hypertension is found in up to 78% of patients who present with acute IMH. Diabetes (in 5% of patients), bicuspid aortic valve (4% of patients), and prior coronary artery bypass grafting (5% of patients) are seen with similar frequencies in patients with IMH as in patients with classic dissection. However, Marfan syndrome and aortic valve disease do not seem to be associated with IMH, contrary to what is seen with classic dissection.

CLINICAL MANIFESTATIONS

The typical symptoms of IMH are chest and back pain, similar to acute dissection, but classically described as even more severe pain.[39] IMH is less likely to present with pulse deficit, aortic insufficiency, or visceral ischemic pain. Because the presentation is somewhat less typical, usually it takes longer to diagnose acute IMH and more imaging studies are performed before final diagnosis is made.

ECG is more likely to be normal in acute IMH than in classic dissection, with up to 46% presenting with normal electrocardiogram. In the IRAD, no patient with IMH had ECG changes consistent with acute infarction. Chest X-ray findings are similar to those seen in classic dissection; widened mediastinum were seen in 51% of patients, abnormal cardiac contour in 15%, and pleural effusion in 14% of patients.

IMH is a dynamic process that can extend progress or regress. Serial imaging studies are warranted if a patient is followed conservatively.[3] Persistent pain, evidence of hypoperfusion, and proximal root involvement with aortic regurgitation have been identified as warning signs. Clinical predictors that have been associated with type A IMH progression include pericardial tamponade, hematoma thickness >1 cm, and initial aortic diameter >50 to 55 mm. Clinical predictors for progression of type B IMH include age >70 years and presence of ulcer like projections in the aorta.

IMH can progress to overt aortic rupture, giving rise to mediastinal, pericardial, or pleural hemorrhage.[2] Contained rupture (where the aortic media disintegrates but the hematoma is maintained intra-aortic by the adventitia) appears to be somewhat more common. IMH can also progress to frank dissection, or it can increase in size, gradually thickening the aortic wall. Owing to remodeling of the diseased aortic segment, IMH can result in contained aneurysm formation, which explains the necessity for imaging follow-up for all patients with IMH.

DIAGNOSIS

As mentioned above, typically it takes longer to make the diagnosis of IMH as compared with diagnosing classic dissection, and more imaging studies are utilized until definitive diagnosis is reached. Echocardiography, CT, and MRI are acceptable techniques for assessing and diagnosing IMH.[39] Both echocardiography (transesophageal) and CT scanning can consistently identify the localized thickening of the aorta and compression of the true lumen (Figure 23.4). However, reliably ruling out a dissection flap and distinguishing between IMH and dissection with thrombosed false lumen can occasionally be challenging. Similar to aortic dissection, CT scan appears to be the most commonly used initial imaging test. MRI may be superior both to TEE and CT scanning in differentiating IMH from classic dissection. Important to note, however, for follow-up on extent and progression of the disease, all the above-mentioned imaging techniques are suitable and can be used based on availability and patient considerations.

MANAGEMENT AND PROGNOSIS

The acute prognosis of IMH seems to be slightly less grim than that of classic dissection. In the IRAD, the overall in-hospital mortality from IMH is 21%. The main determinant of the short-term prognosis, similar to classic dissection, is the location of the process. The overall in-hospital mortality for type A IMH is 39%, whereas for type B IMH it is 8%. Surgically treated patients with type A IMH fare better than those treated medically. However, in other series,[37,38] a strategy of surgical intervention for acute complications only (whether on presentation or during follow-up) and otherwise medical management seems to provide acceptable short- and long-term survival rates. In fact, patients treated with this strategy had comparable survival to those with classic dissection who were treated surgically. Furthermore, in these series of type A IMH, initial aortic diameter and hematoma thickness seemed to be the key predictors of outcome.

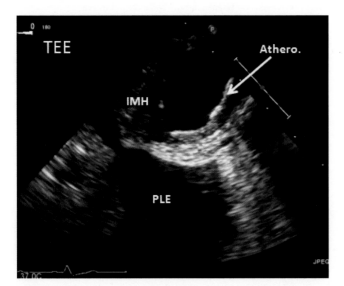

Figure 23.4. Intramural hematoma. Short axis view (on TEE) showing type B intramural hematoma with associated pleural effusion. It appears as a crescent-shaped, thickened aortic wall. Note also the diffuse and the right pleural effusion (PLE). Athero, atherosclerotic plaque; IMH, intramural hematoma; PLE, pleural effusion.

As for type B IMH—resolution has been documented in a significant percentage of patients treated medically (up to 50%), but progression to aneurysm formation or true dissection has also been described in a significant number of patients.[39] Clinical predictors associated with IMH regression include younger age, hematoma thickness of <1 cm, initial aortic diameter of <4 cm, and β-blocker use.

PENETRATING AORTIC ULCER

Penetrating aortic ulcer (PAU) describes a focal area of aortic atherosclerotic plaque that had corroded and penetrated the internal elastic lamina into variable depths of the aortic media.[2,3] The base (or "crater") of these ulcers can fill with debris, thrombotic material, or foam cells. A pseudoaneurysm can form, or there can be rupture in the media or between the media and adventitia resulting in IMH. The IMH can propagate both distally and proximally and seldom can it progress to frank classic dissection. Of note, up to 20% of PAU present without evidence of IMH, likely secondary to fibrotic changes within the aortic media that prevent the formation and propagation of the hematoma.[39] In general, severe atherosclerosis can be seen in the adjacent aortic segments. Most PAUs occur in the descending thoracic aorta, although the process can involve any segment of the aorta. PAUs can occur in multiple. The size of PAU varies significantly and has been described as diameter of 2 to 25 mm and depth of 4 to 30 mm.

EPIDEMIOLOGY

The incidence of PAU is reported to be 2.3% to 11% of AASs. Of note, in autopsy series, up to 5% of aortic dissections seem to originate from PAU.

ETIOLOGY

Patients with PAU tend to be older, have high rates of hypertension (92%), cigarette smoking (77%), and prior evidence of coronary artery disease (46%). There is also a high frequency of concomitant aortic aneurysm (42% to 61%).

CLINICAL MANIFESTATIONS

The commonest clinical manifestation is back pain (seen in 75% of patients). Pleural effusions are also common (seen in 30% of patients).

The natural history of PAU is not well-defined. Many patients do not need urgent surgical intervention on diagnosis, but close follow-up is required owing to potential for progression and complications. The reported complications include the following:

- Progressive aortic remodeling with aneurysm formation.
- Pseudoaneurysm formation from penetration towards the adventitia and containment of the formed hematoma (by the adventitia), essentially creating a contained aortic rupture.
- Complete aortic rupture can rarely occur with resultant mediastinal or pleural hemorrhage.
- PAU can progress to frank aortic dissection. This type of dissection has distinct clinical characteristics that include localized dissection, calcified and thick dissection flap, and retrograde expansion.

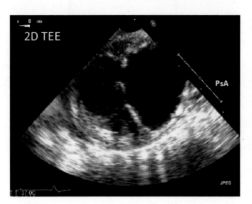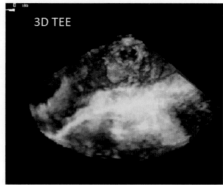

Figure 23.5. Penetrating aortic ulcer. The left panel shows a short axis view of two-dimensional TEE image of a penetrating aortic ulcer with a pseudoaneurysm formation in the descending thoracic aorta. On the right panel, real-time three-dimensional image is shown. The ulcer is seen at an en-face view, from the aortic lumen perspective. Ao, aorta; PAU, penetrating aortic ulcer; PsA, pseudoaneurysm.

DIAGNOSIS

PAUs can be diagnosed by contrast-enhanced CT scan, MRI, and transesophageal echocardiography (Figure 23.5). The ulcer area, the outpouching beyond the expected aortic wall, the surrounding atherosclerosis, and any complications and their extent can be visualized by these techniques.[39,40] Aortography is suboptimal for diagnosis of PAU, because depending on the projection used, the ulcer may not be readily identified.

MANAGEMENT AND PROGNOSIS

The natural history and optimal treatment approach to PAU remains under debate.[39] Some centers advocate early surgical intervention, as the rate of progression, complications, and need for acute aortic surgery were found to be high.[41] However, others demonstrated the safety of watchful expectant management, with serial imaging, and surgical intervention for acute complications with high survival rates for medically managed patients.[42] There is agreement, however, that rupture seen on presentation as well as maximum aortic diameter is predictive of failure of medical management and should be taken into consideration when treatment decisions are made. There is also agreement that should a watchful waiting approach be chosen, the patient should be followed closely at a dedicated aortic center.

TRAUMATIC AORTIC RUPTURE

Traumatic aortic rupture, despite being a life-threatening aortic disease, is not classically considered part of the "AAS" group as it presents in a distinct and unique scenario (Figure 23.6). It is most frequently associated with automobile accidents and results from the shear forces generated by the collision. The mechanism of aortic injury likely involves rapid deceleration and compression of the chest. These in turn induce shearing and torsional forces that can result in aortic transverse tearing at a vulnerable site. The most common site of traumatic aortic rupture is at the aortic isthmus (between the left subclavian origin and the first intercostal arteries). The most-feared complication is complete aortic rupture with mediastinal hemorrhage, which is almost universally fatal.

EPIDEMIOLOGY

Traumatic aortic injury is the second leading cause of death (after head injury) from blunt trauma. Most instances are caused by car accidents. The reported incidence of traumatic aortic rupture is 1.5% to 1.9% of all automobile crashes.[43]

ETIOLOGY

As mentioned above, most of the traumatic aortic injuries occur from car accidents. The persons most vulnerable to aortic injury are those seated close to the side of the impact, even more than those involved in frontal impact crashes.[43] The risk for traumatic aortic rupture is similar for impact from the left and the right sides of the thorax. An important risk factor for aortic injury is high impact injury. Passengers who do not use seat belts are three times as likely to sustain aortic injury compared with those who are belted.

CLINICAL MANIFESTATIONS

For patients who survive to arrival to the emergency room, the most common clinical sign of aortic injury is hemodynamic instability. Of note, in a review of cases of traumatic aortic injuries

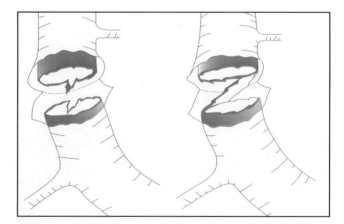

Figure 23.6. Traumatic aortic rupture. Diagram showing shear forces causing complete (left panel) or near-complete (right panel) traumatic aortic rupture.

from a level I trauma center, 23% of cases arrived to the emergency room without vital signs, and the diagnosis was made by postmortem examination.[44] Of those who arrived to the emergency room, 47% were hemodynamically unstable on presentation. Associated injuries were common and included lung injuries in 80% of patients, visceral injuries in 63%, extremities in 60%, and head injury in 50% of the patients.

Chest X-ray may be abnormal in >80% of patients with traumatic aortic injury. Widened mediastinum, tracheal shift, downward displacement of the left main bronchus, opacification of the aortopulmonary space, and pleural effusion are common findings on the initial chest X-ray.

DIAGNOSIS

CT scanning and TEE are the main tools for diagnosing traumatic aortic injury. CT scan is the most widely used technique. Aortic injury can be reliably diagnosed as well as accompanying pulmonary, visceral, and other injuries can be delineated.

TEE can be used as well with the main advantage that it can be used at the bedside or at the operating room. The characteristic finding is a thick and irregular medial flap that appears almost perpendicular to the aortic wall. Of note, other aortic injuries can be diagnosed on TEE as well, including intraluminal clot, classic dissection, or IMHs.

MANAGEMENT AND PROGNOSIS

The prognosis of traumatic aortic rupture is extremely grave.[44] As mentioned, a large percentage of patients die before reaching the hospital, and of those surviving to hospital admission, many present with profound hemodynamic instability with high rates of early mortality (14% early mortality and additional 46% intraoperative mortality). A minority of the patients, those who are hemodynamically stable on presentation, can be managed with medical optimization and delayed repair, with good results. Traditionally, the only treatment option for traumatic aortic rupture was open repair; however over the recent years several reports of successful endovascular repair have been described.[45] Endovascular repairs offer an excellent treatment option for suitable candidates and appear to have lower rates of postoperative mortality.

REFERENCES

1. Vilacosta I, San Román JA. Acute aortic syndrome. *Heart.* 2001;85:365–368.
2. Vilacosta I, Aragoncillo P, Cañadas V, et al. Acute aortic syndrome: a new look at an old conundrum. *Postgrad Med J.* 2010;86:52–61.
3. Lansman SL, Saunders PC, Malekan R, et al. Acute aortic syndrome. *J Thorac Cardiovasc Surg.* 2010;140(6)(suppl):S92–S97.
4. Ahmad F, Cheshire N, Hamady M. Acute aortic syndrome: pathology and therapeutic strategies [review]. *Postgrad Med J.* 2006;82(967):305–312. Wooley CF, Sparks EH, Boudoulas H. Aortic pain. *Prog Cardiovasc Dis.* 1998;40:563–589.
5. Hagan PG, Nienaber CA, Isselbacher EM, et al. The International Registry of Acute Aortic Dissection (IRAD): new insights into an old disease. *JAMA.* 2000;283(7):897–903.
6. Mészáros I, Mórocz J, Szlávi J, et al. Epidemiology and clinicopathology of aortic dissection. *Chest.* 2000;117(5):1271–1278.
7. Tsai TT, Trimarchi S, Nienaber CA. Acute aortic dissection: perspectives from the International Registry of Acute Aortic Dissection (IRAD). *Eur J Vasc Endovasc Surg.* 2009;37(2):149–159. Epub 2008 Dec 20.
8. Nienaber CA, Fattori R, Mehta RH, et al.; International Registry of Acute Aortic Dissection. Gender-related differences in acute aortic dissection. *Circulation.* 2004;109(24):3014–3021. Epub 2004 Jun 14.
9. Mehta RH, Manfredini R, Hassan F, et al.; International Registry of Acute Aortic Dissection (IRAD) Investigators. Chronobiological patterns of acute aortic dissection. *Circulation.* 2002;106(9):1110–1115.
10. Raghupathy A, Nienaber CA, Harris KM, et al.; International Registry of Acute Aortic Dissection (IRAD) Investigators. Geographic differences in clinical presentation, treatment, and outcomes in type A acute aortic dissection (from the International Registry of Acute Aortic Dissection). *Am J Cardiol.* 2008;102(11):1562–1566. Epub 2008 Sep 12.
11. Januzzi JL, Isselbacher EM, Fattori R, et al.; International Registry of Aortic Dissection (IRAD). Characterizing the young patient with aortic dissection: results from the International Registry of Aortic Dissection (IRAD). *J Am Coll Cardiol.* 2004;43(4):665–669.
12. Nistri S, Sorbo MD, Marin M, et al. Aortic root dilatation in young men with normally functioning bicuspid aortic valves. *Heart.* 1999;82(1):19–22.
13. Eagle KA, Isselbacher EM, DeSanctis RW; International Registry for Aortic Dissection (IRAD) Investigators. Cocaine-related aortic dissection in perspective. *Circulation.* 2002;105(13):1529–1530.
14. Hsue PY, Salinas CL, Bolger AF, et al. Acute aortic dissection related to crack cocaine. *Circulation.* 2002;105(13):1592–1595.
15. Park SW, Hutchison S, Mehta RH, et al. Association of painless acute aortic dissection with increased mortality. *Mayo Clin Proc.* 2004;79(10):1252–1257.
16. Nallamothu BK, Mehta RH, Saint S, et al. Syncope in acute aortic dissection: diagnostic, prognostic, and clinical implications. *Am J Med.* 2002;113(6):468–471.
17. Bossone E, Rampoldi V, Nienaber CA, et al.; International Registry of Acute Aortic Dissection (IRAD) Investigators. Usefulness of pulse deficit to predict in-hospital complications and mortality in patients with acute type A aortic dissection. *Am J Cardiol.* 2002;89(7):851–855.
18. Gilon D, Mehta RH, Oh JK, et al.; International Registry of Acute Aortic Dissection Group. Characteristics and in-hospital outcomes of patients with cardiac tamponade complicating type A acute aortic dissection. *Am J Cardiol.* 2009;103(7):1029–1031.
19. Movsowitz HD, Levine RA, Hilgenberg AD, et al. Transesophageal echocardiographic description of the mechanisms of aortic regurgitation in acute type A aortic dissection: implications for aortic valve repair. *J Am Coll Cardiol.* 2000;36(3):884–890.
20. Matsumura N, Yamamoto K, Takenaka H, et al. Hoarseness and aortic arch dissection. *Intern Med.* 2008;47(5):473. Epub 2008 Mar 3.
21. Suzuki T, Mehta RH, Ince H, et al.; International Registry of Aortic Dissection. Clinical profiles and outcomes of acute type B aortic dissection in the current era: lessons from the International Registry of Aortic Dissection (IRAD). *Circulation.* 2003;108(suppl 1):II312–II317.
22. Mehta RH, O'Gara PT, Bossone E, et al.; International Registry of Acute Aortic Dissection (IRAD) Investigators. Acute type A aortic dissection in the elderly: clinical characteristics, management, and outcomes in the current era. *J Am Coll Cardiol.* 2002;40(4):685–692.
23. Von Kodolitsch Y, Schwartz AG, Nienaber CA. Clinical prediction of acute aortic dissection. *Arch Intern Med.* 2000;160(19):2977–2982.
24. Moore AG, Eagle KA, Bruckman D, et al. Choice of computed tomography, transesophageal echocardiography, magnetic resonance imaging, and aortography in acute aortic dissection: International Registry of Acute Aortic Dissection (IRAD). *Am J Cardiol.* 2002;89(10):1235–1238.
25. McMahon MA, Squirrell CA. Multidetector CT of aortic dissection: a pictorial review. *Radiographics.* 2010;30(2):445–460.
26. Shiga T, Wajima Z, Apfel CC, et al. Diagnostic accuracy of transesophageal echocardiography, helical computed tomography, and magnetic resonance imaging for suspected thoracic aortic dissection: systematic review and meta-analysis. *Arch Intern Med.* 2006;166(13):1350–1356.
27. Ranasinghe AM, Bonser RS. Biomarkers in acute aortic dissection and other aortic syndromes. *J Am Coll Cardiol.* 2010;56(19):1535–1541.
28. Suzuki T, Distante A, Zizza A, et al.; IRAD-Bio Investigators. Diagnosis of acute aortic dissection by D-dimer: the International Registry of Acute Aortic Dissection Substudy on Biomarkers (IRAD-Bio) Experience. *Circulation.* 2009;119(20):2702–2707. Epub 2009 May 11.
29. Mehta RH, Suzuki T, Hagan PG, et al.; International Registry of Acute Aortic Dissection (IRAD) Investigators. Predicting death in patients with acute type A aortic dissection. *Circulation.* 2002;105(2):200–206.
30. Trimarchi S, Eagle KA, Nienaber CA, et al.; International Registry of Acute Aortic Dissection Investigators. Role of age in acute type A aortic dissection outcome: report from the International Registry of Acute Aortic Dissection (IRAD). *J Thorac Cardiovasc Surg.* 2010;140(4):784–789. Epub 2010 Feb 21.
31. Rampoldi V, Trimarchi S, Eagle KA, et al.; International Registry of Acute Aortic Dissection (IRAD) Investigators. Simple risk models to predict surgical mortality in acute type A aortic dissection: the International Registry of Acute Aortic Dissection score. *Ann Thorac Surg.* 2007;83(1):55–61.
32. Tsai TT, Evangelista A, Nienaber CA, et al.; International Registry of Acute Aortic Dissection (IRAD). Long-term survival in patients presenting with type A acute aortic dissection: insights from the International Registry of Acute Aortic Dissection (IRAD). *Circulation.* 2006;114(1)(suppl):I350–I356.
33. Trimarchi S, Eagle KA, Nienaber CA, et al.; International Registry of Acute Aortic Dissection (IRAD) Investigators. Importance of refractory pain and hypertension in acute type B aortic dissection: insights from the International Registry of Acute Aortic Dissection (IRAD). *Circulation.* 2010;122(13):1283–1289. Epub 2010 Sep 13.
34. Trimarchi S, Eagle KA, Rampoldi V, et al.; IRAD Investigators. Role and results of surgery in acute type B aortic dissection: insights from the International Registry of Acute Aortic Dissection (IRAD). *Circulation.* 2006;114(1)(suppl):I357–I364.
35. Tsai TT, Fattori R, Trimarchi S, et al.; International Registry of Acute Aortic Dissection. Long-term survival in patients presenting with type B acute aortic dissection: insights from the International Registry of Acute Aortic Dissection. *Circulation.* 2006;114(21):2226–2231. Epub 2006 Nov 13.
36. Evangelista A, Mukherjee D, Mehta RH, et al.; International Registry of Aortic Dissection (IRAD) Investigators. Acute intramural hematoma of the aorta: a mystery in evolution. *Circulation.* 2005;111(8):1063–1070. Epub 2005 Feb 14.
37. Kitai T, Kaji S, Yamamuro A, et al. Clinical outcomes of medical therapy and timely operation in initially diagnosed type A aortic intramural hematoma: a 20-year experience. *Circulation.* 2009;120(11)(suppl):S292–S298.

38. Song JK, Yim JH, Ahn JM, et al. Outcomes of patients with acute type A aortic intramural hematoma. *Circulation.* 2009;120(21):2046–2052. Epub 2009 Nov 9.

39. Sundt TM. Intramural hematoma and penetrating atherosclerotic ulcer of the aorta [review]. *Ann Thorac Surg.* 2007;83(2):S835–S841; discussion S846–S850.

40. Vilacosta I, San Román JA, Aragoncillo P, et al. Penetrating atherosclerotic aortic ulcer: documentation by transesophageal echocardiography. *J Am Coll Cardiol.* 1998;32(1):83–89.

41. Cho KR, Stanson AW, Potter DD, et al. Penetrating atherosclerotic ulcer of the descending thoracic aorta and arch. *J Thorac Cardiovasc Surg.* 2004;127(5):1393–1399; discussion 1399–1401.

42. Tittle SL, Lynch RJ, Cole PE, et al. Midterm follow-up of penetrating ulcer and intramural hematoma of the aorta. *J Thorac Cardiovasc Surg.* 2002;123(6):1051–1059.

43. Fitzharris M, Franklyn M, Frampton R, et al. Thoracic aortic injury in motor vehicle crashes: the effect of impact direction, side of body struck, and seat belt use. *J Trauma.* 2004;57(3):582–590.

44. Duwayri Y, Abbas J, Cerilli G, et al. Outcome after thoracic aortic injury: experience in a level-1 trauma center. *Ann Vasc Surg.* 2008;22(3):309–313. Epub 2008 Apr 14.

45. Xenos ES, Abedi NN, Davenport DL, et al. Meta-analysis of endovascular vs open repair for traumatic descending thoracic aortic rupture [review]. *J Vasc Surg.* 2008;48(5):1343–1351. Epub 2008 Jul 15.

PATIENT AND FAMILY INFORMATION FOR:
Acute Aortic Syndromes

Acute Aortic Syndromes (AAS) are an array of disorders that lead to damage to the wall of the aorta, the main and largest artery that delivers blood from the left ventricle of the heart to the body organs and tissues. These disorders are frequently sudden and are associated with severe chest pain that is sometimes quite intense. The diagnosis is based on clinical impression and has to be confirmed by one or more imaging techniques that can show the nature, site, extent, and complication of the disorder. Early diagnosis and treatment are important, and delay in treatment may lead to further damage, complications, and even death. AAS include, among others, aortic dissection, Intramural Hematoma (IMH), and Penetrating Aortic Ulcer (PAU).

Aortic dissection is a partial tear of the wall of the aorta. The tear results in separation of the layers that make the wall (dissection). Aortic dissection may be the result of high blood pressure or of weakness of the aortic wall. Aortic dissection can cause severe chest pain.

The diagnosis of the condition and the treatment should be started immediately. The treatment depends on the location and the extent of the tear. Tears that are closer to the heart, in the section of the aorta known as the ascending aorta have to be treated by surgery as soon as possible. During surgery, part of the ascending aorta will be replaced by a Dacron tube. This is a major surgery that carries a certain risk. However, it is riskier not to operate. Without surgery, the aortic wall may rupture and cause serious complications such as bleeding around the heart that may compress the heart to a degree that it may not function well. Dissection may also cause occlusion of arteries connected to the aorta and cause damage to organs they supply. Dissection may damage one of the heart valves and cause it to leak. Surgery will deal with these complications.

Dissection of the more distal part (remote, away from the heart) can be handled by medications. Dissection of this part, if uncomplicated, does not require surgery.

Surgery will be performed by a cardiovascular surgeon who specializes in this kind of surgery. At the end of surgery, monitoring in the recovery room and later in a postoperative intensive care unit will be required. The medical treatment includes pain control, aggressive treatment of elevated blood pressure (and thus decrease the pressure on the aortic wall that may be the culprit responsible the tear), and drugs that diminish the intensity of the contraction of the heart with a hope to decrease arterial pulsation that may have deleterious effect on the damaged aortic wall.

IMH is considered by many to be a variant of aortic dissection. The etiology of IMH is the same as that of dissection. In IMH there is a separation within a layer of the aortic wall that fills with a blood clot. Unlike dissection, there is no tear of the layers, and therefore there is no flapping motion of the torn layer seen in dissection. However, nearly one-third of all IMH progresses to classical aortic dissection, whereas another third resolves spontaneously and heals. The symptoms of dissection and IMH may be similar. Treatment is also very similar: urgent surgical repair for ascending aorta IMH and medical watchful waiting with medication to control pain and hypertension for descending aortic IMH.

One of the complications of aortic atherosclerosis is formation of a crater (ulcer) in the innermost layer of the aorta. When this ulcer expands it can rarely penetrate through the outer layers, creating a hole in the wall of the aorta (PAU). This complication of atherosclerosis can lead to severe pain and internal hemorrhage. In some cases, the hole created by the PAU is sealed off by the tissue around the aorta, creating a weak spot prone to complications. The treatment of complicated ulcer is frequently surgical. Here again it is important to control the blood pressure and to arrest the progression of atherosclerosis.

AAS are relatively rare. Most patients and very frequently their family or friends are familiar with the symptoms, the treatment modalities, and the prognosis of coronary heart disease and acute myocardial infarction (or heart attack). These are frequently discussed in public and in the media, and almost always happened to someone they know. When the diagnosis of AAS is made, and the details are discussed with the patients, the initial response will usually be "thank god the heart is OK," or "I am glad it is not a heart attack." This is, of course, a too optimistic response. AAS, on average is more dangerous than coronary artery disease, and the immediate prognosis in many undiagnosed or untreated patients may lead to patient's demise within hours. Acute type A dissection or IMH has a mortality rate of 1% to 2% per hour. In these patients surgery may be lifesaving. It is estimated that 75% to 85% of operated patients will be able to leave the hospital.

Acute aortic transection is even worse. It has extremely poor prognosis—most of the patients with this disorder are dead by the time they are brought to medical attention. Of those who survive the trip to the hospital—supportive care, rapid diagnosis, and surgery may occasionally prevent death.

When a patient reports to a medical facility with severe chest pains, the immediate medical practice challenge is usually "to rule out acute coronary syndrome." This includes history, physical examination, repeat electrocardiograms, and cardiac enzymes evaluation. If deemed necessary stress test is also ordered. Usually, after 12 to 24 hours of monitoring, when all tests are negative and the pain subsides, "Myocardial infarction is ruled out," and the patient is reassured and frequently discharged.

Every year, 5 to 6 people per every 100,000 individuals suffer from acute aortic dissection, which means approximately 15,000 cases in the United States alone. It is estimated, that in spite of the increasing and improving diagnostic technology available, 20% to 25% of dissection patients are discharged without diagnosis after "an MI was ruled out." Some are readmitted, other die as outpatients, and a few develop chronic dissection that may be discovered later during unrelated medical evaluation. The medical and nonmedical literature has many stories describing how dissection was missed. The annals of legal medicine also describe many such cases, where failure to diagnose dissection led to malpractice suit.

AAS should always remain in the differential diagnosis of patients with chest pain, regardless of their age and their coronary risk factors. Dissection or IMH cannot be ruled out by normal EKG or normal cardiac enzymes (although signs of myocardial ischemia and even infarction may be the result of aortic dissection that involves the coronary arteries).

Unless the reason for the chest pain is very clear, echocardiograms and chest X-ray should be reviewed in each case of suspicious chest pain. The nature of the pain may suggest the diagnosis. In dissection or IMH, it is more than just chest discomfort, usually described as intense, sharp, and tearing. Occasionally the pain follows the route of intimal tear and changes its location. Occasionally it waxes and wanes.

The threshold to perform diagnostic tests to evaluate the possibility of dissection should be quite low in patients with chest pains, risk factors, and physical findings that increase the likelihood of dissection. These include, among others, severe hypertension, murmur of aortic insufficiency, symptoms and signs of acute arterial occlusion, connective tissue disorder, bicuspid aortic valve and dilated aorta by history, chest X-ray findings, or TTE.

When AAS is clinically suspected, the patient and his family should immediately be told and should become aware of the seriousness of the condition and the need to further explore for accurate diagnosis. Each diagnostic modality (TEE, CT, and MRI) carries a small risk that has to be clarified.

When indicated, aortic surgery or interventional procedure has to be performed immediately. The patient and/or his family have to be approached as soon as possible and informed consent obtained. The discussion has to be as detailed as possible, and all questions should be answered. However, everyone has to be aware that procrastination and hesitation may be dangerous. Requests by the patient and his/her family to wait and see ("He/she is already feeling better," "His/her sister is coming from Europe," etc.) need to be discussed patiently, disclosing how unsafe watchful waiting can be in these conditions.

As noted earlier in this review, surgery for AAS carries a significant risk that depends, among other factors on the age of the patient, the type, the site and the extent of the lesion, the involvement of the aortic valve, the presence of cardiac tamponade, and mediastinal bleeding. All these issues should be disclosed as soon as possible with the party who consents for the surgery (patient and/or his legal representative).

It should be borne in mind that AAS is frequently associated with very severe pains that require treatment by narcotics and tranquilizers. At this stage, the patient may be not legally responsible for his/her decisions and further discussion and family consent should be advisable, if possible.

Anuj Mediratta
Vera H. Rigolin

Pericardial Effusion and Tamponade

Disease processes involving the pericardium are encountered in a variety of clinical settings. Pericardial effusions and cardiac tamponade are the most commonly encountered pericardial disorders and are often seen in general medical clinics or wards, emergency rooms, and intensive care units. A high degree of clinical suspicion is required as the diagnosis of pericardial disorders can be subtle and is easily confused with other intrathoracic processes. Although many patients can be managed as outpatients or on medical wards, appropriate triage is essential as intensive care may be required, as some patients can rapidly decline and may require urgent interventions.

Specific management of pericardial disease as a whole is quite limited within the cardiovascular literature. There is paucity of randomized controlled trials, minimal advances in diagnosis or treatment over the last several decades, and for years, a lack of guidelines for the management of these conditions.

This review will focus on presentation, physiology, diagnostic testing, and management of patients with pericardial effusions and cardiac tamponade.

NORMAL PERICARDIUM

In the normal heart the pericardium consists of a mostly avascular membrane with both visceral and parietal layers separated by a fluid-containing potential space. The visceral pericardium, a thin one-cell layer of mesothelial cells is directly attached to the epicardium, whereas the parietal pericardium, a 2-mm layer comprising mostly of collagen and elastin is separated from the visceral layer by 5 to 15 ml of pericardial fluid. The reflection of the visceral pericardium is near the junction of the inferior and superior vena cavae to the right atrium. Portions of the caval vessels therefore lie within the pericardial sac.[1] The left atrium, however, is mostly outside the pericardium. The pericardium serves several functions—anchors the heart and great vessels within the mediastinum, acts as a barrier to infection, and minimizes friction—however, congenital absence and/or surgical removal does not cause any specific pathologic process. The pericardium is well innervated acting with sensory input (i.e., pain) and autonomic involvement with vagal tone and secretion of prostaglandins with cardiac reflexes.[2,3]

PERICARDIAL EFFUSIONS AND CARDIAC TAMPONADE

In the normal heart, the pericardial fluid is present to lubricate the pericardium during the cardiac cycle and reduce friction between the membranes. A pericardial effusion is present when a greater than normal amount of pericardial fluid is present. Pericardial effusions can be caused by increased fluid production, decreased resorption of fluid, or changes in fluid content with or without foreign substances within the space. Pericardial effusions range from small, clinically insignificant effusions to medical emergencies as in cardiac tamponade. Multiple classifications systems are used for describing pericardial effusions based on the cause of the effusion, type of fluid, and the size. It is important to note that the effect of an effusion on intrapericardial pressure relates to compliance, rate of accumulation, and volume of fluid in space. Thus, the pericardium can often accommodate large, slowly growing effusions although it may not be able to do so for rapidly accumulating effusions.[2–5]

Cardiac tamponade, a potentially life-threatening medical emergency, results when fluid within the pericardium results in elevated pericardial pressure that, in turn, results in compression of cardiac structures. By definition cardiac tamponade is a spectrum of diseases that can range from clinically insignificant to state of decompensation with collapse of cardiac structures that can rapidly progress to cardiogenic shock or death if not treated.[2–4]

HEMODYNAMICS OF PERICARDIAL EFFUSIONS AND TAMPONADE

Fluid within the pericardial space provides a unique set of changes in the cardiovascular system. As mentioned previously, the compensatory response of the pericardium to the accumulation of fluid is an important factor in the ability of the heart to tolerate the increased fluid. Other factors contributing to the compensatory mechanism include the presence of other comorbidities, hydration status, and medications, specifically β-blocking agents.

The initial response to pericardial effusion is adrenergic stimulation with withdrawal of parasympathetic stimulation leading to increased contractility and tachycardia as a way to maintain cardiac output. Of note, this response is blunted in patients with β-blockade.[2]

As the intrapericardial pressure increases, right heart filling becomes impaired, leading to decreased right heart stroke volume, a downstream decrease in left heart preload, and subsequent stroke volume. This effect is most pronounced during inspiration when there is an increase in right heart filling owing to a decrease in intrathoracic pressure.[6] The increased right heart filling causes the septum to bulge towards the left. Because of the constraints of the pericardium and the effusion, the left heart cannot expand to compensate for the volume loss caused by the shift in the septum. Left-sided filling and stroke volume is therefore impaired. The opposite effect is seen during expiration. Left heart filling is further impaired since intrapericardial pressure falls less than intrathoracic pressure during inspiration in tamponade. This results in a decrease in the left ventricular filling gradient during inspiration. The hemodynamic effect of the increased pericardial pressure is seen clinically as a decline in the Korotkoff sounds during inspiration during measurement of the pulsus paradoxus.[2,4]

ETIOLOGY

Pericardial effusions can be caused by a variety of conditions including both inflammatory and noninflammatory processes of the pericardium (Table 24.1). It not completely clear which specific causes of effusion lead to tamponade; however malignancy as well as bacterial, mycobacterial and fungal, and HIV infections have a predisposition to cause large clinically significant effusions.[2–4]

PATIENT HISTORY

As with most disease processes, the patient's history is essential for the diagnosis of pericardial effusion—specifically looking for systemic diseases known to involve the peri-/myocardium such as autoimmune diseases, malignancy, renal, or thyroid disease. Also important are historical details such as trauma, surgery, previous radiation, travel, exposures, or recent illness. Patients typically present with intrathoracic symptoms such as chest discomfort that can have positional or pleuritic component, dyspnea, orthopnea, or cough. Systemic symptoms such as generalized fatigue or weakness, lightheadedness or dizziness,

TABLE 24.1	Etiology of Pericardial Disease
Idiopathic	
	Acute idiopathic pericarditis
	Chronic idiopathic pericardial effusion
Infectious	
	Viral
	Fungal
	Mycobacterial
	Bacterial
	Protozoal
Immune-mediated	
	Post-myocardial infarction: early or late
	Drug-induced
	Connective tissue disease
	Vasculitis
Malignancy/neoplasm	
	Direct invasion
	Secondary to lymphatic obstruction
Metabolic	
	Uremia
	Hypothyriod
	Cirrhosis
	Amyloidosis
Miscellaneous	
	Trauma
	Radiation
	Postsurgical
	Congenital

abdominal distension, and/or peripheral edema are also common presenting symptoms. Less common symptoms are with compression of adjacent structures such as dysphagia, hoarseness, or hiccups. On the contrary, patients can be asymptomatic.[2,3]

Patients with tamponade are generally more symptomatic than those with uncomplicated effusions. Signs of cardiogenic shock such as mental status changes or decreased urine output may be the presenting symptom. In addition, syncope or pulseless electrical activity (PEA) arrest may be the presenting symptom depending on degree of compression. Patients with severe tamponade may present with frank cardiogenic shock.[2–4]

PHYSICAL EXAMINATION

Physical exam should focus on vital signs and the cardiopulmonary exam. Findings can be nonspecific such as tachycardia or hypotension or can be more specific to pericardial effusions. Specific physical findings such as pulsus paradoxus, friction rub, distant heart sounds, loss of apical impulse, and/or dullness at loss of heart sounds at left lung base ("Ewart's sign") may be present. Findings specific to heart failure should be examined, including examination of jugular venous pulse, hepatojugular reflex, lung exam, and peripheral exam for edema. Physical exam may be normal in patients with pericardial effusion without hemodynamic compromise.

Signs such as elevated jugular venous pulsations, tachycardia, hypotension, pulsus paradoxus >10 mm Hg (see below), muffled heart sounds, pericardial rub, altered mental status, peripheral edema or cold, and clammy extremities should alert the clinician of possible tamponade. Classically patients with tamponade present with the constellation of symptoms known as "Beck's triad" with decreased heart sounds, hypotension, and increased central venous pressure.[2,3]

Pulsus paradoxus or paradoxical pulse is actually an exaggeration of normal blood pressure changes that occur with inspiration, rather than a true paradox. By definition, pulsus paradoxus is a >10 mm Hg drop in systolic blood pressure that occurs during inspiration where normal inspiratory change is <10 mm Hg. This can be determined best at the patient's bedside using a sphygmomanometer and a stethoscope. To assess for pulsus, the patient should be instructed to breathe normally. The clinician should then evaluate the systolic blood pressure at which the first Korotkoff sound is auscultated only during expiration (sound appears during expiration and disappears during inspiration). Then the cuff should be slowly deflated until the first Korotkoff sound is heard throughout the respiratory cycle. The difference between these two numbers is the degree of pulsus paradoxus given as a pressure in mm Hg. If tamponade is severe, peripheral pulses may disappear during inspiration. Of note, pulsus paradoxus may not be present when left ventricular ejection fraction is reduced, in presence of septal defects or with aortic regurgitation; conversely it can be seen without pericardial effusions as in pulmonary embolism, chronic lung disease, and constrictive pericarditis.[2–4]

DIAGNOSTIC TESTS

Diagnostic testing typically follows if a pericardial effusion or tamponade is suspected based on the history and physical examination. The diagnostic evaluation usually begins with basic

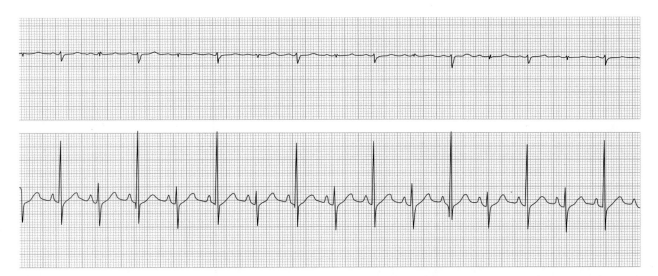

Figure 24.1. Rhythm strip showing electrical alternans caused by swinging movement of the heart within pericardial sac. (Courtesy of Dr James E. Rosenthal, Associate Professor of Medicine, Northwestern University Feinberg School of Medicine, Bluhm Cardiovascular Institute.)

blood tests, ECG, and chest radiograph (Figures 24.1 and 24.2). Transthoracic echocardiography (TTE) is the test of choice to visualize the effusion and should be done urgently if concern for tamponade physiology is present.[2-4]

The echocardiogram is useful to demonstrate the size, location, and extent of the effusion. The echo can also demonstrate the degree of hemodynamic compromise caused by the fluid. Typical echo signs of tamponade include early diastolic collapse of the right ventricle and early systolic collapse of the right atrium, which occur because pericardial pressure transiently exceeds the intracavitary pressure[2,7,8] (Figures 24.3 and 24.4).

Elevated right atrial pressure is demonstrated by plethora of the inferior vena cava (Figure 24.5). The hemodynamic alterations in right- and left-sided filling are demonstrated by respiratory flow variation in the mitral and tricuspid spectral Doppler signals (Figure 24.6). Computerized tomography (CT) and magnetic resonance imaging (MRI) are generally used if

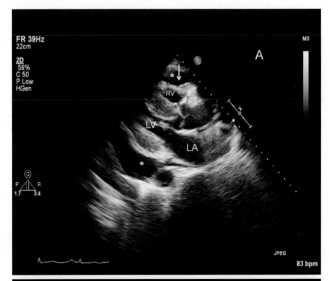

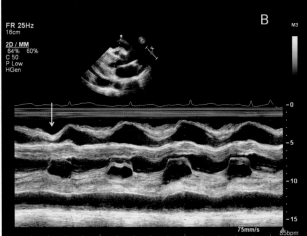

Figure 24.3. Transthoracic echocardiogram showing the parasternal long axis view (**Panel A**) and the corresponding M mode view (**Panel B**). There is a large pericardial effusion (*) with evidence collapse of right ventricle during diastole *(arrow)*. LA, left atrium; LV, left ventricle; RV, right ventricle.

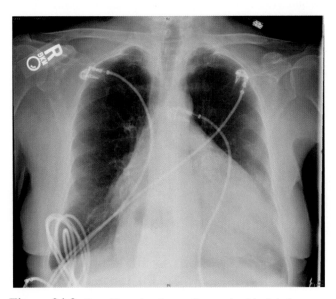

Figure 24.2. Chest X-ray showing cardiomegaly with globular "water bottle" appearance.

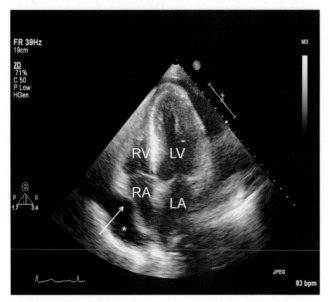

Figure 24.4. Transthoracic echocardiogram showing the apical four-chamber view. There is collapse of the right atrium *(arrow)* owing to the large effusion (*). LA, left atrium; LV, left ventricle; RA, right atrium; RV, right ventricle.

previous tests are inconclusive or if further visualization of specific structures (epicardial fat, loculation, left ventricular pseudoaneurysm, or pericardial thickening) is indicated. Transesophageal echocardiogram can be helpful if TTE is nondiagnostic.[7,8]

LABORATORY TESTING

All patients with pericardial effusions should have initial serum analysis with basic and cardiac-specific labs (Table 24.2). Other individuals require further evaluation with testing as indicated by clinical presentation and risk factors.[2–4]

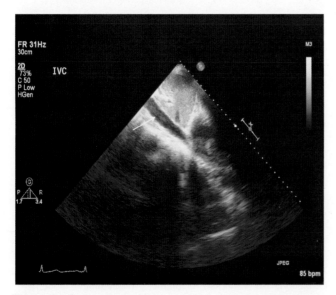

Figure 24.5. Transthoracic echocardiogram showing the subcostal view of inferior vena cava (IVC) *(arrow)*. The IVC is dilated and noncompressible during inspiration, suggesting an increase in right atrial pressure.

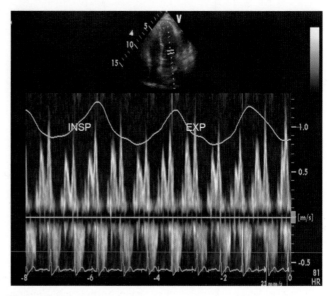

Figure 24.6. Doppler imaging of transmitral valve flow velocities with respiratory cycle and ECG. Note the decrease in the E wave velocity during inspiration (INSP) and increase during expiration (EXP). This corresponds to pulsus paradoxus in this patient. The reverse is true for tricuspid velocities measured during expiration and inspiration.

In addition to serum testing, specific analysis of pericardial fluid should be pursued if pericardiocentesis is to be performed, including cell count and differential, bacterial, and mycobacterial culture, and staining and cytology. If tuberculous (TB) pericarditis is suspected, adenosine deaminase and TB polymerase chain reaction should be performed.[2]

DESCRIPTION AND CLASSIFICATION

Pericardial effusions can be classified by the type of effusion, size, chronicity, and presence or absence of loculations. Evaluation of the fluid can define whether the effusion is transudative, exudative, purulent ("pyopericardium"), or bloody ("hemopericardium"). In addition, pericardial effusions can be classified based on posterior echo-free space on parasternal long-axis view during diastole[2–4]:

TABLE 24.2	Diagnostic Testing for Patients with Pericardial Effusions
EKG	Low voltage, axis change, electrical alternans, ST elevations, PR depression
CXR	Cardiomegaly, globular shape
Echocardiogram	RA notching, RV collapse, IVC noncompressibility, inspiratory variation in TV and MV velocities
CT	Evidence of loculation
TEE	For nondiagnostic TTE
Pericardiocentesis	
Pericardial biopsy	
Serum labs	CBC, chemistry, cardiac biomarkers in all patients. In select patients: HIV, ESR, CRP, LDH, ANA, Lyme disease antibody

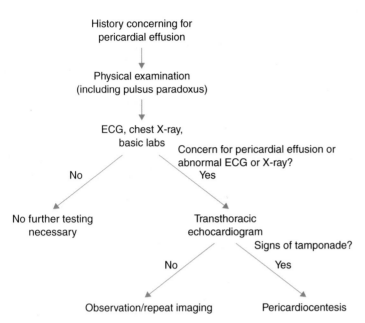

History concerning for
pericardial effusion

↓

Physical examination
(including pulsus paradoxus)

↓

ECG, chest X-ray,
basic labs

Concern for pericardial effusion or
abnormal ECG or X-ray?

No — Yes

No further testing
necessary

Transthoracic
echocardiogram

Signs of tamponade?

No — Yes

Observation/repeat imaging — Pericardiocentesis

Figure 24.7. Pericardial effusion algorithm showing diagnostic evaluation and workup when pericardial effusion/tamponade is suspected.

1. Physiologic <10 mm, seen in systole only
2. Small <10 mm, in both systole and diastole
3. Moderate—10 to 20 mm, can be seen anteriorly
4. Large—≥20 mm, seen anteriorly and apically
5. Very Large—large with compression of the heart.

There is a role for diagnostic pericardiocentesis and/or pericardial biopsy if diagnosis is uncertain and suspicion for malignancy is high. Fluid cytology and biopsy can be positive individually and in combination greatly improve sensitivity of malignant effusion.[2–4]

TREATMENT

Treatment is generally aimed at treating the etiology of the pericardial effusion. Nonsteroidal anti-inflammatory agents are often used to treat the pain and inflammation of pericarditis. Patients with potential tamponade are preload-dependent; therefore, intravenous fluids are essential in treating pericardial effusions. Blood pressure should be supported with inotropic agents such as norepinepherine, dobutamine, or dopamine if any evidence of poor end-organ perfusion (renal or liver failure, mental status changes, and decreased urine output) is seen. Mechanical ventilation should be avoided if possible as positive pressure ventilation further reduces preload and can worsen tamponade or can precipitate it in patients with large pericardial effusions. If possible, cessation of β-blocking agents should be pursued in early stages to allow for compensatory tachycardia response. Hemodynamic monitoring with pulmonary artery balloon catheter can be helpful; however it should not delay definitive treatment.[2–4]

Cardiac tamponade requires urgent identification and drainage of effusion regardless of etiology. Certain cases of refractory, chronic, or known malignancy may benefit from symptomatic management with catheter drainage, percutaneous balloon pericardiotomy, or surgical approaches if previous approaches fail.

A clinical algorithm for the pericardial effusions is outlined in Figure 24.7.

CONCLUSION

The normal pericardium serves to prevent infection, minimize friction, and maintain the structures within the mediastinum. Diseases of the pericardium can present with positional chest pain, dyspnea, symptoms of heart failure, or other nonspecific symptoms. Pericardial effusion can result from any cause of pericarditis and is often caused by infections (most often viral), autoimmune processes, and malignancy. A detailed physical examination should be performed for signs of circulatory compromise, including examination for pulsus paradoxus. If suspicion for hemodynamically significant pericardial effusion is present, urgent evaluation with echocardiogram should be performed focusing on specific echocardiographic findings of tamponade. If hemodynamic compromise is present emergent pericardiocentesis should be performed.

REFERENCES

1. Johnson, D. The pericardium. In: Standring S, Ellis H, Collins P, Wigley C, Berkovitz BKB. Gray's Anatomy: The Anatomical Basis of Clinical Practice. 39th ed. Edinburgh; New York: Elsevier Churchill Livingstone; 2005: 995–996.
2. LeWinter MM. Pericardial diseases. In: Libby P, Bonow RO, Mann DL, et al., eds. *Braunwald's Heart Disease: A Textbook of Cardiovascular Medicine.* 8th ed. Philadelphia, PA: Saunders; 2007:1829–1852.
3. Ewer SM. Diseases of the pericardium. In: Cuculich PS, Kates AM, eds. *The Washington Manual Cardiology Subspecialty Consult.* 2nd ed. Philadelphia, PA: Lippincott Williams & Wilkins; 2009:139–151.
4. Maisch B, Seferovic PM, Ristic AD, et al. Guidelines on the diagnosis and management of pericardial diseases executive summary; The task force on the diagnosis and management of pericardial diseases of the European Society of Cardiology. *Eur Heart J.* 2004;25:587–610.
5. Spodick DH. Acute cardiac tamponade. *N Engl J Med.* 2003;349(7):684–690.
6. Robb JF, Laham RJ. Profiles in pericardial disease. In: Baim DS, ed. *Grossman's Cardiac Catheterization, Angiography & Intervention.* 7th ed. Philadelphia, PA: Lippincott Williams & Wilkins; 2006:731.
7. Feigenbaum H, Armstrong WF, Ryan T. Pericardial diseases. In: *Feigenbaum's Echocardiography.* 7th ed. Philadelphia, PA: Lippincott Williams & Wilkins; 2010:241–262.
8. Oh JK, Seward JB, Tajik AJ. Pericardial diseases. In: *The Echo Manual.* 3rd ed. Rochester, MN: Lippincott Williams & Wilkins; 2006:289–309.

PATIENT AND FAMILY INFORMATION FOR:
Pericardial Effusion and Tamponade

The heart and the blood vessels connected to the heart are surrounded by a sac called the pericardium which normally contains a small amount of fluid. The pericardium functions to keep the heart anchored within the chest, helps to lubricate it as it pumps and protects it from infection. At times the pericardium can become inflamed—from viruses, cancer, autoimmune processes, or other reasons such as a previous heart attack or heart surgery—leading to increased irritation and fluid buildup. Some symptoms of irritation of this area may be chest discomfort/pain, painful or difficult breathing, or simply feeling lightheaded, tired, or weak. Diseases relating to the pericardium are most often self-limited; however some may require specific testing, hospitalization, or procedures as they can be life-threatening.

When the pericardium becomes inflamed, the condition is called pericarditis. If a greater than normal amount of fluid is present around the heart, the condition is called a pericardial effusion. Fluid around the heart is not harmful in itself because the heart can still function normally with a certain amount of fluid. However, too much fluid around the heart may result in increased pressure around the heart resulting in a decrease in the heart's pumping function. This condition is called cardiac tamponade and needs to be closely managed in a hospital and may require drainage of the fluid.

TESTING

There are a variety of tests that can be done to determine whether the pericardium is inflamed or contains too much fluid. These include basic and specialized blood tests. Other tests that help to evaluate the heart and the pericardium include a chest X-ray and an electrocardiogram. An echocardiogram (heart ultrasound) is a painless test using sound waves to visualize the heart, the pericardium, and any fluid. The echocardiogram can tell if parts of the heart are being compressed by fluid (Figure 24.4). Other tests may be used such as CT scans, MRI, or right heart catheterization.

TREATMENT

Treatment with anti-inflammatory medications such as ibuprofen may be beneficial for reducing the inflammation in the pericardium if pericarditis is present. Other treatments are aimed at treating the cause of the fluid such as treating an infection, cancer, or other processes. Many of these conditions require no specific treatment because the body can absorb the fluid over time; however if cardiac tamponade is present, a procedure called pericardiocentesis may be required to drain the fluid around the heart. If a diagnosis cannot be made, it is possible that some fluid may need to be removed or a biopsy of the pericardium may need to be taken.

Pericardiocentesis is a safe procedure done at the bedside or in a cardiovascular procedure room to remove the extra fluid from the pericardium. The procedure is typically performed with the aid of either a heart ultrasound or an X-ray technology and involves draining the fluid with a needle, often leaving a small drain in place. Although the procedure is invasive, major complications are reported <2% of the time. Pericardial biopsy (called pericardioscopy) involves a flexible or rigid camera that directly looks at the pericardium so that small samples can be obtained. As with pericardiocentesis, the complication rate is very low for these procedures.

SUMMARY

The pericardium is a sac surrounding the heart that occasionally becomes inflamed or filled with too much fluid. Typical symptoms include chest discomfort, difficulty in breathing, or feeling weak. Certain tests need to be performed to diagnose problems with the pericardium and may include blood tests, ECG, X-ray, or heart ultrasound. The diseases of the pericardium range widely from mild diseases requiring little to no treatment to life-threatening illness that requires hospitalization and urgent testing and treatment procedures.

Decompensated Valvular Disease in the Cardiac Care Unit

Muhamed Saric

The prevalence of valvular heart disease is strongly influenced by the patient's age. In the United States and other developed countries, significant valvular disease tends to cluster at age extremes; in the young it results primarily from congenital heart disease (CHD) and in the elderly from degenerative wear-and-tear valve changes.

The combined prevalence of moderate and severe CHD is approximately 5 in 1,000 live births.[1] The prevalence of congenital valvular disease is much lower as the bulk of the CHD is accounted for by nonvalvular lesions such as ventricular and atrial septal defects, and patent ductus arteriosus. The prevalence of valvular disease among the elderly ≥75 years of age is approximately 13.3%. This is in contrast to the prevalence rate of 0.7% in the 18- to 44-years age group.[2] Between the age extremes, valvular disease is encountered mostly in the survivors of CHD or in immigrants with rheumatic valvular disease.

Thus a patient in an adult coronary care unit (CCU) in the United States usually falls into one of the following three categories: elderly patients, patients with CHD, and immigrants with rheumatic heart disease. The last two groups often include pregnant women.

Valvular disease presents either as valvular stenosis or valvular regurgitation. When valvular disease is the primary reason for a CCU admission, the patient usually presents with severe degrees of stenosis, regurgitation, or a combination thereof. Among the elderly CCU patients typical valvular disorders include aortic stenosis (AS) and mitral regurgitation; in addition, there is often secondary tricuspid regurgitation. In younger CCU patients, typical valvular disorders include rheumatic mitral stenosis, tricuspid valve endocarditis, and severe pulmonic insufficiency arising as a long-term complication of CHD surgeries performed in childhood.

In general, medical therapy of severe valvular disease is limited to symptom relief and hemodynamic stabilization in preparation for definitive treatment performed by interventional cardiologists and cardiac surgeons. Unfortunately, there is a paucity of solid randomized trial data to support any form of treatment of valvular disease.[3] In the latest joint guidelines of the American Heart Association and the American College of Cardiology, most of the recommendations for the management of valvular disease are based on either nonrandomized trials or expert opinions.[4]

ANTIBIOTIC PROPHYLAXIS OF VALVULAR HEART DISEASE

Routine antibiotic prophylaxis in no longer recommended for acquired valvular disease in a nontransplanted heart unless there is a prior history of endocarditis. For congenital forms of valvular disease in the setting of surgically repaired CHD, antibiotic prophylaxis is recommended only if (1) there is prosthetic material or device, whether placed by surgery or by catheter intervention, during the first 6 months after the procedure, and (2) there are residual defects at the site or adjacent to the site of a prosthetic patch or prosthetic device (which inhibit endothelialization).[5]

AORTIC STENOSIS

ETIOLOGY AND PATHOPHYSIOLOGY

AS in a typical adult CCU patient arises from calcific degeneration of either a previously normal trileaflet aortic valve (TAV) or a congenitally bicuspid aortic valve (BAV). Calcification process is often enhanced by disorders of perturbed calcium phosphate metabolism such as end-stage renal disease and Paget's disease.[6]

Calcific TAV stenosis is typically encountered among the elderly and calcific BAV stenosis in middle-aged patients (Figure 25.1). It is estimated that AS is present in 2% of all Americans, 65 years of age or older.[2] TAV stenosis may be a manifestation of generalized atherosclerosis. BAV is the commonest congenital heart defect occurring in approximately 1% to 2% of all live births.[7] BAV may present as stenosis or regurgitation and may be associated with aortopathies such as aortic aneurysm, aortic dissection, and coarctation.[8]

The major cardiovascular adaptation to pressure overload caused by AS is left ventricular hypertrophy (LVH). Because of LVH the left ventricular chamber becomes smaller and its wall thicker; both these changes lower the wall stress and allow for preservation of left ventricular ejection fraction (LVEF) for very long periods. When LVEF starts to decrease it is often due to an afterload-LVH mismatch (not enough LVH for the degree of AS) rather than cardiomyopathy.

CLINICAL PRESENTATION

AS is usually asymptomatic unless severe. Patients with severe AS typically present with angina, syncope, sudden death, or heart failure. Physical diagnosis may establish the diagnosis of AS but is often incapable of precisely grading AS. Classic auscultatory findings of AS include a systolic crescendo–decrescendo ejection murmur over the precordium that radiates to the neck, and an occasional absence of the valve closing S2 sound.[9] Carotid upstroke is often weak and delayed (pulsus parvus & tardus).

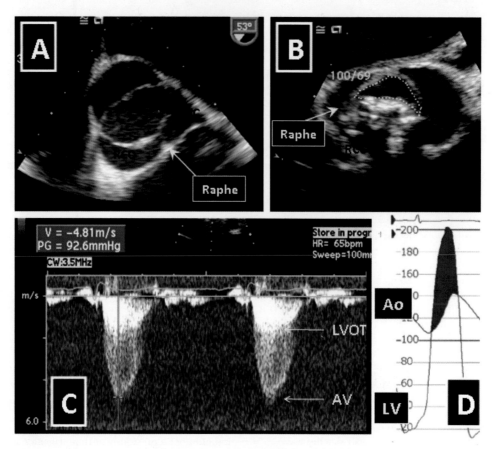

Figure 25.1. Aortic stenosis. **Panel A** and **Panel B** show bicuspid aortic valve on transesophageal echocardiography. In **Panel A**, the bicuspid valve is not significantly stenotic. This is in contrast to **Panel B**
which shows a severely calcified and markedly stenotic bicuspid aortic valve. **Panel C** shows continuous
wave Doppler recording of blood flow across the aortic valve in systole. Note the wide separation between
the normal left ventricular outflow tract (LVOT) velocity and the markedly elevated velocity across the aortic valve (AV). **Panel D** shows simultaneous pressure recordings from the left ventricle (LV) and the aortic
root (Ao). Note the wide separation between the aortic pressure and the markedly elevated LV pressure.

DIAGNOSIS

Electrocardiogram (EKG) often shows signs of LVH and left
atrial enlargement. Chest X-ray (CXR) rarely provides specific
evidence of AS; occasionally aortic valve calcifications are seen
on CXR.

Echocardiography is the primary means of diagnosing and
grading AS. Aortic valve area (AVA) is the primary criterion
of AS. When the flow across the aortic valve is not diminished,
the magnitude of the peak and mean gradient across the aortic
valve in systole is inversely related to AVA (Table 25.1). Other
typical echocardiographic findings of AS include LVH, left
atrial enlargement, and often a normal LVEF.

A low transvalvular gradient (mean gradient ≤30 mm Hg)
does not exclude severe AS. Patients with AS may have low transvalvular gradients for two reasons: (1) Afterload-hypertrophy
mismatch and (2) concomitant cardiomyopathy (such as ischemic heart disease). Differentiating between these two groups
is extremely important as the patients in the first group will
benefit from aortic valve surgery, whereas those in the second
group may not.

Differentiation between the two groups is made after measuring aortic valve parameters (AVA and the gradients) at rest
and following intravenous infusion of increasing amounts of

dobutamine (starting at 5 μg/kg/minute and escalating up
to 20 μg/kg/minute).[10] Aortic valve parameters are usually
measured by echocardiography (modified dobutamine stress
echo). However, these measurements may also be performed
during cardiac catheterization.

Changes in the following three parameters are measured
during dobutamine stress testing in patients with low-gradient
AS: left ventricular stroke volume, AVA, and the mean gradient. If there is an increase in stroke volume of ≤20%, the
patient likely has severe cardiomyopathy and is usually not
a candidate for aortic valve surgery. If the stroke volume increases by 20% or more than two scenarios are possible: (1)
AVA remains essentially the same but the mean gradient increases above 30 mm Hg, and (2) AVA increases by 0.2 cm²
or more but the gradient remains essentially unchanged.
The patients in the first group have true severe AS and will
benefit from aortic valve surgery. The patients in the second
group have pseudosevere AS in the setting of left ventricular
cardiomyopathy; they are unlikely to benefit from aortic valve
surgery (Table 25.2).

For routine diagnosis of AS cardiac catheterization is usually
not necessary. However, coronary angiography is commonly
performed in patients with AS who are scheduled to undergo

TABLE 25.1	Grades of Aortic Stenosis				
	Valve Area	Valve Area Indexed For Body Surface Area	Peak Velocity	Peak Gradient	Mean Gradient
	cm^2	cm^2/m^2	m/sec	mm Hg	mm Hg
Normal	2.0-4.0		< 2.5	< 25	
Mild Aortic Stenosis	> 1.5		2.5-3.0	25-36	< 25
Moderate Aortic Stenosis	1.0-1.5		3.1-4.0	37-64	25-40
Severe Aortic Stenosis	< 1.0	< 0.6	> 4.0	>64	> 40

aortic valve surgery as coronary artery disease is common in the typical age group of patients with AS. When comparing aortic gradients obtained by cardiac catheterization, it is important to emphasize that it is the mean but not the peak aortic gradient that correlates well with echocardiography.

MEDICAL THERAPY

There are no proven medical therapies for prevention or treatment of AS. Antibiotic prophylaxis of bacterial endocarditis in patients with AS is no longer recommended; for details see section on Antibiotic Prophylaxis of Valvular Heart Disease in this chapter's introduction.

Patients with severe AS often present to CCU with clinical signs of heart failure. Diuretics, angiotensin converting enzyme (ACE) inhibitors, and digitalis may be used with caution. Although historically the use of intravenous vasodilators was contraindicated in patients with severe AS, a small study in CCU patients have demonstrated that intravenous nitroprusside actually relieves symptoms of heart failure in patients with severe AS and severely reduced left ventricular systolic function.[11] In that study, intravenous nitroprusside was started at a mean dose of 14 ± 10 μg per minute, and the dose was increased to a mean of 103 ± 67 μg per minute at 6 hours and 128 ± 96 μg per minute at 24 hours.

SURGICAL AND PERCUTANEOUS INTERVENTIONAL THERAPY

AS is a mechanical problem that requires a mechanical solution. Surgical aortic valve replacement (AVR) is currently the preferred therapeutic choice in patients with AS as it improves symptoms and survival. Major indications for AVR are listed in Table 25.3.

Percutaneous interventions for AS include aortic valve balloon valvuloplasty and percutaneous AV replacement. Balloon valvuloplasty is an effective form of therapy for congenital

AS. However, balloon valvuloplasty in calcific TAV or BAV aortic stenosis has been rather ineffective (valve area seldom increases above 1.0 cm² and there is a high rate of restenosis), and it has significant morbidity and mortality. At present, typical indications for balloon valvuloplasty in calcific AS include temporary relief of AS in patient undergoing noncardiac surgery (such as hip replacement) or in those with terminal illness (such as cancer).

Percutaneous valve replacement is a new and promising therapy for AS. Although the first percutaneous implantation of an aortic prosthetic valve has been reported in 2002, such a procedure in the United States is gradually moving from an investigational use within clinical trials to clinical practice.[12]

IMPACT ON PREGNANCY

Patients with calcific AS are seldom of child-bearing age. In patients of child-bearing age, AS is usually caused by noncalcific congenital abnormalities (such as unicuspid aortic valve). Young patients with moderate-to-severe AS should be advised against conception until AS is relieved. Those who nonetheless become pregnant may or may not develop severe symptoms. Pregnant patients with AS and mild symptoms may be managed conservatively during pregnancy with bed rest, oxygen, and β-blockers. Pregnant patients with severe symptoms may need percutaneous or even surgical intervention. These procedures carry significant risk to both the mother and the unborn child.

AORTIC REGURGITATION

ETIOLOGY AND PATHOPHYSIOLOGY

Aortic regurgitation (AR) may be due to disorders of the aortic root or the aortic valve leaflets. BAV, ascending aortic aneurysm, aortic dissection, and endocarditis are common

TABLE 25.2	Dobutamine Stress Test: Differentiating True From Pseudo Aortic Stenosis			
	Stroke Volume Change			
	< 20%		> 20%	
	< 0.2 cm²	Valve Area Change	< 0.2 cm²	> 0.2 cm²
	Remains < 30 mm	Mean Gradient	Becomes > 30 mm Hg	Remains < 30 mm
Conclusion	Severe LV dysfunction		True severe AS	Pseudo-severe AS
AVR Recommendation	No		Yes	No

Abbreviations: AS, aortic stenosis; AVR, aortic valve replacement

TABLE 25.3	Major Indication for Aortic Valve Surgery in Patients with Aortic Stenosis	
	Severe AS	*Moderate AS*
Symptomatic	Class I	Patient with moderate AS are usually not symptomatic
Asymptomatic AND one of the following:		
LVEF < 50%	Class I	No AVR
Patient referred for CABG or other heart surgery	Class I	Class IIa
Patient referred for surgery of the aorta	Class I	Class IIa

causes of AR. Conditions that predispose patient to aortopathies and AR include systemic hypertension and connective tissue disorders (such as Marfan syndrome, Ehlers–Danlos syndrome, and ankylosing spondylitis). In the less developed countries, rheumatic heart disease and tertiary syphilis remain important causes of AR.

In AR, a regurgitant volume flows back into the ventricle through the aortic valve during diastole. There it joins the systemic volume that had entered the left ventricle through the mitral valve. During subsequent systole the two volumes leave the aortic valve together; the systemic volume continues into the aorta and its branches, whereas the regurgitant volume flows back into the ventricle. The cycle then repeats itself. Subsequent pathophysiology depends on whether AR is chronic or acute.

In chronic AR, there is a progressive enlargement of the left ventricle to accommodate the combined systemic stroke volume and the regurgitant volume. This remodeling often prevents significant elevation of left heart pressures. It may take years if not decades for patients with chronic AR to develop congestive heart failure owing to progressive left ventricular systolic dysfunction.

This is in sharp contrast to acute AR where there is sudden volume overload of a nondilated left ventricle, marked elevation of left ventricular and left atrial pressures, life-threatening pulmonary edema, and even cardiogenic shock.

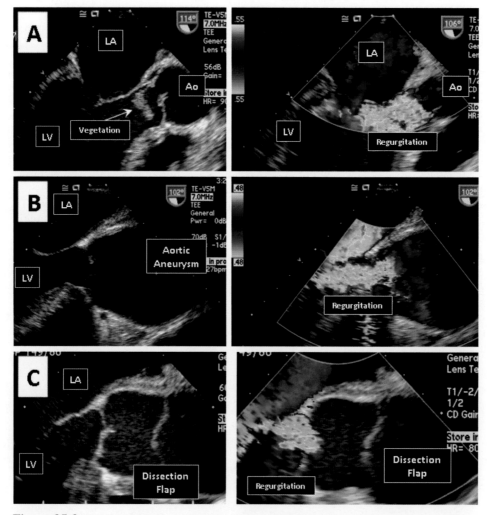

Figure 25.2. Aortic regurgitation. Causes of severe aortic regurgitation include aortic valve endocarditis **(Panel A)**, ascending aortic aneurysm **(Panel B),** and type A aortic dissection **(Panel C)**. LA, left atrium; LV, left ventricle; Ao, ascending aorta.

TABLE 25.4	Grades of Aortic Regurgitation			
	Mild	*Moderate*	*Moderate-Severe*	*Severe*
	(1+)	(2+)	(3+)	(4+)
Regurgitant orifice area (cm²)	<0.1	0.10-0.19	0.20-0.29	>0.3
Regurgitant Fraction	<30%	30-39%	40-49%	>50%
Regurgitant Volume (mL)	30	30-44	45-59	>60
Vena contracta (cm)	<0.3	0.3 - 0.6	>0.6	

Although severe acute AR represents only a minority of AR cases, its often fulminant and life-threatening course necessitates CCU admission. The rest of the AR section will be devoted to severe acute AR.

CLINICAL PRESENTATION

Among the most common causes of severe acute AR are chest trauma, bacterial endocarditis, and the dissection of the ascending aorta (type A aortic dissection). Patients with severe acute AR frequently present with fulminant pulmonary edema and cardiogenic shock. Patient with endocarditis will also have general signs and symptoms of a systemic bacterial illness. Patient with acute type A aortic dissection will usually complain of severe chest pain, often in the setting of uncontrolled systemic hypertension.

DIAGNOSIS

In severe acute AR, there may be few or no auscultatory findings of AR per se; the diastolic murmur of AR is often soft, short, or even absent because there is rapid equilibration of aortic and left ventricular pressures during diastole. There is usually marked tachycardia and S3 gallop. Wide pulse pressure—the hallmark of severe chronic AR—is routinely absent in severe acute AR.

CXR in severe acute AR frequently shows signs of pulmonary congestion. EKG may show tachycardia; there may also be signs of myocardial ischemia (owing to high myocardial demand brought on by very elevated left ventricular pressures or when acute aortic dissection extends into the coronary artery ostia). When endocarditis leads to periaortic valve abscess, EKG may demonstrate varying degrees of atrioventricular conduction block.

Transthoracic and transesophageal echocardiography are the primary means of evaluating AR. Echocardiography may establish the etiology, mechanism, and severity of MR (Figure 25.2). The diagnostic criteria for grading the severity of AR are listed in Table 25.4.

MEDICAL THERAPY

Severe acute AR is a life-threatening medical emergency that necessitates highest levels of CCU care. Endotracheal intubation, oxygen administration, and diuretic therapy are used to treat pulmonary edema. Afterload reduction may be achieved with the use of intravenous vasodilators (such as nitroprusside). Disease-specific therapies, if available, should also be administered (such as antibiotic therapy for endocarditis).

SURGICAL AND PERCUTANEOUS INTERVENTIONAL THERAPY

At present, there are no effective percutaneous interventions for the treatment of AR. Furthermore, intra-aortic balloon pump (IABP) is absolutely contraindicated when significant AR is present. Diastolic counterpulsations—which are the hallmarks of IABP function—worsen AR. In severe acute AR, aortic valve surgery should be performed as soon as possible especially in cases of type A aortic dissection.

IMPACT ON PREGNANCY

Severe AR, whether acute or chronic, is one of the valvular heart lesions that may be associated with high maternal and/or fetal risk during pregnancy. Pregnant women with AR who have New York Heart Association functional class III–IV symptoms, severe pulmonary hypertension (pulmonary pressure >75% of systemic pressures), and/or LV systolic dysfunction are at particular risk for maternal and fetal complications. The same is true for pregnant women having Marfan syndrome with or without AR.

MITRAL STENOSIS

ETIOLOGY AND PATHOPHYSIOLOGY

Rheumatic heart disease is by far the most frequent cause of acquired mitral stenosis (MS). Acquired narrowing of the mitral valve may also be caused by mitral annular calcifications or cardiac tumors such as myxomas (Figure 25.3). However, these nonrheumatic etiologies seldom cause severe MS. Congenital causes of MS are rare (1% of all MS patients) and include obstructive membranes either immediately proximal to the mitral orifice (supravalvular mitral ring) or within the left atrium (cor triatriatum).

Rheumatic heart disease may be conceptualized as a bacteria-triggered autoimmune inflammatory disorder that leads to progressive lifelong valve damage. The rheumatic process starts as acute rheumatic fever usually in childhood following pharyngitis caused by group A β-hemolytic streptococci ("strep throat"). As streptococcal proteins share antigenic properties with certain connective tissue proteins in the human host, the immune response that is mounted against the streptococci also leads to valvular damage.

Rheumatic mitral valve disease is characterized by leaflet thickening, commissural fusion, chordal fusion, and shortening as well as valve calcifications. MS is the primary manifestation of rheumatic heart disease. Women are more affected than men;

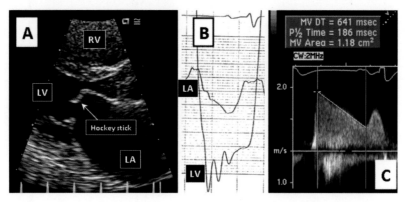

Figure 25.3. Mitral stenosis. **Panel A** shows a 2D transthoracic echocardiogram in the parasternal long-axis view of a patient with rheumatic mitral valve disease. The anterior mitral leaflet has the characteristic hockey stick appearance. **Panel B** represents simultaneous left atrial and left ventricular pressure recordings during cardiac catheterization. Note the marked separation between left ventricular diastolic pressure and the markedly elevated left atrial pressures indicative of severe mitral stenosis. **Panel C** demonstrates the echocardiographic pressure half-time method of determining the mitral valve area in a patient with moderate mitral stenosis. LA, left atrium; LV, left ventricle; RV, right ventricle.

the ratio is approximately 2:1 in favor of women. Rheumatic heart disease is still prevalent worldwide except in the developed countries where most cases are seen in immigrant populations.

Normal mitral valve area in an adult measures approximately 4 to 6 cm^2; this is approximately the area of an American or Canadian 25-cent coin. It takes decades for the valve area decreases to approximately 2.5 cm^2 and for the patient to start developing symptoms. Over the subsequent decades, the mitral valve area diminishes and the diastolic gradient across the mitral valve increases (Table 25.5). Left atrial (LA) enlargement, atrial arrhythmias, and systemic thromboembolism are major complications of rheumatic MS.

CLINICAL PRESENTATION

Dyspnea and other signs and symptoms of congestive heart failure owing to elevated left atrial and pulmonary pressures are the primary manifestations of MS. The degree of symptoms is directly related to the transvalvular mitral gradient in diastole. In turn, the magnitude of the mitral gradient is the result of interplay between the mitral valve area and the blood flow. Doubling the blood flow will quadruple the gradient.

Thus a patient with any degree of MS may become symptomatic if the blood flow is substantially increased such as during exercise, pregnancy, hyperthyroid crisis, fever, or tachyarrhythmia (such as atrial fibrillation). Left atrial enlargement is the primary

cardiac adaptation to MS; left ventricular systolic function is typically normal. Atrial fibrillation, left atrial thrombus formation, and systemic thromboembolism (such as strokes) are important contributors to morbidity and mortality of rheumatic MS.

DIAGNOSIS

Classic auscultatory findings of MS include loud first heart sound (S$_1$), an opening snap (OS) after the second heart sound (S$_2$), and a diastolic rumble. The duration of the S$_2$–OS interval is inversely related to the severity of MS (a shorter interval suggests more severe MS). In patients with normal sinus rhythm, there is also an end-diastolic ("presystolic") accentuation of the rumble.

EKG may demonstrate signs of LA enlargement characterized by wide, saddle-shaped P wave in leads I and II (so-called P *mitrale*) as well as late, deep P-wave inversion in lead V1. Atrial fibrillation is frequently present and there may be signs of right ventricular hypertrophy.

Chest X-ray usually demonstrates LA enlargement with straightening of the left cardiac silhouette. Right ventricular enlargement, signs of pulmonary venous congestion, and mitral valve calcification are frequently observed.[13]

Echocardiography is the primary means of diagnosing MS. By echocardiography one can determine the morphology of the mitral valve, its cross-sectional area, and the mean diastolic transvalvular pressure gradient. In addition, the size and function of cardiac chambers as well as the pulmonary artery pressures can be measured. Cardiac catheterization is not necessary for the diagnosis of MS in most instances.

MEDICAL THERAPY

Patients with MS often present to CCU with clinical signs of heart failure, frequently in the setting of atrial fibrillation. The goal of medical therapy in MS is to alleviate symptoms and prevent systemic thromboembolism. Congestion is treated with diuretics and the heart rate is controlled with β-blockers, certain calcium channel blockers (such as verapamil and diltiazem), and digitalis. Patients are initially anticoagulated with heparin then transitioned to warfarin. Specific therapies for atrial fibrillation may also be necessary.

TABLE 25.5	Grades of Mitral Stenosis		
	Valve Area	Mean Gradient	Pulmonary Artery Systolic Pressure
	cm^2	mm Hg	mm Hg
Normal	4.0-6.0		
Mild Mitral Stenosis	> 1.5	< 5	< 30
Moderate Mitral Stenosis	1.0-1.5	5-10	30-50
Severe Mitral Stenosis	< 1.0	> 10	> 50

These criteria are applicable when the heart rate is between 60 and 90 beats per minute.

TABLE 25.6	Major Indications For Percutaneous Mitral Balloon Valvuloplasty (PMBV)

General Prerequisites For PMBV

Moderate or severe mitral stenosis
Valve morphology favorable for PMBV
Absence of left atrial thrombus
Absence of moderate or severe mitral regurgitation

Appropriate Candidates

Symptomatic patients
Asymptomatic patients with pulmonary hypertension (PASP > 50 mm Hg at rest; > 60 mm Hg with exertion)
Patients with new-onset atrial fibrillation

When appropriate, patients should receive antibiotics for prevention of rheumatic fever recurrence according to the national guidelines.[4] In contrast, antibiotic prophylaxis of bacterial endocarditis in patients with MS is no longer recommended; for details see section on Antibiotic Prophylaxis of Valvular Heart Disease in this chapter's introduction.

SURGICAL AND PERCUTANEOUS INTERVENTIONAL THERAPY

MS is a mechanical problem that requires a mechanical solution. The 10-year survival of patients with MS receiving only medical therapy is unfavorable (50% to 60% overall and below 15% once significant limiting symptoms develop).[4]

When the morphology of the mitral valve is deemed favorable on echocardiography, percutaneous mitral balloon valvuloplasty (PMBV) is the preferred form of invasive treatment of MS. Major indications for PMBV are given in Table 25.6. If PMBV is unavailable or unfeasible, appropriate patients are referred for surgical intervention that may entail surgical commissurotomy, valve repair, or mitral valve replacement.

IMPACT ON PREGNANCY

Often pregnancy is the first time that a patient with MS becomes symptomatic because intravascular volume, cardiac output, and heart rate increase physiologically during pregnancy. PMBV can be performed during pregnancy as it has low risk of complications to the mother or the fetus.

MITRAL REGURGITATION

ETIOLOGY AND PATHOPHYSIOLOGY

According to the French cardiac surgeon Carpentier, all causes of mitral regurgitation (MR) fall into one of the following three categories: (1) *Annular dilatation* (as seen in dilated cardiomyopathy); (2) *excessive leaflet motion* (as seen in mitral valve prolapse, papillary muscle rupture, or endocarditis); and (3) *restricted leaflet motion* (as seen in rheumatic valve disease and ischemic cardiomyopathy).[14]

In MR, blood exits the left ventricle both antegrade—through the left ventricular outflow tract (systemic stroke volume) and retrograde—through the mitral valve (regurgitant volume). During diastole the regurgitant volume meets in the left atrium the systemic volume returning through the pulmonary veins. The combined volume then enters the left ventricle through the mitral valve. The process leads to volume overload of the left heart.

In chronic MR, there is progressive enlargement of the left atrium and the left ventricle to accommodate the combined systemic stroke volume and regurgitant volume. This remodeling often prevents significant elevation of left heart pressures; consequently it may take years if not decades for the patient to develop congestive heart failure (owing to progressive left ventricular systolic dysfunction) and atrial fibrillation (owing to left atrial enlargement).

This is in sharp contrast to acute MR where there is sudden volume overload of nondilated left heart chambers, marked elevation of left atrial pressures, life-threatening pulmonary edema, and even cardiogenic shock.

It is estimated that there are approximately 2.5 million patients with moderate-to-severe or severe MR in the United States at present.[15] Although acute MR represents only a minority of these cases, every health care professional working in the CCU setting should become proficient in diagnosing and managing this often life-threatening form of MR. The remainder of this section will be devoted to severe acute MR.

CLINICAL PRESENTATION

The leading causes of acute MR are bacterial endocarditis, papillary muscle rupture (traumatic or following myocardial infarction), and chordal rupture in the setting of pre-existing myxomatous valve degeneration and mitral valve prolapse.

Irrespective of the cause, patients with severe acute MR frequently present with fulminant pulmonary edema and cardiogenic shock. Patient with endocarditis will present with general signs and symptoms of a systemic bacterial illness. Nontraumatic papillary muscle rupture is a mechanical complication that usually occurs 3 to 5 days after acute myocardial infarction. Posteromedial papillary muscle (which usually has solitary blood supply from either the right coronary or the left circumflex artery) ruptures more frequently that the anterolateral one (which is usually supplied by both the left anterior descending and circumflex arteries).

DIAGNOSIS

In severe acute MR, there may be few or no auscultatory findings of MR per se; the systolic murmur is often soft, short, or even absent because there is rapid equilibration of left ventricular and left atrial pressures during systole. There is frequently tachycardia and S_3 gallop.

CXR in severe acute MR routinely shows signs of pulmonary congestion. EKG may show tachycardia; there may also be signs of myocardial infarction when acute MR is caused by papillary muscle rupture.

Measurement from a pulmonary artery catheter—which is often placed at bedside in the CCU—usually reveals a marked elevation of the systolic V wave in the pulmonary artery wedge pressure tracings (Figure 25.4). Cardiac output is often low.

Transthoracic and transesophageal echocardiography are the primary means of evaluating MR. Echocardiography can

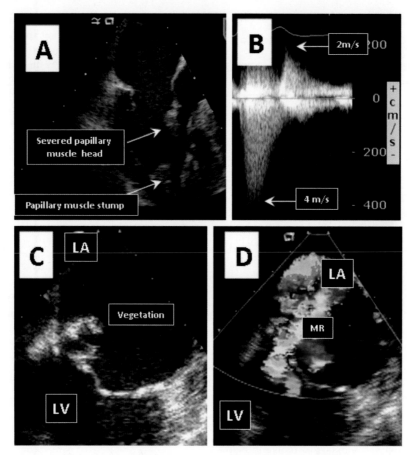

Figure 25.4. Mitral regurgitation. **Panel A** demonstrates anterior papillary muscle rupture in a patient with recent myocardial infarction. **Panel B** shows spectral Doppler tracing in a patient with severe acute mitral regurgitation. Note the relatively low peak velocity of the mitral regurgitant jet (4 m per second in this patient compared with approximately 5 m per second in normal people) indicative of systemic hypotension. The jet also decelerates rapidly towards the baseline indicative of rapid equilibration between LV and LA pressures toward the end of systole. Note also the relatively high antegrade velocity (2 m per second in this patient; normal is approximately 1 m per second) indicative of severe mitral regurgitation and a large regurgitant volume. **Panels C and D** show transesophageal echocardiographic findings in a patient with *Staphylococcus aureus* mitral valve endocarditis. **Panel C** is a 2D image showing large vegetation on the atrial side of the anterior mitral leaflet. **Panel D** demonstrates a very large regurgitant jet originating from the perforated anterior mitral leaflet. LA, left atrium; LV, left ventricle; MR, mitral regurgitation.

establish the etiology, the mechanism, and severity of MR. The diagnostic criteria for grading the severity of MR are listed in Table 25.7.

TABLE 25.7	Grades of Mitral Regurgitation			
	Mild	*Moderate*	*Moderate-Severe*	*Severe*
	(1+)	*(2+)*	*(3+)*	*(4+)*
Regurgitant orifice area (cm²)	<0.2	0.20-0.29	0.30-0.39	>0.4
Regurgitant Fraction	<30%	30-39%	40-49%	>50%
Regurgitant Volume (mL)	30	30-44	45-59	>60
Vena contracta (cm)	<0.3	0.3 - 0.7		>0.7

Note: Vena contracta is the narrowest portion of the regurgitant jet.

MEDICAL THERAPY

Severe acute MR is a life-threatening medical emergency that requires highest levels of care in the CCU. Endotracheal intubation, oxygen administration, and diuretic therapy are used to treat pulmonary edema. Afterload reduction may be achieved with the use of intravenous vasodilators (such as nitroprusside). Disease-specific therapies, if available, should also be administered (such as coronary revascularization and anti-ischemic medical therapy).

SURGICAL AND PERCUTANEOUS INTERVENTIONAL THERAPY

Severe acute MR often requires percutaneous insertion of the IABP, which is threaded through the femoral artery into the descending thoracic aorta with its tip just distal to the origin of the left subclavian artery. Significant coexisting aortic regurgitation is a contraindication for IABP insertion. IABP and the medical therapies described above are usually only palliative; the patient frequently requires urgent surgery to repair or replace the mitral valve.

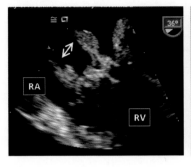
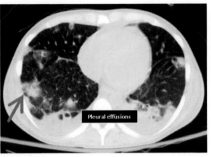

Figure 25.5. Tricuspid regurgitation. **Panel A** shows very large vegetation on the atrial side of the tricuspid valve on transesophageal echocardiogram in an intravenous drug user having *Staphylococcus aureus* bacteremia. **Panel B** shows septic emboli to the lung *(arrow)* in the same patient. RA, right atrium; RV, right ventricle.

IMPACT ON PREGNANCY

Severe MR, whether acute or chronic, is one of the valvular heart lesions that may be associated with high maternal and/or fetal risk during pregnancy. Pregnant women with MR who have New York Heart Association functional class III–IV symptoms, severe pulmonary hypertension (pulmonary pressure >75% of systemic pressures), and/or LV systolic dysfunction are at particular risk for maternal and fetal complications.

TRICUSPID REGURGITATION

ETIOLOGY AND PATHOPHYSIOLOGY

Tricuspid regurgitation (TR) is very prevalent. It is estimated that at present there are approximately 1.6 million individuals in the United States who have at least moderate-to-severe TR.[15] There are numerous causes of severe TR ranging from right ventricular dilatation to congenital leaflet abnormalities (such as Ebstein's anomaly),[16] trauma, carcinoid tumor and endocarditis. TR is frequently a complication of left heart disorders (such as left ventricular dysfunction, mitral and aortic valve disease, etc.).

Severe TR may be chronic or acute. The impact of severe chronic TR on the right heart is equivalent to the impact of severe MR on the left heart (see above). Among the most common causes of severe acute TR are chest trauma and infective endocarditis (often in the setting of intravenous drug use, central venous catheterization, or pacemaker and defibrillator lead placement).

CLINICAL PRESENTATION

Severe TR presents with jugular venous distension, hepatomegaly, ascites, and peripheral edema. Unlike severe acute MR or AR, severe acute TR is usually not a medical emergency.

DIAGNOSIS

In severe chronic TR there is a systolic murmur that augments with inspiration. Such a murmur is often soft or absent in severe acute TR owing to rapid equalization of right ventricular and right atrial pressures. EKG frequently reveals tachycardia.

CXR may reveal coin lesions in the lungs indicative of pulmonary septic emboli. Transthoracic and transesophageal echocardiography are the primary means of evaluating TR. Echocardiography can establish the etiology, mechanism, and severity of TR (Figure 25.5).

MEDICAL THERAPY

Appropriate antibiotic therapy should be administered to patients with tricuspid valve endocarditis. Disease-specific therapies should be administered whenever possible.

SURGICAL AND PERCUTANEOUS INTERVENTIONAL THERAPY

Tricuspid valve is not essential for life; in the past it was a frequent practice to treat tricuspid endocarditis with surgical excision of the tricuspid leaflet. Nowadays, the tricuspid valve should be surgically repaired whenever possible. If valve replacement is required, a bioprosthesis is the preferred option because of high rate of thromboembolic complications with mechanical tricuspid valve prostheses.

IMPACT ON PREGNANCY

Isolated severe TR regurgitation, unless acute, usually does not present a significant problem during pregnancy.

REFERENCES

1. Warnes CA, Libertshson R, Danielson GK, et al. Task Force 1: the changing profile of congenital heart disease in adult life. *J Am Coll Cardiol.* 2001;37:1170–1175.
2. Lloyd-Jones D, Adams RJ, Brown TM, et al.; American Heart Association Statistics Committee and Stroke Statistics Subcommittee. Heart disease and stroke statistics_2010 update: a report from the American Heart Association. *Circulation.* 2010;121:e46–e215.
3. Tricoci P, Allen JM, Kramer JM, et al. Scientific evidence underlying the ACC/AHA clinical practice guidelines. *JAMA.* 2009;301(8):831–841. Erratum in: *JAMA.* 2009;301(15):1544.
4. Bonow RO, Carabello BA, Chatterjee K, et al. ACC/AHA 2006 guidelines for the management of patients with valvular heart disease: a report of the American College of Cardiology/American Heart Association Task Force on Practice Guidelines (Writing Committee to Revise the 1998 Guidelines for the Management of Patients With Valvular Heart Disease). *Circulation.* 2006;114:e84–e231.
5. Nishimura RA, Carabello BA, Faxon DP, et al. ACC/AHA 2008 guideline update on valvular heart disease: focused update on infective endocarditis: a report of the American College of Cardiology/American Heart Association Task Force on Practice Guidelines endorsed by the Society of Cardiovascular Anesthesiologists, Society for Cardiovascular Angiography and Interventions, and Society of Thoracic Surgeons. *J Am Coll Cardiol.* 2008;52(8):676–685.
6. Saric M, Kronzon I. Aortic stenosis in the elderly. *Am J Geriatr Cardiol.* 2000;9:321–329, 345.
7. Saric M, Kronzon I. Congenital heart disease in adults. In: Lang RM, Vannan MA, Khanderia BK, eds. *Dynamic Echocardiography: A Case-Based Approach.* 1st ed. Springer; Saunders, an imprint of Elsevier, Inc., St. Louis, Missouri. 2010:Chap 105:438–439.
8. Saric M, Kronzon I. Aortic dissection. In: Lang RM, Vannan MA, Khanderia BK, eds. *Dynamic Echocardiography: A Case-Based Approach.* 1st ed. Springer; 2010:Chap 37:171–175.
9. Selzer A, Lombard JT. Clinical findings in adult aortic stenosis—then and now. *Eur Heart J.* 1988;9(suppl E):53–55.

10. deFilippi CR, Willett DL, Brickner ME, et al. Usefulness of dobutamine echocardiography in distinguishing severe from nonsevere valvular aortic stenosis in patients with depressed left ventricular function and low transvalvular gradients. *Am J Cardiol.* 1995;75:191–194.

11. Khot UN, Novaro GM, Popovic ZB, et al. Nitroprusside in critically ill patients with left ventricular dysfunction and aortic stenosis. *N Engl J Med.* 2003;348:1756–1763.

12. Cribier A, Eltchaninoff H, Bash A, et al. Percutaneous transcatheter implantation of an aortic valve prosthesis for calcific aortic stenosis. *Circulation.* 2002;106:3006–3008.

13. Kronzon I, Saric M, Lang RM. Mitral stenosis. In: Lang RM, Vannan MA, Khanderia BK, eds. *Dynamic Echocardiography: A Case-Based Approach.* 1 ed. Springer; 2010:Chap 9:38–45.

14. Carpentier A, Deloche A, Dauptain J, et al. A new reconstructive operation for correction of mitral and tricuspid insufficiency. *J Thorac Cardiovasc Surg.* 1971;61(1):1–13.

15. Stuge O, Liddicoat J. Emerging opportunities for cardiac surgeons within structural heart disease. *J Thorac Cardiovasc Surg.* 2006;132(6):1258–1261.

16. Saric M, Kronzon I. Ebstein's anomaly. In: Lang RM, Vannan MA, Khanderia BK, eds. *Dynamic Echocardiography: A Case-Based Approach.* 1st ed. Springer; 2010:Chap 111:462–464.

PATIENT AND FAMILY INFORMATION FOR:
Decompensated Valvular Disease

GENERAL CONCEPTS OF VALVULAR HEART DISEASE

The heart has four valves: two on the left side (called mitral and aortic valves) and two on the right side (called tricuspid and pulmonic valves). Normally, the blood flows across the valves without problem and only in forward direction. Normal valves prevent the backflow of the blood through the heart.

Valve disease occurs when the valves become either narrowed or leaky. When a valve is narrowed, the blood has trouble crossing it. When the valve is narrowed the doctors called that condition stenosis. When a valve is leaky, the blood flows backwards, something that should not happen in a healthy heart. When the valve is leaky the doctors call that condition regurgitation or insufficiency.

AORTIC STENOSIS

WHAT IS MY ILLNESS?

One of the valves in your heart called the aortic valve is narrowed; the doctors call this condition aortic stenosis. The aortic valve connects the main pumping chamber of the heart to the main blood vessel that leaves the heart called the aorta. Because of the narrowing, the blood has trouble crossing the aortic valve; this exerts strain on the main pumping chamber of the heart. This is similar to what happens when a highway lane is closed and all the cars now have to go through the remaining lanes; a traffic jam develops.

The narrowing gets worse over time; it usually takes many years for the narrowing to become severe. As the narrowing of the aortic valve gets worse, the walls of the main pumping chamber get thicker but the pumping action of the heart chamber usually remains normal. When the narrowing is very severe, you may experience the following symptoms: chest pain, shortness of breath, or you may pass out. In rare instances you may die suddenly.

HOW WILL I BE TREATED?

Medications may help relieve your symptoms but they cannot cure the narrowing. Once the aortic valve is severely narrowed and you experience above symptoms, the only solution is to have the valve replaced. This requires heart surgery. Depending on your age and other factors, the surgeon will replace the narrowed valve with either a metal prosthesis or a tissue prosthesis. The advantage of a metal prosthesis is that can last for the rest of your life. The downside of a metal prosthesis is that you have to take a pill for blood thinning for the rest of your life. A tissue prosthesis is made of either pig or cow tissue and looks quite like your valve. If you receive a tissue prosthesis you will not need to take blood thinners. However, a tissue prosthesis usually lasts about only 10 years or so.

WHAT IF I AM PREGNANT OR THINKING OF BECOMING PREGNANT?

If you have severe narrowing of the aortic valve you may need to delay pregnancy until the narrowing is relieved—usually through the use of balloon catheter inserted through you groin, threaded to your heart, and blown up inside the valve to make it larger. If you are already pregnant and you have symptoms (such as shortness of breath or chest pain) you may need to take certain medications that are effective for you but not harmful to the child. If your symptoms during the pregnancy are severe you may need the balloon catheter treatment or even open heart surgery. These procedures carry significant risk to both you and your unborn child.

AORTIC REGURGITATION

WHAT IS MY ILLNESS?

One of the valves in your heart called the aortic valve is leaky; the doctors call this condition aortic regurgitation or aortic insufficiency. The aortic valve connects the main pumping chamber of the heart to the main blood vessel that leaves the heart called the aorta. Because of the leaky valve, with each heartbeat some amount of blood goes from the heart into the aorta (as it should). Unfortunately some amount of blood in you also leaks back from the aorta into the heart. This puts strain on the main pumping chamber of the heart that has to pump much harder. A heart with a leaky valve is like a leaky pail of water. If you carry a leaky pail you will not be able to carry as much water as if you were carrying a pail with no hole in it.

The valve leak may develop over many years or may develop suddenly. If the leak develops over time, you heart has time to adapt. It gets bigger and bigger but over time may weaken. It is more dangerous if the leak develops suddenly. When the leak is sudden and severe, you experience shortness of breath, swelling of your legs, and other symptoms. Sudden and severe leakage is life-threatening and in that instance you will most likely need to be in an intensive care unit.

HOW WILL I BE TREATED?

Medications may help relieve your symptoms but they cannot cure the leak. If your leak is sudden and severe, you will most likely need to undergo open heart surgery to have the valve repaired or replaced by the surgeon. If the surgeon cannot repair the valve, he or she will replace the valve with a prosthesis.

Depending on your age and other factors, the surgeon will use either a metal prosthesis or a tissue prosthesis. The advantage of a metal prosthesis is that can last for the rest of your life. The downside of a metal prosthesis is that you have to take a pill for blood thinning for the rest of your life. A tissue prosthesis is made of either pig or cow tissue and looks a lot like your valve. If you receive a tissue prosthesis you will not need to take blood thinners. However, a tissue prosthesis usually lasts about only 10 years or so.

WHAT IF I AM PREGNANT OR THINKING OF BECOMING PREGNANT?

Severe leakage of the aortic valve may not be well tolerated during pregnancy and the condition may harm the unborn child. Women with severe leakage who are considering pregnancy may need to delay it until the condition is treated. If you are already pregnant, you may experience significant heart problems during your pregnancy.

MITRAL STENOSIS

WHAT IS MY ILLNESS?

When the mitral valve is narrowed, the doctors call this condition mitral stenosis. The mitral valve connects the left upper chamber of the heart (called the left atrium) to the main pumping chamber of the heart (called the left ventricle). The upper chamber is like an entryway into the main room.

Because of the narrowing, the blood has trouble crossing the mitral valve and filling the main pumping chamber of the heart. This exerts strain on the left upper chamber of the heart. This is similar to what happens when a highway lane is closed and all the cars now have to go through the remaining lanes; a traffic jam develops.

The narrowing gets worse over time; it usually takes many years for the narrowing to become severe. As the narrowing of the mitral valve gets worse, the left upper chamber gets bigger and the pressures in the lungs get higher. As the upper chamber gets larger, it loses its ability to conduct electricity correctly. This results in abnormal heartbeat called atrial fibrillation. This abnormal heartbeat makes the heart work inefficiently and also allows for blood clots to form inside the heart (something that does not happens in healthy hearts). The clot may shatter and send pieces travelling through the blood stream. If the pieces are big enough they may clog smaller blood vessels throughout the body; it is particularly bad when they end up in the brain where they will cause a stroke. If you develop this abnormal heartbeat you might need to take blood thinners for the rest of your life.

When the narrowing is very severe, you may experience the following symptoms: shortness of breath, difficulty in walking upstairs and uphill as well as swelling of your legs.

HOW WILL I BE TREATED?

Medications may help relieve your symptoms but they cannot cure the narrowing. Once the mitral valve is significantly narrowed and you experience above symptoms, and the only solution is to open or replace the valve. In many patients, the narrowed mitral valve can be opened by small balloons mounted on plastic tubes called catheters. You will first undergo ultrasound imaging of the heart. If the ultrasound doctor thinks that you are a good candidate, you will be sent to the cath lab. There a special cardiologist will insert the catheter into your veins, thread it to you heart, make a small hole between the right and the left upper chambers of your heart to bring the catheter above the narrowed valve. In the next step, the balloon will be passed across the mitral valve and blown up. This procedure, when successful, can make the narrowed orifice much bigger if not normal.

If you are not a candidate for the balloon procedure, you may need open heart surgery. Depending on your age and other factors, the surgeon will replace the narrowed valve with either a metal prosthesis or a tissue prosthesis.

WHAT IF I AM PREGNANT OR THINKING OF BECOMING PREGNANT?

If you have severe narrowing of the mitral valve you may need to delay pregnancy until the narrowing is relieved—usually through the use of balloon catheter inserted through you groin, threaded to your heart, and blown up inside the valve to make it larger. If you are already pregnant and you have symptoms (such as shortness of breath or chest pain) you may need to take certain medications that are effective for you but not harmful to the child. If your symptoms during the pregnancy are severe you may need the balloon catheter treatment or even open heart surgery. These procedures carry significant risk to both you and your unborn child.

MITRAL REGURGITATION

WHAT IS MY ILLNESS?

When the mitral valve is leaky, the doctors call this condition mitral regurgitation or mitral insufficiency. The mitral valve connects the left atrium to the left ventricle. The atrium is like an entryway into the main room.

As the atrium gets larger, it loses its ability to conduct electricity correctly. This may result in abnormal heartbeat called atrial fibrillation. This abnormal heartbeat makes the heart work inefficiently and also allows for blood clots to form inside the heart (something that does not happens in healthy hearts). The clot may shatter and send pieces travelling through the blood stream. If the pieces are big enough they may clog smaller blood vessels throughout the body causing strokes. If you develop this abnormal heartbeat you might need to take blood thinners for the rest of your life.

Because of the leaky valve, the blood flows backwards into the atrium of the heart. This puts strain on the main pumping chamber of the heart which has to pump much harder. A heart with a leaky valve is like a leaky pail of water. If you carry a leaky pail you will not be able to carry as much water as if you were carrying a pail with no hole in it.

The valve leak may develop over many years or may develop suddenly. If the leak develops over time, you heart has time to adapt. It grows bigger and over time may weaken. It is much more dangerous if the leak develops suddenly. When the leak is sudden and severe, you experience shortness of breath, swelling of your legs, and other symptoms.

HOW WILL I BE TREATED?

Medications may help relieve your symptoms but they cannot cure the leak. If your leak is sudden and severe, you will most likely need to undergo open heart surgery to have the valve repaired or replaced by the surgeon. If the surgeon cannot repair the valve, he or she will replace the valve with a prosthesis.

While you are waiting for your open heart surgery, your intensive care doctors may place a special balloon pump through your groin into aorta. After the balloon is securely placed in the aorta, you will have to be lying of your back all the time until the balloon pump is removed.

Depending on your age and other factors, the surgeon will use either a metal prosthesis or a tissue prosthesis.

WHAT IF I AM PREGNANT OR THINKING OF BECOMING PREGNANT?

Severe leakage of the mitral valve may not be well tolerated during pregnancy and the condition may harm the unborn child. Women with severe leakage who are considering becoming pregnant may need to delay their pregnancy until the condition is treaded. If you are already pregnant, you may experience significant heart problems during your pregnancy.

TRICUSPID REGURGITATION

WHAT IS MY ILLNESS?

One of the valves in your heart called the tricuspid valve is leaky; the doctors call this condition tricuspid regurgitation or tricuspid insufficiency. The tricuspid valve connects the right upper chamber of the heart called the right atrium to a pumping chamber on the right side of the heart called the right ventricle. The upper chamber is like an entryway into the main room.

Because of the leak, you may notice that your neck veins have gotten big and that you have pain under the right rib cage where the liver is. You may also have swelling in your legs.

A very common cause of a leaky tricuspid valve is infection of the valve when germs in the bloodstream eat up the valve tissue. The germs can get into your blood stream if you shoot drugs or have catheters or pacemakers placed in your veins by your doctors.

HOW WILL I BE TREATED?

Medications cannot repair the leak but antibiotics can stop further damage if the leakage is caused by an infection. Even with severe leakage of the tricuspid valve you can live for many years before the heart muscle gives up.

If your leak is severe, you may need to undergo open heart surgery to have the valve repaired or replaced by the surgeon. If the surgeon cannot repair the valve, he or she will replace the valve with a prosthesis. Most likely the surgeon will place a tissue rather than a metal prosthesis. A tissue prosthesis is made of either pig or cow tissue and looks a lot like your own valve. If you receive a tissue prosthesis you will not need to take blood thinners. However, a tissue prosthesis usually lasts about only 10 years or so.

WHAT IF I AM PREGNANT OR THINKING OF BECOMING PREGNANT?

Severe leakage of the tricuspid valve is usually well tolerated during pregnancy unless there are other heart problems.

Tracy Zivin-Tutela
Bruce Polsky

Infective Endocarditis

Infective endocarditis (IE) is a disease that is associated with significant morbidity and mortality. Antimicrobial resistance among common bacterial pathogens has created management issues for physicians.

The three major bacterial causes of IE are streptococci, staphylococci, and enterococci. *Staphylococcus aureus* has now surpassed *Streptococcus viridans* as the leading cause of bacterial endocarditis in the United States.[1–3] We are also now faced with multi drug-resistant *S. viridans* and oxacillin-resistant *S. aureus* (community acquired as well as health care associated).[4–6] The development of intermediate and high-level resistance to vancomycin has also been documented. Vancomycin and aminoglycoside resistance among enterococci is also a common finding in health-care-associated infections.[7]

DIAGNOSIS

The classic clinical manifestation of IE includes bacteremia or fungemia, acute valvulitis, immunologic phenomena, and peripheral emboli. Immunologic and vascular phenomena are a more common presentation in subacute IE. Right-sided endocarditis may also present with septic pulmonary emboli. The modified Duke criteria were developed to aid in the diagnosis of IE.[8] It stratifies patients with suspected endocarditis into "definite," "possible," and "rejected." Definite IE includes microorganisms demonstrated by culture or histopathology of vegetation, vegetation that has embolized or an intracardiac abscess, or two major criteria, or one major and three minor criteria, or five minor criteria. Possible IE includes one major criterion and one minor criterion, or three minor criteria. Rejected diagnosis of endocarditis includes an alternative diagnosis or resolution of IE syndrome with antibiotic therapy for <4 days or no pathological evidence at time of surgery or autopsy.

OUTLINE OF THE DUKE CRITERIA

See Figure 26.1.

THE MAJOR AND MINOR CRITERIA OF THE DUKE CRITERIA

The major criteria include the following (Figure 26.2):

1. Positive blood culture from two separate blood cultures with typical organisms for IE
2. Persistently positive blood cultures
3. Single positive blood culture for *Coxiella burnetii* or IgG antibody titer >1:800
4. Echocardiogram positive for oscillating intracardiac mass on valve or supporting structures or on implanted material in the absence of an alternative anatomic explanation or abscess or new partial dehiscence of prosthetic valve or new valvular regurgitation.

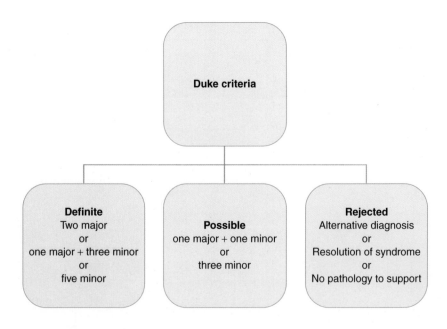

Figure 26.1. Outline of the Duke criteria.

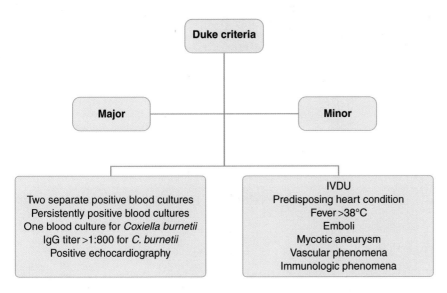

Figure 26.2. The major and minor criteria of the Duke criteria.

The minor criteria include the following:

1. Predisposing heart condition or intravenous drug use
2. Fever >38°C
3. Vascular phenomena, arterial emboli, septic pulmonary infarcts, mycotic aneurysm, intracranial hemorrhage, conjunctival hemorrhage, or Janeway lesions
4. Immunologic phenomena such as glomerulonephritis, Osler's nodes, Roth's spots, and rheumatoid factor
5. Microbiologic evidence such as a blood culture that does not meet a major criterion

THE USE OF ECHOCARDIOGRAPHY IN INFECTIVE ENDOCARDITIS

DIAGNOSIS AND MANAGEMENT WITH ECHOCARDIOGRAPHY: TTE VERSUS TEE

All suspected cases of IE should undergo an echocardiogram. If the clinical suspicion is low then it is reasonable to perform a transthoracic echocardiogram (TTE; Figure 26.3). In a patient with chronic obstructive pulmonary disease, previous thoracic surgery, obesity, or moderate-to-high clinical suspicion for IE, a transesophageal echocardiogram (TEE) should be performed. Moreover, patients with prosthetic valves, staphylococcal bacteremia, or new atrioventricular block should have a TEE performed first, as a TTE will definitely not rule out

endocarditis.[9–11] TEE has been shown to be more sensitive than TTE for the detection of vegetations and abscesses.[12] TEE has also been shown to be cost-effective as the first examination in those with moderate-to-high clinical suspicion of endocarditis. False negative results of echocardiography may occur if vegetations are small or have already embolized. Perivalvular abscess may be missed as well in the patient's early illness. Therefore, repeat echocardiography may be essential several days later. An echocardiogram should be done at the completion of therapy for endocarditis to establish a new baseline for valve function as well as ventricular size and function.

TREATMENT OF ENDOCARDITIS

TREATMENT OF STREPTOCOCCI VIRIDANS ENDOCARDITIS

Native valve highly penicillin-susceptible viridans group streptococci.[13–15] Aqueous crystalline penicillin (pcn) G sodium 12 to 18 million units per day continuous or every 4 hours for *4 weeks duration* (Figure 26.4) or

Ceftriaxone 2 g per day for a *4-week duration*

Vancomycin 30 mg/kg/day divided twice daily for *4 weeks* for those unable to tolerate the above antibiotics

A *2-week* regimen can be done if there is no evidence of cardiac or extracardiac abscess or evidence of decreased renal

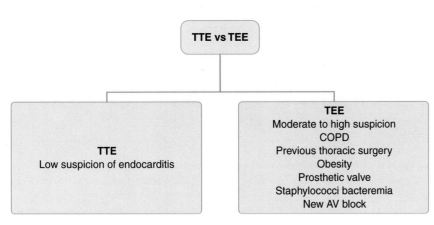

Figure 26.3. The use of echocardiography in infective endocarditis.

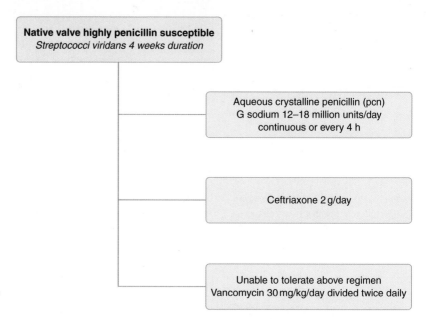

Figure 26.4. Treatment of *Streptococci viridans* endocarditis.

function. However, addition of gentamicin at 3 mg/kg/day in one dose should be added for the entire *2 weeks*.

TREATMENT OF RELATIVELY RESISTANT STREPTOCOCCUS BOVIS OR VIRIDANS ENDOCARDITIS

Relatively resistant Streptococcus bovis or viridians group. Aqueous crystalline pcn G sodium 24 million units per day continuous or every 4 hours for a *4-week duration* (Figure 26.5)

or

Ceftriaxone 2 g per day for a *4-week duration* plus gentamicin at 3 mg/kg/day in one dose for *2 weeks*

Vancomycin 30 mg/kg/day divided twice daily for *4 weeks* for those unable to tolerate the above antibiotics.

Prosthetic valve endocarditis viridans group streptococci. Above regimens for a *6-week duration* of therapy.

TREATMENT OF NATIVE VALVE STAPHYLOCOCCI OXACILLIN-SENSITIVE ENDOCARDITIS

Staphylococci endocarditis without prosthetic involvement. Nafcillin or oxacillin 12 g per day divided equally every 4 hours for *6 weeks* (Figure 26.6)

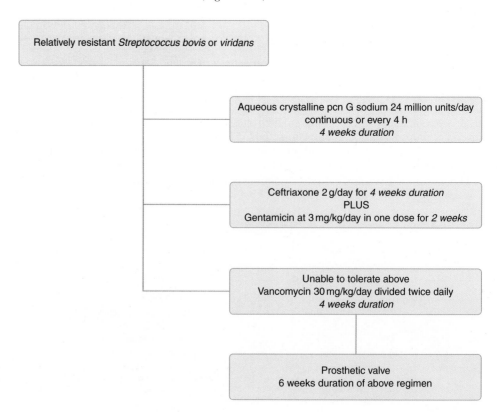

Figure 26.5. Treatment of relatively resistant *Streptococcus bovis* or *viridans* endocarditis.

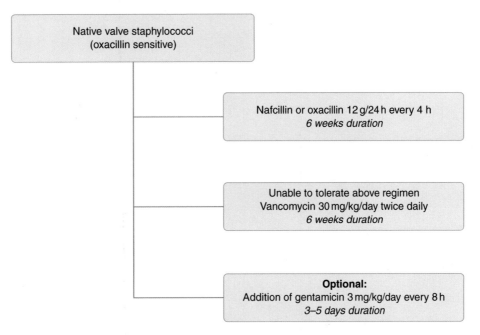

Figure 26.6. Treatment of native valve staphylococci oxacillin-sensitive endocarditis.

Optional addition of gentamicin 3 mg/kg/day divided in two or three equal doses for *3 to 5* days[16]

Vancomycin 30 mg/kg/day divided twice daily for those unable to tolerate the above antibiotics for *6 weeks.*

TREATMENT OF NATIVE VALVE STAPHYLOCOCCI OXACILLIN-RESISTANT ENDOCARDITIS

Oxacillin resistant strains. Vancomycin 30 mg/kg/day divided twice daily for *6 weeks* or daptomycin 6 mg/kg/day (not FDA-approved for left-sided endocarditis; Figure 26.7).

TREATMENT OF PROSTHETIC VALVE STAPHYLOCOCCI ENDOCARDITIS

Staphylococci endocarditis with prosthetic involvement. Nafcillin or oxacillin 12 g per day divided equally every 4 hours plus rifampin 900 mg per day divided in three equal doses for at least *6 weeks* plus gentamicin 3 mg/kg/day divided in two or three equal doses for *2 weeks* (Figure 26.8).[16,17]

Oxacillin-resistant strains. Vancomycin 30 mg/kg/day divided twice daily plus rifampin 900 mg per day divided in three equal doses for at least *6 weeks* plus gentamicin 3 mg/kg/day divided in two or three equal doses for *2 weeks.*[16,17]

TREATMENT OF ENTEROCOCCAL ENDOCARDITIS

Enterococcal endocarditis native or prosthetic valve. Ampicillin 12 g per day every 4 hours in divided doses (Figure 26.9)

or

Aqueous crystalline pcn G 18 to 30 million units per day either continuously or every 4 hours in divided doses

plus

Gentamicin 3 mg/kg/day in three equally divided doses.[18,19]
All for a *4- to 6-week duration*

If pcn allergy to above then vancomycin 30 mg/kg/day divided twice daily plus gentamicin as above.

Endocarditis caused by strains resistant to penicillin, aminoglycoside, or vancomycin should be treated in consultation with an infectious diseases specialist.

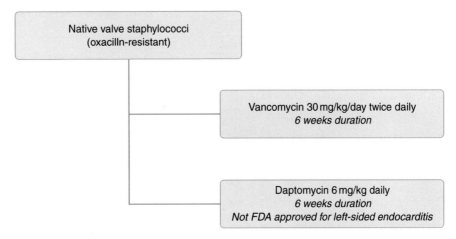

Figure 26.7. Treatment of native valve staphylococci oxacillin-resistant endocarditis.

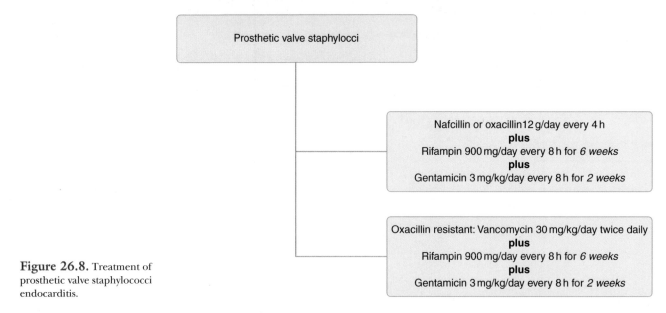

Figure 26.8. Treatment of prosthetic valve staphylococci endocarditis.

SPECIAL CASES OF ENDOCARDITIS

Endocarditis with HACEK group. (*Haemophilus parainfluenzae, Haemophilus aphrophilus, Actinobacillus, Cardiobacterium, Eikenella, Kingella*)

Ceftriaxone 2 g per day for *4 weeks* (Figure 26.10)

or

Ampicillin 12 g per day divided every 4 hours PLUS gentamicin 1 mg per kg divided in three doses for a *total duration of 4 weeks.*

Bartonella species endocarditis. Ceftriaxone 2 g per day for *6 weeks* plus gentamicin 1 mg per kg divided in three doses plus doxycycline 100 mg twice daily for *6 weeks.*

Coxiella brunetii Q-fever endocarditis. Doxycycline 100 mg orally twice a day plus hydroxychloroquine 600 mg per day for *1.5 to 3 years.*

CULTURE-NEGATIVE ENDOCARDITIS

Culture-negative endocarditis. Should be treated in consultation with infectious diseases specialist (Figure 26.11).

Consider ampicillin 12 g per day divided every 4 hours plus gentamicin 1 mg per kg divided in three doses for a *total duration of 4 weeks.*

If pcn allergy to above then vancomycin 30 mg/kg/day divided twice daily plus gentamicin and ciprofloxacin 800 mg per day in two equally divided doses.

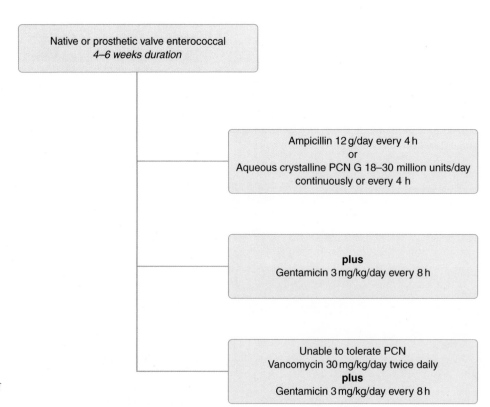

Figure 26.9. Treatment of enterococcal endocarditis.

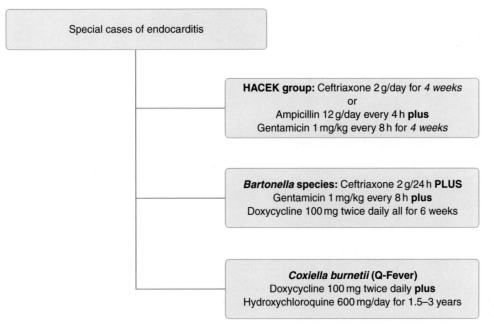

Figure 26.10. Special cases of endocarditis.

CULTURE-NEGATIVE PROSTHETIC VALVE ENDOCARDITIS

Culture-negative prosthetic valve endocarditis. Less than 1 year post-surgery: Vancomycin 30 mg/kg/day divided twice daily plus gentamicin 3 mg/kg/day in three equally divided doses plus cefepime 6 g per day in three divided doses plus rifampin 900 mg per day in three divided doses. *All for 6 weeks except gentamicin for 2 weeks only* (Figure 26.12).

Surgery >1 year. Consider ampicillin 12 g per day divided every 4 hours plus gentamicin 1 mg per kg divided in three doses plus rifampin 900 mg per day in three divided doses for *6 weeks*.

Surgical consultation is advised when endocarditis is associated with the following[20–24]:

Heart failure
S. aureus infection
Fungal infection
Prosthetic dehiscence
Valvular abscess

Multi drug-resistant organism
Left-sided infection with gram-negative bacteria
Persistent infection with positive blood cultures after 1 week of antibiotic therapy
One or more emboli resulting from large vegetation
Emboli during the first 2 weeks of antibiotic therapy
Prosthetic valve endocarditis especially <1 year postoperative.

COMPLICATIONS OF INFECTIVE ENDOCARDITIS

Congestive heart failure (CHF) is more frequent in aortic valve IE than mitral valve and indicative of a worse prognosis (Figure 26.13).[20,23,24]

Embolization occurs in 22% to 50% of patients, most commonly in the lungs, coronary arteries, spleen, bowel, and extremities although 65% of emboli involve the CNS.[25–30] Embolic events occur most commonly in infection with *S. aureus, Candida,* and HACEK organisms. Emboli can occur at anytime during

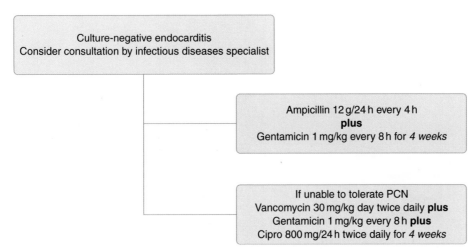

Figure 26.11. Culture-negative endocarditis.

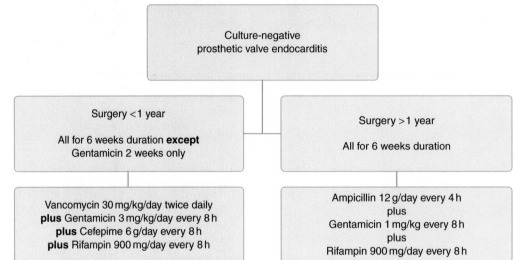

Figure 26.12. Culture-negative prosthetic valve endocarditis.

infection; however, the rate decreases after the first 2 to 3 weeks of successful antimicrobial therapy.[31]

Splenic abscess is more common in left-sided endocarditis and associated more commonly with viridans streptococci and *S. aureus* infections.[32–34]

Mycotic aneurysms result from septic emboli to the arterial or intraluminal space with spread of infection out from the vessel. This occurs most commonly in the intracranial arteries followed by the visceral arteries and least commonly in the extremities.[33]

DISCHARGE THERAPY

Oral antibiotic therapy is unreliable in absorption and not recommended for endocarditis.

Outpatient intravenous antimicrobial therapy may be considered when the following has been achieved[35]:

Medically stable
Low risk for complications for CHF or emboli
No evidence of cardiac conduction abnormalities
Resolved fever
Negative blood cultures
No evidence of valve ring abscess
Reliable and secure home support system
Easy access to physician should a complication arise
Access to regular visits by a home infusion nurse to monitor for adherence and antibiotic toxicity
Regular visits with physician to assess clinical status and monitor for complications.

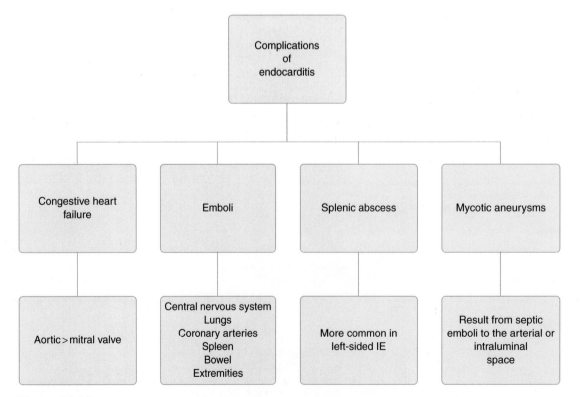

Figure 26.13. Complications of infective endocarditis.

CONCERNS AFTER COMPLETION OF TREATMENT

Concerns after completion of treatment include:

Relapse of infection

Development or worsening CHF

Antibiotic toxicity such as *Clostridium difficile*, audiologic and vestibular toxicity.

REFERENCES

1. Cabell CH, Jollis JG, Peterson GE, et al. Changing patient characteristics and the effect on mortality in endocarditis. *Arch Intern Med.* 2002;162:90–94.

2. Hoen B, Alla F, Setton-Suty C, et al.; Association pour l'Etude et la Prevention de l'Endocardite Infectieuse (AEPEI) Study Group. Changing profile of infective endocarditis: results of a one year survey in France. *JAMA.* 2002;288:75–81.

3. Roder BL, Wandall DA, Frimodt-Moller N, et al. Clinical features of *Staphylococcus aureus* endocarditis. *Arch Intern Med.* 1999;159:462–469.

4. Chambers HF. The changing epidemiology of *Staphylococcus aureus*. *Emerg Infect Dis.* 2001;7:178–182.

5. Naimi TS, LeDell KH, Boxrud DJ, et al. Epidemiology and clonality of community acquired methicillin-resistant *Staphylococcus aureus* in Minnesota, 1996–1998. *Clin Infect Dis.* 2001;33:990–996.

6. Salgado CD, Farr BM, Calfe DP. Community-acquired methicillin-resistant *Staphylococcus aureus*: a meta-analysis of prevalence and risk factors. *Clin Infect Dis.* 2003;36:131–139.

7. Tsakris A, Pournaras S, Maniatia AN, et al. Increasing prevalence of high-level gentamicin resistance among enterococci isolated in Greece. *Chemotherapy.* 2001;47:86–89.

8. Li JS, Sexton DJ, Mick N, et al. Proposed modifications to the Duke criteria for the diagnosis of infective endocarditis. *Clin Infect Dis.* 2000;30:633–638.

9. Daniel WG, Mugge A, Grote J, et al. Comparison of transthoracic and transesophageal echocardiography for detection of abnormalities of prosthetic and bioprosthetic valves in the mitral and aortic positions. *Am J Cardiol.* 1993;71:210–215.

10. Heidenreich PA, Masoudi FA, Maini B, et al. Echocardiography in patients with suspected endocarditis: a cost-effectiveness analysis. *Am J Med.* 1999;107:198–208.

11. Lindner JR, Case RA, Dent JM, et al. Diagnostic value of echocardiography in suspected endocarditis: an evaluation based on the pretest probability of disease. *Circulation.* 1996;93:730–736.

12. Reynolds HR, Jagen MA, Tunick PA, et al. Sensitivity of transthoracic versus transesophageal echocardiography for the detection of native valve vegetations in the modern era. *J Am Soc Echocardiogr.* 2003;16:67–70.

13. Francioli P, Etienne J, Hoigné R, et al. Treatment of streptococcal endocarditis with a single daily dose of ceftriaxone sodium for 4 weeks: efficacy and outpatient treatment feasibility. *JAMA.* 1992;267:264–267.

14. Wilson WR. Ceftriaxone sodium therapy of penicillin G-susceptible streptococcal endocarditis. *JAMA.* 1992;267:279–280.

15. Francioli P, Ruch W, Stamboulian D. Treatment of streptococcal endocarditis with a single daily dose of ceftriaxone and netilmicin for 14 days: a prospective multicenter study. *Clin Infect Dis.* 1995;21:1406–1410.

16. Chuard C, Herrmann M, Vaudaux P, et al. Successful therapy of experimental chronic foreign-body infection due to methicillin-resistant *Staphylococcus aureus* by antimicrobial combinations. *Antimicrob Agents Chemother.* 1991;35:2611–2616.

17. John MD, Hibberd PL, Karchmer AW, et al. *Staphylococcus aureus* prosthetic valve endocarditis: optimal management and risk factors for death. *Clin Infect Dis.* 1998;26:1302–1309.

18. Wilson WR, Wilkowske CJ, Wright AJ, et al. Treatment of streptomycin-susceptible and streptomycin-resistant enterococcal endocarditis. *Ann Intern Med.* 1984;100:816–823.

19. Rice LB, Calderwood SB, Eliopoulous GM, et al. Enterococcal endocarditis: a comparison of prosthetic and native valve disease. *Rev Infect Dis.* 1991;13:1–7.

20. Sexton DJ, Spelman D. Current best practices and guidelines: assessment and management of complications in infective endocarditis. *Cardiol Clin.* 2003;21:273–282.

21. Erbel R, Rohmann S, Drexler M, et al. Improved diagnostic value of echocardiography in patients with infective endocarditis by transoesophageal approach: a prospective study. *Eur Heart J.* 1988;9:43–53.

22. Mills J, Utley J, Abbott J. Heart failure in infective endocarditis: predisposing factors, course and treatment. *Chest.* 1974;66:151–157.

23. Stinson EB. Surgical treatment of infective endocarditis. *Prog Cardiovasc Dis.* 1979;22:145–168.

24. Vikram HR, Buenconsejo J, Hasbun R, et al. Impact of valve surgery on 6-month mortality in adults with complicated, left-sided native valve endocarditis: a propensity analysis. *JAMA.* 2003;290:3207–3214.

25. Lutas EM, Roberts RB, Devereux RB, et al. Relation between the presence of echocardiographic vegetations and the complication rate in infective endocarditis. *Am Heart J.* 1986;112:107–113.

26. DeCastro S, Magni G, Beni S, et al. Role of transthoracic and transesophageal echocardiography in predicting embolic events in patients with active infective endocarditis involving native cardiac valves. *Am J Cardiol.* 1997;80:1030–1034.

27. Heiro M, Nikoskelainen J, Engblom E, et al. Neurologic manifestations of infective endocarditis: a 17-year experience in a teaching hospital in Finland. *Arch Intern Med.* 2000;160:2781–2787.

28. Sanfilippo AJ, Picard MH, Newell JB, et al. Echocardiographic assessment of patients with infectious endocarditis: prediction of risk for complications. *J Am Coll Cardiol.* 1991;18:1191–1199.

29. Rohmann S, Erbel R, Gorge G, et al. Clinical relevance of vegetation localization by transoesophageal echocardiography in infective endocarditis. *Eur Heart J.* 1992;13:446–452.

30. Mugge A, Daniel WG, Frank G, et al. Echocardiography in infective endocarditis: reassessment of prognostic implications of vegetation size determined by the transthoracic and the transesophageal approach. *J Am Coll Cardiol.* 1989;14:631–638.

31. Vilacosta I, Graupner C, San Roman JA, et al. Risk of embolization after institution of antibiotic therapy for infective endocarditis. *J Am Coll Cardiol.* 2002;39:1489–1495.

32. Johnson JD, Raff MJ, Barnwell PA, et al. Splenic abscess complicating infectious endocarditis. *Arch Intern Med.* 1983;143:906–912.

33. Mansur AJ, Grinberg M, da Luz PL, et al. The complications of infective endocarditis: a reappraisal in the 1980s. *Arch Intern Med.* 1992;152:2428–2432.

34. Ting W, Silverman NA, Arzouman DA, et al. Splenic septic emboli in endocarditis. *Circulation.* 1990;82:IV-105–IV-109.

35. Baddour LM, Wilson WR, Bayer AS, et al. Infective endocarditis: diagnosis, antimicrobial therapy, and management of complications: a statement for healthcare professionals from the Committee on Rheumatic Fever, Endocarditis, and Kawasaki Disease, Council on Cardiovascular Disease in the Young, and the Councils on Clinical Cardiology, Stroke, and Cardiovascular Surgery and Anesthesia, American Heart Association: endorsed by the Infectious Diseases Society of America. *Circulation.* 2005;111:e394–e434.

PATIENT AND FAMILY INFORMATION FOR:
Infective Endocarditis

Infective endocarditis is described as an infection of the heart and/or heart valves. It is usually caused by infectious agents that are bacterial in origin. The most common bacterial causes of endocarditis are *Staphylococcus aureus,* streptococci, and enterococci. We are now concerned with drug resistance among these infectious agents; therefore proper diagnosis and treatment is of utmost importance.

DIAGNOSIS

The mainstay of diagnosing infective endocarditis is blood cultures and echocardiogram. All patients suspected of endocarditis should have blood cultures drawn from at least two different sites preferably during a documented fever and always before starting antibiotics. An echocardiogram should be obtained as soon as the diagnosis of endocarditis is suspected. If the echocardiogram is negative and no other diagnosis is established over the next several days, a repeat exam may be necessary.

TREATMENT

Treatment of infective endocarditis varies based on the infectious agent. All cases of endocarditis require intravenous antibiotics. Oral antibiotics are not useful in this disease. If the agent causing the infection is viridans group streptococci, then the treatment will be penicillin, ceftriaxone, or vancomycin. Based on the data obtained from the microbiology lab, the physician will decide which of these antibiotics is best. The treatment will be for 4 weeks unless the patient has a prosthetic heart valve, and then the antibiotics will be needed for at least 6 weeks.

If the infection is caused by staphylococci then the treatment is initiated with nafcillin, oxacillin, vancomycin, or daptomycin. The decision will be based on the presence of resistant or sensitive strains of the staphylococci. Another antibiotic namely gentamicin may be added for the first 3 to 5 days to help clear the infection quicker. These antibiotics will be needed for at least 6 weeks. If the staphylococci infection is associated with a prosthetic heart valve, then the addition of rifampin will be necessary.

Endocarditis caused by enterococci will require treatment with ampicillin, penicillin, or vancomycin with the addition of gentamicin for a duration of 4 to 6 weeks. If the infection is resistant to common antibiotics then consultation with an infectious diseases specialist is recommended.

Some patients with endocarditis do not have a bacterial agent identified. This may result from prior antibiotic use or an unusual agent that is difficult to identify. These cases are referred to as culture-negative endocarditis. All cases of culture-negative endocarditis should have a consultation with an infectious diseases specialist for further investigation. After appropriate blood work is obtained consideration of treatment with ampicillin along with gentamicin, or vancomycin along with gentamicin and ciprofloxacin should be considered for a 4-week duration.

If a patient has a prosthetic valve along with a culture-negative endocarditis, the antibiotic choice is based on when the surgery took place. If the surgery was <1 year prior to infection then treatment should include vancomycin, gentamicin, cefepime, and rifampin. If surgery was >1 year prior to infection then ampicillin, gentamicin, and rifampin should be used. Patients with prosthetic valves should undergo consultation with a surgeon.

Surgical consultation for infective endocarditis is advised in the following situations:

Heart failure
Staphylococci aureus infection
Fungal infection
Prosthetic dehiscence
Valvular abscess
Multi drug-resistant organism
Left-sided infection with gram-negative bacteria
Persistent infection with positive blood cultures after 1 week of antibiotic therapy
One or more emboli resulting from large vegetation
Emboli during the first 2 weeks of antibiotic therapy
Prosthetic valve endocarditis especially <1 year postoperative.

COMPLICATIONS OF INFECTIVE ENDOCARDITIS

The most common complication of endocarditis is congestive heart failure manifested with fluid in the lungs. Other common problems include embolization that comes from bacterial infections. This is when infected tissue from one part of the body migrates to another, by the bloodstream. Emboli can cause strokes and can affect the lungs, spleen, intestines, arms or legs by causing decreased blood flow to these organs. The risk of emboli is highest during the first 1 to 2 weeks of treatment.

DISCHARGE THERAPY

Oral antibiotics are unreliable and not recommended for endocarditis. Outpatient intravenous therapy may be considered when the patient is:

Medically stable
Low risk for complications with CHF or emboli
No evidence of electrical heart abnormalities
Resolved fever
Negative blood cultures
No evidence of valve ring abscess
Reliable and secure home support system
Easy access to physician should a complication arise
Access to regular visits by a home infusion nurse to monitor for adherence and antibiotic toxicity

Regular visits with physician to assess clinical status and monitor for complications

The concerns after completion of treatment include relapse of infection, development or worsening CHF, antibiotic toxicity such as diarrhea with *Clostridium difficile*, hearing loss, or problems with balance and equilibrium. Follow-up with a physician during and after treatment is very important to detect any potential problems.

SECTION V

Intensive Critical Care Therapy

Vishal P. Patel
Janet M. Shapiro

Mechanical Ventilation in the Cardiac Care Unit

OBJECTIVES AND INDICATIONS FOR MECHANICAL VENTILATION

GOALS OF MECHANICAL VENTILATION

Mechanical ventilation is the process by which a device supports the partial or total transport of oxygen and carbon dioxide between the environment and the pulmonary capillary bed. Mechanical ventilation itself is not a treatment modality, but rather a measure to restore effective gas exchange and reduce the patient's work of breathing as the underlying pathology is being treated. The goals of mechanical ventilation are listed in Table 27.1.

INDICATIONS FOR MECHANICAL VENTILATION

The indications for ventilatory support are best understood after one characterizes the causes of respiratory failure into either hypoxemic or hypercapnic categories (Table 27.2).

Most of the patients being admitted to a cardiac care unit (CCU) will fall into the category of hypoxemic respiratory failure caused by cardiogenic pulmonary edema, which leads to decreased lung compliance, ventilation–perfusion mismatching, and diffusion impairment. Hypoxemia of mild to moderate severity can often be managed by the administration of oxygen through delivery systems ranging from nasal cannula to face masks. However, it can be increasingly difficult to maintain adequate oxygenation and oxygen delivery with more severe hypoxemia, and these patients may require positive-pressure ventilation as they are commonly in considerable distress.

Physiologic derangements and clinical findings will determine the need for mechanical ventilation, which should be considered early in the course and not be delayed until the need becomes emergent. Patients suffering from cardiogenic shock will have an increased respiratory workload and reduced cardiac output delivered to the muscles of respiration. They are often described as "tiring out" or developing respiratory muscle fatigue and may show physical exam findings such as nasal flaring, tracheal tug, recruitment of accessory muscles of respiration (sternocleidomastoids or intercostals), paradoxical or asynchronous movements of the rib cage and abdomen, and an increased pulsus paradoxus. If the mechanical workload progressively increases, the breathing demand at some point will exceed the capabilities of respiratory pump. The patient will be unable to sustain adequate levels of ventilation to effectively eliminate carbon dioxide, and progressive hypercapnia will ensue.

A substantial proportion of patients who require mechanical ventilation have relatively normal arterial blood gases but show the other signs of respiratory failure mentioned earlier. Therefore,

TABLE 27.1.	Objectives of Mechanical Ventilation

Physiologic objectives
- Improve pulmonary gas exchange by supporting alveolar ventilation and arterial oxygenation
- Decrease the metabolic cost of breathing by unloading the muscles of respiration
- Reduce the risk of Ventilator Associated Lung Injury (VALI)

Clinical objectives
- Improve hypoxemia
- Improve acute respiratory acidosis
- Ease respiratory distress and respiratory muscle fatigue
- Prevent or improve atelectasis
- Allow sedation and/or neuromuscular blockade
- Reduce systemic or myocardial oxygen consumption

TABLE 27.2	Causes of Respiratory Failure

Hypercapnic respiratory failure
- Increased respiratory workload caused by
  - Airway resistance (asthma, airway obstruction)
  - Elastic workload (pulmonary fibrosis, pneumonia, congestive heart failure)
  - Severe metabolic acidosis
  - Carbon dioxide production
  - Copious secretions in the airways
- Diminished central respiratory drive caused by
  - Sedative or analgesic medications
  - Central nervous system injury
- Diminished respiratory muscle function caused by
  - Mechanical disadvantage from
    - Chest wall deformities
    - Dynamic hyperinflation (COPD)
  - Respiratory muscle weakness from
    - Electrolyte abnormalities
    - Myopathies or neuropathies
    - Deconditioning

Hypoxemic respiratory failure
  - Ventilation–perfusion mismatching
  - Right-to-left shunt
  - Alveolar hypoventilation
  - Diffusion impairment
  - Reduced inspired oxygen concentration

the decision to place a patient on mechanical ventilation should not be determined by abnormalities of the arterial blood gas.

Moreover, increased respiratory work may increase the oxygen cost of breathing to as much as 50% of total body oxygen consumption. When this occurs, the respiratory muscles disproportionally consume oxygen at the expense of aerobic metabolism of other vital organs such as the heart, brain, and kidneys. Under these circumstances, mechanical ventilation decreases the work of breathing, decreases the oxygen cost of breathing, and redistributes oxygen delivery to the respiratory system thereby improving oxygen delivery to other bodily organs.[1,2]

If the underlying pathology is only transient or readily reversible, ventilation may be achieved through noninvasive modes. However, those patients who are postcardiac arrest, undergoing therapeutic hypothermia, experiencing ongoing cardiac ischemia, demonstrating cardiac or airway instability, exhibiting altered mental status, or having copious secretions, are poor candidates for noninvasive ventilation (NIV) and they require endotracheal intubation with positive-pressure ventilation.

NONINVASIVE VENTILATION

NIV refers to a method of delivering ventilatory assistance with the use of a mask interface rather than with an invasive interface, such as an endotracheal tube (ETT) or tracheostomy. NIV may provide respiratory support to selected patients while avoiding complications of invasive mechanical ventilation.[3,4] The modes that are most commonly used in the critical care setting are continuous positive airway pressure (CPAP) and bilevel positive airway pressure (BPAP).

COMPONENTS OF THE NONINVASIVE VENTILATOR

The application of NIV requires a nasal or oronasal mask interface and a device that is capable of delivering sustained high-flow positive air pressure. These systems are much more susceptible to air leaks than is endotracheal intubation. For the purpose of the intensive care unit (ICU), the oronasal mask confers the greatest physiologic improvements with the least amount of airflow resistance and of air leakage from the mouth.[5–9] This mask is secured to the patient's face by the use of adjustable Velcro straps.

NIV can be delivered via the standard type of ventilator found in most ICUs or by a portable ventilator. CPAP is a mode that is often used for patients with acute respiratory failure because of cardiogenic pulmonary edema. BPAP ventilators are capable of delivering very high flow rates and are best suited for use in critically ill patients with concomitant hypoxemia and hypercarbia. They have built-in oxygen blenders and more sophisticated monitoring capabilities and alarm functions. Bilevel machines are pressure-limited and allow for selection of separate inspiratory and expiratory pressure targets.

PHYSIOLOGIC EFFECTS OF NIV

In recent years, there has been a great expansion in the use of NIV in patients with respiratory failure caused by cardiogenic pulmonary edema. NIV reduces respiratory muscle work and facilitates

TABLE 27.3	Potential Indicators of Success with NIV

- Younger patient
- Lower severity of illness (APACHE score)
- Ability to cooperate, coordinate breathing with ventilator, less air leaking
- Moderate degree of hypercarbia ($PaCO_2$ >45 mm Hg, <92 mm Hg)
- Moderate degree of acidemia (pH >7.1, <7.35)
- Improved gas exchange, heart rate, and respiratory rate within 2 h

a slower and deeper pattern of breathing, thus resulting in increased minute ventilation (MV_E) and alveolar ventilation. NIV has been shown to improve gas exchange, normalize arterial carbon dioxide, increase arterial oxygen, increase pH, increase tidal volume (V_T), and decrease respiratory muscle work in acute and chronic respiratory failure.[10–14] It has also been reported to stabilize certain metabolic parameters such as heart rate, respiratory rate, and blood pressure. Details regarding the systemic hemodynamic and cardiovascular effects of positive-pressure ventilation will be discussed in the section *Invasive Mechanical Ventilation*.

SELECTING PATIENTS FOR NIV

Selecting a proper patient is critical to the use of NIV. Successful application of NIV may obviate the need for endotracheal intubation in some patients. A trial of NIV is therefore worthwhile in most patients that do not require emergent intubation, assuming that they have no contraindications. Some potential indicators of success with NIV use are listed in Table 27.3.

The clinician must exclude patients in whom the use of NIV would be unsafe. NIV is an absolute contraindication in patients at risk of imminent respiratory or cardiac arrest or in those who have already suffered so, and these patients should be promptly intubated. Those with unstable conditions such as shock, myocardial ischemia, or life-threatening cardiac arrhythmias should not be managed with NIV. Patients with altered mental status caused by conditions such as meningitis, stroke, or intracranial hemorrhage (with the exception of hypercapnic encephalopathy), and those who are comatose, agitated or uncooperative also cannot undergo NIV. Ideally, patients being considered for NIV should be able to manage their secretions and those with copious amounts should be considered for intubation. Facial surgery, trauma, or deformities that may prevent adequate fitting of the mask interface, and patients with gastric distension and vomiting are relative contraindications.

NIV IN ACUTE CARDIOGENIC PULMONARY EDEMA

Cardiogenic pulmonary edema and COPD exacerbation are the two acute disorders for which NIV has proven beneficial. In acute cardiogenic pulmonary edema, both CPAP and BPAP have been shown to reduce the work of breathing and intubation rates.

CPAP rapidly improves oxygenation by reexpanding flooding alveoli, increasing functional residual capacity, and positioning the lung more favorably on its compliance curve.[15] These effects lead to a reduced work of breathing and improved cardiac performance.[15-17] A number of randomized, controlled studies have shown that CPAP is effective in treating acute pulmonary edema. Rasanen et al.[18] demonstrated rapid improvement in oxygenation and respiratory rate compared to conventional face mask. Lin and Chiang[19] showed a significantly reduced rate of intubation as compared to standard oxygen therapy, but no difference in mortality. Bersten et al.[20] and Lin et al.[21] subsequently showed similar evidence, however, the latter did show a trend toward improved in-hospital mortality.

Several uncontrolled trials support the use of BPAP for patients with acute pulmonary edema by demonstrating low intubation and complication rates.[22-26] However, one of these studies noted a high mortality rate in patients experiencing acute myocardial infarction and cautioned using BPAP in these patients.[26] Evidence produced by Masip et al.[27] in a randomized trial showed significantly reduced intubation rates in patients treated with BPAP compared to standard oxygen therapy. A randomized trial comparing the use of CPAP to BPAP in the treatment of patients with acute pulmonary edema showed significantly more rapid reductions in respiratory rate, dyspnea score, and hypercapnia in the BPAP group compared to the CPAP group, although the trial was aborted because of a greater myocardial infarction rate in the BPAP group.[28] This had been attributed to unequal randomization, however, the results still raise concern for the safety of ventilatory techniques used to treat pulmonary edema complicated by cardiac ischemia or myocardial infarction. A study by Nava et al.[29] did not confirm the increased risk of myocardial ischemia with the use of BPAP as seen in prior studies. However, patients with concomitant hypercapnia experienced more rapid relief of respiratory distress, better gas exchange, and reduced intubation rates, whereas mortality was not affected. A more recent trial compared standard oxygen therapy with NIV (CPAP or BPAP) and found no significant difference in 7- or 30-day mortality between the two groups.[30] In addition, no difference in intubation rate or mortality was seen between the CPAP and BPAP groups. However, the NIV group did achieve more rapid improvement in respiratory distress and metabolic disturbances than did oxygen therapy alone.

For patients with acute cardiogenic pulmonary edema who are hemodynamically stable and meet criteria for NIV, we recommend BPAP as the initial ventilatory mode.

INITIATING NONINVASIVE VENTILATION AND MACHINE SETTINGS

Once the patient has been selected to receive a trial of NIV, it should be initiated as soon as possible. Any delays may result in further deterioration of the patient and increase the likelihood of failure. The oronasal mask should be selected for most patients. Parameters that need to be set with the BPAP mode of ventilation include inspiratory positive airway pressure (IPAP), expiratory positive airway pressure (EPAP), fraction of inspired oxygen (FiO$_2$), and a backup respiratory rate.

IPAP is used synonymously with the term *pressure support* and EPAP is variably labeled as positive end-expiratory pressure (PEEP). Therefore, an IPAP of 15 cm water and an EPAP of 5 cm water are equivalent to a pressure support of 10 cm water

and a PEEP of 5 cm water. The initial target of IPAP and EPAP should be selected on the basis of bedside observation and determined primarily by patient tolerance. Although a universal approach to establishing the initial settings for BPAP has not been established, a minimum IPAP of 10 cm water and EPAP of 5 cm water is usually appropriate as giving the patient higher initial pressures may result in early failure. The V_T being delivered with this mode depends on the difference between IPAP and EPAP. For example, the V_T will be greater while using an IPAP of 15 cm water and an EPAP of 5 cm water (difference of 10 cm water) compared to an IPAP of 10 cm water and an EPAP of 5 cm water (difference of 5 cm water). The goal V_T to be delivered in most patients is usually between 8 and 10 mL per kilogram of ideal body weight. If the physician desires to give the patient higher V_T IPAP can be titrated up. On the other hand, if the goal is to increase PEEP, EPAP can be increased.

The BPAP machine is a pressure-limited device that supports a spontaneous mode of ventilation. That is, the breath will be delivered only if there is a recognized patient effort. If the physician wishes to add a mandatory minimum machine-directed breath, he can set a backup rate of 10 to 12 breaths per minute. However, these forced breaths are commonly not synchronized with the patient's effort.

The initial FiO$_2$ setting should be decided according to the nature of the patient's respiratory failure and baseline arterial blood gas. In severe hypoxemia, oxygen concentrations of up to 100% can be delivered. Patients with respiratory muscle fatigue and increased work of breathing without severe hypoxemia may require much lower oxygen concentrations. A practical approach is to set the initial FiO$_2$ to 100%. Arterial blood gas analysis should then be performed after 1 to 2 hours of initiation of BPAP, and the FiO$_2$ can be titrated down if the PaO$_2$ is at an acceptable level. It is then reasonable to further titrate down the FiO$_2$ in small decrements based on the patient's oxygen saturation on pulse oximetry (usually to a goal greater than or equal to 90%). Table 27.4 shows a protocol to guide the initiation of NIV.

TABLE 27.4	Protocol for Initiation of NIV

1. Appropriately monitored location, with monitoring of pulse oximetry and vital signs

2. Patient in bed or chair at >30° angle

3. Connect all tubing, turn on ventilator, and select and fit mask interface

4. Start with low pressure with backup rate; 8–12 cm water IPAP; 3–5 cm water EPAP; backup rate of 12 breaths/min

5. Gradually increase IPAP (10–20 cm water) as tolerated to achieve alleviation of dyspnea, decreased respiratory rate, increased V_T, and good patient–ventilator synchrony

6. Provide FiO$_2$ supplementation as needed to keep oxygen saturation >90%

7. Check for air leaks and readjust straps if needed

8. Consider mild sedation in agitated or anxious patients

9. Monitor initial blood gas (1–2 h after initiation) and then as needed

10. Encouragement, reassurance, and frequent checks and adjustments as needed

MONITORING AND TROUBLESHOOTING

As a general rule, patients that are started on NIV should be monitored in the same way as patients who are mechanically ventilated through an ETT. Patients should be observed closely for the first hours after initiation to troubleshoot, provide reassurance, and monitor for deterioration. If there is no stabilization or improvement over this time, NIV should be considered a failure and the patient should be promptly intubated. If the patient is clearly failing immediately after initiation, the clinician should not wait but should proceed to intubation. Some clinical signs that suggest failure include worsening gas exchange, worsening encephalopathy or agitation, inability to clear secretions, inability to tolerate any of the mask interfaces, persistent signs and symptoms of respiratory fatigue, and hemodynamic instability. Reductions in respiratory rate and accessory muscle use, coupled with improvement in thoracoabdominal synchrony and gas exchange suggest a favorable response and good prognosis if seen within 2 hours.

Many patients cannot tolerate BPAP, and this is usually because of patient–ventilator asynchrony (when the phases of inspiration and expiration do not match that of the patient). This may be related to the mode of ventilation being used; however, this should not be the only consideration as the possibility of a mask leak is fairly common and should always be investigated. Waveform displays of breath-by-breath delivered flow, volume, and pressure are available on most ICU ventilators (Figure 27.1). If the alarms for these parameters are triggered (i.e., low V_T or pressures), this is most likely because of a mask leak. Patients can often be satisfactorily ventilated despite such leakage as most pressure-limited ventilators are able to compensate for leaks by sustaining airflow to maintain mask pressure. If the leak is sufficient enough to interfere with ventilatory support, readjusting the position of the mask on the face with tightening of the Velcro straps may help. In addition, the mask itself may have to be upsized or downsized to ensure a proper fit. Air leaks may also be present if ventilator tubing becomes disconnected from the ventilator or face mask, or if nebulization ports remain open to the atmosphere.

In addition to addressing the possibility of air leaks, asynchrony may also be seen if nonoptimal pressures are being delivered. Increasing or decreasing IPAP can adjust for inadequate V_T. PEEP can be adjusted by increasing or decreasing the EPAP. Extreme tachypnea, agitation, and anxiety may be alleviated by the conservative use of sedative agents, such as opiates or benzodiazepines.

Some of the other problems that may be encountered with NIV are nasal congestion or dryness, nasal bridge redness or ulceration produced by excessive mask tension, irritation of the eyes causing conjunctivitis, and gastric insufflation leading to distension or flatulence. Simple efforts such as the use of in-line heated humidification, nasal saline sprays, the application of foam rubber spacers or mask pillows, reduction in inflation pressures, or the addition of oral simethicone may help alleviate these problems. Major complications such as aspiration, hypotension, and pneumothorax are seldom seen, and these events can be prevented by carefully selecting patients for NIV.

PATIENTS WITH DO NOT INTUBATE ORDER

NIV is frequently used in patients who have a directive for no intubation but have a potentially reversible cause of respiratory failure such as cardiogenic pulmonary edema. These patients may be good candidates for NIV as their short-term prognosis may be significantly improved. In contrast, NIV is also initiated in patients with advanced stage diseases who have poor prognosis. It is a life support measure and its use should be guided by the goals of care, as it may still offer benefits in alleviating respiratory distress or suffering. More information regarding this topic can be found in the chapter 31 on *End of Life Care in the CCU*.

INVASIVE MECHANICAL VENTILATION

Invasive mechanical ventilation is usually initiated in the CCU for patients with respiratory failure, cardiogenic shock, and

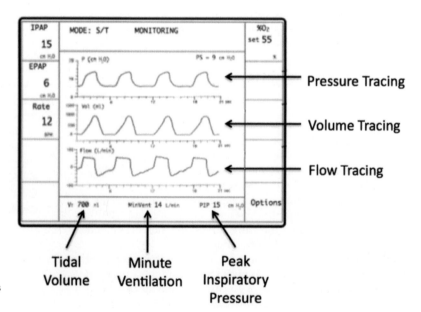

Figure 27.1. Waveform display in NIV (Philips Respironics BiPAP Vision).

cardiac arrest. If a patient with pulmonary edema has a contraindication to or fails NIV, he should be promptly intubated.

UNDERSTANDING THE MECHANICAL VENTILATOR

A basic understanding of the mechanism of ventilation is useful. The term *cycling* or *control* refers to the means by which the ventilator determines that the inspired breath is complete. It is the signal that stops inspiration. This can be sensed either by volume (inspiration stops once the target volume is delivered), pressure (inspiration stops once the target pressure is reached), flow (when flow decreases to a given level, inspiration is terminated), or time (inspiration stops after a preset time interval). The term *limit* refers to a factor that limits the rate at which gas flows into the lungs and causes inspiration to end before cycling is complete. A limit can be pressure, volume, or flow. *Triggering* is the signal that opens the inspiratory valve, allowing air to flow into the patient. To initiate a breath, the ventilator must recognize that a set value has been reached. The trigger can be set to time, volume, pressure, or flow. For example, when a patient's effort reaches the preset pressure value of 1 to 5 cm of water, the machine will deliver a breath.

Breath types can be classified in several different ways. If the patient determines the beginning, duration, and end of a breath, it is said to be *spontaneous*. If the ventilator controls any of these aspects, the breath is considered to be either *assisted* or *mandatory (controlled)*. V_T is the amount of air delivered with each breath. The normal V_T in a 70-kg person is roughly 500 mL. MV_E is the product of V_T and the respiratory rate, and is the amount of air inhaled or exhaled in 1 minute. The normal MV_E is 5 to 8 L per minute. Fraction of inspired oxygen (FiO_2) is the percentage of oxygen in the inspired air, and can range from 21% (room air) to 100%. Positive end-expiratory pressure (PEEP) is the pressure set on the ventilator to prevent expiratory alveolar collapse.

MODES OF INVASIVE POSITIVE-PRESSURE VENTILATION

The selection of ventilator mode for a critically ill patient is generally based on the experience of the clinician and institutional preference.[31–33] There is little evidence that any particular mode affects clinical outcome.

All basic modes of mechanical ventilation are either volume controlled or pressure controlled.[34] In *Volume control (volume preset* or *volume cycled)* ventilation, the machine delivers a preset volume determined by the physician and, within limits, delivers that volume irrespective of the pressure generated within the system. The amount of pressure necessary to deliver this volume will fluctuate from breath to breath based on the resistance and compliance of the patient and ventilator circuit. If the V_T is set at 500 mL, the ventilator will continue to inspire gas until it reaches this goal. Upon completion of the inspired volume, the ventilator will open a valve allowing the patient to passively exhale. It is therefore referred to as *volume-controlled, pressure variable* ventilation.

In *Pressure control (pressure preset* or *pressure cycled)* ventilation, the ventilator applies a predefined pressure target set by the physician. The ventilator will flow gas into the patient until this set pressure is reached. Upon reaching the preset pressure, the ventilator allows for passive exhalation. The resulting V_T will vary according to airways resistance and lung compliance, and is therefore referred to as *pressure controlled, volume variable* ventilation.

The mode is also classified based on how the breath is initiated—whether by the ventilator, the patient, or both.[34] In controlled mechanical ventilation (CMV), the MV_E is determined entirely by the set respiratory rate and the set control (volume or pressure control). The patient does not initiate additional MV_E above that set by the ventilator (i.e., there is no ventilator triggering by the patient). For example in volume-controlled CMV, if the set respiratory rate is 12 breaths per minute and the preset V_T is 500 mL, the patient will be guaranteed an MV_E of 6 L per minute (no lower and no higher). Patients are unable to alter their MV_E if the clinical situation changes such as hypoxemia or worsening acidosis, and acid–base maintenance is solely the responsibility of the physician. This mode does not require any patient effort and should only be used in patients who are apneic caused by brain injury, heavy sedation, or paralysis. If placed on this mode, patients that are awake or spontaneously triggering may generate asynchronous respiratory efforts that may contribute to increased work of breathing, patient discomfort, and worsening gas exchange.

During assist control (AC) ventilation, the physician determines the minimum MV_E by setting the respiratory rate and control (volume or pressure control). The patient can increase his own MV_E by triggering additional breaths (by flow or pressure) above the set respiratory rate. Each time the patient triggers, the ventilator will generate a fully supported breath according to the volume or pressure preset. For example in volume-controlled AC, if the respiratory rate is set to 12 breaths per minute and the V_T to 500 mL, the minimum MV_E will be 6 L per minute. If the patient triggers an additional 8 breaths per minute, the MV_E then becomes 10 L per minute. This mode is the most commonly used mode of ventilation in ICUs and is best suited for those who are awake or still have spontaneous respiratory efforts, and can even be used in those who do not generate any respiratory efforts.

Many manufacturers have incorporated features from volume and pressure controlled AC ventilation to accommodate patients' needs. Pressure-regulated volume control (PRVC) is a dual-control mode available on many newer ventilators. Its basic features are similar to AC ventilation, with the main difference being that the ventilator is able to autoregulate the inspiratory time and flow in order to deliver the preset V_T at the lowest possible plateau airway pressure.

Intermittent mandatory ventilation (IMV) is similar to AC for two reasons. First, the physician decides the minimum MV_E by setting the respiratory rate and volume or pressure preset. Second, the patient is still able to increase his or her own MV_E. The difference between IMV and AC is that in IMV, the increased MV_E is achieved through spontaneous breathing rather than through fully supported patient-triggered ventilator breaths. For example, in volume-controlled IMV, if the set respiratory rate is 12 breaths per minute and the preset V_T is 500 mL, the minimum MV_E will be 6 L per minute. If the patient initiates another 8 breaths per minute, the V_T for each additional breath will depend on how strong the effort is and will vary, though it will be some value greater than 6 L per minute. The spontaneous breaths created by the patient can be unsupported or pressure supported (see below). IMV can also be synchronized according to the patient's inspiratory efforts, called *Synchronized IMV.*

ADDITIONAL MODES OF VENTILATORY SUPPORT

Pressure support ventilation (PSV) differs from the other modes of mechanical ventilation discussed above, in that it is a flow-cycled mode and is intended to support spontaneous respiratory efforts. The ventilator delivers inspiratory pressure until the inspiratory flow decreases to a predetermined percentage of its peak value (usually 25%). In this mode, the physician sets the pressure support level, PEEP, and FiO_2. The patient must trigger each breath because there is no set respiratory rate. Work of breathing is inversely proportional to pressure support level and inspiratory flow rate. V_T is, therefore, determined by a combination of PSV settings, the patient's effort, and underlying pulmonary mechanics. An adequate MV_E cannot be guaranteed and it is thus not recommended for use in patients who are heavily sedated, paralyzed, or who cannot generate spontaneous efforts. In addition, PSV is poorly suited to provide full or near-full ventilatory support.

CPAP is a mode of support that is also applied to spontaneously breathing patients. During the respiratory cycle, a constant pressure is applied to the airway throughout inspiration *and* expiration. The ventilator does not cycle during CPAP, and all breaths must be initiated by the patient. CPAP is commonly combined with PSV or may be used alone in patients weaning from mechanical ventilation to prevent small airways collapse and atelectasis, and functionally is similar to PEEP.

Airway pressure release ventilation (APRV), biphasic airway pressure ventilation (Bi-Vent) and high-frequency ventilation (HFV) are more complicated modes of ventilation that are mainly used for patients with acute respiratory distress syndrome (ARDS) and are beyond the scope of this discussion.

ENDOTRACHEAL INTUBATION

Endotracheal intubation should only be performed by an experienced clinician or anesthesiologist. Patients are often intubated using an induction agent (i.e., propofol, thiopental, or etomidate) and in some instances undergo rapid sequence intubation with the addition of neuromuscular blocking agents. The most commonly used neuromuscular blocking agent, succinylcholine, may cause a sudden release of potassium into the bloodstream and should be avoided in patients with renal failure or hyperkalemia as it may lead to sudden cardiac arrest. Induction agents have a common problem of causing peripheral vasodilation. This effect may become even more pronounced if there is significant dehydration, hypovolemia, or underlying acidosis present. Critically ill patients in a state of compensated shock maintain their circulation by vasoconstriction and tachycardia. The use of a vasodilating induction agent can blunt this response and reduce systemic blood pressure by reducing peripheral vascular resistance.

When positive pressure is applied to the airway, intrathoracic pressure increases and venous return to the heart decreases causing reductions in ventricular filling pressures, stroke volume, and cardiac output. The effects of initiating Positive-pressure ventilation (PPV) on blood pressure and cardiac output can usually be treated with the administration of saline boluses. Intravenous

fluid preparations should always be prepared for the intubation process in the anticipation of such adverse effects. If the effects of vasodilation caused by induction agents cannot be reversed with saline infusion, the temporary use of vasoconstrictor agents (i.e., phenylephrine, norepinephrine, or dopamine) may be required. More details regarding systemic hemodynamic and cardiovascular effects of PPV will be discussed later.

Some of the other complications that may arise during Endotracheal Tube (ETT) placement include nasal trauma, tooth avulsion, or oral and pharyngeal laceration. Injuries occurring to the larynx (i.e., glottic contusion and vocal cord laceration) and trachea (i.e., tracheal laceration, perforation, and rupture) may also occur but are extremely uncommon. Aspiration of gastric contents during intubation can take place.

Once the ETT is advanced through the vocal cords, the tube is secured and the cuff is inflated. Placement is clinically confirmed by the symmetric rise and fall of the chest wall, the presence of bilateral breath sounds, and end-tidal carbon dioxide measurement during manual bag ventilation. If placement is adequate and oxygen saturation is sufficient, the patient can then be attached to the mechanical ventilator. ETT cuff inflation pressure should not exceed more than 30 cm water to avoid complications such as tracheal rupture, pressure necrosis, or tracheo-innominate artery erosion and fistula. A chest radiograph should be obtained in order to ensure ideal location of the tip of the ETT which should be between 3 and 5 cm above the carina.

PHYSIOLOGIC AND PATHOPHYSIOLOGIC CONSEQUENCES OF PPV

SYSTEMIC HEMODYNAMIC AND CARDIOVASCULAR EFFECTS OF PPV

PPV results in an increased mean intrathoracic pressure; the clinical effect on cardiac output is variable and depends on the patient's intravascular volume status/ventricular filling pressures, underlying left ventricular compliance, and ejection fraction. The extent to which the hemodynamic effects occur also varies according to chest wall and lung compliance. Transmission of airway pressure is greatest when there is low chest wall compliance (e.g., fibrothorax) or high lung compliance (e.g., emphysema). Transmission of airway pressure is lowest when there is high chest wall compliance (e.g., sternotomy) or low lung compliance (e.g., ARDS and congestive heart failure).

Increases in intrathoracic pressure can decrease venous return to the right heart. The amount of venous return is determined by the pressure gradient from the extrathoracic veins to the right atrium. The intrathoracic and right atrial pressures increase during positive-pressure ventilation, which reduces the gradient for venous return. This effect may be overexaggerated by increases in PEEP or in those with intravascular volume depletion. Right ventricular output can also be reduced by increased alveolar inflation and compression of the pulmonary vascular bed, resulting in increased pulmonary artery pressures and pulmonary vascular resistance. In addition, left ventricular output may be compromised from shifting of the interventricular septum toward the left ventricle leading to impaired diastolic filling.[35–37]

In contrast to the above adverse effects, positive-pressure ventilation can be beneficial in patients with left ventricular failure and pulmonary edema. Transmyocardial pressures can be reduced by increases in intrathoracic pressure, resulting in a decreased left ventricular afterload and overall improved left ventricular performance. This effect is most likely to be seen when filling pressures are high and ventricular performance is poor. These systemic hemodynamic and cardiovascular effects of PPV can be seen with both noninvasive and invasive PPV, although more evident with the latter.

Positive-pressure ventilation can also affect hemodynamic measurements. This is most pronounced when PEEP is applied, because most hemodynamic measurements are performed at the end of expiration when PEEP is the primary source of positive airway pressure. The pulmonary capillary wedge pressure (PCWP) value may be falsely elevated in patients receiving PPV and not reflective of the true transmural filling pressure of the left ventricle. The true filling pressure can be estimated by subtracting one-half of the PEEP level from the PCWP if lung compliance is normal. If lung compliance is reduced, it can be estimated by subtracting one-quarter of the PEEP from PCWP.[38]

PULMONARY EFFECTS OF PPV

Interpreting the relationship of resistance, lung compliance, and work of breathing is essential for appropriate ventilator management. Measurements of pressure, airflow, and volume can reveal basic physiologic properties of the respiratory system (Figure 27.2).

Peak inspiratory pressure (PIP) is the maximal airway pressure recorded in the patient–ventilator circuit. It represents the total pressure needed to overcome resistance related to the ventilator tubing, ETT, and patient airways in addition to the elastic recoil of the lungs and chest wall. In a relaxed patient without any airway obstruction or resistance from tubing, PIP may represent alveolar pressure. However, if small-bore ETTs are used, if secretions are present in the tubing or airways, or if there is significant airway obstruction or bronchospasm, PIP may not represent alveolar pressures but may be much higher (Table 27.5).

The end-inspiratory pressure is measured by applying an inspiratory pause at the end of passive inflation; this will result in an immediate drop in airway opening pressure to a lower initial value, followed by a gradual decrement until a *plateau airway pressure* is reached. Since plateau pressure is measured when there is no airflow, it reflects the static compliance of the respiratory

TABLE 27.5	Causes of Respiratory Distress in the Patient on Mechanical Ventilation

Ventilator issues
- Inadequate MV_E (V_T or respiratory rate), FiO_2, inspiratory flow rate, PEEP, or trigger sensitivity
- Ventilator circuit leak
- Ventilator malfunction

Increased PIPs with unchanged plateau pressures
- ETT problems
  - Examples: patient biting, increased resistance in tubes by heat and moisture exchange, obstruction by secretions, blood, or foreign object
- Bronchospasm (asthma or COPD)
- Obstruction of lower airways (secretions, blood, or foreign object)
- Aspiration of oropharyngeal or gastric contents

Increased PIPs with increased plateau pressures
- Pneumonia
- Atelectasis
- ARDS and pulmonary edema
- Migration of ETT into a mainstem bronchus
- Pneumothorax
- Abdominal distension

Extrapulmonary issues
- Delirium, anxiety, or pain
- Acute neurologic event
- Sepsis

system. Increases in plateau pressures can be seen in patients with decreased lung compliance (i.e., ARDS, congestive heart failure, multilobar pneumonia, and severe atelectasis) or decreased chest wall compliance (i.e., morbid obesity, kyphoscoliosis, abdominal distension, tension pneumothorax) (Table 27.5).

Normally, a transpulmonary pressure of 35 cm water would inflate the lungs to almost total lung capacity. In patients with ALI or pulmonary edema, total lung capacity may be reduced because of alveolar collapse. Therefore, V_T delivered with each assisted breath may result in heterogeneous ventilation and overdistention of the more compliant regions of the lungs, and subsequent increased plateau/alveolar pressures. This may cause *volutrauma* to the alveoli or cyclic atelectasis as a result of

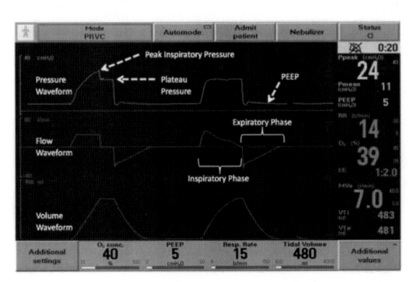

Figure 27.2. Waveform and pressure analysis on the invasive mechanical ventilator (Maquet Servo-*i*).

the shear mechanical forces applied to the alveoli as they are repeatedly opened and closed. This damage is termed ventilator-associated lung injury (VALI) and is often indistinguishable from other causes of ALI clinically and radiographically. Primary interventions to reduce this injury include preventing alveolar overdistension through the use of smaller V_T (6 ml per kilogram of ideal body weight) and keeping plateau pressures to a goal of less than 30 cm water.[39]

Pneumothorax, subcutaneous emphysema, pneumomediastinum, and other forms of extraalveolar air are generally referred to as *barotrauma*. Barotrauma is usually the result of disruption of the pulmonary parenchyma and alveolar rupture from elevated airway pressures or volumes. Lower plateau airway pressures have been associated with a lower incidence of pulmonary barotrauma.[40]

Extrinsic PEEP is generally added to prevent alveolar collapse, and increasing levels may be required depending on the clinical situation. In the setting of respiratory failure from ARDS or congestive heart failure, decreased lung compliance may lead to significant alveolar collapse and refractory hypoxemia caused by increased shunt fraction. In these settings, extrinsic PEEP has been used as an adjunctive treatment to prevent alveolar collapse, recruit alveoli, and improve oxygenation.

Intrinsic PEEP (*PEEP$_i$*, *auto-PEEP*, or *breath stacking*) is present when alveolar pressure exceeds atmospheric pressure at the end of expiration in the absence of a set ventilator PEEP level. When inspiration is initiated before expiratory flow from the preceding breath has ceased, air trapping will occur. Auto-PEEP can develop for numerous reasons including high minute volume (due to high V_T, respiratory rate, or high trigger sensitivity), prolonged inspiratory times (leading to obligatory decrease in expiratory time), and expiratory flow resistance or limitations (due to small-bore ETT, ventilator tubing, or obstructive airways disease). Auto-PEEP can be identified by performing an end-expiratory breath hold while measuring airway pressure. It can also be identified by examining flow and pressure waveforms on the ventilator or by auscultation, which will show continued expiratory airflow from the previous breath when the next breath is triggered. Consequentially, it may potentiate the aforementioned hemodynamic effects of PPV by further increasing intrathoracic pressure.[35] Auto-PEEP will also increase the risk of pulmonary barotrauma and the work of breathing by making it more difficult for the patient to trigger a ventilator assisted breath.[41] Similar effects can also be seen with the addition of extrinsic PEEP. Treatment for auto-PEEP involves adjusting ventilator settings (decreasing inspiratory time, increasing inspiratory flow rate, decreased V_T, decreasing respiratory rate, decreasing trigger sensitivity), maintaining adequate anxiolysis and analgesia to reduce ventilatory demand, and reducing expiratory flow resistance (suctioning, bronchodilators, or changing to a larger diameter ETT).

Although supplemental oxygen is valuable in many clinical situations, inappropriate or excessive therapy can be detrimental. The effects of normobaric hyperoxia on the respiratory system have been extensively studied, showing effects ranging from mild tracheobronchitis to diffuse alveolar damage or ARDS. Hyperoxia appears to produce cellular injury through increased production of reactive oxygen species, which can ultimately result in cell death. In addition, a deleterious inflammatory response may be promoted leading to cellular apoptosis and lung parenchymal and airway injury.[42,43] It is still unclear at what level oxygen

becomes toxic, particularly in critically ill patients. In general, attempts are made to decrease the FiO_2 to less than 60% to a goal PaO_2 of 60 to 65 mm Hg or SpO_2 greater than or equal to 90% as soon as patients are able to tolerate it. Optimal selection of PEEP may also help to decrease oxygen requirements.

INITIAL SETTINGS FOR THE MECHANICAL VENTILATOR

This section will cover the basic initial settings for the volume-controlled AC mode. The settings that need to be considered with this mode include the trigger, V_T, respiratory rate, extrinsic PEEP, and FiO_2.

In the AC mode of ventilation, the physician determines the minimum MV_E required. This is done by setting the V_T and respiratory rate. The appropriate V_T depends on numerous factors, most importantly the disease for which the patient requires mechanical ventilation. In the past, larger V_T (up to 10 to 15 mL per kilogram) was traditionally used to ventilate patients. However, because of complications such as alveolar overdistension, alveolar fracture, and VALI, it is reasonable to use V_T of 8 mL per kilogram ideal body weight in patients that are being ventilated for reasons other than ALI/ARDS.[44,45]

When setting the respiratory rate, it is important to take into account the patient's spontaneous rate and the anticipated ventilatory requirements. For most patients, an initial rate of 12 breaths per minute is reasonable. Higher rates may be required, for example, in patients with severe underlying acidosis or patients being ventilated for ARDS.

A typical initial PEEP of 5 cm of water is often applied to prevent atelectasis. Higher levels of PEEP may be required to recruit alveoli and improve gas exchange; however, attention must be paid to airway pressures to avoid complications of alveolar overdistension. More details concerning specific disease-oriented strategies and the use of PEEP in congestive heart failure and ARDS will be discussed later.

The lowest possible FiO_2 necessary to meet oxygenation goals should be used. Immediately following intubation and the initiation of mechanical ventilation, the FiO_2 should be set to 100%. Arterial blood gas analysis should then be performed after 1 hour to ensure adequate oxygenation. FiO_2 should then be rapidly titrated down (by 10% to 20% every 30 minutes) to a goal PaO_2 of 60 mm Hg or SpO_2 greater than or equal to 90% to avoid complications of high inspired oxygen concentration. V_T or respiratory rate can also be incrementally increased or decreased to alter MV_E and achieve the optimal arterial pH and $PaCO_2$ while monitoring auto-PEEP and airway pressures.

Since volume-controlled AC ventilation provides a fully supported V_T if the patient provides an adequate respiratory effort, the ventilator trigger must also be set. Pressure triggering will deliver a supported breath if the demand valve senses a negative airway pressure deflection greater than the trigger sensitivity. This is usually set to 1-to -3 cm of water. If a flow trigger is used, values of 1 to 3 L per minute are usually adequate.

MONITORING PATIENTS ON INVASIVE MECHANICAL VENTILATION

Patient–ventilator asynchrony is commonly manifested as respiratory distress with "bucking" or "fighting" the ventilator. This happens when the phases of the breath delivered by the ventilator do not match that of the patient. Clinical signs include anxiety, agitation, tachypnea, tachycardia, use of accessory muscles of respiration, and uncoordinated thoracic wall and abdominal movements. Asynchrony can lead to dyspnea and increased work of breathing, and may prolong the duration of mechanical ventilation.[46,47] Bedside observation and examination of ventilator waveforms can help detect the presence and identify the cause of asynchronous ventilation.

Asynchrony or respiratory distress may signify a life-threatening complication, and so rapid assessment is required. In addition to clinical examination, the clinician must monitor ventilator parameters such as V_T, respiratory rate, PIP, plateau airway pressure, and auto-PEEP values. It should be noted that patient–ventilator asynchrony need not be present for possible pulmonary complications associated with mechanical ventilation to arise. In addition, extrapulmonary processes such as fever, pain, delirium, and anxiety may also increase respiratory drive and lead to patient–ventilator asynchrony. Figure 27.3 offers an algorithmic approach to the mechanically ventilated patient in respiratory distress.

Chest radiographs should be followed daily to ensure proper positioning of the ETT (optimal 3 to 5 cm above the carina), as cephalad or caudad migration is very common. Daily radiographs will also allow a more objective assessment of the patient's underlying pathologic process and the development of pneumonia or barotrauma.

Arterial blood gas analysis is usually performed on a daily basis to ensure adequate acid–base balance and oxygenation but is required more frequently if severe hypoxemia or acidosis is present. Acid–base disturbances may require adjustments of MV_E, as they can lead to significant and potentially life-threatening cellular dysfunction or hemodynamic consequences. FiO_2 will be adjusted to ensure adequate oxygenation and avoid potential oxygen toxicity.

Of special importance is the interpretation of arterial blood gases in patients undergoing therapeutic hypothermia after cardiac arrest. The solubility of oxygen and carbon dioxide in the blood increases as temperature decreases. Hypothermia will cause the oxyhemoglobin dissociation curve to shift to the left, that is, oxygen saturation is achieved at lower partial pressures of oxygen. Moreover, carbon dioxide tension is decreased because of a reduced metabolic rate, causing the pH to be higher.[48] Laboratory analysis of arterial blood gases are performed by two different methods. The more common alpha-stat method measures blood gases without temperature correction, whereas the pH-stat method corrects for temperature. If the institution's laboratory uses the alpha-stat method to measure oxygen and carbon dioxide tension in the blood, the reported values may be falsely increased and ventilator settings may be incorrectly adjusted. This can cause an accidental hyperventilation that can lead to cerebral vasoconstriction and further ischemia. For this reason, blood gases should be corrected according to the following equation: for every 1°C below 37°C, the PaO_2 should be subtracted by 5 mm Hg, the $PaCO_2$ should be subtracted by 2 mm Hg, and 0.12 should be added to the pH.[48] Therefore, for patients undergoing therapeutic hypothermia at 33° C, the temperature-corrected PaO_2 would be 20 mm Hg lower whereas the $PaCO_2$ would be 8 mm Hg lower than laboratory reports.

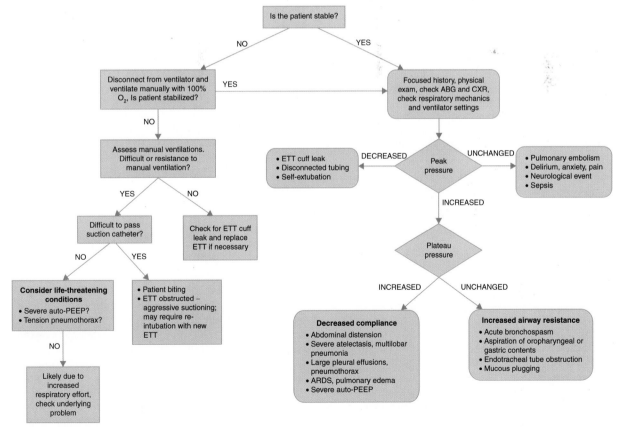

Figure 27.3. Approach to the ventilated patient in respiratory distress.

DISEASE-ORIENTED STRATEGIES— ARDS AND CARDIOGENIC PULMONARY EDEMA

In principle, the ventilatory management of patients with cardiogenic shock and pulmonary edema is similar to that of patients with noncardiogenic pulmonary edema (ARDS). Many of the recommendations regarding ventilatory strategies for these groups of patients are based on avoiding the pulmonary complications of alveolar overdistension and barotrauma. These strategies are called *lung protective strategies*. Because of the overwhelming evidence that inflating the lungs to almost or above total lung capacity can damage normal lung units in patients with ARDS and worsen mortality, the current recommendations are to set the V_T to 6 mL per kilogram of ideal body weight to target plateau airway pressures below 30 cm water.[39,44,45]

PEEP is applied to raise lung volume by the recruitment of collapsed and flooded alveoli, to prevent cell abrasion in the small conducting airways, and to improve oxygenation.[49,50] PEEP is most useful in the treatment of patients with pulmonary edema resulting from increased alveolo-capillary membrane permeability (ARDS) or increased hydrostatic pressure (cardiogenic pulmonary edema).[51] It increases PaO_2 by diminishing intrapulmonary shunting of blood and improving ventilation–perfusion mismatching, and it may also redistribute intraalveolar edema. In conjunction with the lung protective strategies mentioned above, an *open lung approach* using higher levels of PEEP and lower amounts of FiO_2 in patients with ARDS showed improved survival; however, it was unclear whether the benefit seen was because of lower V_T or higher PEEP.[52] A subsequent landmark trial tested lower V_T with higher PEEP and found no further improvement in survival with higher PEEP.[53] In the absence of data proving superiority of lower or higher PEEP, the physician may choose to use lower PEEP to avoid VALI in patients who demonstrate high airway pressures or signs of overt barotrauma. On the contrary, clinicians may use higher PEEP if patients do not have these limiting factors, and oxygenation and lung compliance improve when higher levels of PEEP are applied. If high PEEP is used, careful monitoring of airway pressures and hemodynamic parameters is required. PEEP above 20 cm water should not be used because it is almost impossible to deliver sufficient alveolar ventilation at such high levels.

Since low V_T is recommended as part of ventilatory strategy in pulmonary edema, higher respiratory rates will be required to overcome the resulting hypoventilation and hypercapnia. Typically, the respiratory rate should be set to 20 to 30 breaths per minute.

Once sufficient oxygenation goals have been met, FiO_2 should be titrated down as tolerated to a goal PaO_2 60 to 65 mm Hg or SpO_2 greater than or equal to 90%. If the patient is tolerating an FiO_2 of 60% or less, PEEP should then be slowly titrated down by decrements of 2 to 3 cm water with similar oxygen goals in mind.

SEDATION IN THE MECHANICALLY VENTILATED PATIENT

A majority of patients who are being mechanically ventilated will require sedation and/or analgesia in order to facilitate ventilator synchrony, and alleviate pain and discomfort from critical care procedures and treatments. A number of different agents can be used alone or in combination to achieve consistent sedation, anxiolysis, and analgesia. Common medication classes include benzodiazepines, opioid analgesics, and neuroleptic agents. A neuroleptic agent may be used if medication for delirium is indicated. Each class differs in the amount of anxiolysis, analgesia, amnesia, and hypnosis provided. Elimination of half-life, volume of distribution, and drug clearance may be significantly altered in critically ill patients. No single agent is sufficiently superior to other agents to recommend its standard use in all patients. Selection must, therefore, be individualized according to the patient's distress, physiologic parameters, expected duration of therapy, and potential interactions with other medications. Careful attention should also be paid to the possible development of adverse reactions. Brief descriptions regarding drug classes, effects, and pharmacokinetics are presented in Table 27.6.

A goal depth of sedation should be determined prior to initiating sedative-analgesic regimens and the goal should be individualized according to the clinical situation. Patients expected to have a shorter duration of mechanical ventilation may require lighter sedation or no sedation at all. However, patients who are being mechanically ventilated for severe hypoxemia or ARDS may require deeper sedation. The goal depth of sedation should be frequently assessed and titrated using validated and reliable scales for mechanically ventilated patients as sedation requirements change (e.g., Richmond Agitation-Sedation Scale).[54] Evidence indicates that continuous infusions of sedative-analgesic medications prolong the duration of mechanical ventilation.[55] The most recent clinical practice guidelines suggest the initial use of intermittent boluses, with the initiation of continuous infusions with daily interruptions in patients who require intermittent boluses more often than every 2 hours.[56]

SPECIAL CONSIDERATIONS DURING MECHANICAL VENTILATION

Invasive mechanical ventilation for more than 48 hours is a risk factor for clinically important upper gastrointestinal hemorrhage caused by stress ulceration.[57] Patients are also at risk if they have a previous history of upper gastrointestinal hemorrhage or bleeding diathesis. Clinical trials have demonstrated that histamine-2 receptor antagonists, proton pump inhibitors, and antacids reduce the frequency of overt upper gastrointestinal hemorrhage in ICU patients when compared to no prophylaxis.[58] The current recommendation is to administer an oral proton pump inhibitor for patients who are able to receive enteral medications, or an intravenous H_2 blocker for those that cannot receive enteral medications.

Ventilator-associated pneumonia (VAP) refers to pneumonia that develops at least 48 hours after the initiation of mechanical ventilation. VAP is estimated to affect 30% of all patients receiving mechanical ventilation and carries a mortality rate of 25% to 50%.[59,60] The most likely cause of VAP is aerodigestive tract colonization, followed by aspiration of contaminated secretions into the lower airways. VAP should be considered in patients that develop new or increased fevers, new alveolar infiltrates on chest radiograph, respiratory secretions, leukocytosis, or respiratory abnormalities on examination coupled with increased ventilator demands. Proper specimens should be

TABLE 27.6	Characteristics of Sedative Medications Commonly Used in the ICU Setting			
Drug	Onset	Duration	Effects	
Opioids				
• Morphine	5–10 min	4 h	Potent sedative/analgesic effects, without causing anxiolysis, hypnosis, or amnesia	
• Fentanyl	<0.5 min	30–60 min		
Benzodiazepines				
• Lorazepam	5–20 min	6–8 h	Sedative anxiolytic, hypnotic, and amnestic effects without analgesic effects; diazepam also used as skeletal muscle relaxant	
• Midazolam	1–5 min	30 min		
• Diazepam	1 min	20–60 min		
Neuroleptic				
• Haloperidol	30–60 min	0.5–6 h	Potent sedative anxiolytic with minimal hypnotic and amnesic effects; no analgesia provided	
Anesthetic-sedative				
• Propofol	<1 min	3–10 min	Potent sedative hypnotic, with minimal amnesic effects; anxiolysis seen at low doses; no analgesia provided	
Central α_2 agonist				
• Dexmedetomidine	5–10 min	1–2 h	Sedative sympatholytic with moderate anxiolysis and analgesia; no hypnosis or amnesia; no significant effect on respiratory drive	

collected prior to beginning empiric antibiotic coverage. Steps to reduce the risk and prevent development of VAP should be employed routinely in mechanically ventilated patients. These include semirecumbent positioning, subglottic drainage techniques, and compliance with strict hand washing and other infection control protocols.

WEANING AND EXTUBATION

Weaning patients from mechanical ventilation remains one of the most challenging aspects of intensive care medicine. In general, the approach taken should be a two-step process.

Readiness testing refers to the use of objective clinical criteria to determine whether a patient is ready to begin weaning. The reason for the patient's respiratory failure should have been identified and the patient should have shown a favorable response to the treatment. Chest radiograph should demonstrate improvement in pulmonary edema. Oxygenation should be satisfactory: arterial blood gas analysis showing PaO_2/FiO_2 ratio greater than 200 or SpO_2 greater than or equal to 90% while receiving less than or equal to 50% FiO_2 and PEEP less than or equal to 5 cm water. Patients should be hemodynamically stable with minimal or no need for vasopressor support, and without the presence of myocardial ischemia or unstable cardiac arrhythmias. The absence of sepsis or hyperthermia should be confirmed, as these may lead to an increased respiratory drive and subsequent failure if the patient is extubated. Sedative drugs and neuromuscular blocking agents should be discontinued, and the patient should be awake and alert, or easily arousable, and be able to manage secretions. In addition, significant fluid, electrolyte, and metabolic disorders should be corrected before weaning attempts.

Since predicting readiness to wean on the basis of clinical criteria can sometimes be inaccurate, physiologic tests can be used to refine predictions of weaning success. One such popular predictor, the rapid shallow breathing index (RSBI), is the ratio of respiratory frequency to V_T. Values over 105 breaths/minute/L predict weaning failure but fare no better than other parameters.[61,62] Other physiologic predictors such as MV_E, maximal inspiratory pressure, respiratory system compliance, and oxygen cost of breathing have been studied, but none appear to be superior to objective clinical criteria in predicting a patient's readiness to wean (Table 27.7).

Common methods of weaning include T-piece trials, IMV, and PSV. A T-piece trial involves removing the ventilator with the ETT in situ connected to oxygen and monitoring spontaneous respirations. Studies of efficacy and superiority have been conflicting.[63,64] In addition, once daily spontaneous breathing trials compared to more frequent daily trials did not result in quicker extubation. We prefer using the PSV approach over T-piece since PSV provides reassurance of ventilator alarm features and backup ventilatory assistance in case of apnea, extreme tachypnea, or inadequate MV_E. In addition, PSV overcomes the increased work of breathing from resistance of the ETT that may be seen with T-piece trials. A successful weaning trial meets the criteria outlined in Table 27.7. If the patient meets all of the weaning criteria, the patient may be extubated. If the patient fails to meet all of the criteria, ventilatory support should be resumed and another weaning trial should be attempted the following day. In the case

TABLE 27.7	Criteria for a Successful Weaning Trial

- Pressure support ≤8 cm water (ideally <5 cm water)
- PEEP ≤5 cm water
- SpO_2 >92% while breathing ≤50% FiO_2
- Respiratory rate <35 breaths/min
- Heart rate <140 beats/min
- Systolic blood pressure <180 mm Hg but >90 mm Hg
- No diaphoresis or signs of respiratory fatigue
- Tolerated for at least 30 min–2 h

of cardiogenic pulmonary edema, the administration of diuretics prior to extubation may be beneficial even if the patient is not in overt heart failure, as the cardiovascular effects of PPV discussed earlier will be reversed once positive pressure is removed.

In preparation for extubation, the patient should be placed in the upright position with suctioning of both the oropharynx and ETT performed. The ETT cuff is then deflated as the patient is exhaling and the ETT is removed. Immediately after removal, any secretions that are coughed up and present in the oropharynx should be promptly suctioned and supplemental oxygen via a simple face mask should be provided. Physical examination including auscultation of the lungs to confirm bilateral air entry and the upper airway to exclude the presence of inspiratory stridor and laryngeal edema should be performed.

Respiratory distress following extubation may be caused by airways disease, recurrent pulmonary edema, secretions, or laryngeal edema. In many cases, early and aggressive management with suctioning, bronchodilator therapy, diuresis, or NIV can prevent reintubation. If laryngeal edema is present, the administration of intravenous glucocorticoids and inhaled racemic epinephrine may lessen the need for reintubation. In patients with respiratory distress following extubation, NIV may prevent reintubation if applied early.[65–68] If the patient fails a trial of NIV or meets any of the contraindications to the use of NIV discussed earlier in this chapter, he should be promptly reintubated followed by a thorough evaluation and treatment of the cause of the postextubation respiratory failure.

REFERENCES

1. Cohen CA, Zagelbaum G, Gross D, et al. Clinical manifestations of inspiratory muscle fatigue. *Am J Med.* 1982;73:308–316.
2. Gil A, Carrizosa F, Herrero A, et al. Influence of mechanical ventilation on blood lactate in patients with acute respiratory failure. *Intensive Care Med.* 1998;24:924–930.
3. Squadrone E, Frigerio P, Fogliati C, et al. Noninvasive vs. invasive ventilation in COPD patients with severe acute respiratory failure deemed to require ventilatory assistance. *Intensive Care Med.* 2004;30:1303–1310.
4. Paus-Jenssen ES, Reid JK, Cockroft DW, et al. The use of noninvasive ventilation in acute respiratory failure at a tertiary care center. *Chest.* 2004;126:165–172.
5. Navalesi P, Fanfulla F, Frigerio P, et al. Physiologic evaluation of noninvasive mechanical ventilation delivered with three types of masks in patients with chronic hypercapnic respiratory failure. *Crit Care Med.* 2000;28:1785–1790.
6. Girault C, Briel A, Benichou J, et al. Interface strategy during noninvasive positive pressure ventilation for hypercapnic acute respiratory failure. *Crit Care Med.* 2009;37:124–131.
7. Soo Hoo GW, Santiago S, Williams AJ. Nasal mechanical ventilation for hypercapnic respiratory failure in chronic obstructive pulmonary disease: determinants of success or failure. *Crit Care Med.* 1994;22:1253–1261.
8. Liesching T, Kwok H, Hill NS. Acute applications of noninvasive positive pressure ventilation. *Chest.* 2003;124:699–713.
9. Hess, D. Noninvasive positive pressure ventilation: predictors of success and failure for adult acute care applications. *Respir Care.* 1997;42:424–431.
10. Brochard L, Isabey D, Piquet J, et al. Reversal of acute exacerbations of chronic obstructive lung disease by inspiratory assistance with a facemask. *N Engl J Med.* 1990;323:1523–1530.
11. Meduri GU, Conoscenti CC, Menashe P, et al. Noninvasive facemask ventilation in patients with acute respiratory failure. *Chest.* 1989;95:865.
12. Elliot MW, Steven MH, Phillip GD, et al. Noninvasive mechanical ventilation for acute respiratory failure. *Br Med J.* 1990;300:358–360.
13. Pennock BE, Kaplan PD, Carlin BW, et al. Pressure support ventilation with a simplified ventilatory support system administered with a nasal mask in patients with respiratory failure. *Chest.* 1991;100:1371–1376.
14. Meduri, GU, Abou-Shala N, Fox RC, et al. Noninvasive face mask mechanical ventilation in patients with acute hypercapnic respiratory failure. *Chest.* 1991;100:445–454.
15. Katz JA, Marks JD. Inspiratory work with and without continuous positive airway pressure in patients with acute respiratory failure. *Anesthesiology.* 1985;63:598–607.
16. Bradley TD, Holloway RM, McLaughlin RP, et al. Cardiac output response to continuous positive airway pressure in congestive heart failure. *Am Rev Respir Dis.* 1992;145:377–382.
17. Baratz DM, Westbrook PR, Shah PK, et al. Effect of nasal continuous positive airway pressure on cardiac output and oxygen delivery in patients with congestive heart failure. *Chest.* 1992;102:1397–1401.
18. Rasanen J, Heikkila J, Downs J, et al. Continuous positive airway pressure by face mask in acute cardiogenic pulmonary edema. *Am J Cardiol.* 1985;55:296–300.
19. Lin M, Chiang HT. The efficacy of early continuous positive airway pressure therapy in patients with acute cardiogenic pulmonary edema. *J Formos Med Assoc.* 1991;90:736–743.
20. Bersten AD, Holt AW, Vedig AE, et al. Treatment of severe cardiogenic pulmonary edema with continuous positive airway pressure delivered by face mask. *N Engl J Med.* 1991;325:1825–1830.
21. Lin M, Chiang HT, Chang MS, et al. Reappraisal of continuous positive airway pressure therapy in acute cardiogenic pulmonary edema: short term results and long-term follow up. *Chest.* 1995;107:1379–1386.
22. Meduri GU, Turner RE, Abou-Shala N, et al. Noninvasive positive pressure ventilation via face mask: first-line intervention in patients with acute hypercapnic and hypoxemic respiratory failure. *Chest.* 1996;109:179–193.
23. Meduri GU, Conoscenti CC, Menashe P, et al. Noninvasive face mask ventilation in patients with acute respiratory failure. *Chest.* 1989;95:865–870.
24. Lapinsky SE, Mount DB, Mackey D, et al. Management of acute respiratory failure due to pulmonary edema with nasal positive pressure support. *Chest.* 1994;105:229–231.
25. Hoffman B, Welte T. The use of noninvasive pressure support ventilation for severe respiratory insufficiency due to pulmonary oedema. *Intensive Care Med.* 1999;25:15–20.
26. Rusterholtz T, Kempf J, Berton C, et al. Noninvasive pressure support ventilation (NIPSV) with face mask in patients with acute cardiogenic pulmonary edema (ACPE). *Intensive Care Med.* 1999;25:21–28.
27. Masip J, Betbesé AJ, Páez J, et al. Non-invasive pressure support ventilation versus conventional oxygen therapy in acute cardiogenic pulmonary oedema: a randomised trial. *Lancet.* 2000;356:2126–2132.
28. Mehta S, Jay GD, Woolard RH, et al. Randomized, prospective trial of bilevel versus continuous positive airway pressure in acute pulmonary edema. *Crit Care Med.* 1997;25:620–628.
29. Nava S, Carbone G, Dibatista N, et al. Noninvasive ventilation in cardiogenic pulmonary edema. *Am J Respir Crit Care Med.* 2003;168:1432–1437.
30. Gray A, Goodacre S, Newby D, et al. Noninvasive ventilation in acute cardiogenic pulmonary edema. *N Engl J Med.* 2008;359:142–151.
31. Rappaport SH, Shpiner R, Yoshihara G, et al. Randomized, prospective trial of pressure-limited versus volume-controlled ventilation in severe respiratory failure. *Crit Care Med.* 1994;22:22–32.
32. Prella, M, Feihl F, Domenighetti G. Effects of short term pressure-controlled ventilation on gas exchange, airway pressures, and gas distribution in patients with acute lung injury/ARDS: comparison with volume-controlled ventilation. *Chest.* 2002;122:1382–1388.
33. Chiumello D, Pelosi P, Calvi E, et al. Different modes of assisted ventilation in patients with acute respiratory failure. *Eur Respir J.* 2002;20:925–933.
34. Irwin RS, Rippe JM. Mechanical ventilation part I: invasive. In: *Irwin and Rippe's Intensive Care Medicine.* 6th ed. Philadelphia, PA: Lippincott Williams and Wilkins; 2008:643–659.
35. Pinksy MR. Cardiovascular issues in respiratory care. *Chest.* 2005;128:592S–597S.
36. Qvist J, Pontoppidan H, Wilson RS, et al. Hemodynamic responses to mechanical ventilation with PEEP: the effect of hypovolemia. *Anesthesiology.* 1975;42:45–55.
37. Fougères E, Teboul JL, Richard C, et al. Hemodynamic impact of positive end-expiratory pressure setting in acute respiratory distress syndrome: importance of volume status. *Crit Care Med.* 2010;38:802–807.
38. Marini JJ, O'Quin R, Culver BH, et al. Estimation of transmural cardiac pressures during ventilation with PEEP. *J Appl Physiol.* 1982;53:384–391.
39. The Acute Respiratory Distress Syndrome Network. Ventilation with lower tidal volumes as compared with traditional tidal volumes for acute lung injury and the acute respiratory distress syndrome. *N Engl J Med.* 2000;342:1301–1308.
40. Boussarsar M, Thierry G, Jaber S, et al. Relationship between ventilatory setting and barotrauma in the acute respiratory distress syndrome. *Intensive Care Med.* 2002;28:406–413.
41. Gurevitch MJ, Gelmont D. Importance of trigger sensitivity to ventilator response delay in advanced chronic obstructive pulmonary disease with respiratory failure. *Crit Care Med.* 1989;17:354–359.
42. Barazzone C, Horowitz S, Donati YR, et al. Oxygen toxicity in mouse lung: pathways to cell death. *Am J Respir Cell Mol Biol.* 1998;19:573–581.
43. Mantell LL, Lee PJ. Signal transduction pathways in hyperoxia-induced lung cell death. *Mol Genet Metab.* 2000;71:359–370.
44. Dreyfuss D, Soler P, Basset G, et al. High inflation pressure pulmonary edema. Respective effects of high airway pressure, high tidal volume, and positive end-expiratory pressure. *Am Rev Respir Dis.* 1988;137:1159–1164.
45. International consensus conferences in intensive care medicine: ventilator-associated lung injury in ARDS. Cosponsored by American Thoracic Society, The European Society of Intensive Care Medicine, and The Societe de Reanimation de Langue Francaise, approved by the ATS Board of Directors. *Am J Respir Crit Care Med.* 1999;160:2118–2124.
46. Hansen-Flaschen JH. Dyspnea in the ventilated patient: a call for patient-centered mechanical ventilation. *Respir Care.* 2000;45:1460–1464.
47. Georgopolous D, Prinianakis G, Kondili E. Bedside waveforms interpretation as a tool to identify patient-ventilator asynchronies. *Intensive Care Med.* 2006;32:34–47.
48. Polderman KH. Mechanisms of action, physiological effects, and complications of hypothermia. *Crit Care Med.* 2009;37:S186–S202.
49. Lachmann B. Open up the lung and keep the lung open. *Intensive Care Med.* 1992;18:319–321.
50. Muscedere JG, Mullen JB, Gan K, et al. Tidal ventilation at low airway pressures can augment lung injury. *Am J Respir Crit Care Med.* 1994;149:1327–1334.
51. Barbas, CS, de Matos GF, Pincelli MP, et al. Mechanical ventilation in acute respiratory failure: recruitment and high positive end-expiratory pressure are necessary. *Curr Opin Crit Care.* 2005;11:18–28.
52. Amato MB, Barbas CS, Medeiros DM, et al. Effect of a protective-ventilation strategy on mortality in the acute respiratory distress syndrome. *N Engl J Med.* 1998;338:347–354.
53. The Acute Respiratory Distress Syndrome Network. Higher vs. lower end-expiratory pressure in patients with the acute respiratory distress syndrome. *N Engl J Med.* 2004;351:327–336.
54. Ely EW, Truman B, Shintani A, et al. Monitoring sedation status over time in ICU patients: reliability and validity of the Richmond Agitation-Sedation Scale (RASS). *JAMA.* 2003;289:2983–2991.

55. Kollef MH, Levy NT, Ahrens TS, et al. The use of continuous IV sedation is associated with prolongation of mechanical ventilation. *Chest.* 1998;114:541–548.

56. Jacobi J, Fraser GL, Coursin DB, et al. Clinical practice guidelines for the sustained use of sedatives and analgesics in the critically ill adult. *Crit Care Med.* 2002;30:119–141.

57. Cook DJ, Fuller HD, Guyatt GH, et al. Risk factors for gastrointestinal bleeding in critically ill patients. *N Engl J Med.* 1994;330:377–381.

58. Cook, DJ, Reeve BK, Guyatt GH, et al. Stress ulcer prophylaxis in critically ill patients. Resolving discordant meta-analyses. *JAMA.* 1996;275:308–314.

59. Chastre J, Fagon JY. Ventilator-associated pneumonia. *Am J Resp Crit Care Med.* 2002;165:867–903.

60. Guidelines for the management of adults with hospital acquired, ventilator associated, and health care associated pneumonia. *Am J Resp Crit Care Med.* 2005;171:388–416.

61. Meade M, Guyatt G, Cook D, et al. Predicting success in weaning from mechanical ventilation. *Chest.* 2001;120:400S–424S.

62. Tobin MJ, Jubran A. Variable performance of weaning-predictor tests: role of Bayes' theorem and spectrum and test-referral bias. *Intensive Care Med.* 2006;32:2002–2012.

63. Brochard L, Rauss A, Benito S, et al. Comparison of three methods of gradual withdrawal from ventilatory support during weaning from mechanical ventilation. *Am J Respir Crit Care Med.* 1994;150:896–903.

64. Esteban A, Frutos F, Tobin MJ, et al. A comparison of four methods of weaning patients from mechanical ventilation. Spanish Lung Failure Collaborative Group. *N Engl J Med.* 1995;332:345–350.

65. Nava S, Gregoretti C, Fanfulla F, et al. Noninvasive ventilation to prevent respiratory failure after extubation in high-risk patients. *Crit Care Med.* 2005;33:2465–2470.

66. Ferrer M, Valencia M, Nicolas JM, et al. Early noninvasive ventilation averts extubation failure in patients at risk: a randomized trial. *Am J Respir Crit Care Med.* 2006;173:164–170.

67. Esteban A, Frutos-Vivar F, Ferguson ND, et al. Noninvasive positive-pressure ventilation for respiratory failure after extubation. *N Engl J Med.* 2004;350:2452–2460.

68. Keenan SP, Powers C, McCormack DG, et al. Noninvasive positive-pressure ventilation for postextubation respiratory distress: a randomized controlled trial. *JAMA.* 2002;287:3238–3244.

PATIENT AND FAMILY INFORMATION FOR:
Mechanical Ventilation

A mechanical ventilator is a machine that helps patients breathe when they are not able to breathe enough on their own. It is commonly referred to as a *breathing machine or respirator*. Most patients who require help breathing with mechanical ventilators are cared for in a hospital's ICU or CCU. Many people think of mechanical ventilators as a way to treat breathing-related issues. However, patients are placed on ventilators in order to support their breathing function while giving time for treatments to improve their condition. Being on a respirator means the patient is critically ill—it is life support.

WHY MECHANICAL VENTILATORS ARE USED

Mechanical ventilators help support the patient by pushing breaths with oxygen into the lungs, as well as removing carbon dioxide from the lungs. There are some patients who are in an CCU in whom breathing is difficult—they may feel short of breath and tired from the work that their breathing requires. This is called *respiratory failure* and is often caused by the cardiac disease where poor pumping leads to fluid buildup in the lungs. Some patients also have pneumonia, COPD or asthma, or too much mucus present in the windpipe or airways and these conditions make it even more difficult to breathe. Mechanical ventilators can help ease the work of breathing for these people and prevent their condition from getting worse. If a patient does not get help early enough, the condition can worsen very quickly and ultimately cause the heart and lungs to stop.

Other patients may not be breathing at all because they are in a coma, have brain damage or injury, very weak muscles, or because they suffered a cardiac arrest. In this case, a ventilator must be used to breathe for the patient.

HOW MECHANICAL VENTILATORS WORK

There are two basic types of ventilators that are available. The first is called a *noninvasive ventilator* or *BiPAP machine*. This device pushes air into the lungs through tubing that is connected to the patient by way of a mask, which covers the nose and mouth. It can help improve oxygen levels in the blood and lessen the amount of work that the muscles need to do in order for the patient to breathe. Patients can still speak to their family and friends while on this machine, and they may also be able to eat providing it is safe to do so. This type of ventilator is commonly used in the CCU for patients suffering from shortness of breath caused by heart failure.

For a patient who has started on BiPAP, they have to be monitored very closely. Even with the help of this device, some patients will continue to have a great deal of trouble breathing. If the patient has not improved within a few hours of this device being started, then this machine is not successful and the patient will need a second type of machine, called the *invasive mechanical ventilator*. Moreover, not all patients are good candidates for BiPAP and the doctors may decide that it is more harmful than beneficial to use it.

The invasive mechanical ventilator is connected to the patient through an breathing tube that is placed in the mouth or nose and down into the windpipe. The process of placing the tube into the patient's windpipe is called *intubation*. The device blows air into the lungs and it can help a person by doing all of the breathing for them or just assisting their breaths. The difference between BiPAP and the invasive ventilator is that with the invasive ventilator the doctors have more control over a person's breathing and are able to completely rest the muscles used for breathing.

HOW PATIENTS FEEL WHILE ON INVASIVE MECHANICAL VENTILATORS

The ventilators themselves do not cause pain, but most people who require invasive ventilators do not like the feeling of having a tube in their mouth or nose. They cannot talk because the tube passes through the voice box into the windpipe. They also cannot eat when the tube is in place, and so they need a temporary feeding tube from the mouth to the stomach until the breathing tube is removed. Some people will feel some discomfort as air from the machine is being pushed into the lungs and they will try to breathe out while the machine is trying to push air in. This is called *fighting* against the ventilator and makes it more difficult for the ventilator to help. In addition, people undergo many diagnostic tests and therapies that can cause physical discomfort or pain. For these reasons, patients are often given medications such as sedatives or painkillers to make them feel more comfortable.

HOW PATIENTS ARE MONITORED

Anyone on a ventilator will be hooked up to a monitor that measures heart rate, breathing rate, blood pressure, and oxygen levels at regular intervals. Other tests that may be done routinely include chest X-rays and blood tests that will measure the amount of acid, oxygen, and carbon dioxide in the blood. The doctors, nurses, and respiratory therapists use this information to gauge how well the patient is doing and to see if any adjustments need to be made to the ventilator.

RISKS OF MECHANICAL VENTILATION

Some risks of mechanical ventilation do exist. However, if the doctors feel that the patient needs to be on a ventilator, the benefits of placing the patient on one are always greater than these potential risks.

When a person is first placed on a respirator, they may experience a drop in blood pressure. This can usually be reversed with the use of intravenous fluids, but some patients may temporarily require medications to keep their blood pressure normal.

Sometimes, a part of the lung that is weak can become too inflated with air and start to leak. This leaked air collects in an empty space between the lungs and chest wall. Since there is a limited amount of space in the chest, the leaked air starts to take up more space and the lung begins to collapse. This is called a *pneumothorax*. This air needs to be removed as soon as possible because it can result in life-threatening complications. It is drained by a *chest tube*, which is likely to remain until the patient no longer requires the ventilator.

The pressure used to put air into the lungs can also damage the lungs. Doctors try to keep this risk at a minimum by using the lowest amount of pressure that is needed. In addition, very high levels of oxygen may be harmful to the lungs. Unfortunately, patients who already have damaged lungs may need very high levels of oxygen until the lungs start to heal, which makes it difficult to reduce this risk.

Doctors will only give as much oxygen as it takes to make sure the body is getting enough supply to the vital organs.

As mentioned above, many patients on mechanical ventilation will need some level of sedation. Different patients will react to each medication differently. At times, sedation medications can build up and the patient may remain in a deep sleep for hours or days, even after the medication is stopped. The doctors and nurses try to adjust the medications so that the right amount is being delivered at all times.

The breathing tube can allow bacteria from the mouth to get into the lungs more easily. This can cause an infection such as pneumonia that can be a serious problem and could mean that the patient has to stay on the machine longer. People who are very sick can be more prone to infection than others. All members of the medical staff take maximum precautions to prevent this from happening; however, if an infection occurs, it can be treated with antibiotics.

HOW LONG MECHANICAL VENTILATORS ARE USED

Ventilators can be life saving, but they do not fix the primary disease or injury. Ventilators help support a patient until other treatments become effective. The medical team will always try to help patients get off the ventilator at the earliest possible time but will not do so until there has been improvement or reversal of the problem at hand.

Weaning refers to the process of getting the patient off the ventilator. Depending on the patient, this process may take a few hours up to a few days. Specific criteria are used to decide whether a patient is ready to come off of the respirator including blood oxygen levels, chest X-ray results, and physical examination. Some patients will never improve enough to be taken off the ventilator completely and may require long-term support with their breathing.

Not every patient improves just because they are on a ventilator and patients can die even though they are on a respirator. It is hard to predict or know for sure if a person will recover with treatment. Sometimes, doctors feel very sure the ventilator will help and the patient will recover. Other times, the doctors only have a rough idea of the chances a person will survive. For patients who are very sick and at the end of life, mechanical ventilation sometimes only postpones death.

28

Horiana Grosu
Ruth Minkin

Pulmonary Embolism

Pulmonary embolism (PE) is a relatively common disease, with an estimated annual incidence of 23 cases diagnosed per 100,000 persons in the United States.[1] More than 50% of cases are undiagnosed. Untreated PE has a high mortality, although risk for death is reduced significantly with anticoagulation.[2]

PE refers to obstruction of the pulmonary artery or one of its branches by material (e.g., thrombus, tumor, air, or fat) that originated elsewhere in the body. In this chapter we will discuss PE resulting from thrombus.

PATHOPHYSIOLOGY

Although venous thromboembolism (VTE) is a common disease, underlying pathogenic mechanisms are only partially known, particularly in comparison with those of atherothrombosis. During the past decades, progress was made in the identification and characterization of the cellular and molecular mechanisms that interdependently influence Virchow's triad. It is now accepted that the combination of stasis and hypercoagulability, much more than endothelial damage and activation, are crucial for the occurrence of venous thrombosis; venous thrombi are mainly constituted by fibrin and red blood cell, and less by platelets.[3] Most PEs originate from the deep venous system of lower extremities, iliofemoral veins being the source of most clinically significant PEs; however, upper extremities, pelvic and renal veins, and the right heart, could potentially be the embolic source as well.

After reaching the pulmonary circulation, large thrombi may lodge at the bifurcation of the main pulmonary artery or the lobar branches and cause hemodynamic compromise. Smaller thrombi continue traveling distally and are more likely to produce pleuritic chest pain, presumably by initiating an inflammatory response adjacent to the parietal pleura. Only about 10% of emboli cause pulmonary infarction, usually in patients with preexisting cardiopulmonary disease.

PREDISPOSING FACTORS

Most patients with acute PE have an identifiable risk factor at the time of presentation.[4] Immobilization of only 1 or 2 days may predispose to PE.[5] Among patients in whom immobilization was a predisposing factor, 65% were immobilized for more than 2 weeks.[6] Other predisposing factors include surgery within the last 3 months, stroke, paresis or paralysis, history of VTE, malignancy, and central venous instrumentation within the last 3 months.[4,5] Additional risk factors identified in women include obesity (BMI $\geq$29 kg per m^2), heavy cigarette smoking (>25 cigarettes per day), and hypertension.[7] The risk for

PE in patients hospitalized with heart failure is twice that of hospitalized patients who do not have heart failure, and PE is a frequent cause of death in patients hospitalized with heart disease.[8,9] The lower the ejection fraction, the greater the risk for VTE.[10]

Based on the clinical presentation, PE can be classified as massive or submassive.

Massive PE causes hypotension, defined as a systolic blood pressure <90 mm Hg or a drop in systolic blood pressure of $\geq$40 mm Hg from baseline for a period >15 minutes. It is a catastrophic entity that frequently results in acute right ventricular (RV) failure and death. Hypotension results from reduction in cardiac output (CO) owing to increased pulmonary vascular resistance (PVR). PVR is increased from physical obstruction of the vascular bed with thrombus and vasoconstriction, the latter due to the effects of inflammatory mediators and hypoxia. When obstruction of the vascular bed approaches 75%, the right ventricle must generate a systolic pressure in excess of 50 mm Hg and a mean pulmonary artery pressure approximating 40 mm Hg to preserve pulmonary perfusion.[11] The normal right ventricle is unable to accomplish this and may eventually fail. Patients with underlying cardiopulmonary disease experience more substantial deterioration in CO than normal individuals.

When death occurs, it is often within 1 to 2 hours of the event, although patients remain at risk for 24 to 72 hours. All acute PEs not meeting the definition of massive PE are considered submassive PE.

A saddle PE is a PE that lodges at the bifurcation of the main pulmonary artery into the right and left pulmonary arteries. Most saddle PEs are submassive. In a retrospective study of 546 consecutive patients with PE, 14 (2.6%) had a saddle PE. Only two of the patients with saddle PE had hypotension.[12]

DIAGNOSIS

SYMPTOMS/SIGNS

The clinical diagnosis of PE is difficult because symptoms and signs are very nonspecific and occur with similar frequency in patients with and without PE.

In the prospective investigation of pulmonary embolism diagnosis II (PIOPED II), the symptoms and signs were analyzed among patients with PE who did not have preexisting cardiopulmonary disease.[4] Dyspnea at rest or with exertion was most common but not a universal finding, occurring in 73% of patients with PE. The onset of dyspnea occurred over seconds or minutes in 72% of patients. The other common symptoms reported were pleuritic chest pain (44%), calf or thigh pain (44%), calf or thigh swelling (41%), cough (34%), and wheezing (21%).[4]

Tachypnea (respiratory rate >20 breaths per minute) occurred in 54% to 70% of patients who did not have previous cardiopulmonary disease. Tachycardia (heart rate >100 beats per minute) occurred less frequently (24% to 30%). One of the signs of right atrial, RV, or pulmonary artery pressure elevation (neck vein distension, RV lift, accentuated pulmonary component of the second sound) was documented in only 21% of patients who did not have previous cardiopulmonary disease. Lung examination showed abnormalities in 30% of patients with PE. Rales and decreased breath sounds were the most frequently detected abnormalities. Fever can be the presenting physical finding in patients with VTE, occurring with similar frequency in those with PE and pulmonary hemorrhage or infarction, and those with PE who did not have the latter. The fever was usually of low grade.[13]

DIAGNOSTIC TESTS

Because the clinical signs and symptoms of PE are not specific, timely diagnostic testing must be done to confirm the diagnosis (Figure 28.1).

LABORATORY TESTING

Most of routine laboratory tests are nonspecific in the setting of PE. Despite the fact that dyspnea is the main presenting symptom of PE, evaluation of oxygenation by pulse oximetry and arterial blood gas determination has a limited role in establishing the diagnosis.[14]

Arterial blood gas determination usually reveals hypoxemia, hypocapnia, and respiratory alkalosis, but these findings are not always seen. As an example, massive PE with hypotension and respiratory collapse can cause hypercapnia and a combined respiratory and metabolic acidosis (the latter because of lactic acidosis).

In PE, the fibrinolytic system is activated. *D Dimer* is a cross-linked fibrin degradation product that may be used as a marker for ongoing fibrinolysis.[15] Quantitative and semi-quantitative assays for D dimer are used. For quantitative assays, a level >500 ng per ml is considered to be abnormal.[16] The D-dimer level also increases with a number of conditions other than VTE[15] (Table 28.1). Numerous studies have reported on utility of D-dimer assays for the diagnosis of PE. The general consensus is that these are best characterized as having good sensitivity

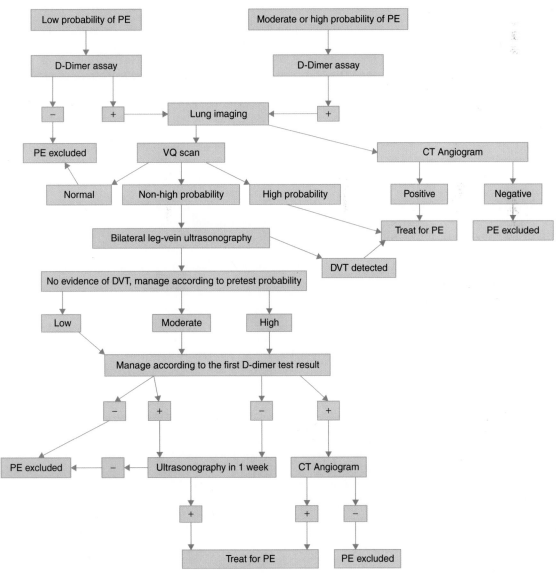

Figure 28.1. Algorithm for diagnosing pulmonary embolism.

TABLE 28.1	Disorders Associated with Increased Plasma Levels of Fibrin D-Dimer
Arterial thromboembolic disease:	Myocardial infarction
	Stroke
	Acute limb ischemia
	Atrial fibrillation
Venous thromboembolism:	Deep vein thrombosis
	Pulmonary embolism
Eclampsia and preeclampsia	
Disseminated intravascular coagulation	
Severe infection: Sepsis	
Systemic inflammatory response syndrome	
Vasooclusive episode of sickle cell disease	
Severe liver disease	
Malignancy	
Renal disease:	Acute renal failure
	Nephrotic syndrome
	Chronic renal insufficiency
Normal pregnancy	
Congestive heart failure	

Adapted from UpToDate Version 18.1, January 2010.

and negative predictive value but poor specificity and poor positive predictive value. In patients with suspected PE, D dimer is elevated in approximately 95% of cases when measured by enzyme-linked immunosorbent assay (ELISA), quantitative rapid ELISA, or semi-quantitative ELISA.[16] D-dimer levels are normal in 40% to 68% of patients without PE, regardless of the assay used owing to high frequency of the positive D-dimer levels in patients without thromboembolic disease.[16] The specificity decreases even further in patients with renal disease and/or increased age.[17]

The ability of a normal or negative D-dimer assay to exclude acute PE depends on both the type of D-dimer assay and the clinical pretest probability for acute PE. In patients with a normal D-dimer concentration independent of the clinical probability of PE, the 3-month VTE risk is 2.3%; whereas, in patients with a high clinical probability of PE despite a normal D-dimer concentration, approximately 1 in 10 patients will still have PE.[18,19] In patients with an unlikely clinical probability and a normal D-dimer concentration the risk of VTE, if the patient is untreated, is approximately 1%.[19]

In conclusion, the evidence indicates that a D-dimer level <500 ng per ml by quantitative ELISA or semi-quantitative latex agglutination is sufficient to exclude PE in patients with a low or moderate pretest probability of PE.

Troponin. Serum troponin I and T are frequently elevated in patients with PE, mainly in those with moderate-to-extensive clot burden, which leads to acute right heart pressure overload.[20] Most studies indicate that troponins are not useful for the establishment of PE diagnosis but are a valuable tool in the prediction of adverse outcomes for patients with PE.[21–24]

An elevated brain natriuretic peptide (BNP) or N-terminal pro-brain natriuretic peptide (NT-proBNP) can predict RV dysfunction and mortality related to a PE[25,26]; however, they have limited usefulness as a diagnostic test for PE having sensitivity

and specificity of 60% and 62%, respectively.[27] Some reports suggested that BNP and NT-proBNP have a very high (approaching 100%) negative predictive value with regard to early death, which makes them particularly useful for ruling out massive life-threatening PE.[28–31]

Electrocardiography. ECG abnormalities are common in patients with PE; however, the ECG is of limited diagnostic value[32] with the majority of patients presenting with tachycardia and nonspecific ST-segment and T-wave changes.[33]

The "classic" ECG abnormalities suggestive of PE (S1Q3T3 pattern, RV strain, and new incomplete right bundle branch block [RBBB]) are infrequent during acute PE seen mostly in patients with massive acute PE and cor pulmonale.[34]

ECG changes that have been reported to correlate with poor prognosis include atrial arrhythmias, RBBB, inferior Q-waves, precordial T-wave inversion, and ST-segment changes.[35,36]

Echocardiography. Echocardiographic abnormalities are seen in less than half of the patients presenting with acute PE. The most commonly reported findings include increased RV size, decreased RV function, and tricuspid regurgitation.[37,38] These changes are more common in patients with massive PE, and the echocardiography is often used to guide the use of thrombolytic therapy.[39]

Pulmonary angiogram had been the gold standard for diagnosis, but now CT angiogram is effectively the diagnostic test. A negative pulmonary angiogram excludes the diagnosis of clinically significant PE. Although largely a safe procedure it still carries <2% mortality and approximately 5% morbidity in patients without significant pulmonary hypertension and hemodynamic instability.[40,41] Consequently, alternative, less-invasive testing modalities have been extensively studied in patients with suspected PE.

Ventilation–Perfusion (V/Q) scan is one of the most commonly used tests for PE diagnosis. The PIOPED[42] study evaluated the accuracy of V/Q scanning by comparison with the reference standard, the pulmonary angiogram.

Diagnostic accuracy was greatest when the V/Q scan was combined with pretest clinical probability. The most useful "scenarios" include patients with high clinical probability of PE and high-probability V/Q scan (likelihood of PE 95%), low clinical probability of PE and low-probability V/Q scan (likelihood of PE 4%), and a normal VQ scan that essentially excluded diagnosis of PE. However, most V/Q scans did not fall into these categories, with a diagnostic accuracy ranging from 15% to 86% that was unacceptable to either confirm or rule out the diagnosis of PE.

CT pulmonary angiogram (CT-PA) is currently the initial diagnostic test for PE in the majority of cases. In addition to greater diagnostic yield compared with V/Q scanning, this imaging may also provide an alternative diagnosis in the absence of PE that could explain patients' symptoms.[43]

PIOPED II study is the largest to date assessing the accuracy of CT-PA in diagnosing PE.[44] Among 824 patients with suspected diagnosis of PE, the sensitivity of CTA was 83% and the specificity was 96%.

In patients with a positive CT-PA and a high, intermediate, or low pretest clinical probability the likelihood of PE was 96%, 92%, and 58%, respectively (i.e., positive predictive value). The likelihood that PE was absent in patients with a negative CT-PA and a low, intermediate, or high clinical probability was 96%, 89%, and 60%, respectively (i.e., negative predictive value). This study suggested that CT-PA requires concomitant pretest clinical probability assessment to be an effective diagnostic tool for confirming or excluding PE. Authors calculated pretest clinical probability using the Wells' Criteria[45] (Table 28.2).

The study investigators concluded that the predictive value CTA is high with a concordant clinical assessment, but additional testing is necessary when the clinical probability is inconsistent with the imaging results. Negative CT-PA has excellent negative predictive value for excluding PE. Patients with negative CT-PA combined with negative lower extremity Doppler, and low or intermediate clinical probability have <2% incidence of PE within 3 months follow up.[46]

Numerous studies have evaluated the safety and efficiency of relatively complex combinations of clinical decision rules and diagnostic tests in patients with suspected PE to develop an effective algorithm for evaluation of patients with suspected acute PE.[46-48] The Christopher Study[48] was a prospective multicenter cohort study of 3,306 consecutive patients with clinically suspected acute PE. The authors used modified Wells' criteria to categorize patients as "PE likely" or "PE unlikely" (Table 28.2). All patients were followed up for a period of 3 months after presentation to document the occurrence of subsequent symptomatic VTE.

Patients classified as PE unlikely underwent quantitative D-dimer testing by ELISA. PE was considered excluded in those with a normal D-dimer test. Patients classified as PE likely and patients classified as PE unlikely who had abnormal D-dimer tests underwent CT-PA. The CT-PA confirmed PE, excluded PE, or was inconclusive (seldom). At 3-month follow-up, the following outcomes were reported:

Among 1,028 untreated patients in whom PE was excluded by clinical assessment plus D-dimer testing, there were one deep vein thrombosis (DVT) (0.1%), four nonfatal PE (0.4%), and no fatal PE.

Among 1,436 untreated patients in whom PE was excluded by CT-PA, there were eight DVT (0.6%), three nonfatal PE (0.2%), and seven fatal PE (0.5%).

Among 674 treated patients in whom PE was detected by CT-PA, there were 6 DVT (0.9%), 3 nonfatal PE (0.4%), and 11 fatal PE (1.6%).

This study suggests that an algorithm using clinical assessment, D-dimer testing, and CT-PA can be used to exclude PE.[49]

THERAPY FOR ACUTE PE

Untreated PE has a very high mortality (up to 30%) with most deaths occurring within several hours after the initial event owing to recurrent thromboembolism.[2,50] Therefore the appropriate therapy has to be initiated as soon as possible. The therapeutic interventions can be categorized into general resuscitation measures and anticoagulation.

General resuscitation measures should focus on stabilizing the hemodynamics and oxygenation of the patient. The main concern is development of RV failure owing to acutely raised pulmonary arterial pressure. Hypotension, the most alarming presenting sign of PE, must be treated promptly. In the setting of hypotension (systolic blood pressure <90 mm Hg, or drop from baseline blood pressure over 40 mm Hg) the initial approach must include intravenous fluid resuscitation with isotonic solution. Administration of 500 to 1,000 ml of normal saline is usually sufficient. Physicians must be cautious in administering larger volumes of fluids as this may increase RV wall stress and eventually lead to RV ischemia and worsening of RV failure.[51] If hypotension persists despite intravenous fluid resuscitation, vasopressors should be administered.

There are no randomized controlled trials of PE that show benefit of one vasoactive agent over others. Norepinephrine, dopamine, and dobutamine may be considered. Norepinephrine is the least likely to cause tachycardia. Dobutamine is an excellent choice for an inotrope in a setting of cardiogenic shock as it increases myocardial contractility; however, its vasodilatory properties could potentially worsen hypotension. Therefore, consideration should be given to using a combination of these agents to minimize risk of worsening tachycardia and hypotension.

Anticoagulation therapy should be initiated promptly in patients with confirmed PE. Anticoagulation should be initiated also in those patients with suspected PE and without excessive risk of bleeding while the confirmatory diagnostic tests are in progress. As mentioned earlier this recommendation is based on the fact that untreated PE has mortality of approximately 30%, whereas the risks of major bleeding with anticoagulation is <3%.[50,52] Therapeutic anticoagulation must be achieved within the first 24 hours of the treatment[53] to minimize the chance of recurrent PE and death.

Current available anticoagulation regimens include continuous intravenous unfractionated heparin (IV UFH),

TABLE 28.2	Modified Wells' Criteria for Diagnosis of Pulmonary Embolism
Clinical symptoms of DVT	3.0
Other diagnosis less likely than PE	3.0
Heart rate >100	1.5
Immobilization (≥3 days) or surgery in previous 4 weeks	1.5
Previous DVT/PE	1.5
Hemoptysis	1.0
Malignancy	1.0
Probability	*Score*

TRADITIONAL CLINICAL PROBABILITY ASSESSMENT

High	>6.0
Moderate	2.0–6.0
Low	<2.0

SIMPLIFIED CLINICAL PROBABILITY ASSESSMENT

PE likely	>4.0
PE unlikely	≤ 4.0

Data adapted from Wells PS, Anderson DR, Rodger M, et al. Derivation of a simple clinical model to categorize patients' probability of pulmonary embolism: increasing the model's utility with the SimpliRED D-dimer. *Thromb Haemost.* 2000;83:416–420; van Belle A, Buller HR, Huisman MV, et al. Effectiveness of managing suspected pulmonary embolism using an algorithm combining clinical probability, D-dimer testing, and computed tomography. *JAMA.* 2006;295(2):172–179.

subcutaneous low-molecular-weight heparin (SC LMWH), subcutaneous unfractionated heparin (SC UFH), and subcutaneous fondaparinux. Treatment of massive PE includes use of thrombolytic therapy.

SC LMWH has been found to be at least as effective and safe as IV UFH in patients with PE.[54,55] A meta-analysis of 12 studies analyzing 1,951 patients with either submassive PE or asymptomatic PE in conjunction with symptomatic DVT found that LMWH was associated with less tendency of recurrent thromboembolic events, less major bleeding complications, and comparable all-cause mortality as IV UFH. Therefore for most of the hemodynamically stable patients with PE, LMWH is the preferred initial therapy.

IV UFH may be preferred over LMWH in patients with persistent hypotension due to PE—when thrombolytic therapy is being considered—in patients with increased risk for bleeding complications, or in morbidly obese (>150 kg) when subcutaneous absorption is questionable and unpredictable. In patients with renal insufficiency and creatinine clearance <30 ml per minute IV UFH is the initial therapy as there are no well-studied data on efficacy and safety of LMWH. In patients with mild or moderate renal insufficiency (CrCl of 30 to 80 ml per minute) there is no required dose adjustment for LMWH.

Fondaparinux is a synthetic pentasaccharide, which has a sequence derived from the minimal antithrombin-binding region of heparin. It catalyzes factor Xa inactivation by antithrombin without inhibiting thrombin. Fondaparinux has been compared only with IV UFH but not with LMWH in a large open-label trial of patients with acute PE not requiring thrombolytic therapy.[57] Fondaparinux was associated with a similar frequency of recurrent VTE and major bleeding.

Several formulations of SC LMWH are available including enoxaparin, dalteparin, tinzaparin, nadroparin, ardeparin, and reviparin. Enoxaparin is the most commonly used agent in both inpatient and outpatient setting for initial PE therapy. Enoxaparin is administered subcutaneously at a dose of 1 mg per kg of actual body weight twice per day. Alternative dose of 1.5 mg per kg of actual body weight once daily could be utilized. Twice daily regimen is preferred for patients with cancer, extensive clot burden, and an actual body weight between 101 and 150 kg.

To monitor enoxaparin therapy anti-Xa level may be measured; in most of the patients treated for acute PE this is not necessary. However, it may be warranted in certain cases, such as renal insufficiency, morbid obesity, low body weight, and pregnancy.

Administration of IV UFH requires continuous infusion as intermittent bolusing is associated with greater risk of major bleeding. A weight-based dosing protocol suggested by the 2008 ACCP Antithrombotic and Thrombolytic Therapy guidelines[58] is most commonly used starting with a bolus of 80 units per kg, followed by an infusion at 18 units/kg/hour. Infusion rate should be titrated every 4 to 6 hours to a goal activated partial thromboplastin time (aPTT). In most patients, the therapeutic aPTT is 1.5 to 2.5 times the control aPTT. Therapeutic aPTT range and dose adjustments differ from institution to institution. This is because the level of aPTT that correlates with a specific anti-Xa factor activity varies according to the reagents that are used to measure the aPTT. Therefore, each institution must establish its own protocol for titration of the UFH infusion.

If SC UFH regimen is chosen the most reasonable protocol is suggested in 2008 ACCP Antithrombotic and Thrombolytic.[58]

SC UFH should be initiated at a dose of 17,500 units or 250 units per kg every 12 hours. The dose should then be titrated to achieve therapeutic aPTT range. Dose adjustment should be an increase or decrease of the current dose by 10% to 30%.

As discussed above fondaparinux has been compared with IV UFH and has similar efficacy and complication rate. Fondaparinux dose is weight-based (5 mg for patients <50 kg, 7.5 mg for patients weighing 50 to 100 kg, and 7.5 mg for patients >100 kg) and administered once daily. Fondaparinux is contraindicated in patients with severe renal insufficiency (creatinine clearance <30 ml per minute). Monitoring anti-Xa level is not routinely recommended in patients with normal kidney function.

Thrombolytic therapy for PE remains a controversial issue. Thrombolytic therapy is considered for patients with confirmed massive PE. Available literature demonstrates that thrombolytic therapy followed by anticoagulation is associated with short-term hemodynamic benefits compared with anticoagulation alone. However, to this date there are no conclusive data to demonstrate mortality benefit with thrombolysis.[59–61]

In the case of a confirmed PE, the following clinical scenarios warrant consideration for thrombolysis: persistent hypotension, severe hypoxemia, large perfusion defect on V/Q scans, extensive embolic burden on CT, RV dysfunction, free-floating right atrial or ventricular thrombus, patent foramen ovale. Among all the above situations, hemodynamic compromise due to PE is the only one indication that has been widely accepted for use of thrombolytic therapy.[58] Compared with anticoagulation alone, thrombolytic therapy has demonstrated acceleration of thrombus lysis, reduction of pulmonary arterial pressures, and resolution of RV dysfunction[42,62–64] as well as a trend towards improved clinical outcomes in patients with hemodynamic compromise. The decision to administer thrombolysis must be made promptly, as the reduced cardiac output and inadequate tissue perfusion can lead to irreversible organ damage. The risk of death is very high in the presence of persistent hypotension and shock.[63,64,65]

There are very limited data on successful use of thrombolytic therapy during cardiopulmonary resuscitation efforts in the case of cardiac arrest related to acute PE.[66,67]

Recombinant tissue plasminogen activator is the available thrombolytic agent. It is administered as 100 mg given intravenously over 2 hours. Once the decision is made to administer thrombolytic therapy all invasive interventions should be minimized and anticoagulant therapy discontinued. The agent should be administered through a peripheral intravenous line.[58] Once the thrombolytic infusion is completed aPTT should be measured. Heparin should be restarted without a loading dose after aPTT is less than twice the upper limit of normal. If the aPTT exceeds this value, the test should be repeated every 4 hours until the above value is achieved.

Major contraindications for thrombolytic use include intracranial disease, uncontrolled hypertension at presentation, and recent major surgery or trauma (Table 28.3). However, when making a decision regarding thrombolysis the importance of the specific contraindication should always be weighed against the strength of indication and life-threatening nature of the PE.

The most common adverse effect of thrombolytic therapy is bleeding. Retrospective data analysis of the patients with PE who received alteplase showed 19% major bleeding complications, the commonest being gastrointestinal site (in 30% of patients).[68] Bleeding may commonly occur at the sites of invasive

TABLE 28.3	Contraindications for Thrombolysis in Pulmonary Embolism	
Absolute	*Relative*	
History of hemorrhagic stroke	Bleeding disorder	
Current intracranial neoplasm	Nonhemorrhagic stroke within prior 2 months	
Recent intracranial surgery or trauma (<2 months)	Uncontrolled hypertension (systolic BP over 200 or diastolic BP over 110)	
Active or recent internal bleeding (in prior 6 months)	Surgery within prior 10 days	
	Thrombocytopenia (<100,000 platelets/mm^3)	

procedures.[69] The most devastating bleeding complication associated with thrombolytic therapy use is intracranial hemorrhage. This complication is reported in up to 3% of patients who received thrombolytic therapy for PE, which is higher than the rate of intracranial hemorrhage reported with thrombolysis use for acute coronary event.[70–72]

Inferior vena cava (IVC) filters prevent large thrombi from the lower extremities and pelvic veins from reaching the pulmonary circulation. IVC filters are indicated in the following circumstances: active bleeding or other absolute contraindication for anticoagulation, recurrence of PE despite therapeutic anticoagulation, and may be considered in the presence of hemodynamic or respiratory compromise that is so severe that further VTE could be potentially fatal.[58]

No randomized trials have evaluated IVC filters as a sole therapy for an acute PE. The PREPIC trial evaluated IVC filters as an adjunct to anticoagulation in high-risk patients with proximal DVT. The study showed that IVC filters reduced the incidence of PE, increased incidence of DVT, and did not change the overall frequency of VTE (DVT and/or PE combined).[73,74]

Complications of IVC filters can be related to the insertion procedure (bleeding, thrombosis at the insertion site) or to presence of a filter itself (migration, thrombosis, erosion, and perforation of IVC wall). Currently, routine insertion of IVC filter is not recommended.[58]

Pulmonary embolectomy by surgery or catheter may be considered for treatment of acute PE in patients with hemodynamic compromise who are unable to receive thrombolytic therapy owing to bleeding risk or when the condition of such patient is so critical that it does not allow sufficient time for systemic thrombolysis to reach its effect.[58] Embolectomy should only be performed in centers where such expertise is available.

Catheter embolectomy using rheolytic (injection of pressurized saline to macerate the emboli) or rotational (fragmentation of an embolus through conventional cardiac catheter) mechanisms have been utilized with success, although significant periprocedural mortality has been reported.[74,75,76,77]

Emergency surgical embolectomy has been performed in patients with acute PE who require surgical excision of a right atrial thrombus or impending paradoxical arterial embolism in a setting of patent foramen ovale. It can also be considered to rescue patients in whom thrombolysis has been unsuccessful.[78,79]

LONG-TERM MANAGEMENT OF PULMONARY EMBOLISM

In most of the patients presenting with acute PE, the initial anticoagulation regimen of LMWH, IV UFH, or fondaparinux is transitioned to a long-term therapy with an oral agent. Warfarin, a vitamin K antagonist, is the most commonly used and best-studied agent. Long-term therapy with warfarin is highly effective in preventing further VTE and recurrent PE.[80] Warfarin therapy should begin on the same day or a day after the heparin or fondaparinux is started. It should not be initiated before the heparin or fondaparinux as warfarin administered alone is associated with an increased risk for recurrent VTE. Warfarin should be overlapped with heparin or fondaparinux for at least 5 days and until the international randomized ratio (INR) has remained within therapeutic range (between 2.0 and 3.0) for at least 24 hours.[58] The usual initial dose of warfarin is 5 mg once daily for first 48 to 72 hours; then the dose should be adjusted according to the INR value. Initially INR measurements should be performed daily, then at 2 to 4 week intervals when the dosing has stabilized.

Duration of anticoagulation therapy depends on several factors: (a) first or recurrent PE and (b) presence of risk factors for PE.

With the first episode of PE the treatment duration will depend on the identification of a risk factor for a VTE and whether the specific risk factor is reversible. Patients with first episode of PE and a reversible or a temporary risk factor that has resolved should be treated with warfarin for at least 3 months.[58] Temporary risk factors could include surgical intervention, trauma, and prolonged immobilization. Pregnancy confers increased risk for VTE that extends into early postpartum period. Management of a pregnant patient with acute PE is beyond the scope of this chapter.

Extending anticoagulation for first episode of acute PE with a reversible or a temporary risk factor for more than 3 months does not provide additional benefit.[81,82]

The duration of the anticoagulation therapy for a first episode of unprovoked PE (no reversible or temporary risk factors) is uncertain. The evidence on whether extending therapy for more than 3 months is beneficial is conflicting.[83–85] The 2008 ACCP Antithrombotic and Thrombolytic Therapy guidelines recommend 3 months of warfarin therapy and then reassessment for unprovoked PE. Indefinite anticoagulation is recommended for patients who do *not* have risk factors for bleeding and are willing to continue anticoagulant monitoring.[58]

For patients who have experienced two or more episodes of VTE, indefinite anticoagulation therapy is recommended.

REFERENCES

1. Anderson FA Jr, Wheeler HB, Goldhei RJ, et al. A population-based perspective of the hospital incidence and case-fatality rates of deep vein thrombosis and pulmonary embolism. The Worcester DVT Study. *Arch Intern Med.* 1991;151:933–938.
2. Carson JL, Kelley MA, Duff A, et al. The clinical course of pulmonary embolism. *N Engl J Med.* 1992;326(19):1240–1245.
3. Martinelli I, Bucciarelli P, Mannucci PM. Thrombotic risk factors: basic pathophysiology. *Crit Care Med.* 2010;38(2):S3–S9.
4. Stein PD, Beemath A, Matta F, et al. Clinical characteristics of patients with acute pulmonary embolism: data from PIOPED II. *Am J Med.* 2007;120(10):871–879.
5. Heit JA, O'Fallon WM, Petterson TM, et al. Relative impact of risk factors for deep vein thrombosis and pulmonary embolism: a population-based study. *Arch Intern Med.* 2002;162(11):1245–1248.
6. Stein PD, Terrin ML, Hales CA, et al. Clinical, laboratory, roentgenographic and electrocardiographic findings in patients with acute pulmonary embolism and no pre-existing cardiac or pulmonary disease. *Chest.* 1991;100:598–603.

7. Goldhaber SZ, Grodstein F, Stampfer MJ, et al. A prospective study of risk factors for pulmonary embolism in women. *JAMA.* 1997;277(8):642–645.

8. Beemath A, Stein PD, Skaf E, et al. Risk of venous thromboembolism in patients hospitalized with heart failure. *Am J Cardiol.* 2006;98:793–795.

9. Pulido T, Aranda A, Zevallos MA, et al. Pulmonary embolism as a cause of death in patients with heart disease: an autopsy study. *Chest.* 2006;129(5):1282–1287.

10. Howell MD, Geraci JM, Knowlton AA. Congestive heart failure and outpatient risk of venous thromboembolism: a retrospective, case control study. *J Clin Epidemiol.* 2001;54:810–816.

11. Benotti JR, Dalen JE. The natural history of pulmonary embolism. *Clin Chest Med.* 1984;5(3):403–410.

12. Ryu JH, Pellikka PA, Froehling DA, et al. Saddle pulmonary embolism diagnosed by CT angiography: frequency, clinical features and outcome. *Respir Med.* 2007;101(7):1537–1542.

13. Stein PD, Afzal A, Henry JW, et al. Fever in acute pulmonary embolism. *Chest.* 2000;117:39–42.

14. Rodger MA, Carrier M, Jones GN, et al. Diagnostic value of arterial blood gas measurement in suspected pulmonary embolism. *Am J Respir Crit Care Med.* 2000;162(6):2105–2108.

15. Kelly J, Rudd A, Lewis RR, et al. Plasma D-dimers in the diagnosis of venous thromboembolism. *Arch Intern Med.* 2002;162:747–756.

16. Stein PD, Hull RD, Patel KC, et al. D-dimer for the exclusion of acute venous thrombosis and pulmonary embolism: a systematic review. *Ann Intern Med.* 2004;140(8):589–602.

17. Karami-Djurabi R, Klok FA, Kooiman J, et al. D-dimer testing in patients with suspected pulmonary embolism and impaired renal function. *Am J Med.* 2009;122(11):1050–1053.

18. Righini M, Goehring C, Bounameaux H, et al. Effects of age on the performance of common diagnostic tests for pulmonary embolism. *Am J Med.* 2000;109(5):357–361.

19. Gibson NS, Sohne M, Gerdes VE, et al. The importance of clinical probability assessment in interpreting a normal d-dimer in patients with suspected pulmonary embolism. *Chest.* 2008;134(4):789–793.

20. Meyer T, Binder L, Hruska N, et al. Cardiac troponin I elevation in acute pulmonary embolism is associated with right ventricular dysfunction. *J Am Coll Cardiol.* 2000;36(5):1632–1636.

21. Pruszczyk P, Bochowicz A, Torbicki A, et al. Cardiac troponin T monitoring identifies high-risk group of normotensive patients with acute pulmonary embolism. *Chest.* 2003;123(6):1947–1952.

22. Giannitsis E, Muller-Bardorff M, Kurowski V, et al. Independent prognostic value of cardiac troponin T in patients with confirmed pulmonary embolism. *Circulation.* 2000;102(2):211–217.

23. Konstantinides S, Geibel A, Olschewski M, et al. Importance of cardiac troponins I and T in risk stratification of patients with acute pulmonary embolism. *Circulation.* 2002;106(10):1263–1268.

24. Douketis JD, Crowther MA, Stanton EB, et al. Elevated cardiac troponin levels in patients with submassive pulmonary embolism. *Arch Intern Med.* 2002;162(1):79–81.

25. Klok FA, Mos IC, Huisman MV. Brain-type natriuretic peptide levels in the prediction of adverse outcome in patients with pulmonary embolism: a systematic review and meta-analysis. *Am J Respir Crit Care Med.* 2008;178(4):425–430.

26. Cavallazzi R, Nair A, Vasu T, et al. Natriuretic peptides in acute pulmonary embolism: a systematic review. *Intensive Care Med.* 2008;34(12):2147–2156.

27. Sohne M, Ten Wolde M, Boomsma F, et al. Brain natriuretic peptide in hemodynamically stable acute pulmonary embolism. *J Thromb Haemost.* 2006;4(3):552–556.

28. Kucher N, Printzen G, Doernhoefer T, et al. Low pro-BNP levels predict benign clinical outcome in acute PE. *Circulation.* 2003;22:649–653.

29. Kucher N, Printzen G, Goldhaber SZ. Prognostic role of BNP in acute PE. *Circulation.* 2003;107:1576–1578.

30. Proszczyk P, Kotrubiec M, Bochowicz A, et al. N-terminal pro-BNP in patients with acute PE. *Eur Respir J.* 2003;22:649–653.

31. Ten Wolde M, Tulevski II, Mulder JW, et al. BNP as a predictor of adverse outcome in patients with PE. *Circulation.* 2003;107:2082–2084.

32. Rodger M, Makropoulos D, Turek M, et al. Diagnostic value of the electrocardiogram in suspected pulmonary embolism. *Am J Cardiol.* 2000;86(7):807–809.

33. Stein PD, Saltzman HA, Weg JG. Clinical characteristics of patients with acute pulmonary embolism. *Am J Cardiol.* 1991;68:1723.

34. Panos RJ, Barish RA, Whye DW Jr, et al. The electrocardiographic manifestations of pulmonary embolism. *J Emerg Med.* 1988;6(4):301–307.

35. Geibel A, Zehender M, Kasper W, et al. Prognostic value of the ECG on admission in patients with acute major pulmonary embolism. *Eur Respir J.* 2005;25(5):843–848.

36. Ferrari E, Imbert A, Chevalier T, et al. The ECG in pulmonary embolism. Predictive value of negative T waves in precordial leads—80 case reports. *Chest.* 1997;111(3):537–543.

37. Come PC. Echocardiographic evaluation of pulmonary embolism and its response to therapeutic interventions. *Chest.* 1992;101(4)(suppl):151S–162S.

38. Gibson NS, Sohne M, Buller HR. Prognostic value of echocardiography and spiral computed tomography in patients with pulmonary embolism. *Curr Opin Pulm Med.* 2005;11(5):380–384.

39. Goldhaber SZ. Echocardiography in the management of pulmonary embolism. *Ann Intern Med.* 2002;136(9):691–700.

40. Stein PD, Athanasoulis C, Alavi A, et al. Complications and validity of pulmonary angiography in acute pulmonary embolism. *Circulation.* 1992;85(2):462–468.

41. Hofmann LV, Lee DS, Gupta A, et al. Safety and hemodynamic effects of pulmonary angiography in patients with pulmonary hypertension: 10-year single-center experience. *AJR Am J Roentgenol.* 2004;183(3):779–786.

42. The PIOPED Investigators. Value of the ventilation/perfusion scan in acute pulmonary embolism. Results of the prospective investigation of pulmonary embolism diagnosis (PIOPED). *JAMA.* 1990;263(20):2753–2759.

43. Hall WB, Truitt SG, Scheunemann LP, et al. The prevalence of clinically relevant incidental findings on chest computed tomographic angiograms ordered to diagnose pulmonary embolism. *Arch Intern Med.* 2009;169(21):1961–1965.

44. Stein PD, Fowler SE, Goodman LR, et al. Multidetector computed tomography for acute pulmonary embolism. *N Engl J Med.* 2006;354(22):2317–2327.

45. Wells PS, Anderson DR, Rodger M, et al. Derivation of a simple clinical model to categorize patients' probability of pulmonary embolism: increasing the model's utility with the SimpliRED D-dimer. *Thromb Haemost.* 2000;83:416–420.

46. Musset D, Parent F, Meyer G, et al. Diagnostic strategy for patients with suspected pulmonary embolism: a prospective multicentre outcome study. *Lancet.* 2002;360(9349):1914–1920.

47. Wells PS, Anderson DR, Rodger M, et al. Excluding pulmonary embolism at the bedside without diagnostic imaging: management of patients with suspected pulmonary embolism presenting to the emergency department by using a simple clinical model and d-dimer. *Ann Intern Med.* 2001;135(2):98–107.

48. van Belle A, Buller HR, Huisman MV, et al. Effectiveness of managing suspected pulmonary embolism using an algorithm combining clinical probability, D-dimer testing, and computed tomography. *JAMA.* 2006;295(2):172–179.

49. Wells PS, Ginsberg JS, Anderson DR, et al. Use of a clinical model for safe management of patients with suspected pulmonary embolism. *Ann Intern Med.* 1998;129(12):997–1005.

50. Horlander KT, Mannino DM, Leeper KV. Pulmonary embolism mortality in the United States, 1979–1998: an analysis using multiple-cause mortality data. *Arch Intern Med.* 2003;163(14):1711–1717.

51. Kucher N, Goldhaber SZ. Management of massive pulmonary embolism. *Circulation.* 2005;112:e28.

52. Schulman S, Beyth RJ, Kearon C, et al. Hemorrhagic complications of anticoagulant and thrombolytic treatment: American College of Chest Physicians Evidence-Based Clinical Practice Guidelines (8th Edition). *Chest.* 2008;133:257S.

53. Raschke RA, Reilly BM, Guidry JR, et al. The weight-based heparin dosing nomogram compared with a "standard care" nomogram. *Ann Intern Med.* 1993;119(9):874–881.

54. Quinlan DJ, McQuinlan A, Eikelboom JW. Low molecular weight heparin compared with intravenous unfractionated heparin in the curative treatment of pulmonary embolism: a meta-analysis of randomized controlled trials. *Ann Intern Med.* 2004;140:175–183.

55. Prandone P, Carnovali M, Marchiori A. Subcutaneous adjusted-dose unfractionated heparin vs fixed dose low molecular weight heparin in the initial treatment of venous thromboembolism. *Arch Intern Med.* 2004;164:1077–1083.

56. Buller HR, Davidson BL, Decousus HL, et al. Subcutaneous fondaparinux versus intravenous unfractionated heparin in the initial treatment of pulmonary embolism. *N Engl J Med.* 2003;349:1695–1702.

57. Kearon C, Kahn SR, Agnelli G, et al. Antithrombotic therapy for venous thromboembolic disease: American College of Chest Physicians Evidence-Based Clinical Practice Guidelines (8th Edition). *Chest.* 2008;133:454S.

58. Thabut G, Thabut D, Myers RP, et al. Thrombolytic therapy of pulmonary embolism: a meta-analysis. *J Am Coll Cardiol.* 2002;40(9):1660–1667.

59. Goldhaber SZ, Visani L, De Rosa M. Acute pulmonary embolism: clinical outcomes in the International Cooperative Pulmonary Embolism Registry (ICOPER). *Lancet.* 1999;353(9162):1386–1389.

60. Dong B, Jirong Y, Liu G, et al. Thrombolytic therapy for pulmonary embolism. *Cochrane Database Syst Rev.* 2006;(2):CD004437.

61. Dalla-Volta S, Palla A, Santolicandro A, et al. PAIMS 2-alteplase combined with heparin versus heparin in the treatment of acute pulmonary embolism: plasminogen Activator Italian Multicenter Study 2. *J Am Coll Cardiol.* 1992;20:520–526.

62. Goldhaber SZ, Haire WD, Feldstein ML, et al. Alteplase versus heparin in acute pulmonary embolism: randomized trial assessing right ventricular function and pulmonary perfusion. *Lancet.* 1993;341:507–511.

63. Konstantinides S, Giebel A, Heusel G, et al. Heparin plus alteplase compared to heparin alone in patients with submassive pulmonary embolism. *N Engl J Med.* 2002;347:1143–1150.

64. Kucher N, Rossi E, De Rosa M, et al. Massive pulmonary embolism. *Circulation.* 2006;113:577–582.

65. Bailen MR, Cuadra JA, Aguayo De Hoyos E. Thrombolysis during cardiopulmonary resuscitation in fulminant pulmonary embolism: a review. *Crit Care Med.* 2001;29(11):2211–2219.

66. Kurkciyan I, Meron G, Sterz F, et al. Pulmonary embolism as a cause of cardiac arrest: presentation and outcome. *Arch Intern Med.* 2000;160(10):1529–1535.

67. Fiumara K, Kucher N, Fanikos J, et al. Predictors of major hemorrhage following fibrinolysis for acute pulmonary embolism. *Am J Cardiol.* 2006;97(1):127–129.

68. Meyer G, Gisselbrecht M, Diehl JL, et al. Incidence and predictors of major hemorrhagic complications from thrombolytic therapy in patients with massive pulmonary embolism. *Am J Med.* 1998;105(6):472–477.

69. Gore JM. Prevention of severe neurologic events in the thrombolytic era. *Chest.* 1992;101(4)(suppl):124S–130S.

70. Goldhaber SZ. Modern treatment of pulmonary embolism. *Eur Respir J Suppl.* 2002;35:22s–27s.

71. Kanter DS, Mikkola KM, Patel SR, et al. Thrombolytic therapy for pulmonary embolism. Frequency of intracranial hemorrhage and associated risk factors. *Chest.* 1997;111(5):1241–1245.

72. Decousus H, Leizorovicz A, Parent F, et al. A clinical trial of vena caval filters in the prevention of pulmonary embolism in patients with proximal deep-vein thrombosis. Prevention du Risque d'Embolie Pulmonaire par Interruption Cave Study Group. *N Engl J Med.* 1998;338(7):409–415.

73. Eight-year follow-up of patients with permanent vena cava filters in the prevention of pulmonary embolism: the PREPIC (Prevention du Risque d'Embolie Pulmonaire par Interruption Cave) randomized study. *Circulation.* 2005;112(3):416–422. Epub 2005 Jul 11.

74. Kuo WT, van den Bosch MA, Hofmann LV, et al. Catheter-directed embolectomy, fragmentation, and thrombolysis for the treatment of massive pulmonary embolism after failure of systemic thrombolysis. *Chest.* 2008;134(2):250–254.

75. Schmitz-Rode T, Janssens U, Duda SH, et al. Massive pulmonary embolism: percutaneous emergency treatment by pigtail rotation catheter. *J Am Coll Cardiol.* 2000;36(2):375–380.

76. Eid-Lidt G, Gaspar J, Sandoval J, et al. Combined clot fragmentation and aspiration in patients with acute pulmonary embolism. *Chest.* 2008;134(1):54–60.

77. Leacche M, Unic D, Goldhaber SZ, et al. Modern surgical treatment of massive pulmonary embolism: results in 47 consecutive patients after rapid diagnosis and aggressive surgical approach. *J Thoracic Cardiovasc Surg.* 2005;129:1018–1023.

78. Meneveau N, Seronde MF, Blonde MC, et al. Management of unsuccessful thrombolysis in acute massive pulmonary embolism. *Chest.* 2006;129:1043–1050.

79. Hutten BA, Prins MH. Duration of treatment with vitamin K antagonists in symptomatic venous thromboembolism. *Cochrane Database Syst Rev.* 2006;(1):CD001367.

80. Campbell IA, Bentley DP, Prescott RJ, et al. Anticoagulation for three versus six months in patients with deep vein thrombosis or pulmonary embolism, or both: randomized trial. *BMJ.* 2007;334(7595):674.

81. Pinede L, Ninet J, Duhaut P, et al. Comparison of 3 and 6 months of oral anticoagulant therapy after a first episode of proximal deep vein thrombosis or pulmonary embolism and comparison of 6 and 12 weeks of therapy after isolated calf deep vein thrombosis. *Circulation.* 2001;103(20):2453–2460.

82. Ridker PM, Goldhaber SZ, Danielson E, et al. Long-term, low-intensity warfarin therapy for the prevention of recurrent venous thromboembolism. *N Engl J Med.* 2003;348(15):1425–1434. Epub 2003.

83. Kearon C, Gent M, Hirsh J, et al. A comparison of three months of anticoagulation with extended anticoagulation for a first episode of idiopathic venous thromboembolism. *N Engl J Med.* 1999;340(12):901–907.

84. Agnelli G, Prandoni P, Becattini C, et al. Extended oral anticoagulant therapy after a first episode of pulmonary embolism. *Ann Intern Med.* 2003;139(1):19–25.

PATIENT AND FAMILY INFORMATION FOR:
Pulmonary Embolism

At least 100,000 cases of pulmonary embolism (PE) occur each year in the United States. PE is the third most common cause of death in hospitalized patients. Most of these deaths occur within the first few hours of the happening.

Causes: A PE is a blood clot in the lung. This blood clot typically comes from blood vessels in the leg, pelvis, and arms. A clot that forms in the legs, pelvis, or arms is called deep venous thrombosis. A clot that travels in the bloodstream to different parts of the body is called an embolus.

Risk factors: Blood clots can form in deep veins because of one of the following reasons:

- Damage occurs to the inner lining of the vein as may result from injuries caused by physical, chemical, or biological factors such as surgery, serious injury, inflammation, and an immune response.

- Blood flow is slow as in prolonged immobilization such as postsurgery, being sick and in bed for a long time, or traveling.

- The blood is more likely to clot than normal as in certain inherited conditions (such as factor V Leiden, antithrombin III) or treatment with birth control pills or hormones.

In hospitalized patient we use blood thinners to stop blood clot development.

Deep venous thrombosis symptoms: Swelling of the affected part, gradual onset of pain, redness, warmth to the touch, worsening of leg pain when bending the foot, leg cramps especially at night, and bluish or whitish discoloration of skin (Figure 28.2).

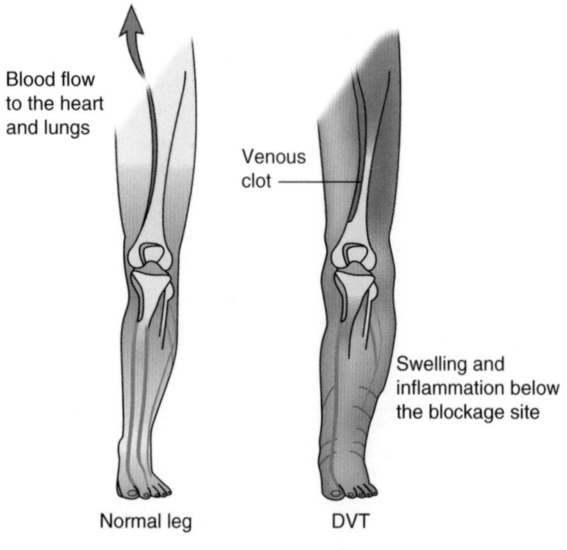

Almost 30% to 50% of patients with DVT do not experience any symptoms.

PE, what is happening? The lung is made of clusters of tiny air sacs and capillaries. The exchange of the air between the lungs and blood are through the arterial and venous systems. Arteries and veins carry and move blood throughout the body, but the process for the two blood vessels is very different. Remember how the blood circulation works, the venous system brings blood low in oxygen from the organs and periphery back to the right side of the heart. Blood then gets pumped through the pulmonary arteries to the lungs for oxygenation.

For the PE to occur the blood clot (embolus) must travel from the veins in the leg, through the heart into the lungs. This blood clot travels inside the vessels of the lung until it reaches the smaller vessels where it becomes stuck or wedged. Once the clot gets wedged it prevents any further blood from traveling to that part of the lung. When no blood reaches a part of a lung that part of the lung suffers an infarct, meaning it dies because no blood or oxygen is reaching it. This is referred to as a pulmonary or lung infarct (Figure 28.3).

When the small arteries of the lung become blocked by a pulmonary embolus they cannot carry as much blood. When this happens, pressure builds up. The heart needs to work harder to force the blood through the vessels against this pressure and the right side of the heart will become enlarged. Consequently, not enough blood flows to the lungs to pick up oxygen and heart failure that involves the right side of the heart occurs (Figure 28.4).

PE symptoms: The symptoms include chest pain, cough, rapid breathing, rapid heartbeat, and shortness of breath. Other symptoms that may occur are anxiety, bluish skin discoloration, sweaty skin, dizziness, leg pain, fainting, low blood pressure, or sudden death.

EXAMS AND TEST

The following laboratory tests and imaging may be done to evaluate how well your lungs are working and where the clot is located (Figure 28.5).

Arterial blood gases (ABG). ABG is done to test how well your lungs move oxygen into the blood and remove carbon dioxide from the blood. Most of the blood tests are performed on venous blood (blood from the vein)—after the blood has already passed through the body's tissues but an ABG test uses blood drawn from an artery, where

Blood flow to the heart and lungs

Venous clot

Swelling and inflammation below the blockage site

Normal leg   DVT

Figure 28.2. Symptoms of deep venous thrombosis. DVT, deep vein thrombosis.

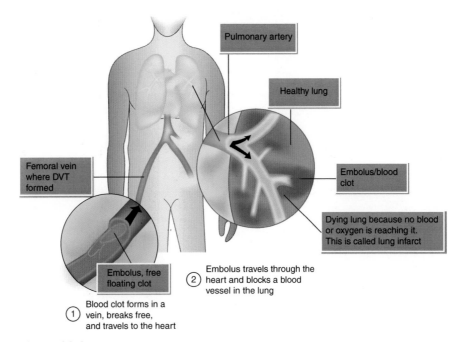

Figure 28.3. Mechanism for development of pulmonary embolism.

the oxygen and carbon dioxide levels can be measured before they enter body tissues.

D-dimer level. This test measures a substance in the blood that is released when a blood clot dissolves. If the test shows high levels of the D dimer, there is a possibility of a deep vein blood clot. If D dimer is normal, DVT is unlikely.

Electrocardiogram (EKG). It is a test that records the heart's activity by measuring electrical currents through the heart muscle. In case of PE, tachycardia (rapid heartbeat) is frequently seen and also several rhythm patterns. These results can help in the diagnosis.

Chest X-ray involves exposing a part of the body to a small dose of ionizing radiation to produce images of the inside of the body. A chest X-ray makes images of the heart, lungs, airways, blood vessels, and the bones of the spine and chest. A PE cannot be seen on the chest X-ray. However, if a part of the lung tissue dies, this can be seen on the X-ray and it is called lung infarct.

CT angiogram of the chest is a special X-ray with sophisticated computers to produce multiple cross-sectional pictures of the inside of the chest used for the diagnosis of PE. The test takes approximately 30 minutes and some of the side effects include allergic reaction to the contrast media and renal failure; however, the benefits of an accurate diagnosis far outweigh the risk. You will be asked to sign a consent form for the CT angiogram.

Pulmonary ventilation/perfusion scans or *V/Q scan.* It is a test that measures air and blood flow in the lungs to diagnose PE. The ventilation scan shows where air flows in the lungs and the perfusion scan shows where blood flows in the lungs. The scans use a low-risk radioactive substance. For the ventilation scan, a small amount of radioisotopic

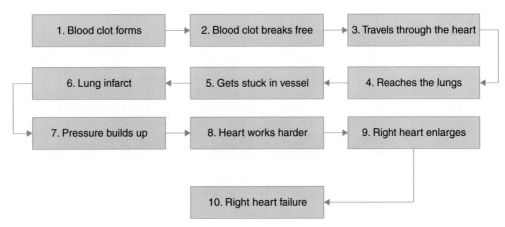

Figure 28.4. Mechanisms involved in the progression of pulmonary embolus and development of heart failure.

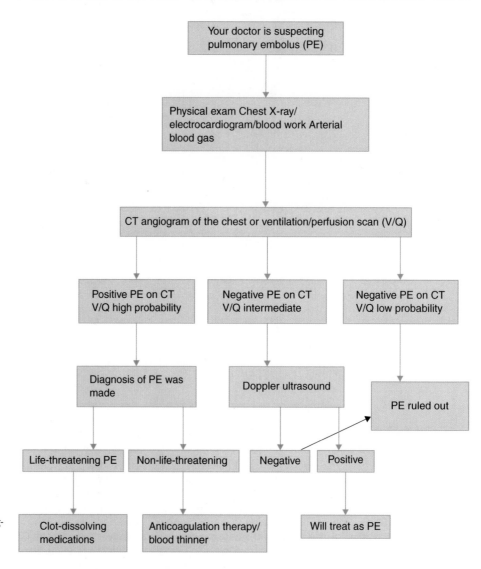

Figure 28.5. Algorithm for diagnosis and treatment of pulmonary embolism.

gas is inhaled and for the perfusion scan, the isotope is injected into a vein in the arm. Special scanners outside of your body create images of air and blood flow patterns in the lungs. The presence of an embolus will show as a mismatch between ventilation of the portion of the lung and its blood perfusion.

Pulmonary angiogram. This is an X-ray test taken after a dye is injected into the blood vessels in the lungs. The test shows areas of blockage in the lungs. It provides a clear picture of the blood flow through the arteries. It is seldom done because of the side effects associated with the use of dye.

Doppler ultrasound exam of an extremity. The test uses ultrasound to examine the blood flow in the veins. A water-soluble gel is placed on a transducer, which directs the high-frequency sound waves to the veins being tested to diagnose deep venous thrombosis.

Echocardiogram is a test in which ultrasound is used to examine the heart motion, shape, and function.

Blood tests check whether you have an inherited blood clotting disorder that can predispose for clots to form.

TREATMENT

The goal is to stabilize the heart and the lung function and to prevent new clots from forming. Oxygen therapy may be required to maintain normal oxygen levels. In cases of severe, life-threatening PE, treatment may involve dissolving the clot and preventing new clots from forming.

Treatment to prevent clots is called anticoagulation therapy or simply use of blood thinners. The most commonly used clot-prevention medicines are heparin and warfarin (Coumadin). Heparin or heparin-type drugs can be given intravenously (into a vein) or as injections under the skin (subcutaneous). These are the first medications to be given and they are transitioned over to warfarin which is given in pill form.

Patients who have reactions to heparin or related medications may need other medications.

For patients who are very ill and at risk of dying, your doctors may want to use a strong medicine to break up the blood clot—called thrombolytic or TPA. Because these medicines are very powerful in breaking up the blood clot in the lung, they can cause bleeding elsewhere—it is most dangerous and worrisome if bleeding occurs in the brain. Although the chance is low, if it does occur, it may be fatal.

Patients who cannot tolerate blood thinners or for whom they may be too risky may need a device called an IVC filter. This device is placed in the main central vein in the belly area. It prevents large clots from traveling into the blood vessels of the lungs (Figure 28.5).

Louis Brusco Jr.

Sedation and Analgesia in the Cardiac Care Unit

Patients in a cardiac care unit (CCU) experience pain, anxiety, stress and, at times, delirium and altered mental status. Sedation and analgesia of these patients is not only a humane way to treat their discomfort but it also is an integral part of their therapy to allow them to tolerate the various other therapies, treatments, and instrumentation that they are subjected to in the critical care setting. It is also integral in reducing the metabolic response and oxygen demands of the critically ill cardiac patient.

Sedatives and analgesic medications carry with them hemodynamic, respiratory, neurologic, and other side effects, so that proper sedation is a balance between adequacy of sedation and minimizing these other effects. In addition, development of delirium in the cardiac care setting is a complication that dramatically affects the survival and quality of life of patients after they have recovered from their illness. Recently, the implication of the very choice of the agent in the development of delirium has led to a reevaluation of the impact of all sedative/analgesic regimens in the context of their propensity to cause or help delirium.

The desired level of sedation in the cardiac care setting can vary widely between the awake, alert, conversant, oriented, and comfortable patient, and the patient who is in a drug-induced coma and therapeutically paralyzed. The precise level of sedation and the agents used are determined by the indications for sedation, whether they are anxiety, insomnia, agitation, coordination with a mechanical ventilator, prevention of removal of tubes or lines, protection against myocardial ischemia, or the need for amnesia during paralysis. Agents are chosen depending on the relative amounts of the different components of analgesia, anxiolysis, amnesia, sleep, and muscle relaxation that are needed.

Although use of pharmacologic agents is the main way to achieve these goals, it cannot be stressed enough that other measures that reduce even the very need for sedation are tremendously beneficial to patients, their comfort, and the avoidance of confusion and delirium. Such measures include orientation, assurance, and communication from the nursing staff; proper environmental controls such as lighting, temperature, and noise control; assessment and management of sensations such as hunger, thirst, and need to void; providing a variety of stimuli, such as visitors and media; and maintenance of a diurnal variation, with, if possible, a window facing the outside.

EVALUATION OF LEVEL OF SEDATION

One goal of management of critically ill cardiac patients is maintaining an optimal level of pain control and sedation. Unfortunately, pain and anxiety are subjective and somewhat difficult to measure consistently from caregiver to caregiver. More than 50% of patients who were interviewed after their ICU stays rated their pain as moderate to severe, during rest as well as during procedures.[1-3] Thus, the assessment of pain and anxiety must be discussed first before moving on to the pharmacology of the agents.

Although patients in a CCU are monitored with highly sophisticated equipment, technological methods of pain and anxiety such as those using electroenphalography (EEG), cerebral function analyzing monitors (CFAM), lower esophageal contractility, combinations of physiologic variables, or serum concentrations of medications, among others, have all proven to be no more reliable and a lot more complicated and expensive as compared to simple, clinically based scoring systems. Properly designed scoring systems can be used not only to assess and record pain and anxiety but also to allow the bedside nurse to titrate therapy more in a more tightly defined window on their own, meeting regulatory requirements without needing repeated orders from a practitioner who is licensed to prescribe the medications.

The most basic of clinical methods of pain assessment is simply asking the patient to rate their pain on a scale of 0 to 10, with zero being no pain at all and 10 being the worst pain one could imagine. Although simple and widely used, and despite those instructions being given, the very fact that not infrequently some patients will answer "11" shows that when pain is being experienced acutely, the overall severity of the pain seems much greater than some historical control. One step up from a simple number scale is the use of a Visual Analog scale (VAS)—which is simply a line that has the above scale marked off in measured intervals. This scale is highly reliable and valid from patient to patient and caregiver to caregiver.[4] It can be further modified to have pictures of happy and unhappy patients or faces on the scale in varying degrees instead of numbers. Unfortunately, it is limited because it ignores qualitative aspects of pain, and many critically ill cardiac patients are not strong enough or awake enough to use such a system.

Measuring sedation and level of consciousness is similarly difficult and requires the assessment of a practitioner observing the patient. The most basic method is to perform a mental status and neurologic exam and report the results. This is not practical on a repeated basis and does not allow the easy determination of changes that would allow titration of medications from time to time. The Glasgow coma scale (GCS) is widely used for the assessment of level of consciousness, but it was designed and validated for patients with neurologic deficits and is not designed for assessment of sedation.

Sedation scales are subjective tools that, in general, measure the patient's responsiveness to verbal, audio, and/or physical stimuli. The ideal scale would determine the degree of sedation and agitation, be applicable in a variety of patient situations, have a well-defined sedation goal, include behavioral descriptors, be easy to measure and score with minimal training, and be reproducible, reliable, and valid across caregivers. Proper use of such as scale can reduce the duration of mechanical ventilation and also the length of stay in both the CCU and the hospital.[5] However, even though this has been known for more than 10 years, the clinical use of scoring systems still remains low.[6] It is therefore imperative that every patient care area or unit that sedates critically ill patients chooses a sedation scale that best fits its patients, trains the caregivers in its use, and develops procedures to use that information in the sedation of the patients in the cardiac care area.

One of the most widespread of the currently used sedation scales is the Ramsay sedation scale (RSS), introduced in 1974 and modified slightly since then. The modified scale is shown in Table 29.1. Although it was primarily designed for use during research into sedative agents and was groundbreaking, it was less than ideal for clinical use. Since its debut, many others have been developed for different reasons. Some of the more commonly referenced or clinically used ones include the sedation–agitation scale (SAS—Table 29.2),[7] the motor activity assessment scale,[8] the Vancouver interactive and calmness scale (VICS),[9] the Richmond agitation–sedation scale (RASS; Table 29.3),[10] the adaptation to intensive care environment (ATICE) instrument,[11] and the Minnesota sedation assessment tool (MSAT).[12]

A thorough review and comparison of the above scales is beyond the spectrum of this chapter.[13] The decision to use one scale or the other is many times a local, multidisciplinary decision. What is important is that a scale is indeed used and that it is performed in a standard and consistent fashion.

ANALGESIC AND SEDATIVE AGENTS

Critically ill cardiac patients are often treated with continuous infusions of potent medications. Some, such as sedative-hypnotics, have sedation as a primary action; whereas others, such as opioids, have a sedative action that is a secondary effect to the primary analgesic effect. Patients require sedatives because of pain, anxiety, delirium, and the desire to keep them from remembering an uncomfortable time in their lives. Most often it is much easier to administer such medications through continuous infusion when patients are on mechanical ventilation. Use of such agents through continuous infusion, however, is associated with prolonged mechanical ventilation and a longer stay in the CCU, whereas daily interruption of sedative treatment has been shown to reduce the duration of mechanical ventilation and CCU duration.[14] Thus it is no longer considered acceptable to sedate patients to a deep state but rather to move to a lighter plane of sedation. This is more difficult and requires the use of sedation scales as above, sedation protocols, and the selection of agents that are somewhat easier to titrate and have shorter durations of action than in use previously. It has also been shown that a shift towards more of an analgesic-based sedation instead of a sedative-hypnotic-based regimen is beneficial.[15,16] We will therefore review the most commonly used agents in the CCU for sedation.

Some definitions are needed to help in the classification and description of the various agents. "Analgesic agents" have as their primary mode of action the reduction of patients' pain. They usually will have the sedation of patients as a side effect, but the sedative effect and the analgesic effect may have different potencies and durations of action. Analgesics can be broadly divided into "opioids," meaning morphine-like in action, and "nonopioids" that are medications such as nonsteroidal anti-inflammatory agents and acetaminophen.

"Sedative-hypnotics" are medications that have as their primary effect the reversible depression of the central nervous system, inducing sleep, allaying anxiety, and causing amnesia.

Other drugs used in sedation are drugs such as "psychotropic medications," for example, haloperidol or risperidone that are antipsychotic medications that interfere with neurotransmitters in the brain, which affect the way the cerebral neurons interact with each other.

OPIOIDS

Opioids are the mainstay of analgesic therapy in the CCU patient. Opioid analgesics, such as morphine, act selectively on neurons that transmit and modulate nociception, leaving other sensory modalities and motor functions intact. Opioid receptors are found in the brain, spinal cord, and peripheral tissues. When bound to receptors, opioids produce analgesia, drowsiness, changes in mood, and mental clouding. An important feature of opioid analgesia is that it is not associated with loss of consciousness except at extremely high doses. When given to a patient who is not in pain, the effect will often be described as unpleasant and troubling.

All opioids depress respiratory drive in a dose-dependent manner, and this depression is increased when opioids are given in conjunction with sedative-hypnotic medications. In general, opioids have minimal hemodynamic effects when given to patients who are not volume depleted but can cause hypotension in patients who are volume depleted owing to venodilatation. The primary problems with long-term administration of opioids are tachyphylaxis, dependence, and withdrawal symptoms on discontinuation of long-term continuous infusion. A dosing summary is presented in Table 29.4.

TABLE 29.1	Modified Ramsay Sedation Scale
Score	*Definition*
1	Anxious and agitated or restless or both
2	Cooperative, oriented, and tranquil
3	Responds to commands only
4	Brisk response to a light glabellar tap or loud auditory stimulus
5	Sluggish response to a light glabellar tap or loud auditory stimulus
6	No response to a light glabellar tap or loud auditory stimulus

Performed using a series of steps: observation of behavior (score 1 or 2), followed (if necessary) by assessment of response to voice (score 3), followed (if necessary) by assessment of response to loud auditory stimulus or light glabellar tap (scores 4–6).

TABLE 29.2	Sedation-Agitation Scale (SAS)	
Score	Term	Descriptor
7	Dangerous Agitation	Pulling at ET tube, trying to remove catheters, climbing over bedrail, striking at staff, thrashing side-to-side
6	Very Agitated	Requiring restraint and frequent verbal reminding of limits, biting ETT
5	Agitated	Anxious or physically agitated, calms to verbal instructions
4	Calm and Cooperative	Calm, easily arousable, follows commands
3	Sedated	Difficult to arouse but awakens to verbal stimuli or gentle shaking, follows simple commands but drifts off again
2	Very Sedated	Arouses to physical stimuli but does not communicate or follow commands, may move spontaneously
1	Unarousable	Minimal or no response to noxious stimuli, does not communicate or follow commands

GUIDELINES FOR SAS ASSESSMENT

1	Agitated patients are scored by their most severe degree of agitation as described
2	If patient is awake or awakens easily to voice ("awaken" means responds through voice or head shaking to a question or follows commands), that's an SAS 4 (same as calm and appropriate—might even be napping)
3	If more stimuli such as shaking is required but patient eventually does awaken, that's SAS 3
4	If patient arouses to stronger physical stimuli (may be noxious) but never awakens to the point of responding yes/no or following commands, that's an SAS 2
5	Little or no response to noxious physical stimuli represents an SAS 1

ETT=Endotracheal Tube

TABLE 29.3	Richmond Agitation–Sedation Scale	
Score	Term	Description
+4	Combative	Overtly combative or violent, immediate danger to staff
+3	Very agitated	Pulls on or removes tube(s) or catheter(s) or exhibits aggressive behavior toward staff
+2	Agitated	Frequent nonpurposeful movement or patient–ventilator dyssynchrony
+1	Restless	Anxious or apprehensive but movements not aggressive or vigorous
0	Alert and calm	
−1	Drowsy	Not fully alert, but has sustained (>10) awakening, with eye contact, to voice
−2	Light sedation	Briefly (<10) awakens with eye contact to voice
−3	Moderate sedation	Any movement (but no eye contact) to voice
−4	Deep sedation	No response to voice but any movement to physical stimulation
−5	Unarousable	No response to voice or physical stimulation

Performed using a series of steps: observation of behaviors (score +4 to 0), followed (if necessary) by assessment of response to voice (score −1 to −3), followed (if necessary) by assessment of response to physical stimulation such as shaking shoulder and then rubbing sternum if no response to shaking shoulder (score −4 to −5).

Morphine. Morphine is the prototypical opioid. It was discovered in 1804 and is the most abundant alkaloid found in opium. It has been sold commercially for almost 200 years and remains a mainstay in the sedation of critically ill cardiac patients, despite the fact that other opioids lack some of the problems associated with morphine, This is primarily because of cost and familiarity factors. The dose required to produce analgesia, as in most opioids, varies and is dependent on factors such as tolerance, tachyphylaxis, and metabolic and excretory ability. Although morphine is metabolized in the liver, 6% to 20% of the

TABLE 29.4	Analgesics Used in the CCU		
Drug	*Elimination Half-Life*	*Peak Effect (IV)*	*Starting Dose*
Morphine	2–4 h	10–30 min	1–4 mg bolus
			1–5 mg/h infusion
Hydromorphone	2–4 h	10–20 min	0.2–1 mg bolus
			0.5–2 mg/h infusion
Fentanyl	2–5 h	2–3 min	25–100 μg bolus
			25–200 μg/h infusion
Remifentanil	4 min	1.5 min	6–9 μg/kg/h infusion
Methadone	12–24 h	30–60 min	5–50 mg every 6–12 h based on previous opioid dose

metabolites are morphine-6-glucoronide, a metabolite that is excreted by the kidneys[17,18] and although the data are variable, this metabolite is anywhere from half as potent to 20 to 40 times more potent than morphine itself[18,19] and can accumulate in case of renal failure. For this reason, the long-acting opioid, hydromorphone, is preferred in renal failure. When given through bolus injection, morphine causes histamine release but this is not a factor when administered through infusion in CCU patients. However, when given by bolus, it was one of the classical treatments for cardiogenic pulmonary edema, as the vasodilation and preload reduction it causes, along with the analgesia, made patients in cardiogenic pulmonary edema much more comfortable.

It is the most hydrophilic opioid and therefore has the longest onset of action. A bolus dose of morphine will act in 5 to 10 minutes and last 2 to 3 hours; after continuous infusion, it does not exhibit prolongations in half-life (known as "context sensitive half-life") as seen with fentanyl and, to a lesser extent, with sufentanil and alfentanil.[20]

Usual doses to start morphine through infusion are 0.5 to 2 mg per hour. Bolus doses of morphine can be given at 2 to 4 mg every 1 to 2 hours as a start, but doses can be increased as tolerance develops. It is not unusual to see patients requiring morphine infusions of 15 mg per hour or more.

Hydromorphone. Hydromorphone, the commonest name for the drug actually called either dihydromorphone or dimorphone, is a semi-synthetic derivative of morphine. It was synthesized and researched in the 1920s. It is slightly more lipophilic than morphine and exhibits superior fat solubility and speed of onset than morphine.[21] It is thought to be three to four times stronger than morphine but with a lower risk of chronic dependency. It lacks the renally excreted active metabolites of morphine. It also has a slightly longer duration of action than morphine—approximately 3 to 4 hours. Its duration of action makes it slightly more cumbersome to adjust through continuous infusion; however, because it does not exhibit the context-sensitive half-life prolongation of fentanyl it is sometimes preferable to fentanyl via infusion for long durations of sedation.

Most clinicians will start with hydromorphone at 0.1 to 0.2 mg per hour and titrate as needed. Bolus doses of 0.5 mg given every 2 to 4 hours can be a starting point for intermittent IV dosing.

Fentanyl. Fentanyl is a fully synthetic opioid that was first developed in 1960 and has served as the parent molecule to the synthetic opioids that have been developed since then—sufentanil, alfentanil, and remifentanil. It is far more potent than morphine—approximately 40 times more potent on a milligram per milligram basis. Similar to other opioids, it works by binding to opioid receptors in the brain, spinal cord and periphery, but its highly lipophilic chemistry causes it to cross the blood–brain barrier very easily, giving it an extremely short onset of action. It does not cause histamine release, and, like other opioids, is neither an arterial vasodilator nor a negative inotrope.[22] It can, however, cause venodilatation and hypotension in a patient who is volume depleted. It is a potent blocker of endogenous catecholamines, which can be beneficial (in preventing a patient from becoming hypertensive and/or tachycardic with procedures) and detrimental (causing hypotension in patients whose hemodynamics are dependent on an elevated level of endogenous catecholamines).

Fentanyl is primarily metabolized in the liver to inactive metabolites, but its cessation of action is primarily through redistribution from the brain to the peripheral tissues rather than metabolism of active drug. Therefore, although a single or a few bolus doses have a shorter duration of action than morphine, on the order of 60 to 90 minutes, when given by infusion, even after 2 hours, the time to decrease by 50% concentration goes from 30 minutes for a bolus dose to 120 minutes with the infusion, and the time to decrease by 80% goes from 60 minutes with a bolus to more than 600 minutes with the infusion.[20] This "context-sensitive half-life" is due to slow release from the fatty compartments that fentanyl has such an affinity for, and causes a greatly prolonged effect for fentanyl when given by infusion—to an effective half-life much longer than morphine after a few hours of infusion.

Fentanyl also has a particular problem in many patients—of having rapidly escalating dosing requirements.[23] It is not uncommon for patients to start out on one dose, and 24 to 48 hours later be requiring four to five times as much as they were just a day or two earlier. This tolerance seems greater for many patients than with the longer-acting opioids and, combined with the context-sensitive half-life prolongation, make fentanyl a less than ideal medication to use for critically ill cardiac patients for any longer than 24 to 48 hours.

Fentanyl dosing usually starts at 50 to 100 μg for a bolus dose or 50 to 100 μg per hour via infusion with titration—it is not uncommon to rapidly (over 24 to 72 hours) require 500 to 750 μg per hour via infusion.

Sufentanil. Sufentanil is similar to fentanyl in every way except that it is more potent—approximately 10 times more potent than fentanyl and almost 400 times more potent than morphine. It does not exhibit quite the same context-sensitive half-life prolongation as fentanyl. It was synthesized in 1974. It is perhaps the most potent sympatholytic opioid in clinical practice. Its use in critically ill cardiac patients has been minimal because it is still under patent protection and is much more expensive than fentanyl when used for sedation in the CCU.

Remifentanil. Remifentanil is a potent ultrashort-acting synthetic opioid.[24] It is unique in that it has a rapid onset of action, and it has an ester linkage that undergoes rapid hydrolysis by nonspecific tissue and plasma esterases, which means that it has an organ-independent metabolism and does not accumulate in either renal or hepatic failure. Its context-sensitive half-life remains at a flat 4 minutes even after prolonged infusions.[25] It is fairly potent—approximately twice as potent as fentanyl and 100 times as potent as morphine. Hemodynamically it is very stable, but unlike fentanyl it does cause histamine release when given as a bolus and many times an antihistamine such as diphenhydramine is given as an adjunct when it is used for sedation. It is a potent respiratory depressant, and practitioners familiar with its use commonly see patients who are awake but will not breathe until it is fully worn off, which happens minutes later.

Remifentanil seems to have all the makings of an ideal sedative agent for critically ill cardiac patients. Although studies have been promising, review of a meta-analysis of studies in critically ill patients[26] shows that although remifentanil use is associated with a reduction in time to tracheal extubation, there was no reduction in mortality, duration of mechanical ventilation, length of intensive care unit stay, or risk of agitation. The other reason it is not currently a viable analgesic for CCU use is that it is still on patent and extremely expensive—recent change in marketing arrangements for the drug have caused the price to double in the United States. Until the price significantly decreases, remifentanil remains a theoretical but not a practical answer to analgesic needs in the CCU.

Methadone. Almost polar opposite in pharmacology to remifentanil is methadone, among the longest-acting opioids.[27] It is a synthetic opioid that is structurally unlike morphine but still acts on opioid receptors and produces many of the same effects. It was developed in 1937 and has been used commonly owing to its long duration of action and low cost. High doses of methadone can block the euphoric effects of other opioids such as heroin and morphine, and it has become a mainstay in the treatment of patients addicted to opioid narcotics. Although that is its most common use, it does have other uses as well, and one of those is in the long-term critically ill patient. Methadone has excellent oral bioavailability (80% to 90%), has an elimination half-life of 12 to 24 hours, and is equipotent with morphine. It can be given as oral tablets or suspension, or intravenously.

Patients who are on long-term opioid infusions may suffer withdrawal symptoms on cessation—others, while not experiencing true withdrawal symptoms, simply need the medication slowly tapered to allow the patient to gradually reach a state of no sedation. Frequently, this will take place when the patient is ready to leave a CCU but is prevented from leaving by the presence of a sedative infusion. Using methadone to transition a patient from a continuous intravenous infusion of opioid

sometimes can be an ideal way to bridge this gap. Commonly, the patient will be given methadone at a dose of 0.5 to 0.75 mg per day of the equivalent amount of morphine the patient is on. The ready availability of methadone as an oral suspension makes it easy to give it even to patients receiving tube feeds. It has been studied in pediatric patients, but the pharmacology is applicable to adult patients as well.[28]

One consideration in patients receiving methadone that does not exist with the other opioids is that methadone is associated with prolongation of the QTc interval in high doses and has been implicated in progressing on to torsade de pointes. The mean daily dose in one study was >350 mg per day, a very, very high dose and in usual use it is easy to limit doses to below that, but, especially in cardiac patients who may be more predisposed to arrhythmias and QT prolongation, this must be considered.[29]

SEDATIVE-HYPNOTICS

In addition to opioids for analgesia, patients in cardiac care settings require sedation for anxiety, restlessness, agitation, and to decrease chances of remembering bad experiences in the CCU. Anxiety is best treated after pain is controlled with analgesics and reversible conditions such as hypoxia, infections, renal or hepatic failure, and metabolic abnormalities are corrected. Most sedative-hypnotics work by binding to the inhibitory γ-aminobutyric acid (BABA) receptor, which counterbalances the action of excitatory neurotransmitters. By themselves, they have minimal respiratory depressant effect unless patients are made unresponsive to outside stimuli, but with even minimal doses of opioids the respiratory depression is significantly augmented. The clinical effects are very similar—so are the differences in pharmacokinetics, cost, and side effects of administration. A dosing summary is contained in Table 29.5.

Lorazepam. Lorazepam is a moderately slow onset long-acting benzodiazepine that is available to be given either through intravenous bolus or infusion or through the oral route. Its initial onset is in 5 to 10 minutes, but a wide therapeutic dosing range means that some patients will be fairly well sedated with a small initial dose and others will require multiple, higher doses.[30] For example, patients who are withdrawing from alcohol will sometimes require very high doses, whereas elderly patients will sometimes become heavily sedated with minute doses. Elderly patients may sometimes also "disinhibit" and become very agitated with all benzodiazepines; therefore, they should be used with caution in the elderly.[31]

Lorazepam is metabolized in the liver to inactive metabolites; it has an elimination half-life of 10 to 20 hours and an effective duration of action of 3 to 6 hours. It is glucuronidated in the liver, and because the glucuronidation system is less affected in liver dysfunction than oxidative system, lorazepam may not be as affected by hepatic dysfunction as other medications, but it should still be used with caution in patients with liver dysfunction. It is not unusual for a patient to receive 24 hours of a moderate dose of lorazepam and take 5 to 7 days to wake up.

Like all members of this class of drugs, lorazepam will cause hypotension through arterial dilatation and will cause a more pronounced hypotension through venodilatation in patients who are volume depleted. Lorazepam is diluted in propylene glycol, and with long-term high-volume infusions propylene

TABLE 29.5	Sedatives Used in the CCU		
Drug	*Elimination Half-Life*	*Peak Effect (IV)*	*Starting Dose*
Midazolam	3–5 h	1–2 min	1–2 mg bolus
			0.5–10 mg/h infusion
Lorazepam	10–20 h	2–20 min	1–2 mg bolus
			0.5–10 mg/h infusion
Propofol	20–30 h	1–2 min	20–70 mg bolus (sedation)
			100–200 mg bolus (intubation)
			25–100 μg/kg/min infusion
Haloperidol	10–24 h	3–20 min	2–10 mg bolus
			2–10 mg/h infusion
Dexmedetomidine	2 h	5–15 min	0.2–1.5 μg/kg/h

glycol toxicity can occur, causing acute tubular necrosis, lactic acidosis, and a hyperosmolar state.[32]

Initial bolus doses of lorazepam are typically from 0.5 to 2 mg, and infusion rates usually start at 0.5 to 1 mg per hour and can go as high as 20 to 25 mg per hour, with rates of >100 mg per hour not unheard of for patients in severe alcohol withdrawal.

Midazolam. Midazolam is a rapid onset, short-acting benzodiazepine. It has the characteristic of causing anterograde amnesia (amnesia after administration) perhaps better than any other sedative. When given in small doses, it is not unusual for the patients to be arousable and talking and later have no recollection of those events. It has a short onset of perhaps 1 to 2 minutes, and although the half-life is 1 to 4 hours, its duration of action after a single bolus dose is <15 minutes. It is water soluble in the bottle and becomes highly lipophilic at body pH. Its short duration of action is due to rapid equilibration and redistribution among the various body compartments. Owing to its lipophilic nature and high volume of distribution in fatty compartments, it has a prolonged context-sensitive half-life and also owing to accumulation of an active metabolite, α_1-hydroxymidazolam.[33] The half-life more than doubles, but, more important, because the short duration of action after bolus dose is due to redistribution, the effective duration of action after infusions of >24 hours approaches that of lorazepam.

Midazolam is the drug of choice for short-term sedation in the nonintubated patient, especially for procedures. It has minimal respiratory depressant effects when given alone, but it highly potentiates the respiratory suppression of opioids. Dosing information is found in Table 29.5.

Propofol. Propofol is a rather unique drug that is not a benzodiazepine and has no other drugs in its class, as alkylphenol. It is highly lipophilic and totally insoluble in water and is thus prepared in a 10% lipid emulsion at a concentration of 10 mg per ml. Similar to the benzodiazepines, it works on the GABA receptor, and it has excellent sedative and hypnotic properties, adequate amnestic properties, and no analgesic properties. By itself, it has minimal respiratory depressant properties at lower doses but will suppress respiration at doses used for induction of general anesthesia, 1.5 to 2 mg per kg. Rapid equilibration across the blood–brain barrier is the reason for its extremely

rapid onset of action.[34] Unlike benzodiazepines, in addition to vasodilatation it is also a myocardial depressant and thus can cause hypotension after large bolus dosing in hemodynamically unstable patients.

Propofol shows a short duration of action after <24 hours of infusion, and infusions of longer than 24 hours show only a slight prolongation of effect; after 24 hours patients wake up much faster than with midazolam or lorazepam. It is metabolized in the liver, but there is extrahepatic metabolism as well;[35] therefore, there is little or no prolongation of effect in renal or hepatic failure.[36]

Because of its formulation, a number of considerations must be mentioned. Because it is an emulsion in lipid, with high volumes of administration fat overload is a concern, especially in patients also receiving lipid formulations as part of total parenteral nutrition. Nutritional lipids should be adjusted downwards to compensate for the lipid administered with the propofol, and patients should be followed for hypertriglyceridemia and, with longer infusions, pancreatitis.[37] The lipid nature of the propofol emulsion makes it an excellent medium to grow bacteria, and to reduce the chances of bacterial overgrowth propofol in the United States has additives to act as bacteriostatic agents. Depending on the formulation, propofol will have ethylenediaminetetraacetic acid (EDTA), sodium metabisulfite, or alcohol. Patients who are sulfite allergic could have an adverse reaction to the propofol solution.[38]

Propofol has also been implicated in a potentially fatal syndrome termed propofol infusion syndrome (PRIS).[39] Because propofol has properties similar to barbiturates such as sodium pentothal and pentobarbital in lowering cerebral metabolic rate for oxygen and decreasing intracranial pressure, it became popular to use it at fairly high doses for prolonged periods in patients with head injury and elevated intracranial pressure from cerebral edema. In 2001, the first series of cases of patients receiving propofol at doses >5 mg/kg/hour developed progressive myocardial failure with dysrhythmias, metabolic acidosis, hyperkalemia, and evidence of muscle cell destruction.[40] Other studies have confirmed a dose-dependent connection, but there have also been some patients with some of the features of PRIS who received it at lower doses for only a few hours. Therefore, anyone receiving propofol infusion must be observed for the signs of PRIS, and most institutions have installed a cap of 5 mg/kg/hour on dosage of propofol for durations >24 hours.

Dexmedetomidine. Dexmedetomidine is another unique medication with a novel mechanism of action. It binds to the α_2 receptors in the brain as an agonist, and the location of the receptors determines the action of the medication. Dexmedetomidine binds to α_2 receptors in the locus ceruleus of the brain stem, giving it its sedative and anxiolytic effects, and in the dorsal horn of the spinal cord, releasing substance P and producing its analgesic effects.[41] It causes less hypotension than clonidine, which also is an α_2 receptor agonist, and much more sedation and analgesia. The hallmark of dexmedetomidine therapy is mild sedation and induction of sleep, anxiolysis, analgesia with minimal respiratory depression, and reduction of stress response to surgery and other stimuli. The type of sleep is also important, as it comes closer than any other sedative to causing a sleep that mimics normal rapid eye movement sleep. Patients sedated with dexmedetomidine appear tranquil and comfortable, yet being readily arousable and interactive and oriented when stimulated, only to fall right back to that tranquil, sleeping state when the stimulus is discontinued.[42]

The dosing of dexmedetomidine is also different from the other sedatives mentioned above. Bolus doses are poorly tolerated, do not have a good clinical effect, and are rarely used. A loading infusion may be used at the start of the therapy, with a dose of 1 mcg per kg of actual body weight given as an infusion over 10 minutes (which translates into 6 mcg/kg/hour rate of infusion for 10 minutes). Alternatively, an infusion may just be started at the desired rate. Although in the United States, the approved dose range is from 0.2 to 0.7 mcg/kg/hour for up to 24 hours, doses higher than that for longer periods have been safely used.[43] Distribution half-life is 6 minutes, and elimination half-life is 2 hours, but effective duration of action is different—after a loading infusion, onset of sleep sensation starts during the loading and is at its peak 10 to 20 minutes after the load is complete. After cessation of therapy, there is a gradual return to baseline mental status—but because the sleep is so mild and so natural, plus other medications are also given, it is very difficult to indeed tell when the effect of the drug has lessened significantly.

The adverse effects of dexmedetomidine include paradoxical hypertension, especially during the bolus dose, followed by hypotension and bradycardia from the sympathetic inhibition. These can be beneficial, but they may also require the adjustment of other medications, such as β-blockers or calcium channel blocker medications.

The biggest drawback in using dexmedetomidine is a practical one. The other sedatives used via infusion in a cardiac care setting can be given through bolus, and, when given through bolus or at high enough rates of infusion, reliably produce a patient who is essentially unresponsive to painful stimuli. This level of sedation is difficult, if not impossible, to attain with dexmedetomidine alone. Thus, other medications often need to be used for sudden breakthroughs of agitation and pain, and the need for those additional medications many times discourages caregivers from gaining extensive experience with dexmedetomidine.

Because of the more natural sleep pattern that is produced by dexmedetomidine, there has been hope that it will reduce the amount of delirium seen in patients in critically ill patients.

Delirium has become an important topic of discussion in critical care, as can be seen in the next section.

DELIRIUM

Over the past 10 years delirium in all types of critically ill patients has become an important area of concern. Even as medical knowledge and technology over time have improved survival of severely ill patients, many times their mental state after such recovery was less than optimal. Patients would recover from their multisystem organ dysfunction, only to be left with a delirious mental status that required long-term sedation, rehabilitation, or institutionalization in a skilled nursing facility. Elderly patients in particular seemed more susceptible to the onset of delirium, and it has been diagnosed in up to 60% to 80% of patients requiring mechanical ventilation.[44] Having delirium in a CCU is associated with a higher reintubation rate, a higher mortality, and a longer length of stay. It also has a high rate of progression to permanent cognitive impairment. Thus, it is no longer a condition that can be expected to clear once the patient leaves the CCU.

Delirium is a disturbance in consciousness with inattention accompanied by a change in cognition or perceptual disturbance that develops acutely over a short period, from a few hours to a few days.[45] It can be further broken down into hyperactive and hypoactive forms.[46] The hyperactive form, commonly mislabeled "ICU psychosis" in the past, is characterized by agitation, restlessness, attempting to remove catheters and tubes, and emotional lability. It has a better long-term prognosis. The hypoactive form is characterized by withdrawal, lethargy, flat affect, apathy, and decreased responsiveness. It is sometimes erroneously termed ICU or critical care "encephalopathy." Making the diagnosis of either type with precision is sometimes difficult and can be done with one of two validated tools that can be found here.[44,47]

For the purposes of this chapter, it is important to recognize a number of aspects of delirium in critically ill cardiac patients. First is to diagnose it, and to rule out other organic causes of the condition. Second is to realize that sedative regimens that are used in the CCU have been implicated in the development of delirium. Sedatives and analgesics work by altering neurotransmitter levels, and the exposure to benzodiazepines and/or opioids are involved in 98% of patients with delirium.[48] Some agents within a class have at times been shown to be more causative of delirium than others. Morphine,[49] fentanyl,[50] midazolam,[50] and lorazepam[51] have all been implicated in the development of delirium, with lorazepam probably being the most consistently implicated. Conversely, the newer, more expensive agents, dexmedetomidine[52] and remifentanil,[53] may have lower incidences of delirium. It has not yet been established, however, if the costs involved in using remifentanil or dexmedetomidine, among the other disadvantages, are worth the reduction in delirium.

Finally, it is important to know what can be used to treat the hyperactive type of delirium and what can be done to prevent delirium in the first place. As far as treatment of the delirium goes, in the past it was thought that patients needed to be "unscrambled;" therefore, potent antipsychotic medications, such as haloperidol or risperidone were used. Indeed, the very initiation of using a delirium assessment tool can increase the use of haloperidol dramatically.[54] Haloperidol is the only parenteral medication available to use in the delirious patient, as benzodiazepines do not seem to be helpful.[55] Use of an atypical antipsychotic, quetiapine, seems to be the best studied and shows promise in treating patients with delirium in combination with haloperidol.[56] We are still in an early phase of this research, and much more work needs to be done.[57] Finally, it is important not to underestimate the importance of nonpharmacologic therapy. Such things as cognitive stimulation, reorientation prompts, a sleep protocol, visual and hearing aids, reminders to prevent volume depletion, and walking/exercise all reduced the incidence of delirium, and although labor-intensive, are absolutely essential in reducing and treating delirium in the CCU.[58]

CONCLUSION

Patients in a cardiac care setting many times need sedative or analgesic medications to help them through their course. These medications have benefits but also side effects that need to be considered before administering the medications. The choice of medications may have long-lasting implications for patients in their recovery phase. Using a method of treating these patients that is balanced between personal professional experience and judgment and an evidence-based approach is the best method of properly choosing the optimal regimen.

REFERENCES

1. Carroll KC, Atkins PJ, Herold GR, et al. Pain assessment and management in critically ill postoperative and trauma patients: a multisite study. *Am J Crit Care.* 1999;8:105–117.
2. Puntillo KA. Pain experiences of intensive care unit patients. *Heart Lung.* 1990;19:526–533.
3. Stanik-Hutt JA, Soeken KL, Belcher AE, et al. Pain experiences of traumatically injured patients in a critical care setting. *Am J Crit Care.* 2001;10:252–259.
4. Chapman CR, Casey KL, Dubner R, et al. Pain measurement: an overview. *Pain.* 1985; 22:1–31.
5. Brook AD, Ahrens TS, Schaiff R, et al. Effect of a nursing implemented sedation protocol on the duration of mechanical ventilation. *Crit Care Med.* 1999;27:2609–2615.
6. Payen JF, Bosson JL, Chanques G, et al. Pain assessment is associated with decreased duration of mechanical ventilation in the intensive care unit: a post hoc analysis of the DOLOREA study. *Anesthesiology.* 2009;111:1308–1316.
7. Riker RR, Picard JT, Fraser GL. Prospective evaluation of the Sedation–Agitation Scale for adult critically ill patients. *Crit Care Med.* 1999;27:1325–1329.
8. Devlin JW, Boleski G, Mylnarek M, et al. Motor Activity Assessment Scale: a valid and reliable sedation scale for use with mechanically ventilated patients in an adult surgical intensive care unit. *Crit Care Med.* 1999;27:1271–1275.
9. De Lemos J, Tweeddale M, Chittock D, et al. Measuring quality of sedation in adult mechanically ventilated critically ill patients: the Vancouver Interaction and Calmness Scale. *J Clin Epidemiol.* 2000;53:908–919.
10. Sessler CN, Gosnell MS, Grap MJ, et al. The Richmond Agitation–Sedation Scale—validity and reliability in adult intensive care unit patients. *Am J Respir Crit Care Med.* 2002;166:1344–1348.
11. De Jonghe B, Cook D, Griffith L, et al. Adaptation to the Intensive Care Environment (ATICE): development and validation of a new sedation assessment instrument. *Crit Care Med.* 2003;31:2344–2354.
12. Weinert C, McFarland L. The state of intubated ICU patients: development of a two-dimensional sedation rating scale for critically ill adults. *Chest.* 2004;126:1883–1890.
13. Sessler CN. Sedation scales in the ICU. *Chest.* 2004;126:1727–1730.
14. Kress JP, Pohlman AS, O'Connor MF, et al. Daily interruption of sedative infusions in critically ill patients undergoing mechanical ventilation. *N Engl J Med.* 2000;342:1471–1477.
15. Karabinis A, Mandragos K, Stergiopoulos S, et al. Safety and efficacy of analgesia-based sedation with remifentanil versus standard hypnotic-based regimens in intensive care unit patients with brain injuries: a randomized, controlled trial. *Crit Care.* 2004;8:R268–R280.
16. Park G, Lane M, Rogers S, et al. A comparison of hypnotic and analgesic based sedation in a general intensive care unit. *Br J Anaesth.* 2007;98:76–82.
17. Hasselström J, Säwe J. Morphine pharmacokinetics and metabolism in humans. Enterohepatic cycling and relative contribution of metabolites to active opioid concentrations. *Clin Pharmacokinet.* 1993;24:344–354.
18. Van Dorp ELA, Romberg R, Sarton E, et al. Morphine-6-glucuronide: morphine's successor for postoperative pain relief? *Anesth Analg.* 2006;102:1789–1797.
19. Frances B, Gout R, Monsarrat B, et al. Further evidence that morphine-6β-glucuronide is a more potent opioid agonist than morphine. *J Pharmacol Exp Ther.* 1992;262:25–31.
20. Shafer SL, Varvrel JR. Pharmacokinetics, pharmacodynamics and rational opioid selection. *Anesthesiology.* 1991;74:53–63.
21. Murray A, Hagen NA. Hydromorphone. *J Pain Symptom Manage.* 2005;29:S57–S66.
22. Stanley TH, Webster LR. Anesthetic requirements and cardiovascular effects of fentanyl-oxygen and fentanyl-diazepam-oxygen anesthesia in man. *Anesth Analg.* 1978;57:411–416.
23. Arnold JH, Truog RD, Scavone JM, et al. Changes in the pharmacodynamic response to fentanyl in neonates during continuous infusion. *J Pediatr.* 1991;119:639–643.
24. Glass PSA, Hardman D, Kamiyama Y, et al. Preliminary pharmacokinetics and pharmacodynamics of an ultra-short-acting opioid: remifentanil (GI87084B). *Anesth Analg.* 1993;77:1031–1040.
25. Hughes MA, Glass PSA, Jacobs JR. Context-sensitive half-time in multicompartment pharmacokinetic models for intravenous anesthetic drugs. *Anesthesiology.* 1992;76:334–341.
26. Tan JA, Ho KM. Use of remifentanil as a sedative in critically ill adults patients: a meta-analysis. *Anaesthesia.* 2009;64:1342–1352.
27. Sim SK. Methadone. *Can Med Assoc J.* 1973;109:615–619.
28. Siddappa R, Fletcher J, Heard AMB, et al. Methadone dosage for prevention of opioid withdrawal in children. *Paediatr Anaesth.* 2003;13:805–810.
29. Krantz MJ, Kutinsky IB, Robertson AD, et al. Dose-related effects of methadone on QT prolongation in a series of patients with torsade de pointes. *Pharmacotherapy.* 2003;23: 802–805.
30. Wagner BK, O'Hara DA. Pharmacokinetics and pharmacodynamics of sedatives and analgesics in the treatment of agitated critically ill patients. *Clin Pharmacokinet.* 1997;33: 426–453.
31. Greenblatt DJ, Sellers EM, Shader RI. Drug disposition in the elderly. *N Engl J Med.* 1982;306:1081–1088.
32. Horinek EL, Kiser TH, Fish DN, et al. Propylene glycol accumulation in critically ill patients receiving continuous intravenous lorazepam infusions. *Ann Phramocther.* 2009;43:1964.
33. Malacrida R, Fritz ME, Suter PM, et al. Pharmacokinetics of midazolam administered by continuous intravenous infusion to intensive care patients. *Crit Care Med.* 1992;20: 1123–1126.
34. Barr J, Egan TD, Sandoval NF, et al. Propofol dosing regimens for ICU sedation based upon an integrated pharmacokinetic-pharmacodynamic model. *Anesthesiology.* 2001;95:324–333.
35. Veroli P, O'Kelly B, Bertrand F, et al. Extrahepatic metabolism of propofol in man during the anhepatic phase of orthotopic liver transplantation. *Br J Anaesth.* 1992;68:183–186.
36. Nathan N, Debord J, Narcisse F, et al. Pharmacokinetics of propofol and its conjugates after continuous infusion in normal and in renal failure patients: a preliminary study. *Acta Anaesthesiol Belg.* 1993;44:77–85.
37. Possidente CJ, Rogers FB, Osler TM, et al. Elevated pancreatic enzymes after extended propofol therapy. *Pharmacotherapy.* 1998;18:653–655.
38. Langevin PB. Propofol containing sulfite-potential for injury. *Chest.* 1999;116:1140–1141.
39. Wong JM. Propofol infusion syndrome. *Am J Ther.* 2010;17:487–491.
40. Cremer OL, Moons KG, Bouman EA, et al. Long-term propofol infusion and cardiac failure in adult head injured patients. *Lancet.* 2001;357:117–118.
41. Kamibayashi T, Maze M. Clinical uses of alpha2-adrenergic agonists. *Anesthesiology.* 2000;93:1345–1349.
42. Coursin DB, Coursin DB, Maccioli GA. Dexmedetomidine. *Curr Opin Crit Care.* 2001;7: 221–226.
43. Tan JA, Ho KM. Use of dexmedetomidine as a sedative and analgesic agent in critically ill adult patients: a meta-analysis. *Intensive Care Med.* 2010;36:926–939.
44. Pun BT, Ely EW. The importance of diagnosing and managing ICU delirium. *Chest.* 2007;132:624–636.
45. American Psychiatric Association. *Diagnostic and Statistical Manual of Mental Disorders.* 4th ed. text revision. Washington, DC: American Psychiatric Association; 2000.
46. Meagher DJ, MacLullich AMJ, Laurila JV. Defining delirium for the International Classification of Diseases, 11th revision. *J Psychosom Res.* 2008;65:207–214.
47. Ely EW, Margolin R, Francis J, et al. Evaluation of delirium in critically ill patients: validation of the Confusion Assessment Method for the Intensive Care Unit (CAM-ICU). *Crit Care Med.* 2001;29:1370–1379.
48. Ely EW, Gautam S, Margolin R, et al. The impact of delirium in the intensive care unit on hospital length of stay. *Intensive Care Med.* 2001;27:1892–1900.
49. Dubois MJ, Bergeron N, Dumont M, et al. Delirium in an intensive care unit: a study of risk factors. *Intensive Care Med.* 2001;27:1297–1304.
50. Granberg Axèll AI, Malmros CW, Bergbom IL, et al. Intensive care unit syndrome/delirium is associated with anemia, drug therapy and duration of ventilation treatment. *Acta Anaesthesiol Scand.* 2002;46:726–731.
51. Parndaripande P, Shintani A, Peterson J, et al. Lorazepam is an independent risk factor for transitioning to delirium in intensive care unit patients. *Anesthesiology.* 2006;104:21–26.
52. Riker RR, Shehabi Y, Bolesch PM. Dexmedetomidine vs midazolam for sedation of critically ill patients: a randomized trial. *JAMA.* 2009;301:489–499.
53. Radtke FM, Franck M, Lorenz M, et al. Remifentanil reduces the incidence of post-operative delirium. *J Int Med Res.* 2010;38:1225–1232.
54. Van den Boogaard M, Pickkers P, van der Hoeven H, et al. Implementation of a delirium assessment tool in the ICU can influence haloperidol use. *Crit Care.* 2009;13:R131.
55. Lonergan E, Luxenberg J, Areosa Sastra A. Benzodiazepines for delirium. *Cochrane Database Syst Rev.* 2009;(4):CD006379.
56. Devlin JW, Roberts RJ, Fong JJ, et al. Efficacy and safety of quetiapine in critically ill patients with delirium: a prospective, multicenter, randomized, double-blind, placebo-controlled pilot study. *Crit Care Med.* 2010;38:419–427.
57. Girard TD, Panharipande PP, Carson SS, et al. Feasibility, efficacy, and safety of antipsychotics for intensive care unit delirium: the MIND randomized, placebo-controlled trial. *Crit Care Med.* 2010;38:428–437.
58. Lundström M, Edlund A, Karlsson S, et al. A multifactorial intervention program reduces the duration of delirium, length of hospitalization, and mortality in delirious patients. *J Am Geriatr Soc.* 2005;53:622–628.

PATIENT AND FAMILY INFORMATION FOR:

Sedation and Analgesia

WHY PATIENTS NEED SLEEP OR PAIN MEDICATIONS IN THE CCU

Patients in a CCU can experience pain, anxiety, stress and, at times, an altered mental status. Quite simply, a CCU is a scary and uncomfortable place to be in for any length of time. Often, it is the most severely ill patient who requires the most sedation.

Patients in a CCU will at the very least have attached to them a number of wires connecting them to the monitor, in addition to some sort of intravenous catheter. Patients who are more seriously and acutely ill may have intravenous catheters in their neck or chest, or larger tubes in their groin supporting their hearts. The most seriously ill patients will have a tube in their mouth—an endotracheal tube—to connect their lungs to an artificial respirator. Usually, more support or monitoring an apparatus provides to the patient, the more uncomfortable it tends to be. The endotracheal tube, being hard plastic in contact with the main airway, is quite possibly the most irritating. Although some patients can tolerate an endotracheal tube without sedation, most patients need some sedation to tolerate the tube.

Treatments given to patients also tend to be, at best, uncomfortable, and, at worst, painful. Critically ill patients in a bed in a CCU do not tend to cough or breathe deeply enough and need help getting phlegm up from their lungs. Sometimes this is done by clapping on their backs, which can be uncomfortable. Sometimes, however, that maneuver is not enough, and a small tube needs to be placed into the patient's nose or mouth and into their lungs to get the phlegm out before the patient develops pneumonia.

In addition to being able to tolerate devices in the CCU, there is also the need for patients to get some sleep. It is very difficult to sleep in a CCU; because things are happening at all hours of the day and night, it is difficult to make it dark enough for people to fall asleep. In addition, the monitors make noises, often with each heartbeat, and the attached cables and tubes frequently pull and wake patients up as they turn. The beds in a CCU are optimized for both durability and to keep from damaging the skin, and may not be the most comfortable for sleeping.

For these and other reasons, many times it is necessary to give patients either pain medications or sleep-inducing medications as part of their treatment in a CCU.

GOALS OF SEDATION AND PAIN MANAGEMENT IN THE CCU

Very often, family members do not have the same goals in mind as their caregivers when it comes to the treatment of pain or of the sedation of a loved one in the CCU. Some families think it is bad for the patient to be sedated and want them to be more awake and interactive, going so far as to overstimulating the patient during visits. They get the mistaken impression that if the patient is not awake, they are in either an unintended or an induced coma and that is a bad thing. They repeatedly ask for the sedation to be turned down. Other families are concerned that the patient is feeling too much discomfort or will remember too much and want them more deeply sedated.

It is important to realize that sedation of patients in the CCU has become an important area of research and concern over the last 15 years. It was always known that patients needed sedation and pain medication in a CCU for them to not pull out their tubes or hurt themselves. It was also felt that sedating patients fairly heavily was a good thing, to reduce the stress of being in the CCU, and, simply, to just be humane to the patient. Although there were always concerns that too much sedation was a bad thing, it was not until 2000 that research publications showed clearly that it was important not to oversedate patients. That one study, and others following it, showed that waking patients up every day—even for a short period—and then reevaluating the need and dose of sedation—leads to less time on the respirator, less time in the CCU, and an improved survival rate. However, it is not an easy thing to do—there is a risk of the patient getting too awake and hurting themselves, and therefore it must be done in the right patients at the right time and speed. It has also become clear through recent research that the type and amount of sedation can have strong influence on the patient's mental state long after they have recovered from their physical ailments and have left the CCU.

Usually some type of rating scale is used that makes it very easy to tell whether the patient is at the desired level of sedation. The scales are generally of two types. In the more basic scale, a patient is asked to rate their pain either on a number scale or by pointing at a line or chart, sometimes with happy or sad faces on it, sometimes with just a line or ruler on it. These are used primarily to rate the patient's pain and will be used before and after every dose of pain medication to try to put a number rating to the pain a patient is feeling. In this way, the doctors caring for the patients can adjust the amount of medication by seeing what dose produces what response.

In the other type of scale, the nurse evaluates a patient and many times will do something like talk to a patient or touch a patient, to see their reaction, then gives the patient a number scale rating to determine their level of sedation. The physicians taking care of the patient, or the CCU nurse, will sedate the patient according to those ratings; therefore the physician will write an order for sedation and it will say "titrate to sedation level X," which means the nurse has to try to adjust the medication to the keep the level at "X," whatever X is.

All this is by way of stating that it is important to have discussions with the physicians and nurses taking care of your family member about the precise goals of sedation. To be able to fully understand the sedation of a family member, ask to see the sedation scale in use in that particular CCU, discuss the desired level of sedation, and ask whether they perform a daily wake-up test. A family can also offer to help in the daily wake-up test, but that takes a progressive staff in the CCU and a family that can avoid getting emotional at the bedside, as the wake-up may not be pleasant sometimes to watch. Once you understand the goals of sedation, then you can help to try to help the staff in the CCU keep the patient at the desired level of sedation.

NONSEDATIVE METHODS OF KEEPING PATIENTS COMFORTABLE

Using medications is not the only method we have of keeping patients comfortable in the CCU. There are a number of other methods that are tried and true. The most important among these it to continually reorient the patient to time, place, and, if necessary, name. The CCU is a very confusing place, and lack of sleep plays havoc on patient's ability to keep track of time. It is not unusual for a patient in a CCU to become confused and not know where they are, or what day it is, or to overestimate the amount of time that has passed since they have seen a family member. This is more common with older patients, but younger patients can also be affected. Families tend to get very depressed and upset at such actions. Some can even get angry at their family member. It is important to remember that this happens all the time and is not at all unusual. It also does not signify any permanent damage. This is probably where family members can be the most helpful to the staff in the CCU and to the patient. It may have to be done more than once on a visit. Another good thing for family members to do is to try to get patients to remember things from outside the CCU—bringing up events, people, foods, clothing, and so on. Bringing pictures to the CCU, especially with the patient in them with other people, is a very good way to aid in this process. By repeatedly reorienting patients, telling them the day, reminding them what day or what hour they last saw you or another family member, you can help the staff in the CCU use less-sedating medications and ultimately help get the patient out of CCU faster and in better mental shape.

SEDATIVE AND PAIN MEDICATIONS IN THE CCU

It is helpful for family to understand the different types of medications that are used in the CCU to promote sleep and treat pain. This is because some of them may have different meanings to the lay person, incorrect meanings that may have a negative connotation to you. Patients in the CCU, most of the time, get either strong pain relievers such as morphine, strong sleep medications such as Ativan (lorazepam), or tranquilizers such as haloperidol. It is important for you to understand why each of those are used.

PAIN MEDICATIONS

Patients in the CCU have pain—if they are on the respirator, just the breathing tube alone causes a fair amount of discomfort and pain. Lying in bed for long periods is also uncomfortable. They may have surgical incisions, and many of the procedures that are done are painful. To treat those pains, most often patients are given medications such as morphine—others might be Dilaudid (hydromorphone), fentanyl, or even methadone. This class of drugs is commonly called opiates or narcotics. They are given through the intravenous line, either continuously or intermittently. They differ primarily in how long they last, and some of the minor side effects. For example, morphine and hydromorphone may have more of a mind-altering quality to their effect than methadone or fentanyl. Fentanyl is the shortest-acting, at about 45 minutes to an hour, then morphine, which lasts 2 to 3 hours, hydromorphone, which lasts 3 to 4 hours, and, finally, methadone that can last 8 to 12 hours. Patients who are less ill may be able to receive pain medications by mouth—these generally last longer, from 6 to 24 hours each dose.

Pain medications such as these have a number of effects. First, they are used to reduce the amount of pain a patient feels. It is important to realize that these medications do not work like when you take something for a headache—1 minute, you have pain, soon afterwards, the pain is totally gone. Most often, the patient will still feel the sensation that was painful, but it will not be as intense, they may not care that they feel it, and they will be more comfortable; they may even say that the sensation is still there but it does not hurt. Second, these medications will have somewhat of a sleep-inducing effect, but this effect is shorter than the pain-relieving effect and if small enough doses are given may be minimal if present at all. The commonest side effect regarding these medications is that they interfere with the patient's desire to breathe—so, if they go to sleep, they may not breathe, which is why they are monitored after they receive the medications. The other major side effect these medications have is that they can cause nausea and vomiting. So when these medications are given, physicians and nurses have to balance the desirable effects with the undesirable side effects.

When to give these medications is usually decided in a number of ways. If the patient is awake, it might be given only when they ask for them and not otherwise. Sometimes, a patient might be connected to a patient controlled analgesia pump where the patient gets small amounts of pain medication through the intravenous line whenever they push the button. The safety mechanism with both of these is that if the patient is too sleepy to either ask for the medication or push the button—he or she won't get too much and won't get too sleepy. This is why you might hear a nurse say that the patient has to ask for the medication himself or herself and that they cannot give it just because a family member wants the patient to get more medication because he or she is grimacing or has a look on the face that looks like pain—it might be dangerous to give the patient pain medication in that state. For patients who are more sick, the nurse might be instructed by the physicians to use a pain scale such as described above to administer medications. Finally, patients, especially those on mechanical ventilators, may be on a continuous amount of the medications so that they are getting a small amount every minute to provide constant comfort, and the rate at which they give the pain medication is determined by the scales mentioned above.

SEDATIVE (SLEEP) MEDICATIONS

In addition to medications to treat pain, to treat patients' anxiety and help them sleep, patients may also get sedative medications such as midazolam (Versed) or lorazepam (Ativan), which are modern versions of a similar drug many people know about called diazepam (Valium). These medications have a wide range of effects that depend on dose, ranging from treating anxiety and making a patient feel calm, to inducing a comfortable sleep, to rendering a patient unconscious. Even low doses can cause amnesia, and the patient may not remember things that happen while under the influence of these medications. Although this may many times be a beneficial effect, as the CCU can be a scary place, it can also make it more difficult for the family to reorient the patient as discussed earlier. Furthermore, elderly patients can sometimes get wild and agitated with these medications and lose control of inhibitions—a side effect called dis-inhibition. When combined with the pain medications described above, they can enhance the pain medication's ability to depress patients breathing; therefore they have to be used with caution when used together. Moreover, the combination of the deep sleep of the sedatives and the nausea and vomiting from the pain medications can be dangerous as patients can have stomach contents go into the lungs and cause pneumonia. This is not at all to say that they cannot be used together, just that these are concerns that need to be watched for. Both lorazepam and midazolam can either be given intermittently or continuously through the intravenous line. They differ only in that midazolam, when given once or twice, is very short-acting, of the order of 15 to 30 minutes, where lorazepam can last for 2 to 4 hours. When given continuously, depending on what dose is required and how long the infusion is running for, it can take a few hours to a few days to wear off.

Another medication that can be used continuously, usually in patients who are on mechanical ventilation, is called propofol. Propofol is easy to remember as it is a milky white liquid, sometimes nicknamed "milk of anesthesia." It is a powerful sleep-inducing agent and is usually not used to just treat anxiety, but, rather to go further and either makes patients very sleepy or even unconscious. Its ability to cause amnesia is not quite as much as for lorazepam or midazolam; so patients need to be more asleep with this medication if the goal is to keep them from remembering things. It is very short-acting, which is why it is usually used only continuously. Similar to lorazepam or midazolam, it can cause blood pressure to drop and when given with the narcotic pain relievers it can cause a patient to stop breathing.

Furthermore, a different type of medication used in these settings is a relatively new drug called dexmedetomidine (Precedex). This drug causes a very natural and restful sleep and does not work like other drugs to depress the patient's drive to breathe. The sleep it causes is totally different from other medications—the patient will appear to be asleep, not responsive to verbal stimulation, yet, with gentle touch, will wake up and be totally coherent and appropriate, only to drift back to sleep when the stimulus is removed. It also has very nice pain-relieving qualities and treats pain in a different manner than narcotics, so the combination of the two is a very effective way to treat pain. It does not have any amnesia effects; therefore it is not useful to make patients not remember their time in the CCU. It has a ceiling effect, so that it never will produce the deep sleep or near coma condition as midazolam, lorazepam, or propofol will produce, and it cannot be given intermittently but only continuously and takes some time both to work and stop working, about 20 to 30 minutes on either end. It is most useful in combination with the other medications. Its main advantage is that it recently has been shown to cause less delirium in the CCU, as discussed below.

DELIRIUM

When a patient is in the CCU and is subject to all the stresses of being there—the constant stimulation, the lights, the noise, the lack of natural sleep, and the administration of the above medications—can all sometimes result in the patient developing a state of altered consciousness called delirium. Delirium is an acute state of confusion. It is characterized by a combination of drowsiness, disorientation, hallucination, a sudden inability to focus attention, sleeplessness, and severe agitation and irritability. When it develops it carries with it a longer time in the CCU and the hospital and a higher rate of complications such as infections and death. It is more common in older patients, and one out of four elderly patients admitted to the hospital will suffer from some form of delirium. Preventive measures include the daily wake-up and lessening the use of sedatives, and the reorientation and helping the patient focus also help tremendously. Use of dexmedetomidine for sedation, with its more natural sleep tendencies, has been shown in some studies to decrease the incidence of delirium. Once it starts, it may require the use of tranquilizers that act on the chemicals in the brain that are out of balance and help straighten them out again. A number of tranquilizers can be used. If it is decided that the patient needs to get the medication fast, a medication called haloperidol (Haldol) can be given either intravenously or subcutaneously. If they are given orally, in addition to haloperidol, another common one is risperidone, and there are others as well. Tranquilizers such as these will cause a dazed and stunned look, and the patient will frequently be awake, answer questions in a rather flat toned voice, show little emotion, and have a very slow reaction to any stimuli. This is just a phase the patient will go through on their way to recovery, but it can last for some time, sometimes days or weeks, until the patient is back to the usual state of mind.

ADDICTION

A very common reaction of families to hearing that their relative is getting these medications, some of them whose names they associate with drug abuse, is "will they become addicted?" Strong pain killers such as morphine cause two types of dependence, commonly termed "addiction." Patients may get chemically or physically dependent, where their bodies cannot tolerate a sudden withdrawal of the drug, and it needs to be reduced slowly over time, otherwise the patient can get withdrawal symptoms. This is easily treated with slow tapering of the medication over time, and the risk for it goes up depending on the dose and the duration of medications the patient received in the CCU, which is another reason to give as little as possible. However, people mistake this for psychological dependency, in which the patient mentally craves the drug and needs it from a mental standpoint. Only a minute fraction of patients receiving morphine-like drugs in the CCU ever become psychologically dependent on the medications, and the risk is considered small for the benefit most patients get from these important medications. The sedative drugs such as lorazepam are much less likely but can still cause a physical dependence.

CONCLUSION

It is important to understand the choice of medications and why each is used. The doctors and nurses must balance the need to treat pain and the need to reduce stress and anxiety with the very real side effects these medications can cause. By discussing with your relative's doctors and nurses exactly what medications your relative is receiving, and what the goals of therapy are, you can both understand better the treatment plan and also be more helpful to both the staff and to the patient, because the best calming effect usually use a calm family member being at the bedside working with the staff of the CCU to keep a patient oriented, calm, and tranquil. It will also allow the family member to endure the stay of their relative in the CCU with less stress to themselves as well.

Anip Bansal
Gagangeet Sandhu
James P. Jones

CHAPTER

30

Renal Failure in the Cardiac Care Unit

DEFINITIONS

Acute kidney injury (AKI), previously called acute renal failure, is a common problem in the cardiac care unit (CCU) that is associated with increased morbidity and has an independent effect on the risk of short-term mortality. Traditionally, AKI has been defined as a rapid (i.e., over hours to weeks) and usually reversible decline in glomerular filtration rate (GFR). In an effort to standardize this subjective definition, numerous attempts have been made to define AKI more objectively. The most commonly accepted definitions are the RIFLE classification[1] and the acute kidney injury network (AKIN) criteria[2] that are listed in Table 30.1.

A new terminology, *cardiorenal syndrome*,[3] has recently been proposed to define the spectrum of disorders seen because of the hemodynamic interdependence between the heart and the kidneys. It includes those disorders of the heart and kidneys where acute or chronic dysfunction in one organ may induce acute or chronic dysfunction of the other. Five subtypes have been defined:

Type 1 acute cardiorenal syndrome: Acute worsening of cardiac function leading to renal dysfunction
Type 2 chronic cardiorenal syndrome: Chronic abnormalities in cardiac function leading to renal dysfunction
Type 3 acute renocardiac syndrome: Acute worsening of renal function causing cardiac dysfunction
Type 4 chronic renocardiac syndrome: Chronic abnormalities in renal function leading to cardiac disease
Type 5 secondary cardiorenal syndrome: Systemic conditions causing simultaneous dysfunction of the heart and kidney

EPIDEMIOLOGY AND RISK FACTORS

The incidence of AKI varies, with an average incidence of 5% in hospitalized patients and 25% in the intensive care unit.[4–6] The incidence of AKI requiring renal replacement therapy (RRT) was 4% in a large, multicenter study.[5] The incidence varies significantly owing to the lack of standardized definitions used in the literature. In a large, tertiary center CCU, characteristics such as older age, African American race, diabetes, hypertension, previous coronary disease, and heart failure were incrementally more common across increasing renal dysfunction strata.[7] Decompensated heart failure, shock, use of iodinated contrast media, aggressive diuresis, and use of nephrotoxic medications are common precipitants of AKI.

PATHOPHYSIOLOGY AND APPROACH TO ACUTE KIDNEY INJURY

The kidney plays a key role in maintenance of fluid balance and excretion of waste products. Volume depletion is initially compensated by various systemic mechanisms in an attempt to restore tissue perfusion. Hypovolemia, for any reason, reduces release of atrial natriuretic peptide, increases production of antidiuretic hormone (ADH), and increases sympathetic (and decreases parasympathetic) activity through the baroreceptor reflex. In the kidney, the combination of hypotension and sympathetic activation leads to reduced perfusion pressure in the afferent arteriole and a decrease in the GFR. A decrease in tubular sodium chloride

TABLE 30.1	Comparison of RIFLE Classification and AKIN Criteria for AKI				
RIFLE Criteria	*Serum Creatinine*	*Glomerular Filtration Rate*	*Urine Output*		*AKIN*
Risk	1.5× Upper limit of normal (ULN)	>25% decrease	<0.5 ml/kg/h for 6 h	Stage 1,	serum creatinine 1.5–2× baseline (or rise by >0.3 mg/dl)
Injury	2× ULN	>50% decrease	<0.5 ml/kg/h for 12 h	Stage 2,	2–3× baseline
Failure	3× ULN (also rise by 0.5 mg/dl if baseline level >4 mg/dl)	>75% decrease	<0.3 ml/kg/h for 24 h or anuria for 12 h	Stage 3,	>3× baseline (also if on renal replacement therapy)
Loss	Persistent acute kidney disease >4 weeks				Not defined
ESRD	End stage renal disease (requiring dialysis >3 mo)				Not defined

AKIN, Acute Kidney Injury Network; ESRD, end-stage renal disease.

(due to slower transit and increased proximal reabsorption) is sensed by the macula densa in the distal convoluted tubule, and this causes the juxtaglomerular apparatus to release renin. Renin activates angiotensin, which is converted peripherally to angiotensin II. Apart from being a potent vasoconstrictor, it also acts on the adrenal cortex to produce aldosterone, which increases salt and water reabsorption in the kidney. In addition to these mechanisms, the kidney possesses the ability to autoregulate, that is, maintain its perfusion pressure despite changes in mean blood pressure over a wide range of 80 to 180 mm Hg.

As a consequence of this compensatory mechanism, the renal tubules remain intact despite renal hypoperfusion. When normal renal perfusion is restored, urine flow returns to normal.

A concept that is important in understanding the pathophysiology of AKI in the CCU is that of effective circulating volume (ECV). ECV is the arterial blood volume effectively perfusing tissue. ECV is a dynamic quantity and not a measurable distinct compartment that normally varies directly with extracellular fluid (ECF). The ECV may not vary directly with the extravascular fluid volume in certain diseases, such as congestive heart failure (CHF) or hepatic cirrhosis; therefore, in these clinical settings, renal hypoperfusion may occur despite apparent volume excess.

In contrast to prerenal AKI, if the hypovolemia is severe or sustained owing to other toxic injuries, the renal tubules can become necrotic and lose their ability to conserve salt and water. Tubular obstruction by necrotic cells at the pars recta (where the proximal tubule narrows into the descending loop of Henle) leads to rise in the intraluminal pressure, decreasing the glomerular tubular gradient. This reduction in GFR may persist even after restoration of normal hemodynamics. Furthermore, injury to the tubular basement membrane can result in back leak of tubular fluid into the interstitial tissue. In this situation, urine flow may not be restored despite restoration of normal renal perfusion.

Based on this pathophysiology of renal adaptation to injury, the approach to AKI is the same in every clinical setting:

delineation into the three pathophysiological categories of prerenal, intrinsic renal, or postrenal AKI (Table 30.2). Prerenal azotemia results from ineffective renal perfusion and is the commonest cause of AKI in patients presenting to the emergency room. Renal or intrinsic AKI is secondary to an intrinsic renal disease and in the CCU most commonly results from ischemic or toxic acute tubular necrosis (ATN). The prerenal and intrinsic renal categories are not mutually exclusive but rather represent a continuum of renal injury where persistence of the ischemic insult may deteriorate into ATN. A prerenal state also sensitizes the kidney to nephrotoxic insults thus accounting for the increase in the incidence of AKI owing to nephrotoxic agents in hypovolemic states. Postrenal AKI owing to obstruction in the urinary collecting system is an uncommon cause of AKI in the CCU but should always be ruled out promptly because of its reversibility.

CLINICAL EVALUATION

Either a rise in the blood urine nitrogen (BUN) and serum creatinine or a drop in the urine output should alert the clinician to the presence of AKI. One of the earliest signs of AKI may be oliguria that is conventionally defined as urine output <400 ml per day. In the CCU, oliguria means insufficient urinary output for that particular patient, usually <0.5 ml/kg/hour. However, a patient who is fluid overloaded or with a high catabolic rate may require a urine flow rate considerably higher than this minimum standard. A number of etiologies of AKI present with nonoliguric rises in the BUN and creatinine; therefore absence of oliguria does not preclude an evaluation of renal injury.

The history should be focused on identification of risk factors for AKI, determination of baseline renal function to ascertain presence of chronic kidney disease (CKD) if possible, careful assessment of symptoms and precipitants of volume depletion (careful review of the intake and output), careful review of vital signs to identify episodes of hypotension, and a

TABLE 30.2	Common Etiologies of Acute Kidney Injury in the CCU

PRERENAL AKI

1. Hypovolemia, e.g., renal (diuretics) or extra renal fluid loss (bleeding, diarrhea, vomiting, sequestration)

2. Decreased renal perfusion: decreased forward flow secondary to low cardiac output, renal vasoconstriction, systemic vasodilation, hepatorenal syndrome, impairment of renal autoregulation (NSAIDS, ACE inhibitors, angiotensin receptor blockers [ARBs])

RENAL AKI

1. Acute tubular necrosis
   a. Ischemic
   b. Toxic, e.g., use of radiocontrast media, aminoglycosides, amphotericin B, calcineurin inhibitors, mannitol, hemolysis, rhabdomyolysis
   c. Infection, with or without sepsis

2. Glomerular diseases or vasculitis
   a. Glomerulonephritis, e.g., as a complication of bacterial endocarditis, lupus nephritis
   b. Thrombotic microangiopathies, e.g., malignant hypertension, scleroderma crisis

3. Interstitial nephritis commonly related to antibiotic use

4. Renovascular obstruction, e.g., atheroembolic disease, arterial dissection

POST RENAL AKI

Urinary retention owing to use of anticholinergic agents, obstruction, and compression by hematoma or mass

NSAID, Nonsteroidal anti-inflammatory drugs; ACE, angiotensin converting enzyme; ARB, angiotensin II receptor blocker.

thorough review of all home medications as well as all recently administered in-hospital medications to identify possible nephrotoxins. The history is essential in determining the etiology of AKI as it may lead the clinician to prevent further exposure to ongoing nephrotoxic insults.

Another important historical feature is the temporal correlation between the possible nephrotoxic insult and the clinical course of AKI. The serum creatinine rises rapidly (within 24 to 48 hours) in patients with AKI following renal ischemia and radiocontrast exposure. Peak serum creatinine concentrations are usually seen after 3 to 5 days with contrast nephropathy and return to baseline after 5 to 7 days. In contrast, serum creatinine concentrations usually peak later (7 to 10 days) in ATN and sometimes even later in atheroembolic disease. The rise in serum creatinine seen with many tubular epithelial cell toxins (e.g., aminoglycosides) or in the setting of drug-induced acute interstitial nephritis usually happens 7 to 10 days after onset of therapy.

"Information from the physical examination is invaluable and must be integrated with the historical and laboratory data.

The patient's volume status must be carefully assessed by examination of skin turgor, edema, jugular venous distension, orthostatic hypotension, and pulmonary vascular congestion. In addition, certain findings on physical examination can be diagnostic, for example, the presence of a distended bladder in a patient with urinary retention, a skin rash in suspected drug-induced interstitial nephritis, papilledema in malignant hypertension, or retinal cholesterol plaques in a patient with atheroembolic disease.

DIAGNOSTIC EVALUATION

Even with a careful history and examination, the etiology of AKI may be challenging. Figure 30.1 is a clinical pathway that will simplify the diagnostic approach to AKI. Microscopic examination of the urine and urinary indices can be informative. Certain findings on urinalysis can point towards specific diagnoses as shown in Table 30.3. In prerenal or postrenal AKI, the urinalysis should be devoid of cells, casts, and protein.

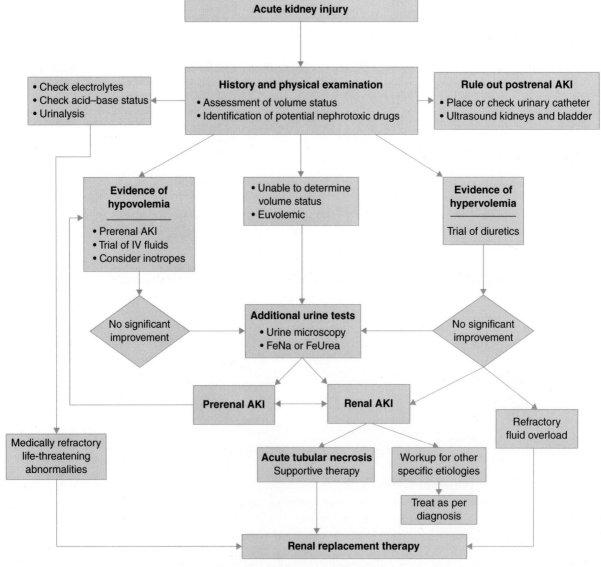

Figure 30.1. Acute kidney injury pathway. FeNa, fractional excretion of sodium.

TABLE 30.3	Urinalysis in Acute Kidney Injury
Finding	*Possible Diagnosis*
Muddy brown granular casts or epithelial cell casts	Acute tubular necrosis
RBC casts, dysmorphic RBCs	Acute glomerulonephritis
WBC casts, eosinophils	Acute interstitial nephritis
Large blood on dipstick with no RBCs	Hemoglobinuria or myoglobinuria
Specific crystals	Crystalline nephropathies, e.g., indinavir, bactrim or acyclovir associated, urate nephropathy

TABLE 30.4	Diagnostic Indices to Differentiate Prerenal and Renal Acute Kidney Injury	
Diagnostic Index	*Prerenal AKI*	*Renal AKI*
Serum BUN to creatinine ratio	>20	<10–15
Urine Na (mEq/L)	<10	>20
Urine/serum creatinine ratio	>50	<20
Urine osmolality	>500	Variable
Urine specific gravity	>1.020	~1.010
Fractional excretion of sodium (FeNa) (%)	<1	>1
Fractional excretion of urea (FeUrea) (%)	<35	>50
Fractional excretion of uric acid (%)	<12	>20

BUN, blood urine nitrogen.

Various urinary indices are commonly used to differentiate prerenal AKI from renal AKI in oliguric AKI. They cannot be used reliably in the setting of nonoliguric AKI. The most commonly used index is the fractional excretion of sodium (FeNa). FeNa is the percentage of the sodium filtered by the kidney and excreted in the urine. It is measured in terms of plasma and urine sodium rather than by the interpretation of urinary sodium concentration alone, as urinary sodium concentrations can vary with water resorption. FeNa is calculated as FeNa = [(Urine sodium/Plasma sodium)/(Urine creatinine/Plasma creatinine)] × 100. An FeNa <1% is indicative of a prerenal etiology. It is important to remember that diuretics inhibit tubular sodium reabsorption so that in the CCU, patients receiving diuretics can have an FeNa >1% despite intravascular volume depletion. A fractional excretion of urea nitrogen may be more helpful in this setting. Similarly, the FeNa can be >1% despite volume depletion in patients with underlying CKD secondary to impaired tubular function at baseline. Also, prerenal states are not the only causes of low FeNa; it can also be low in acute glomerulonephritis, early obstructive nephropathy, liver failure, contrast nephropathy, pigment-induced nephropathy, and normal renal function. Some of the other diagnostic indices in this regard are listed in Table 30.4.

Because the most commonly used marker of AKI, that is, serum creatinine rises 24 to 48 hours after the inciting injury, there is active research towards identifying newer serum and urine biomarkers for the early diagnosis of AKI. Some of the most promising markers are serum and urine neutrophil gelatinase associated lipocalcin (NGAL),[8,9] interleukin 18 (IL-18),[10] kidney injury molecule-1 (KIM-1),[11] and cystatin C. Further research is needed before these markers replace serum creatinine as a marker of AKI in the clinical setting.[12]

Although glomerular diseases are an uncommon cause of AKI in the CCU, the finding of RBC casts or dysmorphic casts should prompt further evaluation. Estimation of urinary protein excretion is an important adjunct to further classify these patients. The use of random, spot urine protein/urine creatinine ratio as an estimate of 24-hour protein excretion has simplified this task by eliminating the need for cumbersome and often inaccurate 24-hour urine collections. A random urine protein/creatinine ratio >1 g protein per g of creatinine is usually seen in the presence of glomerular diseases. This should be used only when the patient is in steady state as the results may not be accurate in the setting of AKI. A number

of serological tests for secondary etiologies could help narrow the differential diagnosis; however, a definite diagnosis would require a kidney biopsy.

All patients with AKI should have periodic monitoring of serum electrolytes (sodium, potassium, magnesium, calcium, and phosphorus) and acid–base status as these are frequently abnormal and can become life-threatening, for example, severe hyperkalemia or severe metabolic acidosis.

Even though postrenal AKI is relatively uncommon in the CCU, a renal ultrasound should be obtained in all cases of unexplained AKI. A false negative study may be due to concomitant volume depletion or extrinsic compression, for example, secondary to a retroperitoneal hematoma. In the latter scenario, a CT scan of the abdomen may be diagnostic.

DRUG DOSING

AKI affects renal drug elimination and other pharmacokinetic processes involved in drug disposition (e.g., absorption, drug distribution, metabolism). Drug dosing errors are common in patients with renal impairment and can cause adverse effects and poor outcomes. Dosages of drugs cleared renally should be adjusted according to estimated creatinine clearance. The most commonly used formulas are listed in Table 30.5. The authors recommend the CKD–EPI formula that can be easily found on the Internet. However, all these formulas were studied in patients with CKD with stable creatinine clearances and not in patients with AKI who have day-to-day variations in the GFR. The actual GFR is much lower than the estimated GFR (usually <10 ml per minute) for patients who are developing AKI and higher than the estimated GFR in patients who are in the recovery phase of AKI.

Loading doses of medications should not be decreased in patients with AKI or CKD. Recommended methods for maintenance dosing adjustments are dose reductions, lengthening the dosing interval, or both. Physicians should be familiar with commonly used medications that require dosage adjustments; however it is impossible to be aware of all the subtle

TABLE 30.5	Common Formulas Used to Estimate Glomerular Filtration Rate
Name	Formula
MDRD formula	eGFR (ml/min/1.73 m^2) = 175 × [serumcreatinine(μmol/L) × 0.0113]$^{-1.154}$ × Age (years)$^{-0.203}$ (0.742 if female)
Cockcroft–Gault	eGFR = (140-age) × (Wt in kg) × (0.85 if female) / (72 × Cr)
CKD-EPI*	eGFR = 141 × min(Scr/κ,1)$^\alpha$ × max(Scr/κ,1)$^{-1.209}$ × 0.993^{Age} × 1.018 [if female] × 1.159 [if black]

*Scr is serum creatinine (mg/dL), κ is 0.7 for females and 0.9 for males, α is –0.329 for females and –0.411 for males, min indicates the minimum of Scr/κ or 1, and max indicates the maximum of Scr/κ or 1.

adjustments that are often needed. Before prescribing any new medication, dosing in AKI/CKD should be verified using any reliable print or electronic resource. Careful monitoring of drug levels, when available, can ensure therapeutic efficacy while minimizing toxicity.

In patients who are on RRT especially those on intermittent hemodialysis (IHD), the drug dosing for those drugs that are significantly dialyzed should be scheduled to be given postdialysis.

PREVENTION OF ACUTE KIDNEY INJURY

Because very few specific treatments are available for renal AKI, the key is prevention. This is especially true for patients who are at higher risk for developing AKI, for example, patients with advanced age, preexisting renal impairment, diabetes, hypertension, congestive heart failure, sepsis, or hypovolemia.

In addition to patients with prerenal azotemia, specific groups of patients may benefit from fluid administration to prevent AKI i.e. patients with early sepsis, rhabdomyolysis and; those receiving drugs such as amphotericin B and contrast media, or drugs associated with crystal deposition such as acyclovir and sulfonamides. However, overaggressive fluid resuscitation should be avoided to prevent complications of fluid overload.

Maintenance of a mean arterial blood pressure >65 mm Hg with optimization of volume status and use of vasoactive agents is critical to maintain optimal renal perfusion. In the setting of decompensated heart failure, the judicious use of inotropes can be necessary to prevent AKI. Low-dose dopamine does increase renal plasma flow; however, clinical studies do not support the use of "renal dose" dopamine to prevent AKI or reduce the requirement of RRT.[13,14] The use of dopamine (or of fenoldopam,[15] a short-acting dopamine receptor-1 agonist) for this objective is not recommended at present.

When using potentially nephrotoxic antimicrobials, attention to drug levels, adjusted dosing, and dose interval may minimize the risk of drug-induced nephrotoxicity. Furthermore, daily assessment of continued need for broad spectrum antibiotics based on culture results is essential. Early identification of drug-induced AKI and discontinuation of the offending agent can prevent further renal injury.

CONTRAST-INDUCED NEPHROPATHY

Contrast-induced nephropathy (CIN) is generally defined as an increase in serum creatinine concentration of >0.5 mg per dl or 25% above baseline within 48 hours after contrast administration. Risk factors for CIN include advanced age, preexisting CKD, dehydration, hypotension, intra-aortic balloon pump, concomitant administration of nephrotoxic drugs, sepsis, diabetes mellitus, and congestive heart failure requiring active diuretic use. Various scoring systems are available to quantify this risk.[16] In patients with established AKI, consideration should be made to avoid the use of contrast media if possible until AKI has resolved. Certain measures such as the following may be useful in minimizing the risk of CIN:

1. The use of low-osmolar or iso-osmolar contrast media and use of lowest possible volume (e.g., avoiding left ventriculograms in patients at risk).
2. Optimization of volume status: Discontinuation of diuretics and ACEI/ARBs if possible. Use of isotonic saline starting 6 to 8 hours before contrast administration to ensure adequate hydration is a commonly used strategy.
3. Isotonic sodium bicarbonate has been shown to be superior to isotonic saline in some studies but the evidence is equivocal.[17]
4. Another agent commonly used is N-acetyl cysteine (NAC). Evidence for the preventive efficacy of NAC is equivocal, but in the absence of significant side effects it is widely used.[18]
5. All other potential nephrotoxins should be discontinued if possible.
6. Periprocedural hemodialysis has no role in the prevention of CIN.[19]

AKI POST-CARDIAC SURGERY

AKI is a common complication in postcardiac surgery also. The risk factors most commonly associated with AKI in this setting include female sex, left ventricular dysfunction, diabetes, peripheral vascular disease, chronic obstructive pulmonary disease, emergent surgery, use of intra-aortic balloon pump, cardiopulmonary bypass time, and, most important, preoperative elevations in serum creatinine.[20] The avoidance of cardiopulmonary bypass has been shown to be associated with lower incidence of postoperative AKI and should be considered if possible.[21] Recently, nesiritide[22] and fenoldopam have shown some promise in preventing postcardiac surgery AKI.

TREATMENT OF AKI

The treatment of AKI depends on the etiology of AKI. In postrenal AKI, rapid relief of obstruction will treat the AKI. Prerenal AKI owing to hypovolemia should be managed with prompt restoration of the effective circulatory volume usually by administration of crystalloid solutions. Hypovolemia can be caused by renal or extrarenal causes, and careful history and examination as outlined above is essential to determine absolute or effective hypovolemia. The adequacy of restoration of intravascular volume can be guided by periodic assessment of the central venous pressure (CVP). However, the possibility that right-sided heart failure, pulmonary arterial hypertension, or positive pressure ventilation can elevate the CVP to normal levels despite intravascular hypovolemia should always be kept in mind while interpreting the results. The use of Swan–Ganz catheter-guided therapy has fallen out of favor after trials showed that additional use of these catheters increased anticipated adverse events but did not have any effect on overall mortality and hospitalization.

In decompensated CHF, preload and afterload reduction with diuretics and vasodilators are the cornerstones of therapy. The judicious use of diuretics with close monitoring of hemodynamics and renal parameters can increase cardiac output and lower renal venous hypertension, thereby improving renal perfusion. Appropriate use of inotropes may restore normal renal perfusion especially in patients with acute systolic heart failure or advanced left ventricular systolic dysfunction. The temporary discontinuation of ACE inhibitors or angiotensin receptor blockers and avoidance of NSAIDs may also help increase renal perfusion.

The management of intrinsic AKI depends on the underlying etiology. The management of individual diseases, especially the glomerular diseases, is beyond the scope of this chapter. We are going to focus on the special considerations in patients with ATN, which is a common cause of renal AKI in the CCU. In case of any doubt regarding whether the patient has prerenal AKI or established ATN secondary to sustained renal hypoperfusion, an adequate trial of crystalloids and/or the use of vasoactive agents may be the only differentiating feature; rapid reversibility indicates a prerenal mechanism. While fluid resuscitation is ongoing, frequent monitoring of respiratory status in patients with heart failure is essential to avoid pulmonary edema. Withdrawal of all possible nephrotoxic agents to avoid further injury to the kidney should be done concurrently.

Once ischemic or nephrotoxic ATN is established, there is no specific therapy. The only goal of treatment is to avoid complications secondary to AKI and prevent further injury.

A number of drugs have been tried to reduce the requirement for RRT and to accelerate renal recovery but none has shown a conclusive benefit. Diuretics are commonly used in oliguric AKI to convert it to nonoliguric AKI. The theory is that diuretics wash out the tubules, which may be partially blocked with necrotic debris; improve blood flow (when vasoconstriction is inappropriate) by renal cortical vasodilation; and prevent fluid overload. However, randomized controlled trials have shown an increased risk of adverse events with this strategy with no reduction in the need for RRT. Similarly, the use of selective renal vasodilators such as dopamine or fenoldopam is not supported by current clinical evidence and thus is not recommended.[12]

RENAL REPLACEMENT THERAPY

Conventional indications for initiation of RRT include refractory fluid overload, refractory hyperkalemia, refractory metabolic acidosis, and uremic syndrome. Other indications include uremic pericarditis, uremic encephalopathy, uremic neuropathy, and suspected drug/toxic overdose with a dialyzable substance; the optimal time to initiate RRT in these patients is not

known. Traditional triggers for treatment were based on studies in CKD patients, whereas patients with AKI who are critically ill may have a reduced tolerance of metabolic derangements. Furthermore, the identification that iatrogenic fluid overload may play a role in perpetuating the multiorgan dysfunction in critically ill patients has led to the belief that early initiation of RRT in this population may have beneficial effects on overall morbidity and mortality.

The available modalities for RRT include Intermittent Hemodialysis (IHD), continuous renal replacement therapy (CRRT), hybrid therapies such as sustained low-efficiency dialysis and peritoneal dialysis. The choice of modality depends on institutional availability, physician preference, patient hemodynamic status and the presence of other comorbidities. CRRT has been postulated to be more physiological owing to its continuous nature. It is especially useful in the hemodynamically unstable patients with AKI where use of IHD could lead to further ischemic insult and delay in renal recovery. However, no randomized study has proven this theoretical benefit over conventional, intermittent dialysis.

One modality of CRRT, especially useful in the CCU is slow continuous ultrafiltration that can allow removal of large amounts of fluid from the patient while minimizing the risk of hemodynamic instability. It can be considered as a therapeutic option in the management of a fluid overloaded patient with diuretic resistance even in the absence of AKI.

RECOVERY FROM ACUTE TUBULAR NECROSIS

Recovery from ATN is the rule rather than the exception. More than 90% of patients with ATN recover renal function sufficient to discontinue dialysis. The timing of this recovery varies among individual patients and can happen even after weeks of AKI. A post-ATN diuresis can commonly be seen in the recovery phase owing to osmotic diuresis. It is important to monitor these patients closely as they are often at the risk of developing new prerenal azotemia and electrolyte derangements if volume intake does not match urinary losses.

REFERENCES

1. Bellomo R, Ronco C, Kellum JA, et al. Acute renal failure—definition, outcome measures, animal models, fluid therapy and information technology needs: the Second International Consensus Conference of the Acute Dialysis Quality Initiative (ADQI) Group. *Crit Care.* 2004;8:R204–R212.
2. Mehta RL, Kellum JA, Shah SV, et al. Acute Kidney Injury Network: report of an initiative to improve outcomes in acute kidney injury. *Crit Care.* 2007;11:R31.
3. Ronco C, Haapio M, House AA, et al. Cardiorenal syndrome. *J Am Coll Cardiol.* 2008;52(19):1527–1539.
4. Tillyard A, Keays R, Soni N. The diagnosis of acute renal failure in intensive care: mongrel or pedigree? *Anaesthesia.* 2005;60:903–914.
5. Uchino S, Kellum JA, Bellomo R, et al. Acute renal failure in critically ill patients: a multinational, multicenter study. *JAMA.* 2005;294:813–818.
6. Hoste EA, Kellum JA, Katz NM, et al. Epidemiology of acute kidney injury. *Contrib Nephrol.* 2010;165:1–8.
7. McCullough PA, Soman SS, Shah SS, et al. Risks associated with renal dysfunction in patients in the coronary care unit. *J Am Coll Cardiol.* 2000;36(3):679–684.
8. Mishra J, Dent C, Tarabishi R, et al. Neutrophil gelatinase associated lipocalin (NGAL) as a biomarker for acute renal injury after cardiac surgery. *Lancet.* 2005;365:1231–1238.
9. Haase M, Bellomo R, Devarajan P, et al. Accuracy of neutrophil gelatinase-associated lipocalin (NGAL) in diagnosis and prognosis in acute kidney injury: a systematic review and meta-analysis. *Am J Kidney Dis.* 2009;4(6):1012–1024.
10. Parikh CR, Abraham E, Ancukiewicz M, et al. Urine IL-18 is an early diagnostic marker for acute kidney injury and predicts mortality in the intensive care unit. *J Am Soc Nephrol.* 2005;16:3046–3052.

11. Han WK, Bailly V, Abichandani R, et al. Kidney injury molecule-1 (KIM-1): a novel biomarker for human renal proximal tubule injury. *Kidney Int.* 2002;62:237–244.

12. Brochard L, Abroug F, Brenner M, et al. Prevention and management of acute renal failure in the ICU patient: an international consensus conference in intensive care medicine. *Am J Respir Crit Care Med.* 2010;181(10):1128–1155.

13. Lauschke A, Teichgräber UK, Frei U, et al. "Low-dose" dopamine worsens renal perfusion in patients with acute renal failure. *Kidney Int.* 2006;69(9):1669–1674.

14. Friedrich JO, Adhikari N, Herridge MS, et al. Meta-analysis: low dose dopamine increases urine output but does not prevent renal dysfunction or death. *Ann Intern Med.* 2005;142:510–524.

15. Landoni G, Biondi-Zoccai GG, Tumlin JA, et al. Beneficial impact of fenoldopam in critically ill patients with or at risk for acute renal failure: a meta-analysis of randomized clinical trials. *Am J Kidney Dis.* 2007;49:56–68.

16. McCullough PA, Adam A, Becker CR, et al.; CIN Consensus Working Panel. Risk prediction of contrast-induced nephropathy. *Am J Cardiol.* 2006;98(6A):27K–36K.

17. Hoste EA, De Waele JJ, Gevaert SA, et al. Sodium bicarbonate for prevention of contrast-induced acute kidney injury: a systematic review and meta-analysis. *Nephrol Dial Transplant.* 2010;25(3):747–758.

18. Briguori C, Colombo A, Violante A, et al. Standard vs double dose of N-acetylcysteine to prevent contrast agent associated nephrotoxicity. *Eur Heart J.* 2004;25:206–211.

19. Cruz DN, Perazella MA, Bellomo R, et al. Extracorporeal blood purification therapies for prevention of radiocontrast-induced nephropathy. *Am J Kidney Dis.* 2006;48:361–371.

20. Suen WS, Mok CK, Chiu SW, et al. Risk factors for development of acute renal failure (ARF) requiring dialysis in patients undergoing cardiac surgery. *Angiology.* 1998;49(10):789–800.

21. Massoudy P, Wagner S, Thielmann M, et al. Coronary artery bypass surgery and acute kidney injury—impact of the off-pump technique. *Nephrol Dial Transplant.* 2008;23(9):2853–2860.

22. Mentzer RM Jr, Oz MC, Sladen RN, et al.; on behalf of the NAPA Investigators. Effects of perioperative nesiritide in patients with left ventricular dysfunction undergoing cardiac surgery: the NAPA trial. *J Am Coll Cardiol.* 2007;49:716–726.

PATIENT AND FAMILY INFORMATION FOR:
Renal Failure

WHAT ARE THE KIDNEYS?

The kidneys are two bean-shaped organs that are located in the middle of the back, one on each side. Each measures about the size of a fist. These are vital organs and are made up of about 2 million nephrons (filters) and tubules that process approximately 4 L of blood every 5 minutes.

WHAT ARE THE FUNCTIONS OF THE KIDNEYS?

The human body consists of 60% to 70% water. This water also contains a variety of dissolved materials such as different salts (sodium chloride, potassium chloride, sodium bicarbonate, etc.). All the water in the body is distributed between three spaces—the intracellular compartment (in the cells), interstitial (between the cells), and intravascular (the blood). In an ideal setting, there is a perfect balance of water and salts in between all these compartments. If any deregulation occur, for instance, if we get dehydrated (e.g., diarrhea) or if we get fluid overloaded (e.g., in patients with heart failure), the kidneys jump into action to restore the equilibrium. Therefore, control of fluid and salt balance is an essential function of the kidneys.

Another important function of the kidneys is to excrete toxic wastes (such as urea, acid, etc.) produced by the body on a daily basis. The kidney does this by filtering the blood that flows through it. In other words, the urine is actually a filtered form of blood that has all the waste material in it (urea, extra water, acid, salts, etc.).

The third function of the kidney is to act as an endocrine organ. The main hormone that the kidneys produce is erythropoietin. This is required by the body to produce red blood cells (that carry oxygen in the blood). In addition, the kidneys also activate other inactive products such as vitamin D (helps to maintain healthy bones).

WHAT ARE THE TYPES OF KIDNEY FAILURE?

Depending on the duration of onset, kidney failure can be acute, chronic, or acute on chronic.

Acute: Such patients may have normal functioning kidneys at baseline. Acute kidney failure is a potentially life-threatening condition and may require intensive care treatment. Acute Tubular Necrosis (ATN) is one of the commonest subtypes of acute renal failure in a critically ill patient. In ATN, the kidney tubules get damaged owing to various reasons (infections/pneumonia, low blood pressure resulting from heart failure/heart attack, etc.). With time, and if the underlying etiology is fixed, the tubules may start functioning again as before.

Chronic (when decrease in function takes place gradually over time): Common causes are hypertension and diabetes. Such patients may have Chronic Kidney Disease (CKD). Those who have had regular follow-up with their primary doctors may be aware of their underlying CKD. However, as kidney failure is usually painless, it is not uncommon for patients to know of their underlying CKD until the disease is in an advanced stage.

Acute on chronic: Such patients have acute worsening of their CKD owing to critical illness, for example, pneumonia, heart attack, heart failure, and so on.

WHAT ARE THE COMMON CAUSES OF ACUTE KIDNEY FAILURE?

A failure of the kidneys is generally because of another disease process. Sometimes there may be more than one cause, and therefore it may be impossible to pinpoint the exact cause of acute kidney failure. Death is most common when acute kidney failure is caused by surgery, trauma, or severe infection in someone with heart disease, lung disease, or recent stroke. Old age, infection, loss of blood from the intestinal tract, and progression of kidney failure also increase the risk of death.

Listed below are some of the common causes of acute kidney failure:

Shock: Shock is a life-threatening condition that may accompany severe injury or illness, whereby the body suffers from insufficient blood flow to its vital organs. This can therefore result in decreased oxygen delivery to the organs (hypoxia) leading to organ failure, for example, kidney failure, heart attack (cardiac arrest), and so on. Shock may be of different types/causes: Septic (owing to any infection in the body, pancreatitis, etc.), hemorrhagic (owing to acute blood loss—like in a patient with gastrointestinal bleed from an ulcer), cardiogenic (owing to heart failure from a weak heart or acute heart attack) and hypovolemic (e.g., after severe diarrhea).

Damage from medicines/dyes: Unfortunately many of the medications used to treat patients, may themselves cause kidney damage. People who have serious, long-term health problems are more likely than others to have such adverse effects. Some examples of such medications are as follows:

Antibiotics used to treat life-threatening infections
Pain medicines such as ibuprofen
Some blood pressure medicines and ACE inhibitors (such as enalapril)
The contrast/dyes used in imaging (CAT scan as discussed below) to diagnose life-threatening conditions
Some of the HIV medications, for example, tenofovir.

Urinary tract obstruction: This may happen in patients who have a known history of kidney stones, benign prostate hypertrophy, or seldom in patients with cancer that invade or press on the urinary tract system.

WHAT ARE THE SIGNS AND SYMPTOMS OF KIDNEY FAILURE?

Kidney failure is almost always painless. In the setting of an intensive care unit, the following signs and symptoms may point towards a failing kidney.

Accumulation of fluid/water: Because the failing kidneys are unable to excrete water, accumulation of water in the body manifests as swelling of the feet, lower legs, face, and/or the hands. Sometimes when the kidneys fail, a lot of protein is lost in the urine, which can also cause worsening edema and labored breathing owing to accumulation of fluid in the lungs. If this is severe, the patient may require intubation (whereby the patient is sedated and a breathing tube is inserted in the wind pipe) and breathing support with the help of a machine (ventilator).

Irregular heart rate: Owing to the accumulation of toxins and electrolyte imbalance (hyperkalemia or high potassium), the heart rhythm may become irregular or dangerously slow, leading to cardiac arrest.

Symptoms resulting from accumulation of toxins/waste products such as urea: Loss of appetite, nausea vomiting, fatigue, sleepiness, itching, twitching, and a metallic taste in the mouth. They often indicate that the person is accumulating dangerous amounts of waste products (urea) because the kidneys are not working to excrete them.

Abnormal blood tests suggesting impaired kidney function: Sometimes the patient may be totally asymptomatic but the blood tests may suggest severe kidney failure, for example, hyperkalemia (high potassium), high creatinine, and blood urea nitrogen levels.

HOW TO DIAGNOSE KIDNEY FAILURE?

Nephrologists are specialists in kidney diseases. When a patient has evidence of kidney failure, the intensive care team will seek the help of nephrologists for managing kidney failure. The following tests will help to determine the severity and cause of kidney failure.

Blood test: In most cases, two parameters in the blood namely the BUN and creatinine can give a fair assessment as to the degree of kidney failure. Urea is a byproduct of protein breakdown, and creatinine is a byproduct of normal muscle functioning. In a normal person, the level of creatinine is 0.7 to 1.2 mg per dl and that of BUN is 12 to 24 mg per dl. In addition, blood level of some important electrolytes such as potassium is also taken into consideration while treating a patient of kidney failure.

Urine tests: Microscopic analysis of patient's urine can give some indication as to the type of renal failure (e.g., acute renal failure owing to ATN). Other urine tests such as urine protein concentration and urine electrolytes (sodium, creatinine) can also prove helpful in making the diagnosis, for example, a high protein and blood concentration in the urine with acute renal failure may be suggestive of lupus nephritis (owing to an autoimmune disease called systemic lupus nephritis).

Imaging tests: Noninvasive procedures such as ultrasound and CAT scan help in assessing the condition of the kidneys.

Ultrasound. It is a painless, harmless (uses sound waves that bounce off structures in the body and give images), and quick way to assess for the size and texture of the kidneys. Kidneys are usually normal in size in patients with acute renal failure; unless the patient also has some underlying CKD. Ultrasound is also the procedure of choice to diagnose any obstruction of the urinary tract as it is important to rule it out as the cause of kidney failure in all patients.

Computed axial tomography scan. A CAT scan uses X-rays to produce pictures in crosswise slices. CAT scans can detect kidney stones, blockage, tumors, cysts, and so on. In addition to the kidneys, an abdominal CAT scan can also be used to assess other abdominal organs. Sometimes CAT scans require using contrast dye, which itself carries the risk of causing renal failure, especially in people who already have reduced kidney function.

Kidney biopsy: Very rarely would a nephrologist decide to do a kidney biopsy in a patient with acute renal failure. He/she may decide on doing this if conventional analysis is unable to provide sufficient clue as to the underlying cause of acute renal failure and/or if the treatment modality would require the exact diagnosis rather than the most probable cause of acute renal failure. In kidney biopsy, a piece of kidney tissue is taken out under guidance of CAT scan. This tissue is then analyzed by experts to provide the exact cause of renal failure. Kidney biopsy unfortunately carries a high risk of bleeding (10%) and even death in 1% of the patients.

HOW TO MANAGE A PATIENT WITH KIDNEY FAILURE (HEMODIALYSIS)?

The most definitive treatment of kidney failure is to fix the underlying cause. For example, if the patient is having severe heart failure, the optimization of the heart failure will most likely help in resolving acute renal failure. However, treating the underlying disease may take time, thus necessitating the initiation of Renal Replacement Therapy (RRT). The decision to start RRT may be taken if the patient's serum potassium levels are dangerously high and/or if the patient has mental status changes, and/or if the patient has too much fluid, and/or if the patient develops pericarditis (inflammation of the heart covering owing to high urea).

RRT basically implies the use of artificial methods (dialysis) to carry out the functions of kidneys. The commonly used technique for acute renal failure is hemodialysis.

Hemodialysis is the most common intermittent method of artificial RRT. In hemodialysis, the blood is allowed to flow through a special filter that removes wastes and extra fluids. The clean blood is then returned back to the body. For hemodialysis, the patient needs to have a large bore catheter (VasCath or PermCath) in one of the deep veins of the body. It is therefore placed either in the neck or in the groin. Each session of hemodialysis lasts for 3 to 4 hours and is given either daily or three times a week. However the frequency may be adjusted based on the blood tests, degree of edema, and so on.

HOW LONG WILL THE PATIENT NEED HEMODIALYSIS?

Acute kidney failure is a potentially life-threatening condition and may require intensive care treatment. However, the kidneys usually start working again within several weeks to months after the underlying cause has been treated. Such patients may therefore require hemodialysis temporarily.

The recovery also depends on the state of kidney function at baseline, the underlying cause of acute renal failure, and the type of acute renal failure. In some cases, chronic renal failure or end-stage renal disease may develop, thus requiring hemodialysis lifelong.

Janet M. Shapiro

End-of-Life Care in the Cardiac Care Unit

Patients in the cardiac care unit (CCU) often undergo intensive and heroic treatments intended to save and prolong life. However, such patients managed in an intensive care unit (ICU) are at high risk of death. Many patients do undergo intensive care at the end of life; it has been projected that one in five Americans die in the ICU or subsequently during that hospitalization.[1] The CCU has evolved over the past several decades such that the current CCU provides care to patients with advanced age and illness. Examination of recent temporal trends involving approximately 30,000 CCU patients revealed increases in noncardiovascular critical illness, including sepsis, acute renal injury, and acute respiratory failure as well as increasing use of procedures such as mechanical ventilation.[2] Thus the CCU clinician is faced with critically patients who are on life support measures, some of whom may be at the end of life.

Decision making about end-of-life care in the CCU is a challenge for several reasons. Many patients do not have an advance directive. Even in cardiac patients with advanced interventions, including implantable electronic devices, discussions about advance directives are uncommon.[3] Clinicians face difficulty in prognostication for critically ill patients. In patients with heart failure, variability in the course makes identifying the end of life especially challenging. The guidelines of the Heart Failure Society of America and the American College of Cardiology/American Heart Association promote consideration of end-of-life care in patients with advanced heart failure including decisions about inactivation of implantable defibrillators.[4,5]

It is notable that despite the recommendations of cardiology societies to encourage provision of supportive and palliative care, cardiology journals and textbooks have little end-of-life content compared with other specialties.[6,7] Physicians in the CCU must be knowledgeable about end-of-life care; therefore, the goal of this chapter is to provide practical information about end-of-life decision-making and the process of withdrawal of life-sustaining treatments in the CCU.

DECISION MAKING AT THE END OF LIFE

As clinicians, our goals for patients are to save lives, restore health to a desirable existence, alleviate suffering, and provide the dying with a peaceful and dignified death.

The transition of the goal from curative treatment to comfort care is one of the most challenging aspects of critical care. People want to live; this is most exemplified by studies showing that patients would undergo mechanical ventilation for a

1% chance of ICU survival,[8] and 70% of ICU survivors would undergo intensive care again for a chance to live one more month.[9]

Palliative care may even be provided in conjunction with lifesaving treatments in patients at risk for death. The goals of palliative care are control of symptoms such as pain, dyspnea, and discomfort; effective communication about appropriate goals of treatment and concordance of treatment with patient preferences; and enhancing quality of life. Adopting a palliative care approach and involving a palliative care service may be of great benefit in managing cardiac patients at the end of life.

Effective communication is the means to achieving patient preferences in end-of-life care. The landmark SUPPORT study revealed that the wishes of dying patients were often unexplored by physicians, and those patients received potentially undesired treatments at the end of life.[10] Clinicians must also recognize that their own wishes may not coincide with those of their patients; a large multicenter study of European ICUs found that when asked about preferences at the end of life, physicians and nurses were less likely to desire life support than patients and families.[11] Decision making that is shared between the patient/family and the clinicians is the model process supported by American and European critical care societies.[12,13] The evolution of critical care decision-making from a paternalistic model to the current standard of shared decision-making is predicated on respect for patient autonomy and values. In the critical care unit, up to 95% of patients may be unable to participate in decisions owing to the severe illness, need for life support, and sedative medications.[12] Therefore, the legally recognized appropriate surrogate often assumes the decision-making role to represent the patient's values and preferences. The family-centered approach respects the patient's values, and also acknowledges that many patients would want their family members to participate in decision making.

ETHICAL PRINCIPLES IN END-OF-LIFE DECISION-MAKING

Patient *autonomy* is a foundation ethical principle for patient care. U.S. Supreme Court cases such as the Quinlan and Cruzan cases established that patients have a right to determine which medical treatments to accept or refuse, even when refusal leads to death.[14] Often in the critical care unit, the patient is incapable of participating in the decision making. However, the patient may have left guidance in the form of an advance directive, such as a proxy, living will, or oral statements articulating his or her wishes concerning life support at the end of life. The patient may have assigned a health care proxy to make decisions if he or she becomes unable to do so. If no proxy has been assigned, the surrogate decision maker is chosen from the patient's close relatives or friends based on priority. In this way, the patient's values and preferences can still guide the decision-making process when decision-making capacity is lost.

The principle of *beneficence* maintains that physicians will work to provide the best course of treatment for the patient. Physicians see the goal of preserving life, but beneficence also means the support of the patient's informed decision even when refusal of therapy may lead to death. *Nonmaleficence* means not inflicting harm. This principle instructs the physician to weigh potential harms of treatments against potential benefits and not to provide interventions that will not benefit the patient.

Conflict may arise when the patient, family, and clinician disagree about the appropriateness of an intervention. Nonabandonment is an important principle that obliges the physician to help the family understand the situation and support the family's decision. Physicians are not obligated to go against their own beliefs and therefore, if the physician disagrees with the patient and family decision, the principle of nonabandonment requires the physician to try to transfer care to another physician who will pursue the desired plan of care. The hospital administration or ethics committee may be involved to assist in resolution of these complicated situations.

ADVANCE DIRECTIVES

As stated above, patient autonomy is the strongest ethical principle driving medical decision-making, so that patients have the right to make decisions for themselves, and when conscious capacity is lost, this right remains protected. Advance directives, such as the health care proxy and living will, provide for decision making based on patient values and preferences when the patient loses decision-making capacity. Respect for patient autonomy underlies the federal Patient Self-Determination Act of 1990 that requires hospital personnel to ask patients whether they have an advance directive and inform patients of their right to accept or refuse medical treatments and to create an advance directive.[15] A *do not resuscitate* (DNR) order is one kind of advance directive that addresses interventions in the setting of a cardiopulmonary arrest. A DNR order means that if the patient suffers a cardiopulmonary arrest, the interventions of intubation, CPR, and advanced cardiovascular life support will be withheld. A DNR order is often issued for patients at the end of life and in patients with chronic or terminal illnesses. In some patients with DNR orders, the patient may be expected to benefit from and will receive intensive care interventions, but CPR will be withheld in the event of cardiac arrest. A DNR order is often a first step in the family's decision-making process.

COMMUNICATION

The means to decision making is effective communication and understanding. The contributions of the entire team are often invaluable. Most of ICU nurses do want to be involved in end-of-life decision-making; the bedside nurse usually has important insight into the patient's condition and the family understands and desires. It should not be assumed that families grasp the severity of their relative's illness or the ramifications of life support measures. Family understanding of critical illness and intensive care treatments has been shown to be inadequate.[16] Among family members of ICU patients, only 50% could identify a single failing organ or any treatment.[17] Knowledge about cardiopulmonary resuscitation is especially poor, with a prevalent unrealistic expectation of survival among patients with serious medical illness and their families.[18] A prospective study in an urban American ICU found that only half of the surrogates understood basic facets of their family member's care, such as whether the patient was on a respirator or the resuscitation status.[16] Accordingly, assessing family members' understanding of the patient condition is vital and will be part of the communication strategy in a family meeting.

FAMILY MEETING

Communication with the family occurs in several venues: bedside discussions, conversations with the nurse, telephone updates as well as a formal family meeting. A family meeting is an opportunity to present and review the situation and treatments, provide information on short-term and long-term prognosis, answer questions, explore patient and family values and wishes, and assess the family's understanding of the patient's condition.[19] Investigators have examined family meetings and found missed opportunities in time allotted for family speech, articulating a prognosis, emphasizing the process of surrogate decision-making, supporting the decision, and assuring nonabandonment. Family satisfaction with the meeting was associated with increased time for family speech; presumably this is their opportunity to make the patient and his values known. Prognostication is important for family members, but more than one-third of examined deliberations lacked discussion of prognosis for survival. Investigators also found that less information about prognosis was provided to the less educated families.[20] Although families may doubt the accuracy of the prognosis given by physicians, that prognostic information is desired and important in the family's understanding and deliberation.[21]

Here, we can make some points about the family meeting:

1. The medical team should prepare for the family meeting. The clinicians should discuss the goals of the family meeting, review the patient's condition, and achieve consensus concerning prognosis and treatments to be administered. The team should be aware of specific issues or problems related to the family situation. The bedside nurse may have great insight into the patient's condition and family situation and should be included in the meeting.

2. The physician will lead the discussion in a private, quiet place. All participants should be introduced. The family should be asked their understanding of the condition and treatments. The physician should provide information about the illness, treatments including life support measures, and prognosis in a meaningful and compassionate manner by avoiding excessive medical jargon. The clinicians should explain surrogate and shared decision-making.

3. The clinicians should allow time for the family to speak about the patient's values and preferences, to demonstrate their understanding of the situation, and to ask questions.

4. If withdrawal of life support is discussed, the clinicians should emphasize that this does not mean withdrawal of *care* and that supportive and comfort care will be provided.

5. The staff should offer support for the decision of the family, whether the decision is to withdraw or not withdraw life support. The team should assure the family that the patient will not be abandoned and all measures will be taken to prevent suffering.

6. The family cannot be rushed to make a decision. The meeting may conclude with a plan to reconvene in the following days to review the situation.

These discussions require time and experience. In many situations, the family members report that they never discussed end of life with the patient. Some ways to elucidate patient wishes include asking whether they ever had a conversation about the patient's own wishes, in the setting of another family member's illness or even related to a topic in the news; how the patient lived his life, what it may mean to be dependent in all aspects of care; what they think the patient might say about life support measures if he or she were in this meeting. The leader may ask the family what they believe is a meaningful and acceptable quality of life for the patient.

It is important that clinicians do not relinquish medical decisions to the family. The physicians must provide information, prognosis, and advice on how to proceed. The family provides information about the values and preferences of the patient. The transition from aggressive CCU care to comfort care is often made quickly by clinicians who have the benefit of medical knowledge of disease and prognosis, but families may need time for this adjustment and should not be rushed to make a decision. Planning a follow-up conversation within a specified period allows the clinicians to further assess the patient's trajectory and permits the family to grasp the information and condition. Families need ongoing contact and communication. Families need assurances that all efforts will be made to maintain comfort. Involving the palliative care service may be beneficial in optimizing the medical and nursing treatments for palliation.[22] In one study, family satisfaction was found to be higher among families of ICU nonsurvivors, perhaps because of greater time spent in decision making, communication, and bedside care of patients at the end of life.[23]

Cultural values and beliefs may exert a profound influence on decision making. Domains affecting decisions include attitudes about truth telling concerning illness and prognosis, religious and spiritual beliefs, historical and political context, and the decision-making process in the group.[24] A recent single center study examined illness perceptions among critically ill patients or their surrogates. Perception of illness was greatly affected by race and faith, in which some groups believed that the illness was less serious, and they were less concerned about consequences and more optimistic about treatment effectiveness.[25] The not uncommon clinician impression that the family is not accepting a dire diagnosis and prognosis may therefore at times be explained by cultural factors. Recognizing the influence of cultural factors may lead to enhanced understanding and compassionate and effective communication.

Conflicts may develop between family and physicians, within families as well as among the health care team. Given physicians' inability to be certain of the outcome, the family may be reluctant to accept a poor prognosis. The CCU team may involve other disciplines such as the patient's primary care physician, other involved subspecialties, and chaplaincy and social work. For conflicts that reveal marked differences in desires among the patient, family, and physicians, the hospital ethics committee may be involved. Ethics committee consultations may be beneficial in resolving conflicts, establishing desired care and limiting nonbeneficial life support measures.[26] In addition, legal affairs involvement may be required in rare, complicated situations.

WITHDRAWAL OF LIFE SUPPORT

Ethical principles described previously support the decision to withdraw or withhold life-sustaining treatments. The U.S. Supreme Court cases confirmed that patients or surrogates can refuse life-sustaining therapies.[14] The decision to withdraw life support is based on patient values and preferences as articulated by the patient or his/her proxy or surrogate. Withdrawal of life support would be allowing the patient to die from the underlying disease. Withholding and withdrawing life support are considered equivalent, although clinicians may be more uncomfortable with the withdrawal of treatments.[12] The process of withdrawal of life support may vary depending on the standard of the individual hospital.

Decisions to withhold or withdraw life support are common among critically ill patients; studies have shown that >70% of ICU deaths are preceded by decisions to limit life support.[27] All forms of life support may be withheld or withdrawn, including mechanical ventilation, vasopressors, antibiotics, blood product transfusions, hydration, and nutrition. Sometimes all treatments are discontinued at once, sometimes in a stepwise fashion.[28] With the exception of the withdrawal of mechanical ventilation, withdrawing these other treatments does not often lead to an evident clinical change. The decision to withdraw mechanical ventilation may be a more difficult decision for families as well as for clinicians. With the assurance that withdrawal would be the patient's wish and that medications will be provided for comfort, withdrawal of mechanical ventilation is often desired at the end of life.

At the time of withdrawal of life support, there should be written documentation of the prognosis, discussion, and decision making with the patient/surrogate, goals of care and plan, including orders to discontinue specific therapies. In particular, an order for removal of mechanical ventilation or deactivation of an implantable device should be entered.

WITHDRAWAL OF MECHANICAL VENTILATION

The actual process of withdrawal of life support can be viewed as other critical care procedures comprising multiple steps. Investigators have devised an order form for withdrawal of life-sustaining treatments, which includes all the essential components of the procedure.[29] A protocol organizes the process, supports the clinicians that this is a procedure like all other critical care procedures, and may promote better use of palliative medications at the end of life.

Communication with the family about the process of withdrawing ventilation and what to expect is essential. Although difficult to be certain, the physician should provide an estimation of duration of survival following extubation. Predicting the time until death was addressed in a recent multicenter study of patients who died after the withdrawal of mechanical ventilation (both invasive and noninvasive). The median time until death was 0.93 hours (range of 0 to 6.9 days), with shorter time until death predicted by nonwhite race, number of failing organs, fluid and vasopressor administration. A longer time until death was observed in older patients and women.[30] More than 90% of patients died within 24 hours of withdrawal of mechanical ventilation. The family may want to be present and may desire pastoral care to be present for support. All nonbeneficial treatments, including vasoactive medications, should be discontinued, and alarms should be silenced. Palliative medications should be adjusted prior to extubation while the patient is on a spontaneous breathing mode. The endotracheal tube is removed, and the family should remain with the patient for as long as desired.

WITHDRAWAL OF CARDIOVASCULAR IMPLANTABLE ELECTRONIC DEVICE THERAPY

Implantable defibrillation and pacing devices provide life support that that can be declined or withdrawn based on patient values and preferences.[31] The dying patient or surrogate may request inactivation, if the device effectiveness is outweighed by burdens experienced by the patient: prolonging the dying process, preventing a natural death, and suffering the loss of dignity and quality of life. The Heart Rhythm Society published a consensus statement on the management of cardiovascular implantable electronic devices in patients nearing the end of life.[31] This document sets out the ethical principles, concerns, and practical management of withdrawal of cardiovascular implantable electronic device therapy. Deactivation may prevent uncomfortable shocks in dying patients. In pacemaker-dependent patients, the device sustains life and may, like other life-sustaining treatments such as mechanical ventilation, be discontinued based on the patient's right to decline therapy. If cardiac resynchronization is aiding cardiac function, then inactivation may lead to increased symptom burden.[31] So each therapy must be addressed in light of the overall goals. The Heart Rhythm Society consensus statement offers practical advice for communication, assessing patient understanding of the device, and utilizing the overall care goals to guide management of the cardiac device. The patient's cardiologist and electrophysiologist should be involved in these discussions about deactivation.

NONINVASIVE VENTILATION

Many physicians use noninvasive ventilation for respiratory failure near the end of life.[32] Its use should be guided by the goals of care. A patient who declines mechanical ventilation may receive noninvasive ventilation with the goal of survival: in patients with heart failure, noninvasive ventilation may successfully prevent intubation and the patient may survive the episode. In patients at the end of life, noninvasive ventilation has been used for palliation of dyspnea and as a means to give more time for family to arrive and communicate with the patient. However, if noninvasive ventilation becomes uncomfortable or burdensome, it should be removed. Noninvasive ventilation should be addressed with the patient and family as a life support measure that can be continued or discontinued based on the goals of care.

SYMPTOM MANAGEMENT

Most critically ill patients experience pain and discomfort related to procedures and nursing care in the ICU.[33] The possibility of pain in patients unable to report their symptoms is a great concern for families and clinicians. Dyspnea is a common symptom in critically ill patients. When withdrawal of mechanical ventilation is being discussed, a frequent concern of the family is that the patient will experience respiratory distress. The clinicians should assess the patient with input from the bedside nurse and family. Management is individualized, based on the patient's level of consciousness, underlying disease, and reason for respiratory failure. Because the response to medication will vary, the route of administration and dosages must be adjusted, often with the assistance of the critical care pharmacist.

Opioid analgesia is a basic medication class for patients at the end of life.[12] The desired effects are analgesia and sedation, but there is also a respiratory depressant effect on the medullary respiratory center. Opioid medications are useful in management of the symptoms and signs of respiratory distress. The principle of double-effect justifies the administration of medications given with the intention of providing comfort and relieving suffering, even though the medication may potentially hasten a patient's death.[12] However, studies have demonstrated that the use of palliative medications in the last week of life did not hasten death in a palliative care unit.[34] One study evaluated the use of narcotics or benzodiazepines to manage discomfort following withdrawal of life support; administration of palliative medications was not associated with a shortened time until death.[35] In fact, adequate pain management may mitigate the systemic effects of severe pain and even prolong life.[23] Proper documentation of the clinical indications and goal of the opioid analgesia therapy should always be performed.

In addition to respiratory depression, attention must be directed to several effects of opioid analgesia: inhibition of peristalsis with constipation, nausea, and vomiting; and myoclonus and seizures. Pruritus resulting from morphine can be addressed by switching to a different opioid agonist such as fentanyl.

Benzodiazepine medications provide sedation and anxiolysis. These medications do not provide analgesia but may be useful in combination with an opioid to prevent the anxiety related to pain. Side effects also include depressed level of consciousness and respiratory depression. Delirium, in the form of either an agitated or calm state, is a common symptom in dying patients in the ICU. Although haloperidol is the standard medication for the management of delirium, the team should implement nonpharmacologic measures such as removing restraints, reducing activity and noise, and having family members at the bedside to calm and orient the patient.[12]

AT THE TIME OF DEATH

Notification to the family, optimally in person, using unambiguous language that the patient died is the initial duty. A minority of deaths is determined by brain death criteria and selected patients undergoing withdrawal of life support may be candidates for organ donation following cardiac death. This process requires a specialized protocol for the withdrawal of life support and management in collaboration with the organ donor organization. The staff may assist the family by providing information about the next steps, including autopsy, funeral, and bereavement services.

The critical care unit staff can also benefit from a debriefing about the patient's course, the end-of-life care, and the death. Physicians and nurses have different perspectives on end-of-life decision-making, intensity of interventions, symptom management, and the quality of death and dying.[36] The burdens experienced by ICU nursing staff may lead to burnout, moral distress, and posttraumatic stress disorder. Communication to improve collaboration and the ethical climate may improve the environment for clinicians as well as the care of dying patients.[36]

CONCLUSION

Patients and their families should expect excellence in all treatments in the CCU, including care at the end of life. Patients deserve humanity, compassion, and respect for autonomy. End-of-life care in the CCU requires expertise on many levels: assessing prognosis, communicating information, understanding patient values and preferences for life support, and implementing a patient's end-of-life decision. The CCU team can utilize the expertise of consultants in optimizing end-of-life care. Clinicians' management will be rewarded by alleviating a patient's suffering, facilitating a peaceful and dignified death, and even providing peace and satisfaction for the patient's family.

REFERENCES

1. Angus DC, Barnato AE, Linde-Zwirble WT, et al. Use of intensive care at the end of life in the United States: an epidemiologic study. *Crit Care Med.* 2004;32:638–643.
2. Katz JN, Shah BR, Volz EM, et al. Evolution of the coronary care unit: clinical characteristics and temporal trends in healthcare delivery and outcomes. *Crit Care Med.* 2010;38:375–381.
3. Goldstein NE, Lampert R, Bradley E, et al. Management of implantable cardioverter defibrillators in end-of-life care. *Ann Intern Med.* 2004;141:835–838.
4. Heart Failure Society of America 2006 Guideline Executive Summary: HFSA 2006 Comprehensive Heart Failure Practice Guideline. Disease management in heart failure. *J Card Fail.* 2006;12:10–38.
5. Hunt SA, Abraham WT, Chin MH, et al. 2009 focused update incorporated into the ACC/AHA 2005 guidelines for the diagnosis and management of heart failure in adults: a report of the American College of Cardiology Foundation/American Heart Association Task Force on Practice Guidelines: developed in collaboration with the International Society for Heart and Lung Transplantation. *Circulation.* 2009;119:1977–2016.
6. Mehta NJ, Khan IA, Mehta RN, et al. End-of-life care-related publications in cardiology journals. *Am J Cardiol.* 2001;88:1460–1463.
7. Rabow MW, Hardie GE, Fair JM, et al. End-of-life care content in 50 textbooks from multiple specialties. *JAMA.* 2000;283:771–778.
8. Lloyd CB, Nietert PJ, Silvestri GA. Intensive care decision making in the seriously ill and elderly. *Crit Care Med.* 2004;32:649–654.
9. Danis M, Patrick DL, Southerland LI, et al. Patients' and families' preferences for medical intensive care. *JAMA.* 1988;260:797–802.
10. The SUPPORT Principal Investigators. A controlled trial to improve care for seriously ill hospitalized patients. The study to understand prognoses and preferences for outcomes and risks of treatments (SUPPORT). *JAMA.* 1995;274:1591–1598.
11. Sprung CL, Carmel S, Sjokvist P, et al. Attitudes of European physicians, nurses, patients, and families regarding end-of-life decisions: the ETHICATT study. *Intensive Care Med.* 2007;33:104–110.
12. Truong RD, Campbell ML, Curtis JR, et al. Recommendations for end-of-life care in the intensive care unit: a consensus statement by the American Academy of Critical Care Medicine. *Crit Care Med.* 2008;36:953–963.
13. Davidson JE, Powers K, Hedayat KM, et al. Clinical practice guidelines for support of the family in the patient-centered intensive care unit: American College of Critical Care Medicine Task Force 2004–2005. *Crit Care Med.* 2007;35:605–622.
14. Luce JM. End-of-life decision making in the intensive care unit. *Am J Respir Crit Care Med.* 2010;182:6–11.
15. Patient Self-Determination Act of 1990. Omnibus Budget Reconciliation Act of 1990, Pub Law No. 101–508 (1990).
16. Rodriguez RM, Navarrete E, Schwaber J, et al. A prospective study of primary surrogate decision makers' knowledge of intensive care. *Crit Care Med.* 2008;36:1633–1636.
17. Azoulay E, Chevret S, Leleu G, et al. Half the families of intensive care unit patients experience inadequate communication with physicians. *Crit Care Med.* 2002;28:3044–3049.
18. Heyland DK, Frank C, Groll D, et al. Understanding cardiopulmonary resuscitation decision making. Perspectives of seriously ill hospitalized patients and family members. *Chest.* 2006;130:419–428.
19. Curtis JR, White DB. Practical guidance for evidence-based ICU family conferences. *Chest.* 2008;134:835–843.
20. White DB, Engelberg RA, Wenrich MD, et al. Prognostication during physician-family discussions about limiting life support in intensive care units. *Crit Care Med.* 2007;35:442–448.
21. Zier LS, Burack JH, Micco G, et al. Doubt and belief in physicians' ability to prognosticate during critical illness: the perspective of surrogate decision makers. *Crit Care Med.* 2008;36:2341–2347.
22. Norton SA, Hogan LA, Holloway RG, et al. Proactive palliative care in the medical intensive care unit: effects on length of stay for selected high-risk patients. *Crit Care Med.* 2007;35:1530–1535.
23. Wall RJ, Curtis JR, Cooke CR, et al. Family satisfaction in the ICU. Differences between families of survivors and nonsurvivors. *Chest.* 2007;132:1425–1433.
24. Mularski RA, Puntillo K, Varkey B, et al. Pain management within the palliative and end-of-life care experience in the ICU. *Chest.* 2009;135:1360–1369.
25. Ford D, Zapka J, Gebregziabher M, et al. Factors associated with illness perception among critically ill patients and surrogates. *Chest.* 2010;138:59–67.
26. Schneiderman LJ, Gilmer T, Teetzel HD, et al. Effect of ethics consultations on nonbeneficial life-sustaining treatments in the intensive care setting. *JAMA.* 2003;290:1166–1172.
27. Prendergast TJ, Claessens MT, Luce JM. A national survey of end-of-life care for critically ill patients. *Am J Respir Crit Care Med.* 1998;158:1163–1167.
28. Asch DA, Faber-Langendoen K, Shea JA, et al. The sequence of withdrawing life-sustaining treatment from patients. *Am J Med.* 1999;107:153–156.
29. Treece PD, Engelberg RA, Crowley L, et al. Evaluation of a standardized order form for the withdrawal of life support in the intensive care unit. *Crit Care Med.* 2004;32:1141–1148.
30. Cooke CR, Hotchkin DL, Engelberg RA, et al. Predictors of time to death after terminal withdrawal of mechanical ventilation in the ICU. *Chest.* 2010;138:289–297.
31. Lampert R, Hayes DL, Annas GJ, et al. HRS expert consensus statement on the management of cardiovascular implantable electronic devices (CIEDs) in patients nearing the end of life or requesting withdrawal of therapy. *Heart Rhythm.* 2010;7:1008–1026.
32. Sinuff T, Cook DJ, Keenan SP, et al. Noninvasive ventilation for acute respiratory failure near the end of life. *Crit Care Med.* 2008;36:789–794.
33. Nelson JE, Meier DE, Oei EJ, et al. Self-reported symptom experience of critically ill cancer patients receiving intensive care. *Crit Care Med.* 2001;29:277–282.
34. Sykes N, Thorns A. Sedative use in the last week of life and the implications for end-of-life decision making. *Arch Intern Med.* 2003;163:341–344.
35. Chan JD, Treece PD, Engelberg RA, et al. Narcotic and benzodiazepine use after withdrawal of life support: association with time to death? *Chest.* 2004;126:286–293.
36. Hamric AB, Blackhall LJ. Nurse-physician perspectives on the care of dying patients in intensive care units: collaboration, moral distress and ethical climate. *Crit Care Med.* 2007;35:422–429.

PATIENT AND FAMILY INFORMATION FOR:
End-of-Life Care

The doctors, nurses, and entire CCU team treat patients with the goal of curing disease, prolonging life, and making the patient better. The team also works to relieve pain and suffering. Even with all the medical care, technology, and life support machines, patients may not get better or survive. Sometimes, the patient has an incurable illness such as advanced heart disease that has led to damage of all the vital organs and also led to coma. These patients are in a terminal condition and the use of life support may only postpone death. For patients and families, it is very important to communicate with the CCU team to understand the illness and outlook (prognosis) and to make decisions so that the patient's wishes and values are respected.

HOW ARE END-OF-LIFE DECISIONS MADE?

Decisions in the CCU are based on shared decision-making between the physicians, the patient and family. Communication is the key to decision making for a critically ill patient. The wishes of the patient are most important. If the patient does not want life-sustaining measures, these measures can be stopped. This is respect for the patient's autonomy, which means control over his/her own body. The law states that the patient has a right to agree to or refuse treatments, including life support.

The decision to limit or stop life support measures is based on the wishes of the patient as well as the patient's best interest if the exact wishes are unknown. Often patients in a critical condition cannot communicate or participate in making decisions and trust their closest relatives to make the decisions. The patient may have prepared for this by appointing a health care proxy to make medical decisions if the patient is unable to speak for himself/herself. A surrogate is a close relative or friend who will make decisions if a proxy has not been appointed and the patient is unable to make decisions himself. If the patient has not assigned a proxy, a surrogate is chosen from the patient's close relatives or close friends based on priority. Some patients fill out a proxy or living will; these documents can spell out the care or treatment that the patient wants or does not want in the case of a terminal illness or condition.

Remember that decisions about life support are made based on careful, thorough discussions with doctors, patient, and family/proxy/surrogate. Patients and family members should be sure that the doctors and nurses are aware of wishes concerning the end-of-life care.

FAMILY MEETING

Patients should expect that their physicians will provide information to them and their surrogates about their condition and treatment. A family meeting is often convened to talk about the patient's condition, treatments, and obtain information about the patient's wishes and values. It is often very difficult to be sure of the patient's outcome (prognosis); however, the physicians should give some information about whether the patient is expected to survive and what the function might be if he/she survives. If one member of the family becomes the contact person for the CCU staff, this will help the communication process.

WHAT IS LIFE SUPPORT?

Life support measures are treatments or procedures that support or replace body functions that are failing. When patients have curable or treatable conditions, life support is temporary until the organ function improves. With advanced illness and advanced age, certain diseases lead to a continued decline in function of the organs and of the entire person. Sometimes, the body never recovers and the patient cannot survive without life support.

It is important to understand the benefits and burdens of life support treatments. A treatment may be beneficial if it restores functioning, improves quality of life, and relieves suffering. The same treatment could be a burden if it causes pain, prolongs the dying process, or decreases the quality of life. The decision about whether a treatment is a benefit or a burden is a personal decision based on the patient's preferences and values. If the patient is able to tell the doctors, his/her decision will be respected. If the patient is unable to express his/her wishes, the doctors will meet with the family and proxy/surrogate to learn the patient's preferences and values.

WHAT ARE LIFE SUPPORT MEASURES?

Cardiopulmonary resuscitation (CPR) is a set of treatments given when a patient's heart and breathing stop in order to restart the heart and breathing. It involves breathing for the patient by using a mask or tube placed into the patient's airway. The team will compress the chest and may apply electric shocks to get the heart beating again.

In certain conditions, CPR can be very effective, for example, if a patient has a sudden heart attack. However, in patients at the late stages of a terminal illness who are at the end of life, CPR is usually not successful. Even if the heart does start beating, often the patient remains in a coma or dies within a short time. Making a decision about whether the patient should go through CPR is an important decision. In patients at the end of life, when the heart stops, this would be a natural death. A Do Not Resuscitate (DNR) order means that if the heart stops, CPR will not be done, and the patient would die a natural death.

Mechanical ventilation is the use of a *ventilator* to support the breathing function of the lungs. Ventilator and *respirator* both mean the same machine. A tube is inserted through the mouth into the trachea (windpipe), and this tube is connected to a ventilator that gives the breaths to the patient. Patients on a ventilator are not able to speak, sometimes are awake enough to communicate, and often require sedation so that they are not anxious or uncomfortable. Mechanical ventilation may be used for a short period, such as in heart failure or pneumonia and can also be used for a long time in patients with neurologic disorders, who may still be satisfied with the quality of their life. However, in a dying patient, mechanical ventilation will not improve the condition or the quality of life. In a patient who is dying, being on a respirator may prolong the dying process.

Noninvasive mechanical ventilation is the use of a ventilator machine that is attached to a special face mask. The ventilator will force air through the mask so the patient will feel some pressure of air moving in. Some patients can work well with the mask and even speak; for others, it is uncomfortable. This is a kind of life support that can be used if helpful; if it becomes uncomfortable and is not beneficial, it can be stopped.

Hemodialysis is used to replace the function of failed kidneys, which will clean the blood of wastes that normally accumulate. Dialysis requires placement of a large catheter and long periods on the dialysis machine. Some patients with kidney failure can live for years while receiving dialysis treatments several times each week. For patients at the end of life, dialysis cannot be expected to restore health.

Artificial nutrition and hydration can be given by a feeding tube placed into the stomach, which replaces normal eating and drinking. Artificial feeding may be necessary in some patients undergoing a prolonged illness until their bodies recover. In patients at the end of life, artificial nutrition and hydration still cannot restore health.

WHAT HAPPENS IF THE DECISION IS MADE TO WITHDRAW LIFE SUPPORT?

The decision to withdraw life support is made after careful discussion of the prognosis and patient preferences and values. All forms of life support can be withdrawn. The doctors may suggest placing an order for no CPR—a DNR and not administering certain medications.

The mechanical ventilator can be removed, based on patient desires and values. The physician and nurse will assure that the patient is comfortable. The family can be present during this process if they wish.

HOW WILL THE DYING PATIENT BE TREATED?

The goal of the health care team is to provide the desired and beneficial care. In a dying patient, *pain management and comfort care* will always be provided. Pain and discomfort can be managed by medications and also by factors, such as the family being present. Certain medications such as morphine are used to relieve pain and can also make the patient sleepy. All medications and treatments have other effects so that the overall goal of comfort must be a priority. The physicians and nurses will monitor the patient and also rely on the family to tell the staff whether the patient is comfortable.

There are clinicians who specialize in palliative care and may be consulted to assist the team with care. Patients and families may want the services of pastoral care. If there are questions or disagreements about patient wishes or goals, an ethics committee consultation may be useful.

The overall goal is for the cardiac team to work with the patient and his/her family, proxy, and surrogate to provide care that is beneficial and desired. Comfort and respect are priorities. It is important that there is communication and understanding in the shared responsibility for decision making and care for each patient.

Risk Factors: From the Acute Setting to Chronic Management

Jeanine Albu
Greg Dodell
Aastha Pal
Edgar Argulian
Eyal Herzog

CHAPTER

32

Diabetes Mellitus in the Cardiac Care Unit

DIABETES MELLITUS: GENERAL PRINCIPLES

WHAT IS DIABETES MELLITUS? DIAGNOSIS AND CLASSIFICATION

The defining feature of diabetes mellitus is an inappropriate elevation of blood glucose—hyperglycemia. This could be because of excessive glucose production, impaired glucose clearance, or both. Sustained, chronic hyperglycemia, over several years, leads to tissue injury resulting in chronic micro- and macrovascular complications such as diabetic neuropathy, retinopathy, and nephropathy; and atherothrombotic vascular diseases. "Inappropriate" hyperglycemia has been defined by the experts as the level that, if chronically sustained, will lead to the development of diabetic complications.

The current criteria used to make the diagnosis of diabetes mellitus are listed in Table 32.1.[1] According to the American Diabetes Association 2011 criteria, either random plasma glucose, fasting plasma glucose, an oral glucose tolerance test, or a hemoglobin A1C (% glycosylated hemoglobin, A1C) can be used to diagnose diabetes.[1-2]

Diabetes mellitus is currently classified by etiology as type 1, type 2, gestational, or other specified types (Table 32.2).[1] Type 1 diabetes is characterized by absolute or severe insulin deficiency.[3] Type 2 diabetes is a complex polygenic disease characterized by both insulin resistance and relative insulin deficiency, that is, insulin levels and secretion are inappropriate to the levels of insulin resistance and out of sync with the glucose stimuli (dual defect).[4,5] Gestational diabetes mellitus (GDM) is characterized by onset during pregnancy owing to increased insulin resistance generated by the hormonal milieu. Typically, it resolves at the end of pregnancy; however, women with gestational diabetes are at high risk for developing type 2 diabetes later in life.[6] Other specific types of diabetes listed by etiology are a result of genetic defects in β-cell function and/or insulin action (monogenic diabetes), exocrine pancreatic disease, some endocrinopathies, drug or chemically induced (exogenous corticosteroid administration, etc.), or other rare forms (infections, immune-mediated, etc.). These specific forms could manifest clinically in a similar fashion to either type 1 or type 2 diabetes.

Type 1 diabetes. Certain clinical aspects of diabetes presentation are characteristic of type 1 diabetes: diabetic ketoacidosis; signs of insulin deficiency such as weight loss and/or blood glucose level >250 mg per dl accompanied by nonfasting positive urine ketones acute onset in a child or young adult triggered by

recent infection or viral illness; onset during puberty or association with other autoimmune diseases (thyroiditis, Graves' disease, pernicious anemia, celiac, and Addison disease).

Type 2 diabetes. The pathogenesis of type 2 diabetes is very different from that of type 1 diabetes. As opposed to type 1 diabetes, in type 2 diabetes, insulin resistance is almost universally present, and the defect in insulin secretion is milder—the secretion is just not high enough to overcome the resistance (β-cell dysfunction). Type 2 diabetes is often preceded by a condition called prediabetes characterized either by abnormal fasting glucose levels (impaired fasting glucose or IFG) or by impaired glucose tolerance (IGT; abnormal postprandial glucose) that leads to increased levels of A1C (Table 32.1). During the prediabetes stage, there is a gradual increase in insulin resistance as

TABLE 32.1	**Diagnosis of Diabetes Mellitus**

CRITERIA FOR THE DIAGNOSIS OF DIABETES

1. A1C ≥ 6.5%. The test should be performed in a laboratory using a method that is NGSP certified and standardized to the DCCT assay (http://www.ngsp.org/prog/index.html, accessed 4/13/2010).*

OR

2. FPG ≥ 126 mg/dl (7.0 mmol/l). Fasting is defined as no caloric intake for at least 8 h.*

OR

3. Two-hour plasma glucose ≥200 mg/dl (11.1 mmol/l) during an OGTT. The test should be performed as described by the World Health Organization, using a glucose load containing the equivalent of 75g anhydrous glucose dissolved in water.*

OR

4. In a patient with classic symptoms of hyperglycemia or hyperglycemic crisis, a random plasma glucose ≥200 mg/dl (11.1 mmol/l).

*In the absence of unequivocal hyperglycemia, criteria 1–3 should be confirmed by repeat testing.

CATEGORIES OF INCREASED RISK FOR DIABETES (PRE-DIABETES)*

1. FPG 100–125 mg/dl (5.6–6.9 mmol/l) [IFG]
2. 2-h PG in the 75-g OGTT 140–199 mg/dl (7.8–11.0 mmol/l [IGT]
3. A1C 5.7–6.4%

**For all three tests, risk is continuous, extending below the lower limit of the range and becoming disproportionately greater at higher ends of the range.

Adapted from American Diabetes Association: clinical practice recommendations. Diabetes Care. 2011;34(suppl 1).

TABLE 32.2	Classification of Diabetes Mellitus

TYPE 1 DIABETES

- *Immune Mediated*
- *Idiopathic*

TYPE 2 DIABETES

- *May range from predominately insulin resistant to predominantly insulin deficient*

GESTATIONAL DIABETES
OTHER SPECIFIC TYPES

- Genetic defects of β-cell function
- Genetic defects in insulin action
- Diseases of exocrine pancreas
- Endocrinopathies
- Drug- or chemical-induced diabetes
- Infections
- Uncommon forms of immune-mediated diabetes
- Other genetic syndromes sometimes associated with diabetes

Adapted from Barker JM, Eisenbarth GS. Genetic counseling for autoimmune type 1 diabetes. In: Liebovitz HE, ed. Therapy for Diabetes Mellitus and Related Disorders. 5th ed. Alexandria, VA: American Diabetes Association and Library of Congress Publication; 2009.

a result of various causes (aging, obesity, physical inactivity, or genetics) and, when not accompanied by an increase in insulin secretion, will eventually result in elevated blood glucose levels in the diabetic range. Prediabetes can be identified through the same tests used to diagnose diabetes (Table 32.1). It is now recommended that individuals at risk be screened for the presence of type 2 diabetes (Table 32.3).[1] During this screening, normal glucose tolerance, prediabetes, or full-blown diabetes can be identified. The screening is very important because (1) preventive measures such as weight loss and/or increased physical activity and sometimes pharmacologic measures could deflect the development of type 2 diabetes in the individuals with prediabetes; and (2) early diagnosis and treatment of the clinical manifestation of type 2 diabetes could prevent chronic complications and improve chances of survival.

Prediabetes. It is also part of the metabolic syndrome, defined as a clustering of risk factors that predict the development of both type 2 diabetes and cardiovascular disease (CVD).[7,8] More than 80% of patients with type 2 diabetes have metabolic syndrome and clustering of risk factors for CVD: hypertension, dyslipidemia, and associated inflammation and hypercoagulable state.[7,8] The clustering of these risk factors predicts the development of CVD even independent of the degree of hyperglycemia. The treatment of the risk factors and the underlying pathophysiological causes could prevent both diabetes and CVD. The most prominent underlying modifiable pathophysiological causes are abdominal obesity and insulin resistance.[9] Inflammation and hypercoagulable states are also important to address. The comprehensive treatment of the metabolic syndrome includes smoking cessation, assessment of diabetes risk and implementation of diabetes prevention strategies, control of blood pressure, control of glucose if type 2 diabetes is present, reduction of abdominal obesity, increase in physical activity to at least 30 minutes of activity daily (above usual), decrease in saturated fats to <7% of total calories, elimination of trans

fat, addressing lipid levels such as LDL, triglycerides, and HDL cholesterol according to the 10-year calculated Framingham risk, and eating five servings of fruits and vegetables per day.[8-10]

Inpatient hyperglycemia. Sometimes, when patients are acutely ill, they may develop what is called inpatient hyperglycemia. This can happen in patients who have latent diabetes, prediabetes, or are just at risk for diabetes development but are normally glucose-tolerant. It is unclear how frequently this leads to persistent diabetes after the hospitalization, but inpatient hyperglycemia is a bad prognostic sign that reflects decreased survival in the critical care units.[11] It may be a harbinger of future diabetes if the patient survives. No systematic studies of long-term follow-up for patients with inpatient hyperglycemia have been done.

CLINICAL MANIFESTATIONS OF DIABETES MELLITUS

Clinical manifestations of diabetes mellitus could be acute (diabetic ketoacidosis or hyperosmolar hyperglycemic state) or chronic. The chronic complications manifest as microvascular (retinopathy, neuropathy, or nephropathy) or macrovascular (cerebrovascular disease, coronary artery disease, or peripheral vascular disease) disease. Other complications are susceptibility to infections and connective tissue disorders. Positive correlations were found between glycemic control (as measured by the A1C level) and prevalence and incidence of diabetic microvascular complications. Prospective randomized trials have shown that intensive control of blood glucose significantly reduces the risk of microvascular complications in both type 1

TABLE 32.3	Criteria for testing for diabetes in asymptomatic adult individuals

1) **TESTING SHOULD BE CONSIDERED IN ALL ADULTS WHO ARE OVERWEIGHT (BMI ≥ 25 KG/M²)** * **AND HAVE ADDITIONAL RISK FACTORS:**
   - Physical inactivity
   - First-degree relative with diabetes
   - Members of a high-risk race/ethnicity (e.g., African American, Latino, Native American, Asian American, Pacific Islander)
   - Women who delivered a baby weighing > 9 lb or were diagnosed with GDM
   - Hypertension (≥140/90 mmHg or on therapy for hypertension)
   - HDL cholesterol level <35 mg/dl (0.90 mmol/l) and/or a triglyceride level >250 mg/dl (2.82mmol/l)
   - Women with polycystic ovary syndrome (PCOS)
   - A1C ≥5.7%, IGT, or IFG on previous testing
   - Other clinical conditions associated with insulin resistance (e.g., severe obesity, acanthosis nigricans)
   - History of CVD

2) **IN THE ABSENCE OF THE ABOVE CRITERIA, TESTING FOR DIABETES SHOULD BEGIN AT AGE 45 YEARS**

3) **IF RESULTS ARE NORMAL, TESTING SHOULD BE REPEATED AT LEAST AT 3-YEAR INTERVALS, WITH CONSIDERATION OF MORE FREQUENT TESTING DEPENDING ON INITIAL RESULTS AND RISK STATUS.**

Adapted from American Diabetes Association: clinical practice recommendations. Diabetes Care. 2011;34(suppl 1).
At-risk BMI may be lower in some ethnic groups

TABLE 32.4	Recommendations for Glycemic Control during Chronic Out-patient Management
A1C	<7.0%*
Pre-prandial capillary plasma glucose	90-130 mg/dl
Peak postprandial capillary plasma glucose (Post-prandial glucose measurements should be made 1-2 h after the beginning of the meal)	180 mg/dl

Key concepts in setting glycemic goals are as follows:
- A1C is the primary target for glycemic control
- Goals should be individualized based on:

– duration of diabetes	– known cardiovascular disease or advanced micro-vascular complications
– age/life expectancy	– hypoglycemia unawareness
– co-morbid conditions	– individual patient considerations

- Certain populations (children, pregnant women, and elderly) require special considerations
- More or less stringent glycemic goals may be appropriate for individual patients
- Post-prandial glucose may be targeted if A1C goals are not met despite reaching pre-prandial goals

Adapted from American Diabetes Association: clinical practice recommendations. Diabetes Care. 2011;34(suppl 1).

and type 2 diabetes. The effect of tight glucose control on macrovascular complications in the absence of intensified control of other macrovascular risk factors is presently controversial.[12] It is known, however, that tight control of other CVD risk factors such as hypertension and elevated lipids does significantly reduce risk of fatal and nonfatal macrovascular events in both type 1 and type 2 diabetes patients. This reduction in risk was reported to be 20% to 50% with blood pressure control, 25% to 55% with lipid control, but only 10% to 20% with tight glucose control.[12] A comprehensive approach including tight glucose control and control of other CVD risk factors was reported to lower both micro- and macrovascular complications by 35%.[13] Unintended and adverse tight glucose control effects could be hypoglycemia, weight gain, and possible short-term worsening of proliferative retinopathy, especially and mostly when the patients require insulin, such as patients with type 1 or long-standing type 2 disease. Of particular concern is the effect of hypoglycemia on macrovascular event rates and outcomes.[12]

Treating hyperglycemia to achieve target (outpatient management). It is currently recommended to aim for tight glucose control as early as possible in the course of diabetes treatment (Table 32.4).[1] The target level recommended by the American Diabetes Association (ADA) is A1C<7% or as close to normal as is safely possible to achieve.[1] The A1C should be tested every 6 months if the value is at target or every 3 months when not at target or when treatment changes.

Levels of A1C together with the prevalence of hypoglycemia will dictate the management of glucose control. Correlation of A1C with average glucose level is seen in Table 32.5. If A1C is <7% and the hypoglycemia is not frequent and/or severe, then the treatment can be maintained at the current level. If A1C is between 7% and 8%, this is likely due to 2-hour postprandial elevations; the following need to be reviewed: meal and activity plans, glucose monitoring techniques and frequency, compliance with medication administration and schedule, and sick day management. If A1C is >8%, in addition to previous recommendations, goals setting, assessment of psychosocial issues, diabetes self-management education (DSME workshops) referral and medication adjustments are all likely needed.

Hypoglycemia management. The correct management of hypoglycemia is crucially important in all patients with diabetes who receive insulin or insulin providing medications but especially in those with CVD or advanced complications.[1] The hypoglycemia should be correctly evaluated and treated. It is defined as mild to moderate when levels of blood glucose range from 50 to 70 mg per dl and/or patients can treat it themselves. It can be treated with oral, simple, easily absorbable carbohydrate, such as glucose tablets or gel, orange juice, or soft drinks containing 15 to 20 g of glucose. Glucose levels should be checked again in 15 minutes, and patients must be instructed to carry glucose with them at all times. Severe hypoglycemia is usually when glucose is <50 mg per dl, it is accompanied by altered consciousness, and patients need assistance. They need to take 20 to 30 g of simple glucose by mouth (if able), be given glucagon by intramuscular (IM) injection, or be rescued by emergency medical personnel with intravenous glucose administration. If any severe hypoglycemia

TABLE 32.5	Correlation of A1C with Average Glucose	
	MEAN PLASMA GLUCOSE	
A1C(%)	mg/dl	mmol/L
6	126	7.0
7	154	8.6
8	183	10.2
9	212	11.8
10	240	13.4
11	269	14.9
12	298	16.5

These estimates are based on ADAG data of ~2,700 glucose measurements over 3 months per A1C measurement in 507 adults with type 1, type 2, and no diabetes. The correlation between A1C and average glucose was 0.92. A calculator for converting A1C results into estimated average glucose (eAG), in either mg/dl or mmol/l, is available in http://professional.diabetes.org/eAG.

Adapted fromAmerican Diabetes Association: clinical practice recommendations. Diabetes Care. 2011;34(suppl 1).

episodes occur, then precipitating causes should be assessed, patients should be referred to DSME, use of glucagon IM injections should be taught to family members or care takers, and blood glucose goals should be revised. If patients have frequent severe hypoglycemia or have hypoglycemia unawareness, then families' and friends' support is absolutely needed; patients should wear identifying bracelets; and driving is not recommended.

PHARMACOLOGIC TREATMENT OF HYPERGLYCEMIA: GENERAL PRINCIPLES IN THE OUTPATIENT SETTING

Insulin. Patients with type 1 diabetes are always treated with insulin. In fact, one of the reasons it is very important to make the differentiation between type 1 and type 2 diabetes is to determine whether there is a need for insulin at all times to avoid diabetic ketoacidosis (DKA). Patients with type 2 diabetes may also be insulin requiring for control of blood glucose, although lack of insulin will not produce DKA except in very rare cases. Insulin is used in type 2 patients when it is not possible to achieve glucose level goals with oral agents alone. Insulin treatment should be physiologic and anticipatory. That is, it should include long-acting (basal) insulin to suppress glucose production overnight and normalize fasting glucose and rapid-acting (prandial) insulin to cover meal-related glucose excursions. This physiologic concept is called the basal/bolus concept (Figure 32.1). Examples of different types of insulin and their peak action time and duration of action are shown in Table 32.6. Insulin delivered with a prefilled insulin pen, rather than from a bottle with a syringe and needle, is easier to accurately dose (Figure 32.2A). Similar principles as described above are used for continuous subcutaneous insulin delivery utilizing an insulin pump (Figure 32.2B).

Oral agents. These drugs lower glucose by several mechanisms: improve insulin resistance (sensitizers), improve insulin secretion (secretagogues), improve insulin secretion but also decrease glucagon and gastric emptying through modulation of incretin and gut hormone levels, and those which lower

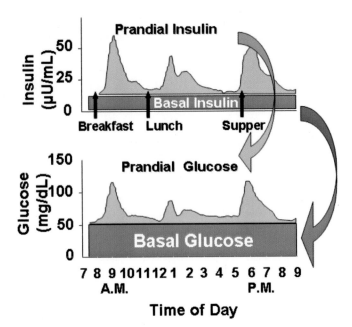

Figure 32.1. Physiologic insulin administration: the basal/bolus concept. The prandial insulin is 50% of the total daily dose administered before each meal to cover the prandial glucose excursions. The basal insulin is 50% of the total daily dose and controls fasting glucose by suppressing glucose production between meals and overnight. (Adapted from the Society for Hospital Medicine Glycemic Control Task Force presentation at www.hospitalmedicine.org)

glucose by decreasing absorption in the gut. The agents that improve insulin resistance are either biguanides or thiazolidinediones. They work through increasing insulin sensitivity in liver, and adipose tissue. The secretagogues work directly on the β-cells (sulfonylureas, amino acids derivatives, and meglitinides). The oral drugs that work through modulating incretin levels (glucagon-like peptide, GLP-1 and others) are dipeptidyl peptidase (DPP-4) inhibitors. GLP-1 analogues,

TABLE 32.6	Insulin preparations by Subcutaneous Administration: Onset, Peak and Duration of Action			
Insulin, Generic Name (Brand)		*Onset*	*Peak*	*Effective*
Rapid-Acting (Prandial or Correction Insulin)				
Aspart (Novolog), Lispro (Humalog), Glulisine (Apidra)		5-15 minutes	30-90 minutes	<5hrs
Short Acting (Prandial or Correction Insulin)				
Insulin Regular (Novolin/Humulin)		30-60 minutes	2-3 hrs	5-8 hrs
Intermediate (Basal Insulin Q12h)				
Insulin NPH (Novolin or Humulin) (OK in pregnancy)		2-4 hrs	4-10 hrs	10-16 hrs
Long-Acting (Basal Insulin Q24h or Q12h)				
Insulin Glargine (Lantus) (avoid in pregnancy)		2-4 hrs	No Peak	20-24 hrs
Insulin Detemir (Levemir) (avoid in pregnancy)		3-8 hrs	No Peak	6-23 hrs
Premixed (Basal and Prandial Mixed)				
75% Lispro Prot. Susp./ 25% Lispro (Humalog Mix 75/25)				
50% Lispro Prot. Susp./ 50% Lispro (Humalog Mix 50/50)				
70% Aspart Prot. Susp./ 30% Aspart (Novolog Mix 70/30)		5-15 minutes	DUAL	10-16 hrs
70% NPH/30% Regular (Novolin or Humulin 70/30)		30-60 minutes	DUAL	10-16 hrs

which produce GLP-1 effects, that is, decrease in glucagon and increases in insulin and amylin secretions, have also been developed but are not administered by the oral route, rather by subcutaneous injections (Figure 32.2A). α-Glucosidase inhibitors decrease glucose absorption in the gut. All these oral agents have potential side effects and have to be used with caution in hospitalized patients particularly when renal and hepatic failure are present, as these increase the risk of hypoglycemia. Combination treatments of different oral drug classes work well and are often used. Such combinations should be tried before insulin treatment is initiated. Insulin should be initiated early, however, if evidence of severe β-cell dysfunction is present, such as rapid weight loss or very high A1C (>9%), despite sustained efforts at diet and exercise, and multiple oral agents' combination.

IDENTIFYING AND TREATING COMPLICATIONS OF DIABETES

The treatment of chronic diabetes complications should be conducted according to published standards of care to ensure early diagnosis and prevent progression. These standards of care are published annually by the ADA.[1] For microvascular disease, retinopathy, nephropathy, and neuropathy are targeted. Retinopathy is one of the eye complications of diabetes mellitus. Retinopathy could be background or proliferative and could lead to retinal detachment, vitreous bleeding, and blindness if not treated. Early laser treatment could prevent blindness. Diabetes is also a risk factor for development of cataracts and glaucoma. Patients should have annual dilated eye examinations after 3 years from onset of type 1 diabetes and at onset of type 2 diabetes. Prevention of background or proliferative retinopathy occurrence or worsening is not only through continuing tight control of blood glucose but also by smoking cessation and control of blood pressure and lipids.

Diabetic nephropathy manifests itself as proteinuria, glomerulosclerosis, and renal failure. Nephropathy should be screened for annually with a urinary microalbumin excretion determination. Goal is <30 mg per g creatinine, which corresponds to approximately 30 mg protein per 24 hours. In addition, glomerular filtration rate (GFR) and creatinine level need to be monitored at least annually. The prevention of nephropathy should be done through tight glucose and blood pressure control and through administration of agents that lower proteinuria, such as angiotensin converting enzyme (ACE) inhibitors and angiotensin receptor blockers (ARB). Treatments of nephropathy presenting with hematuria and nephrotic range proteinuria include dietary protein reduction, blood pressure lowering to <125/75 mm Hg, and revised glucose management for reduced GFR as well as a nephrology consult. If GFR <30, chronic kidney disease (CKD) management principles apply.

Diabetic neuropathy could be peripheral or autonomic and could lead to diabetic foot ulcer, diabetic arthropathy and deformities with pathologic fractures, cellulitis, osteomyelitis, and amputations. The annual screening of feet for diabetes includes a complete assessment of sensation. Inspection of feet should be done at every visit; feet at high risk should be referred for podiatric care and for orthotics.

DIABETES MELLITUS IN THE CARDIAC CARE UNIT

HIGH PREVALENCE OF DIABETES MELLITUS AND/OR HYPERGLYCEMIA IN THE ACUTE CORONARY SYNDROME

The increased prevalence of type 2 diabetes in the United States basically follows the increased prevalence of obesity in the United States in a type of twin epidemics fashion. Patients

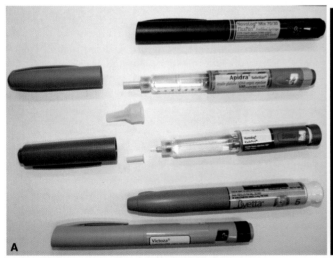 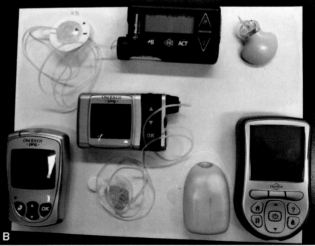

Figure 32.2. A: Insulin injections devices: insulin pens (short-acting, long-acting, and mixed insulins) and pens used to deliver GLP-1 analogues (Byetta and Victoza). Insulin pens are easier to use than syringes, improve patients' attitude and adherence towards the injectable treatment and have accurate dosing mechanisms when used as prescribed. **B:** Insulin pumps and CGMS devices. Insulin pumps deliver insulin subcutaneously through a plastic catheter inserted subcutaneously; they can communicate wirelessly with a glucometer. CGMS devices measure glucose continuously through a sensor inserted subcutaneously. The hope is that in the near future CGMS devices and insulin pumps could be combined to form an artificial pancreas. CGMS, continuous glucose monitoring.

with "the metabolic syndrome," at the center of which are visceral obesity and insulin resistance, are at risk to develop both type 2 diabetes and CVD.[8] Patients with type 2 diabetes and those with associated metabolic syndrome in particular, are at high risk for coronary artery disease (CAD) and CVD events, including nonischemic cardiomyopathy, cerebral and peripheral vascular disease, and death.[14] The underlying abnormalities of the metabolic syndrome in diabetes mellitus are not only in themselves risk factors for CVD but are also associated with pathophysiological states predisposed to acute complications of CVD, that is, the acute coronary syndrome (ACS). Such predisposing factors include increased systemic inflammation, procoagulation, and activation of the renin–angiotensin–aldosterone system with accompanying oxidative stress.[14] Therefore, it is of no surprise that there is a very high prevalence of diabetes in patients acutely admitted to the cardiac care unit (CCU) with ACS. In addition, there are patients with acute hyperglycemia during the ACS (inpatient hyperglycemia) that may or may not resolve after the acute admission to the CCU. In the CRUSADE study 33% of non-ST-segment elevation ACS patients had diabetes,[15] whereas in the United States-based National Registry of Myocardial Infarction, 27% of ST-segment elevation myocardial infarction (STEMI) patients and 34% of NSTEMI patients had diabetes.[16]

DIABETES MELLITUS AND/OR HYPERGLYCEMIA HAVE A NEGATIVE IMPACT ON ACS OUTCOMES

Given the above statistics, it logically follows that diabetes predicts unfavorable outcomes in ACS. Patients afflicted with both conditions (diabetes and ACS) have more frequent hypertension, hypercholesterolemia, and renal failure, regardless of whether the diabetes is a new onset or established. Hyperglycemia affects ACS outcomes as well, and prediabetes tends to worsen ACS outcomes. In fact, admission and consequent glucose levels in patients with ACS are powerful predictors of morbidity and mortality. Along those lines, metabolic syndrome is also predictive of post-ACS morbidity. A retrospective study involving a large number of patients >65 of age demonstrated a clear linear relationship between glucose levels and mortality rate.[17] In addition, hyperglycemia on admission was associated with a higher rise in mortality rate in patients not previously known to have diabetes than in patients with established diabetes.[17]

STRATEGIES FOR IMPROVING OUTCOMES IN ACS COMPLICATED BY DIABETES AND/OR HYPERGLYCEMIA

To counteract acute thrombotic complications in type 2 diabetes, antiplatelet agents, anticoagulation, early invasive strategy in NSTEMI, and prompt reperfusion therapy in STEMI have been employed. In addition to these important lifesaving therapies that are similar to those utilized in nondiabetes patients, glucose-lowering therapies and aggressive use of secondary prevention therapies (i.e., statins, ACE, aldosterone blockers, β-blockers, etc.) will also influence the ACS outcome. Unfortunately, there is no consensus on the most suitable method to measure initial glucose, monitor glucose levels, or even determine the precise glucose value that should be considered abnormal on admission for ACS. Moreover, the benefit for treating hyperglycemia has not been firmly established. Although hyperglycemia is dangerous, hypoglycemia may also

significantly increase mortality rates in ACS, possibly offsetting the beneficial effect of tight glucose control.[18] Therefore it is imperative to closely monitor the intensive glucose control so as to avoid potentially life-threatening hypoglycemia in the inpatient setting, including the CCU.

SUMMARY OF THE CURRENT RECOMMENDATIONS FOR THE MANAGEMENT OF HYPERGLYCEMIA IN THE INPATIENT SETTING, CRITICAL CARE

In general, the awareness that hyper- and hypoglycemia are associated with unfavorable clinical outcomes in the inpatient setting has prompted several societies (ADA, American Association of Clinical Endocrinologists) to develop guidelines for the management of diabetes and hyperglycemia in the inpatient setting, critical care, and noncritical care. The recommendations have evolved through the past 4 years, mainly with changes to the glucose goals recommended and an emphasis on the avoidance of hypoglycemia.[1,19] These guidelines were issued despite the fact that there is no exact consensus on the level of glucose that should be considered abnormal on admission, on the most suitable method to monitor glucose (such as frequency), or on the benefit of tight glucose control in this setting. However, it has been recommended to clearly identify the patient with diabetes or inpatient hyperglycemia, the latter defined as a sustained blood glucose level >180 mg per dl. It should also be taken into consideration that inpatient hyperglycemia could persist posthospitalization (unrecognized diabetes). It is also recommended that the treatment of diabetes and inpatient hyperglycemia in the hospital setting be done through judicious use of an insulin regimen, constructed into protocols that are then tested in the particular institution through continuous quality improvement (QI) processes. We, like others, have developed such a pathway for the management of hyperglycemia in the inpatient setting, critical care, and noncritical care. In the critical care setting, this protocol involves the acute use of intravenous insulin drips with transition to subcutaneous regimens of basal/bolus type in the noncritical care setting. The use of oral agents is not encouraged in the inpatient setting, critical care, as many of the agents have side effects making them contraindicated in acute situations in the hospital setting such as shock, circulatory renal and hepatic failure, NPO status and poor PO intake, and other situations with both increased and decreased insulin action and demands compared with the usual status of the patient. It is also recommended that hypoglycemia treatment be done according to protocols that are to be taught to all nurses and prescribing personnel.

The current blood glucose goal for critical care patients is 140 to 180 mg per dl. This is done for all patients with diabetes or in new onset inpatient hyperglycemia (those who present with glucose persistently >180 mg per dl). Moreover, it is not recommended to lower the blood glucose to <110 mg per dl owing to the risk of hypoglycemia. In the CCU, we have developed a pathway for the use of an IV insulin drip, which was then tested through a QI process (http://www.nycardiologypathways.org). We have taught the pathway to the house staff and prescribing providers, and we designed a flow sheet for the nurses to follow. We also conducted a QI study, where we showed that in the patients treated with the IV insulin drip protocol, there was less hypoglycemia, and glucose levels <180 mg

TABLE 32.7	Insulin Correction Scale				
Blood Glucose	Standard	Low-Dose	Medium-Dose	High Dose	How to Incorporate Prandial Dose (e.g., Using Low-dose Scale)
0–70	Hypo-glycemia Rx	Hypo-glycemia Rx	Hypo-glycemia Rx	Hypo-glycemia Rx	Hypo-glycemia Rx
71–150	No correction	No correction	No correction	No correction	Prandial Dose + no correction
151–200	2 units	1 unit	1 unit	2 units	Prandial Dose + 1 unit
201–250	3 units	2 units	3 units	4 units	Prandial Dose + 2units
251–300	4 units	3 units	5 units	6 units	Prandial Dose + 3units
301–350	5 units	4 units	7 units	8 units	Prandial Dose + 4units
351–400	6 units	5 units	9 units	10 units	Prandial Dose + 5units
>401	6 units + call HO	6 units + call HO	10 units	12 units	Prandial Dose + 6units + call HO

per dl were achieved in shorter time than in patients treated with a subcutaneous regimen consisting mainly of a classic sliding scale. In the CCU, the IV insulin drip (by protocol) that we devised as a hyperglycemia pathway was proven safer than the usual treatment with subcutaneous regimens.

SUMMARY OF CURRENT RECOMMENDATIONS: MANAGEMENT OF HYPERGLYCEMIA IN THE INPATIENT SETTING, NONCRITICAL CARE

Currently, there is no evidence-based glucose goal for noncritical care illnesses. The glucose levels of 140 mg per dl premeal and 180 mg per dl randomly are the goals set, if safely achievable. More stringent goals may be needed in some patients. However, it is very important to avoid hypoglycemia. Insulin, which is the mainstay of treatment, should be adjusted if glucose is <70 mg per dl and be reassessed if values are <100 mg per dl. The subcutaneous (SC) insulin regimens that are recommended involve the basal/bolus type regimen. In this regimen, there are basal insulin and meal insulin (prandial or nutritional), along with correction scale insulin. The scheduled prandial insulin is related to meals. The meal insulin is adjusted according to the point of care blood glucose and is supplemented with the correction insulin to decrease the blood glucose to goal levels. When transitioning from the insulin IV drip to the SC regimen, 75% to 80% of total daily IV insulin dose is used. The total dose is then divided, with 50% to be used for the basal dose and 50% to be equally divided into three doses to be given before meals. In addition, correction insulin is ordered according to the insulin sensitivity of the patient (low dose, medium dose, or high dose) (Table 32.7). The use of a correction insulin scale alone (formerly called sliding scale) is not recommended. After establishing a basal/bolus protocol for our noncritical care inpatients, our own QI process has shown that using the basal/bolus anticipatory schedule pathways was associated with less hypoglycemia. It is imperative that such pathways be taught to the nurses and the prescribing providers thoroughly.

TRANSITION TO OUTPATIENT CARE

It is important that standards of care be established for transition from the inpatient to the outpatient setting for both critical care and noncritical care. In general, length of stay for patients with diabetes, although longer than for those without, has been gradually decreasing just as for all inpatient stays being on average 5 to 6 days. Therefore, the discharge plan for patients with diabetes has to be set from the beginning of the admission. In established diabetes, it is important to determine the goals for the patient's level of glycemic control, but the assessment and management of the microvascular complications must also be addressed. Blood pressure and lipids have to be aggressively controlled. Blood pressure targets are 130/80 mm Hg for diabetics unless there is advanced nephropathy (when 125/75 mm Hg is warranted), LDL <100 mg per dl or <70 mg per dl if acute MI or prior CAD or CVD are present, triglycerides <150 mg per dl, and HDL >40 mg per dl in men and >50 mg per dl in women. In the patients with new onset hyperglycemia, it is important to arrange for follow-up to determine whether the hyperglycemia has persisted, and if not, whether the patient is at risk and needs to be in a diabetes prevention program.

REFERENCES

1. American Diabetes Association: clinical practice recommendations. *Diabetes Care.* 2011;34(suppl 1).
2. The International Expert Committee. International Expert Committee report on the role of the A1C assay in the diagnosis of diabetes. *Diabetes Care.* 2009;32(7):1327–1334.
3. Barker JM, Eisenbarth GS. Genetic counseling for autoimmune type 1 diabetes. In: Liebovitz HE, ed. *Therapy for Diabetes Mellitus and Related Disorders.* 5th ed. Alexandria, VA: American Diabetes Association and Library of Congress Publication; 2009.
4. Lillioja S, Mott DM, Spraul M, et al. Insulin resistance and insulin secretory dysfunction as precursors of non-insulin-dependent diabetes mellitus. Prospective studies of Pima Indians. *N Engl J Med.* 1993;329:1988–1992.
5. Weyer C, Tataranni PA, Bogardus C, et al. Insulin resistance and insulin secretory dysfunction are independent predictors of worsening of glucose tolerance during each stage of type 2 diabetes development. *Diabetes Care.* 2001;24:89–94.
6. Metzger BE, Gabbe SG, Persson B, et al.; International Association of Diabetes and Pregnancy Study Groups Consensus Panel. International association of diabetes and pregnancy study groups recommendations on the diagnosis and classification of hyperglycemia in pregnancy. *Diabetes Care.* 2010;33:676–682.
7. Ford ES, Giles WH, Dietz WH. Prevalence of the metabolic syndrome among US adults: findings from the Third National Health and Nutrition Examination Survey. *JAMA.* 2002;287:356–359.
8. Grundy SM, Cleeman JI, Daniels SR, et al. Diagnosis and management of the metabolic syndrome: an American Heart Association/National Heart, Lung, and Blood Institute Scientific Statement. *Circulation.* 2005;112:2735–2752.
9. Despres JP, Lemieux I. Abdominal obesity and metabolic syndrome. *Nature.* 2006;444:881–887.
10. Grundy SM, Hansen B, Smith SC Jr, et al. Clinical management of metabolic syndrome: report of the American Heart Association/National Heart, Lung, and Blood Institute/American Diabetes Association conference on scientific issues related to management. *Circulation.* 2004;109:551–556.
11. Umpierrez GE, Isaacs SD, Bazargan N, et al. Hyperglycemia: an independent marker of in-hospital mortality in patients with undiagnosed diabetes. *J Clin Endocrinol Metab.* 2002;87:978–982.

12. Skyler JS, Bergenstal R, Bonow RO, et al.; American Diabetes Association, American College of Cardiology Foundation, American Heart Association. Intensive glycemic control and the prevention of cardiovascular events: implications of the ACCORD, ADVANCE, and VA diabetes trials: a position statement of the American Diabetes Association and a scientific statement of the American College of Cardiology Foundation and the American Heart Association. *Diabetes Care.* 2009;32:187–192.

13. Gaede P, Vedel P, Larsen N, et al. Multifactorial intervention and cardiovascular disease in patients with type 2 diabetes. *N Engl J Med.* 2003;348:383–393.

14. Sobel BE. Optimizing cardiovascular outcomes in diabetes mellitus. *Am J Med.* 2007;120(9) (suppl 2):S3–S11.

15. Bhatt DL, Roe MT, Peterson ED, et al. Utilization of early invasive management strategies for high-risk patients with non-ST-segment elevation acute coronary syndromes: results from the CRUSADE Quality Improvement Initiative. *JAMA.* 2004;292:2096–2104.

16. Roe MT, Parsons LS, Pollack CV Jr, et al. Quality of care by classification of myocardial infarction: treatment patterns for ST-segment elevations vs. non-ST-segment elevation myocardial infarction. *Arch Intern Med.* 2005;165:1630–1636.

17. Kosiborod M, Rathore SS, Inzucchi SE, et al. Admission glucose and mortality in elderly patients hospitalized with acute myocardial infarction. Implications for patients with and without recognized diabetes. *Circulation.* 2005;111:3078–3086.

18. Griesdale DEG, Russell J, van Dam RM, et al. Intensive insulin therapy and mortality among critically ill patients: a meta-analysis including NICE-SUGAR study data. *CMAJ.* 2009;180:821–827.

19. Moghissi ES, Korytkowski MT, DiNardo M, et al.; American Association of Clinical Endocrinologists, American Diabetes Association. American Association of Clinical Endocrinologists and American Diabetes Association consensus statement on inpatient glycemic control. *Endocr Pract.* 2009;15:353–369.

PATIENT AND FAMILY INFORMATION FOR:

Diabetes Mellitus

DIABETES MELLITUS: GENERAL PRINCIPLES

WHAT IS DIABETES MELLITUS AND HOW IS IT DIAGNOSED?

Diabetes mellitus means that the level of glucose (blood sugar) in the blood is higher than normal. A higher level of glucose *(hyperglycemia)* in the system over a long period leads to tissue injury, generally affecting the nerves, eyes, and possibly the arteries as well. Table 32.1 presents the current glucose values used to diagnose diabetes mellitus. According to the 2011 ADA criteria, a number of measurements can be used to make the correct diagnosis, such as (1) randomly measured levels of glucose in the blood; (2) the measurement of glucose while fasting; (3) the measurement of blood sugar after a standardized glucose intake is given to the patient orally; or, (4) by measuring the amount of glucose particles attached to blood hemoglobin (AIC) on average over a 3-month period, which is a very consistent indicator of risk for diabetes complications.

WHAT CAUSES DIABETES?

Table 32.2 details various types of diabetes from type 1, type 2, gestational, or other specified types. Type 1 diabetes means that the pancreas (the organ that produces insulin) is not producing enough, or any, insulin to maintain the blood sugar in the normal range. Type 2 diabetes is not only characterized by resistance to the action of insulin for multiple reasons but also by a relative decrease in the body's ability to secrete insulin (insulin is produced but not in sufficient quantities or in an appropriate pattern to overcome the insulin resistance). Increased resistance to insulin, owing to greater quantities of hormones in the blood that occur during pregnancy, is the basis for gestational diabetes. The presence of gestational diabetes constitutes a high-risk factor of developing type 2 diabetes later in the patient's life and therefore these patient's require close follow-up. Other less common types of diabetes could be because of genetic defects affecting insulin's action, pancreatic disease with decreased insulin production, various endocrine dysfunctions, various drugs, rare infections, immune-mediated reactions, and so on. The overall clinical manifestation of these other types are similar to either type 1 or type 2 diabetes.

Type 1 diabetes. Insulin therapy is essential in patients with type 1 diabetes because they do not produce any. DKA is a known complication of type 1 diabetes in patients not receiving insulin injections. This is a very dangerous condition characterized by dehydration, nausea, and vomiting and is so severe that it can lead to coma and even death. It is completely reversible with the appropriate administration of insulin and glucose.

Type 2 diabetes. Basically it means a resistance to insulin and the body' inability to compensate by producing more from the pancreas. Type 2 diabetes is always preceded by a condition called prediabetes. A prediabetes condition is defined by high levels of fasting glucose, reduced tolerance to the higher amounts of glucose, and higher levels of A1C (Table 32.1) but not to the degree seen in full-blown diabetes. A gradual increase in resistance to insulin's action (insulin resistance) occurs with aging, obesity, physical inactivity, and genetic factors. If the insulin resistance is not overcome by producing more insulin then this will lead to increased glucose in the blood (Figure 32.1). It is important to understand that obesity, especially "male-type" abdominal obesity is the central component in developing prediabetes and type 2 diabetes. Prediabetes can be detected through the same tests as full-blown diabetes (Table 32.1). Individuals considered "at risk" should be screened for both prediabetes and type 2 diabetes (Table 32.3). Early detection allows the early implementation of preventive measures aimed at improving insulin resistance (weight loss, increased physical activity, etc.) but early diagnosis and treatment of type 2 diabetes can also prevent chronic complications and can improve chances of survival.

Elevated blood glucose while hospitalized (inpatient hyperglycemia). Sometimes acutely ill patients who are not known to have had diabetes or prediabetes of any kind may develop high blood glucose while admitted to the hospital because the stress on the body from illness causes a state of insulin resistance. This can also happen in patients who have latent diabetes, prediabetes, or just are at risk for diabetes development but are normally glucose-tolerant when not sick. It is unclear how frequently this leads to persistent diabetes after hospitalization, but inpatient elevations of blood glucose have been linked to decreased survival in the critical care units. If the patient survives the critical event but shows signs of IGT (prediabetes), this can be an indication for the future development of diabetes, and it should be addressed by the physician caring for the patient in the outpatient setting. No systematic studies of long-term follow-up for a patient with inpatient elevated blood glucose levels have been done so far.

CLINICAL MANIFESTATION OF DIABETES MELLITUS

Clinical manifestations of diabetes mellitus could be acute (such as DKA) or chronic. The chronic complications may affect the small blood vessels (microvascular) or large blood vessels (macrovascular) in the body. Microvascular complications include worsening vision, nerve dysfunction (neuropathy), and damage to the kidneys. Macrovascular complications include effects on the brain, heart, and other peripheral blood vessels (atherosclerosis and clotting). Other complications include an increased risk of infection and disorders of the skin, joints, and muscles.

TREATING ELEVATED BLOOD GLUCOSE TO ACHIEVE TARGET (OUTPATIENT MANAGEMENT)

Currently it is recommended to aim for tight glucose control early in the course of diabetes (Table 32.4). There are several ways to assess glucose control in diabetes mellitus. One can frequently test blood glucose throughout the day with a glucometer, measure A1C, or measure blood glucose continuously through a subcutaneous catheter (inserted under the skin), that is, continuous glucose monitoring. Glucose monitoring is essential for the patients to achieve the glucose targets. A1C reflects mean glucose over a 2- to 3-month period. Beyond the desirable range, it is a marker for risk of complications. The target level recommended by the ADA is <7% or as close to normal as safely possible to achieve. The A1C should be tested every 6 months if the value is at target or every 3 months when not on target, or when treatment changes. Other glucose targets for tight control have been defined for fasting blood glucose and for glucose checked 2 hours postconsumption of a meal. The fasting glucose target has been defined by the ADA as 90 to 130 mg per dl, whereas 2-hour glucose target has been defined as <180 mg per dl peak value. Glucose monitoring is best demonstrated by a diabetes educator who can also best determine the devices that should be used and how often to test. The glucose should be monitored at least three times per day, before each of the main meals, for patients on insulin injections to guide dosing. Those not on insulin could use self-monitoring as a guide to success.

MANAGEMENT OF LOW BLOOD GLUCOSE (HYPOGLYCEMIA)

The correct management of low levels of blood glucose is crucial in all diabetics but especially in those with cardiac disease, vascular disease, or advanced complications. The low blood glucose levels should be correctly evaluated and treated immediately. The severity of low glucose levels is considered mild to moderate when levels of blood glucose range from 50 to 70 mg per dl and/or patients can treat it themselves. It can be treated with oral, simple, and easily absorbable carbohydrate such as glucose tablets/gel, orange juice, or soft drinks containing 15 to 20 g glucose. Glucose levels should be checked again in 15 minutes and patients must be educated to carry a source of glucose with them at all times. Extremely low blood glucose levels of <50 mg per dl, when accompanied by altered consciousness and requiring the patients to need assistance, is considered to be very severe. They need to take 20 to 30 g of simple glucose orally if able or be given glucagon by intramuscular injection. If not responsive to the previous methods then 911 should be called to have IV glucose administered.

If severe hypoglycemia is consistently present, patients should be referred for a diabetes self-management education workshop, where the use of glucagon injection should be taught to family members or caretakers. In addition, blood glucose goals have to be revised. If patients have frequent episodes of low blood glucose or are unaware of the symptoms that usually accompany these low levels, they need support from family members or friends to prevent them from harm. These at-risk patients should wear identifying bracelets and it is not recommended that they drive.

IDENTIFYING AND TREATING COMPLICATIONS OF DIABETES

The treatment of chronic complications of diabetes should be conducted according to published standards of care to ensure early diagnosis and to prevent progression. These standards of care are published yearly by the ADA. Retinopathy, nephropathy, and neuropathy are the targeted complications. Retinopathy is one of the eye complications of diabetes mellitus. Retinopathy can lead to blindness if not treated early with laser or other methods. Diabetes is also a risk factor for the development of cataracts and glaucoma. Patients should have annual dilated eye examinations after 3 years from the onset of type 1 diabetes and immediately at the time of diagnosis for type 2 diabetes. Prevention of retinopathy is through tight control of blood glucose and also by smoking cessation along with control of blood pressure and blood lipids (cholesterol and triglycerides).

Diabetic nephropathy manifests itself as protein leaking in the urine, which eventually can lead to kidney failure requiring dialysis. The amount of protein leaking in the urine should be checked annually with a random spot urine test. Also the kidney function needs to be monitored at least annually. The prevention of kidney failure should be done through tight glucose and blood pressure control and through administration of agents that lower leakage of protein in the urine. When severe protein leakage is present there may be swelling of the legs, and treatment should include dietary protein reduction, blood pressure lowering to <125/75 mm Hg, and revised glucose management goals.

Diabetic neuropathy can affect the "peripheral" nerves (those going to the feet and legs, hands, etc.) or the nerves that go to the organs. The former can lead to diabetic foot ulcers, damage to the joints, and deformities of the feet with fractures and infections and ultimately even amputations. Inspection of the feet should be done at every visit; feet identified to be at high risk should be referred for podiatric care and for orthotics. Patients should have diabetes self-management education including foot care training.

OTHER ASPECTS OF DIABETES MANAGEMENT

For all newly diagnosed diabetics, essential care should also address the following: (1) Diabetes self-management education and nutrition education; (2) psychosocial screening; (3) pregnancy, contraception, and osteoporosis in women, erectile dysfunction in men; and (4) dental care and vaccinations. A minimum amount of diabetes education (survival skills) should be taught in the hospital before discharge and patients should be referred to an outpatient setting and ADA-certified, diabetes self-management education program. Diabetes self-management nutrition addresses diet and energy balance: weight loss issues if needed, need for carbohydrate counting in insulin-requiring patients, risk of low blood glucose with decreased energy intake, increase in physical activity, increase in dietary fiber (14 g per 1,000 kcal), and alcohol intake (maximum one drink per day for women and two drinks per day for men). Physical activity is recommended to be of both aerobic and resistance type training and should be done in combination. Aerobic activity should be at least 150 minutes per week and it should be of moderate intensity, 50% to 70% of maximum heart rate (220-age). Resistance exercise should be done three times a week if there are no contraindications, such as, the presence of proliferative diabetic retinopathy. A screening is needed to assess the literacy level that is essential for diabetes self-management education of glucose monitoring and medication adherence. Mood disorders such as depression and anxiety must be addressed as they can influence diabetes control as well as coping. Social barriers (family and economic issues) and physical barriers (blindness, amputations, etc.) are all likely to affect diabetes management.

DIABETES MELLITUS IN THE CARDIAC CARE UNIT

HIGH PREVALENCE OF DIABETES MELLITUS AND/OR INCREASED BLOOD GLUCOSE IN THE ACUTE CORONARY SYNDROME

Patients with type 2 diabetes have a very high incidence of obesity and the "metabolic syndrome," and the most common cause of death for these patients is CVD, specifically CAD. Other associated underlying abnormalities of the metabolic syndrome that include inflammation, a tendency to have blood clots in the arteries, and increased oxidative stress in the body are also associated with acute complications of CVD such as ACS ("heart attack"). Numerous studies have shown that there is a very high prevalence of diabetes in patients acutely admitted to the CCU with ACS.

In addition to being frequently present in ACS, diabetes also predicts unfavorable outcomes. Patients afflicted with both conditions (diabetes and ACS) have more frequent high blood pressure, high cholesterol, and kidney failure. This is regardless of whether the diabetes is new onset or established. High blood sugar affects ACS outcomes even if diabetes were not present before the event and is diagnosed in the hospital.

STRATEGIES FOR IMPROVING OUTCOMES IN ACS COMPLICATED BY DIABETES AND/OR HIGH BLOOD GLUCOSE

To counteract complications from cardiac events in type 2 diabetes various blood-thinning medications and early strategies to unblock blood vessels are done as early as possible. In addition to these important lifesaving therapies that are similar to those utilized in nondiabetes patients, glucose-lowering therapies and aggressive use of secondary prevention therapies for control of high blood pressure, cholesterol, and inflammation are also utilized. Currently the consensus is that high blood glucose should be lowered in patients with diabetes and ACS, but the level to be obtained will be dependent on how safe it is to get there without causing too much low blood glucose. Both hyperglycemia and hypoglycemia are harmful and should be avoided in the CCU.

TRANSITION TO OUTPATIENT CARE

It is important that standards of care are established for transition from the inpatient to the outpatient setting for both critical care and noncritical care. In general, length of hospital stay for the patients with diabetes is longer than for those without diabetes but has been gradually decreasing. Therefore a comprehensive and practical plan for discharge for the patients with diabetes has to be done from the beginning of the admission. In established diabetes, it is important not only to determine the goals for the patient's level of sugar control, but the assessment and management of the complications also have to be addressed. In the patients with inpatient hyperglycemia it is important to arrange for follow-up to determine whether the hyperglycemia persists, and if not whether the patient is at risk of developing diabetes.

Obesity, physical activity, and smoking must be addressed in patients with diabetes and heart disease. Blood pressure and cholesterol have to be aggressively controlled. Blood pressure targets are 130/80 mm Hg for diabetics unless there is advanced kidney disease when 125/75 mm Hg is warranted, LDL (bad cholesterol) <100 mg per dl or <70 mg per dl if acute heart attack or prior heart disease is present, triglycerides <150 mg per dl, and HDL (good cholesterol) >40 mg per dl in men and >50 mg per dl in women.

Tiberio M. Frisoli
Eyal Herzog
Franz H. Messerli

Hypertension in the Cardiac Care Unit

We have developed at St. Luke's Roosevelt Hospital Center a novel pathway for the management of arterial hypertension (HTN) in hospitalized patients[1] (Figure 33.1).

The Committee on Public Health Priorities to reduce and control HTN in the U.S. Population concluded that "the CDC's cardiovascular disease program in general, and the HTN program in particular, are dramatically under-funded relative to the preventable burden of disease." The global burden of HTN is tremendous. HTN is a risk factor for essentially every medical condition that would warrant admission to a hospital's cardiac intensive care unit (CCU); in fact, the CCU is where the most severe forms of the HTN burden can be seen.

HTN can be defined as a sustained rise in blood pressure (BP) that increases risk for cerebral, cardiac, and renal events. In industrialized countries, the risk of becoming hypertensive (BP >140 per 90 mm Hg) during a lifetime exceeds 90%. The clinical significance of HTN ranges from it being an innocent bystander, to hypertensive emergencies requiring immediate therapy. Patients may be asymptomatic despite marked elevation in systemic BP, yet end-organ consequences of HTN are typically major causes of morbidity and mortality, hence the designation of HTN as the "silent killer."

HYPERTENSION: DEFINITION AND PATHOPHYSIOLOGY

HTN may be a primary cause for admission to the CCU as in hypertensive emergency. More commonly, however, the CCU patient is admitted for a condition related secondarily to HTN, with high BP as a critical target of therapy and of future risk reduction. For example, while the acute coronary syndrome (ACS) or heart failure (HF) patient is not admitted primarily for HTN, HTN is a mediator of the ongoing myocardial oxygen supply/demand imbalance in ACS, and of pump failure in HF, and thus is a critical target of therapy.

BP is determined by the product of heart rate, stroke volume, and systemic vascular resistance. Heart rate is determined largely by sympathetic activity. Stroke volume depends on cardiac preload and afterload, which in turn depend on multiple variables affecting vascular tone. It follows that BP can be reduced by reducing heart rate, stroke volume, and/or vascular resistance.

HTN can be essential or secondary. Secondary HTN is due to a discernable cause, such as renal or endocrine disease, whereas essential HTN, which is responsible for the most cases, is not. HTN can also be thought of as an elevation of BP caused by one or more abnormalities in cardiac function, vascular function, renal function, and/or neuroendocrine function.

Cardiac: A hyperkinetic circulation caused by excessive sympatho-adrenal activity or increased sensitivity of the heart to baseline neurohormonal regulators increases cardiac output and causes HTN with normal systemic vascular resistance, often in younger patients.

Vascular: Elevated vascular resistance, more common in the elderly, because of abnormal blood vessel responsiveness to sympathetic outflow, endothelial damage which disrupts vasodilatory/vasoconstrictor balance, and ion channel defects will raise BP.

Renal: Renovascular disease leads to increased production of angiotensin II and aldosterone which increase vasomotor tone and sodium/water retention leading to increased cardiac output and systemic vascular resistance.

Neuroendocrine: Neuroendocrine dysfunction as in pheochromocytoma and primary hyperaldosteronism can alter cardiac, vascular, and renal function to cause HTN through a number of various mechanisms.

GENERAL PRINCIPLES ABOUT THE PHARMACOLOGIC MANAGEMENT OF HYPERTENSION

The fundamental concept of HTN treatment is that BP can be decreased by reducing heart rate, stroke volume, and/or systemic vascular resistance. These factors are interrelated, and many pharmacologic agents affect more than one of these determinants of BP. The drugs used to treat HTN are many, but when grouped into classes they are surprisingly few. The armamentarium of drugs used to treat systemic HTN includes those that reduce intravascular volume (diuretics), downregulate sympathetic tone (β-blockers, α-blockers, and central sympatholytics), modulate vascular smooth muscle tone (calcium channel blockers [CCBs] and potassium channel openers), and inhibit the neurohormonal regulators of the circulatory system (angiotensin-converting enzyme [ACE] inhibitors and angiotensin receptor blockers [ARBs]). These drug classes make up the bulk of medications used to treat not only HTN but also the most common disease processes that warrant a CCU admission. β-Blockers, for example, are antihypertensives fundamentally important for reasons that go beyond their antihypertensive effects, in the treatment of HF, ACS, acute neurologic syndrome, and acute aortic syndrome. It is useful to organize drugs in classes and by mechanism of action because an understanding of how the drug class works helps one understand why it is effective for a disease process.

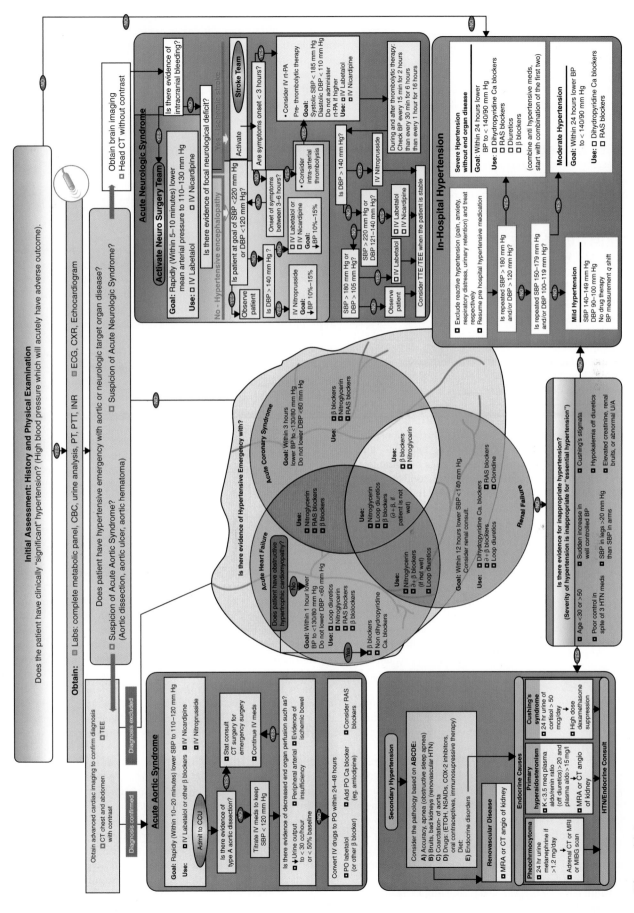

Figure 33.1. Pathway for the management of hypertension for hospitalized patients.

DIURETICS

Diuretics, which function both to reduce intravascular volume and to vasodilate, increase renal excretion of sodium and water. Thiazide diuretics (e.g., chlorthalidone, indapamide, and hydrochlorothiazide) have long duration of action and moderate intensity of diuresis, suiting them more for chronic HTN treatment than for short-term aggressive diuresis. Once considered first-line for HTN, thiazides are now deemed inferior to several other medications in their antihypertensive potency. Loop diuretics (e.g., furosemide) have a relatively short duration of action (4 to 6 hours) and are useful more for brisk diuresis than antihypertensive efficacy, making them critical in the treatment of HF.

ADRENERGIC BLOCKADE: α- AND β-BLOCKERS

β_1 receptors found on myocardial cells, when activated, increase heart rate (chronotropy) and contractility (inotropy). α_1 receptors found on vascular smooth muscle promote contraction and thus vasoconstriction; these receptors on the heart increase inotropy.

β-Adrenergic antagonists (e.g., metoprolol) have negative chronotropic and negative inotropic effects as well as effects on resistance vessels. Not only do β-blockers decrease heart rate and BP, but they protect against the cardiac remodeling imposed by adrenergic stimulation. Some drugs (labetalol, carvedilol) block α- and β-receptors thus mediating vasodilatation (α blockade) and decreased reflex tachycardia. By decreasing heart rate and thus increasing diastolic filling time, these drugs increase preload without compromising cardiac output (decreased afterload and increased preload compensate for decreased heart rate).

CALCIUM CHANNEL BLOCKERS

Calcium ions are major mediators of vascular smooth muscle cell contraction and inotropic and chronotropic function of the heart. Calcium enters vascular smooth muscle cells, cardiomyocytes, and pacemaker cells through voltage-dependent calcium channels.[2] In vascular smooth muscle, the channel allows entry of sufficient calcium for initiation of contraction by calcium-induced intracellular calcium release from the sarcoplasmic reticulum. In addition to these acute regulatory functions, increased intracellular calcium has atherosclerosis-promoting effects.[3]

The dihydropyridine CCBs (e.g., amlodipine, nifedipine, felodopine, isradipine) are highly selective for arterial tissues, including the coronary arteries, where they cause vasodilation. Nicardipine has strong antihypertensive activity; intra-arterially it decreases incidence of vasospasm in subarachnoid hemorrhage, and it is a recommended agent for HTN after acute ischemic stroke and intracerebral hemorrhage.[4] Clevidipine, a new third-generation intravenous dihydropyridine CCB has a high vascular selectivity with a fast onset and offset of BP lowering effect, thus making it easily and rapidly titratable and an especially attractive drug for acute HTN. In perioperative patients requiring HTN treatment, clevidipine compared favorably to nitroglycerin (NTG), nitroprusside, and nicardipine in terms of BP-reducing efficacy and 30-day outcomes (death, MI, stroke, and renal failure).[5]

The nondihydropyridine CCBs (diltiazem and verapamil) bind to different sites and are less selective for vascular smooth muscle; they have negative chronotropic and dromotropic effects on sinoatrial and atrioventricular nodal conducting tissue and negative inotropic effects on cardiomyocytes, making them useful heart rate-controlling agents as in atrial fibrillation with rapid ventricular rate.

Nondihydropyridine CCBs should be used with caution in patients with impaired systolic function or conduction system disease because these agents can exacerbate HF and SA or AV node dysfunction, especially in patients already on β-blocker therapy.

ANGIOTENSIN-CONVERTING ENZYME INHIBITORS

ACE inhibitors prevent the ACE-mediated conversion of angiotensin I to angiotensin II, leading to decreased circulating angiotensin II and aldosterone. Angiotensin II elevates BP and promotes target-organ damage, including atherosclerosis, by various mechanisms: direct effects of angiotensin II on constriction and remodeling of resistance vessels, aldosterone synthesis and release, enhancement of sympathetic outflow from the brain, and facilitation of catecholamine release from the adrenals and peripheral sympathetic nerve terminals.[6,7]

ACE inhibitors decrease levels of vasoconstricting angiotensin II. They also promote natriuresis and reduce intravascular volume. By decreasing bradykinin breakdown, ACE inhibitors promote vasodilatation. They may be nephroprotective because reducing angiotensin II levels reduces renal efferent arteriole constriction thus reducing intraglomerular pressures and limiting glomerular damage over time. For all these reasons, these drugs are particularly useful in the hypertensive diabetic patient and the HF patient.

NITRATES

Organic nitrates are chemically reduced to release nitric oxide (NO), an endogenous signaling molecule that causes vascular smooth muscle relaxation. Although NO can dilate both arteries and veins, venous dilation predominates at therapeutic doses. NO-induced venodilation increases venous capacitance, leading to a decrease in the return of blood to the right side of the heart, and subsequently decreased right ventricular and left ventricular (LV) end-diastolic pressure and volume. This decrease in preload reduces myocardial oxygen demand. At higher concentrations, nitrates may cause arterial vasodilation. In the coronary circulation, NTG preferentially dilates large epicardial arteries rather than smaller coronary arterioles, thus preventing coronary steal phenomenon, encountered with such agents as dipyridamole. It is unclear to what extent the effects of nitrates on coronary vasodilation benefit the patient with angina, because the chronic oxygen deficit in coronary artery disease (CAD) patients causes maximal dilation of coronary arteries, and because atherosclerotic coronary arteries may remain noncompliant even in the face of coronary artery vasodilators. Furthermore, doses of nitrates sufficient to vasodilate epicardial arteries can induce peripheral vasodilation, hypotension, and reflex tachycardia, which harm the delicate supply/demand balance. In patients with HF, however, reflex tachycardia is rare; the venodilation and decreased end-diastolic pressure effects of nitrates make them acceptable at certain doses for decreasing pulmonary congestion in the patient with hypertensive emergency and congestive HF. Side effects related to hypotension include dizziness and syncope; nitrates are contraindicated in hypotension and not advised in diastolic dysfunction and hypertrophic obstructive cardiomyopathy, two disease states for which adequate preload are critical to sustain cardiac output. Moreover, nitrates should not be taken by patients taking phosphodiesterase inhibitors (i.e., Sildenafil [Viagra]).

Sodium nitroprusside is a nitrate that, such as NTG, liberates NO but does so nonenzymatically; as a result nitroprusside does not target specific vessels and consequently dilates both arteries and veins. With rapid onset of action and high efficacy, nitroprusside is useful in hypertensive emergencies but must be infused with continuous BP monitoring. Sodium nitroprusside is metabolized to products which are potentially toxic if they accumulate excessively: cyanide (acid–base disturbance and cardiac arrythmia) is converted to thiocyanate (psychosis, spasms, and convulsions).

HYPERTENSION AND THE CCU

HTN is a risk factor and target of therapy (both short- and long-term) for virtually every condition that warrants a CCU admission. We will review the most common CCU disease states in terms of pathophysiology, diagnosis, and management.

HYPERTENSION AND DISEASES OF THE AORTA

Diseases of the aorta include aortic atheroma, aneurysm, arteritis, and acute aortic syndromes (dissection, intramural hematoma, and penetrating ulcer). These diseases tend to follow an indolent asymptomatic progressive course until they culminate in an acute life-threatening clinical presentation. The most common of these processes is aortic dissection.

Aortic dissection is characterized by an intimal tear and formation of a false lumen within the media of the artery. Repetitive hemodynamic forces produced by the blood ejected into the aorta with each cardiac cycle contribute to the weakening of the aortic intima and to medial degeneration. Sustained HTN intensifies these forces. Acute elevations in heart rate and BP can lead to catastrophic acute worsening of the disease process. The false lumen, as it extends, can obstruct the true lumen leading to such complications as acute myocardial infarction, acute renal failure, and stroke. Many patients with aortic dissection have undermining of the elastic or muscular components of the media which is quantitatively and qualitatively more severe than expected from aging, as seen in such disease processes as Marfan and Ehler-Danlos syndromes, and congenital bicuspid aortic valve.

Patients with aortic syndrome present with acute onset of severe chest pain which typically radiates through the back. The pain is at its most severe at onset, unlike the typically crescendo pain of ACS. Although clearly not diagnostic, terms such as "tearing," "ripping," and "stabbed me in the chest and back" should alert the caregiver to the possibility of dissection. Presentations can vary and thus aortic disease must be considered in any patient presenting with chest pain, especially because some treatments for ACS (thrombolysis) can worsen acute aortic syndrome.

The modalities available for the diagnosis of aortic dissection include CT, MRI, transthoracic echocardiogram (TTE) or transesophageal echocardiogram (TEE), and aortography. The goals of imaging are to establish the diagnosis, determine location of the dissection (ascending, type A dissections are considered surgical emergencies), and determine extent of disease (e.g., coronary or cerebral artery involvement). The choice of modality may be influenced by clinical presentation. The patient with suspected aortic dissection who also presents with physical exam findings suspicious for pericardial effusion or aortic regurgitation may benefit more from a TEE than CT, for example.

Therapy for aortic dissection aims to halt progression; lethal complications arise not because of the tear itself but to extension of the tear such that occlusion or rupture occur. Untreated, aortic dissection will result in death in 25% of patients in 24 hours, 50% in 1 week, and more than 90% in 1 year. As the major etiologic component of the development and progression of aortic dissection, BP is the major target of treatment. Heart rate is also a major target of treatment because BP and heart rate together create hemodynamic force which favors extension of the dissection.

PATHWAY MANAGEMENT

When the dissection involves the ascending aorta, the focus is on surgical management (Figure 33.2). However, whether the dissection is ascending or descending, medical management to reduce BP and heart rate are critical and urgent. Labetalol is an ideal drug as it reduces BP and heart rate, and can be given intrave-

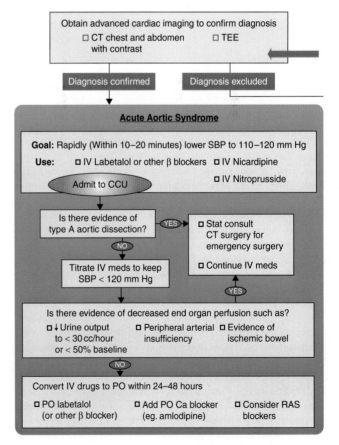

Figure 33.2. Management of hypertension in acute aortic syndrome.

nously for immediate onset of action and titration. We recommend lowering BP within 10 to 20 minutes to a systolic BP level of 110 to 120 mm Hg. Esmolol, with its short half-life, may be a good alternative in those with possible intolerance to β-blockers (reactive airway disease). The CCB nicardipine is an alternative as well. Once the patient is stabilized, whether surgically for ascending or medically for descending dissection, oral forms of the same medications (β-blocker, CCB, and ACE inhibitor) are used for long-term BP control, which is crucial for secondary risk reduction.

HYPERTENSION AND ACUTE NEUROLOGIC SYNDROME

Stroke results from either ischemic or hemorrhagic causes. Ischemic stroke can be categorized by presumed mechanism of ischemia into coagulopathies (protein C deficiency, antiphospholipid antibody), small vessel-lacunar (vasculitis, embolic), large vessel-intracranial (dissection, atherosclerosis), large vessel-extracranial (Takayasu, atherosclerotic), and cardioembolic (atrial fibrillation, ventricular thrombus, infectious endocarditis). Some strokes are cryptogenic, or of undetermined cause. Hemorrhagic stroke can be categorized as intracerebral (bleeding into brain parenchyma, further classified as primary and unrelated to a brain lesion, or secondary and related to a congenital or acquired brain lesion or abnormality), subarachnoid, or intraventricular. HTN is a major risk factor for both ischemic (especially small vessel-lacunar) and hemorrhagic stroke, and thus there is little doubt that treating BP for stroke prevention (both primary and secondary prevention) is justified and very important. However, it is in the treatment of HTN for the patient in the acute phase of a stroke that there has been much controversy and ambiguity; recent data is shedding more light on this important issue.

Stroke is a major cause of morbidity and mortality; it is the third leading cause of death in the United States behind heart disease and cancer. Perhaps more devastating is the morbidity in survivors; stroke is the leading cause of long-term disability in adults. Fifteen to thirty percentage of stroke survivors are permanently disabled, and 20% require institutional care for 3 months.

Timely diagnosis of stroke, greatly dependent on history and physical exam, is critical because early implementation of treatment can improve prognosis; some treatments for ischemic stroke, for example, are only implementable within 3 (intravenous recombinant tissue plasminogen activator rtPA) to 6 hours (intra-arterial thrombolysis) from onset of event. For this reason, the most important piece of history is time of symptom onset. Findings such as focal neurologic deficit, persistent neurologic deficit, acute onset of symptoms, and no history of head trauma favor the diagnosis of stroke; the presence of all four of these findings makes stroke about 80% likely. Symptoms also enable the experienced clinician to determine the vascular distribution (e.g., anterior or posterior) of a stroke. Once stroke is suspected, severity can be assessed with the NIH Stroke Scale, the diagnosis can be further pursued with imaging studies, and tests can be obtained to exclude stroke mimics (tumor, hypertensive encephalopathy, seizure, and migraine variant).

The first imaging test to obtain in the acute stroke patient is a noncontrast CT scan of the brain, because this will identify most intracranial hemorrhage and helps exclude stroke mimickers such as neoplasm. Importantly, CT will not reliably diagnose ischemic stroke when early in its evolution; MRI, on the other hand, will. MRI with diffusion-weighted and perfusion-weighted imaging has a high sensitivity and specificity for ischemic lesions, even within minutes of symptoms onset, and can identify brain tissue that is ischemic but not yet infarcted and therefore amenable to being rescued if successfully revascularized. CT angiogram provides maps of cerebral blood flow thus possibly revealing occlusion or stenosis.

An elevated BP is often detected in the first hours after stroke. For every 10 mm Hg increase above 180 mm Hg, the risk of neurologic deterioration increases by 40% and the risk of poor outcome increases by 23%. Despite this association between elevated BP and poor outcomes, the management of arterial HTN in ischemic stroke has been controversial. Investigators found a U-shaped relationship between death and admission BP; both elevated and low admission levels were associated with high rates of early and late death from stroke.[8] Elevations in mean BP during the first days after stroke had an unfavorable effect on outcomes; death caused by brain injury and brain edema correlated with high initial BP. Theoretical reasons for lowering BP include reducing brain edema, reducing risk of hemorrhagic transformation, and preventing further vascular damage. Conversely, it has been theorized that overly aggressive BP reduction may lead to neurologic worsening.[9] Furthermore, most of the patients experience a drop in BP within the first hour after stroke without any medical treatment. It has thus been suggested that unless thrombolysis is utilized or there is evidence of other BP-related organ dysfunction, there is little scientific evidence and no clinically established benefit for rapid lowering of BP among persons with acute ischemic stroke.[10] Thus, in 2007, an expert panel recommended that antihypertensives should be withheld for acute ischemic stroke, unless BP is more than 220/120 mm Hg[11]; the panel acknowledged that their recommendation was unfortunately not based on very strong or convincing data.

Recent data suggests this "permissive hypertension" may be a mistake. In a study of more than 2,000 ischemic strokes in Mongolia, a systolic BP >200 mm Hg on average 9.3 hours after event onset had an odds ratio of 4.36 for adjusted mortality.[12] In a study of 1,700 patients enrolled 1.0 to 7.9 hours after the event, odds ratios for neurologic impairment at 7 days and functional outcomes at 90 days related to higher SBP at entry, smaller reductions of SBP over the initial 24 hours, and SBP at 24 hours.[13]

PATHWAY MANAGEMENT

If brain imaging confirms intracranial bleeding, neurosurgery must be called for consideration of emergency surgery and BP should be lowered rapidly, within 5 to 10 minutes, to mean 110 to 130 mm Hg with IV Labetalol or Nicardipine. If imaging excludes hemorrhage, the next step is to assess for focal neurologic deficit, commonly present in ischemic stroke and absent in hypertensive encephalopathy. For acute ischemic stroke, according to the expert panel involved in writing the 2007 AHA guidelines, despite some data to suggest systolic BP more than 180 mm Hg should prompt treatment, the consensus at the time was that antihypertensive agents should be withheld unless BP is more than 220/120 mm Hg because of concerns that BP lowering may cause neurologic worsening.[14] This now appears to be incorrect and dangerous. It appears that using 140 to 150 mm Hg as a target SBP may be safe and beneficial,[15] although we do not yet have guidelines incorporating the recent findings. Although often not readily available, a dedicated stroke team should help manage the patient. Part of the reason for this is that for symptoms that persist for less than 3 hours, intravenous rtPA is recommended for selected patients without contraindications (e.g., history of previous intracranial hemorrhage); for symptoms 3 to 6 hours old, intra-arterial thrombolysis may be used. However, BP more than 185/110 mm Hg is a contraindication to IV rtPA. In this setting labetalol and nicardipine may be used. During and after thrombolytic therapy, nitroprusside, labetalol or nicardipine should be used, depending on how high the BP is, to maintain BP below 180/105 mm Hg. For hypertensive encephalopathy on the other hand, the baseline BP must be considered to avoid lowering of excessive BP and prevent cerebral ischemia. Lowering the mean arterial pressure by 25% and the diastolic BP to 100 to 110 mm Hg usually is a safe maneuver because of the pressure autoregulatory cerebral blood flow range.

Patients who were taking antihypertensive medications before their stroke or those who have sustained HTN after their stroke will need long-term antihypertensive treatment. Historically, there was a belief in the medical community that permissive HTN in the long term was protective for patients after an ischemic stroke. In fact, in patients followed from the time of a first ischemic stroke to the time of a second stroke in the same territory, risk was increased rather than decreased with higher BP, a finding driven mainly by systolic BP elevations above 160 mm Hg.[16] It seems that medications such as ARBs can be administered with a reasonable degree of safety when started about 1 day after a stroke.[17] The timing of the reinstitution of treatment and the selection of medications will depend on the patient's neurologic status, the underlying stroke mechanism, the patient's ability to swallow medications, and the presence of concomitant disease. Presumably, most patients with mild to moderate stroke who are not at high risk for increased intracranial pressure may have their prestroke antihypertensive medications restarted 24 hours after their vascular event.

HYPERTENSION AND ACUTE CORONARY SYNDROME

PATHOPHYSIOLOGY

ACS refers to a spectrum of disease that ranges from unstable angina and non-ST-elevation myocardial infaction (NSTEMI) to ST-elevation myocardial infarction (STEMI). Section A of this book provides a detailed description of the pathophysiology and management of ACS patients.

ACS is perhaps best explained in terms of the delicate balance between myocardial oxygen supply and demand. When this balance is disrupted by a disease process that affects coronary blood flow, myocardial ischemia may induce contractile dysfunction precipitating a vicious cycle that includes tachycardia and hypotension, which may further worsen the supply/demand balance.

Myocardial oxygen demand is largely dependent on heart rate, myocardial wall stress (systolic pressure), and LV contractility. Myocardial oxygen supply depends on the coronary circulation. In contrast to most other vascular beds, myocardial oxygen extraction is near-maximal (75% of arterial oxygen content) at rest.[18] Consequently, demand for increased myocardial oxygen consumption must be met primarily by increased oxygen delivery. A twofold increase in any of the determinants of oxygen consumption requires an approximately 50% increase in coronary flow.

HTN increases demand: it increases myocardial wall stress and thus requirements of coronary flow. HTN also may limit

supply: it is a risk factor for vascular remodeling and atherosclerosis, the disease process that limits coronary blood flow. Even at an early age, increased vascular wall tension in persons with high BP leads to thinning, fragmentation, and fracture of elastin fibers, as well as increased collagen deposition in arteries, which results in decreased compliance of these vessels. In addition to these structural abnormalities, the HTN-mediated functional abnormality of increased arterial rigidity because of endothelial dysfunction develops over time because of aging and HTN and contributes to systolic HTN.[19]

Many of the mechanisms that initiate and maintain HTN (increased sympathetic nervous system and renin–angiotensin–aldosterone system activity; deficiencies in release and/or activity of vasodilators, structural and functional abnormalities in conductance and resistance arteries) are also those that mediate damage to target organs, including the coronary vessels and the myocardium.[20] This may be why antihypertensive drugs exert at least some of their beneficial effects on the vasculature by actions that are independent of BP lowering alone.

The medications used to treat ACS can be understood within the framework of the supply/demand balance. β-Blockers work to decrease BP and heart rate, two major determinants of myocardial oxygen demand. Nitrates decrease preload, thus ventricular filling pressures and wall stress (demand). Nitrates also cause coronary vessel dilatation (supply). Morphine decreases pain and therefore heart rate, while also decreasing venous return and filling pressures (demand). Often the ACS patient will need a cardiac catheterization whether for diagnostic or treatment purposes. Cardiac catheterization is the gold-standard for diagnosis of coronary vessel disease, and angioplasty and coronary stenting can relieve the stenosis or occlusion (supply) in a way no medication can.

PATHWAY MANAGEMENT

Our recommendation for antihypertensive therapy in ACS patients includes the following:

β-Blockers are the first-line of treatment based on their ability to reduce both heart rate and BP and thus, myocardial oxygen demand (Figure 33.3). NTG has been a cornerstone of therapy for decades, and in the hypertensive patient, intravenous NTG is effective in the reduction of BP and symptoms. Patients need to be monitored for potential adverse effects, particularly profound hypotension, which can exacerbate ischemia. An ACE inhibitor or an ARB can also be considered for the management of HTN in patients with ACS. In patients with ACS we recommend to lower BP to less than 130/80 mm Hg within 3 hours and we recommend not to lower the diastolic pressure to lower than 60 mm Hg.

HYPERTENSION AND HEART FAILURE

HF can be caused by a decrease in cardiac output such that end-organ perfusion is compromised (systolic dysfunction), or to maintenance of cardiac output at the expense of increased left atrial filling pressures (diastolic dysfunction), or both. Both systolic and diastolic dysfunction can be understood in terms of the determinants of cardiac performance.

The determinants of cardiac performance are preload, afterload, contractility, and heart rate. As the ability of the

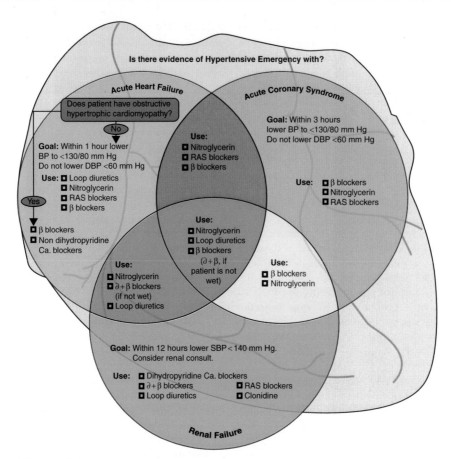

Figure 33.3. Management of hypertension in acute cardiovascular and renal disease.

myocardium to maintain normal forward output fails, compensatory mechanisms are activated to preserve circulatory function. Preload increases to increase stroke volume (Frank-Starling mechanism). Hemodynamic stress that cannot be compensated initiates structural changes at the cellular levels, referred to as myocardial remodeling. If the Frank-Starling and remodeling mechanisms are unable to reestablish cardiac output, neurohormonal systems are also activated. While each of these mechanisms may contribute to maintenance of circulatory function, each may also contribute to development and progression of pump dysfunction.

HTN is intricately linked to both systolic and diastolic dysfunction by affecting each of these mechanisms. The renin–angiotensin system that is so fundamentally linked to HTN and that recruits intravascular volume to sustain end-diastolic filling pressures may elevate preload to the point of putting a patient on the flat or descending portion of the Frank-Starling curve. HTN induces cardiac remodeling and LV hypertrophy; to decrease LV wall stress, contractile proteins are added to myocytes in parallel, thus increasing wall thickness and decreasing cavity size. Increasing thickness and decreasing cavity size relieves the increase in wall stress, but at the expense of LV remodeling and hypertrophy. Finally the sympathetic activation that increases vascular tone also increases myocardial oxygen demand and eventually results in downregulation of β-adrenergic receptors, further impairing the ability of the system to maintain forward output.

The staples of HF treatment are diuretics, β-blockers, and ACE inhibitors. Diuretics, specifically loop diuretics, combat

the increased total body volume that is central to the pathophysiology of HF. β-Blockers and ACE inhibitors/ARBs combat the cardiac remodeling and neurohormonal activation. The CCB Amlodipine, while not first-line, appears to be safe if needed for the treatment of HTN (or angina) in the patient with LV dysfunction.[21]

PATHWAY MANAGEMENT

In our simplified algorithm we recommend a goal of lowering BP to 130/80 mm Hg within 1 hours of treatment (Figure 33.3). One caveat in the management of HTN in the setting of acute HF is the exclusion of hypertrophic cardiomyopathy. In patients with hypertrophic cardiomyopathy we recommend the exclusive use of a β-blocker or a nondihydropyridine CCB (in patients with a contraindication to β-blockers) and avoidance of diuretics or NTG. Our recommended sequence of add-on drugs for treatment of HTN in HF are loop diuretics, NTG, RAS blockers, and β-blockers. In patients with both a diagnosis of ACS and acute HF an alternative sequence of the drug choice is NTG, followed by RAS blockers and β-blockers.

HYPERTENSION AND RENAL FAILURE

Renal failure tends not to be the primary reason for CCU admission but rather a complication or comorbidity of some other disease process requiring CCU care, such as hypertensive emergency or acute decompensated heart failure (AHF). Nonetheless, as renal failure is associated with poor outcomes, preserving or improving the CCU patient's renal function must be a primary objective.

Severe and/or long-standing HTN induces renal microvascular damage. Mechanical stress and endothelial injury lead to increased vascular permeability, activation of the coagulation cascade and platelets, and deposition of fibrin. This fibrinoid necrosis narrows the vessel lumen which causes renal hypoperfusion and triggers massive renin release, generating a vicious cycle of ongoing injury. Renin–angiotensin system activation leads to further vasoconstriction and pressure natriuresis which together lead to end-organ hypoperfusion, ischemia and dysfunction that manifests as a hypertensive emergency. HTN begets renal damage which begets more HTN, which if severe enough causes acute end-organ damage (hypertensive emergency).

Regarding renal failure in the setting of AHF, there is the concept of cardiorenal syndrome, a term used to emphasize the influence that cardiac and renal function have on each other. HF decreases renal perfusion and predisposes to renal failure. Renal failure makes diuretic dose requirements for HF higher; if HF is hemodynamically significant such that renal perfusion is compromised, inotropes or dialysis may be the only effective options. Diuretics increase solute delivery to distal segments of the nephron, resulting in epithelial cell hypertrophy and hyperplasia, which increases the solute resorptive capacity of the kidney. Reduction in extracellular fluid volume also leads to an increase in solute and fluid reabsorption, specifically in the proximal tubule. These mechanisms together result in a state in which HF and renal failure worsen each other and make difficult the treatment of both.

PATHWAY MANAGEMENT

For the hypertensive emergency patient in acute renal failure, we recommend a goal of lowering SBP to 140 mm Hg within 12 hours and considering consultation by a nephrologist (Figure 33.4). A recommended strategy is for a 10% to 20% reduction in mean arterial pressure during the first 1 to 2 hours, and then further 10% to 15% reduction during the next 6 to 12 hours.

Some physicians advocate the use of fenoldopam, which is unique among the parenteral BP agents because it mediates peripheral vasodilation by acting on peripheral dopamine-1 receptors. Fenoldopam has onset of action within 5 minutes, peak action by 15 minutes, and duration of action from 30 to 60 minutes. No adverse effects have been reported. Fenoldopam improves creatinine clearance, urine flow rates, and sodium excretion in severely hypertensive patients with both normal and impaired renal function.[22]

Our recommended sequence of add-on drugs are dihydropyridine CCB (nicardipine: onset 5 to 15 minutes, duration 4 to 6 hours, increases stroke volume and reduces both cardiac and cerebral ischemia), $\alpha + \beta$-blocker (labetalol: liver metabolism, onset in 2 to 5 minutes, peak at 5 to 15 minutes, duration 2 to 4 hours, maintains cardiac output because of α-blocking effect), loop diuretics, RAS blocker, and clonidine.

Regarding long-term management, it is important to note that chronic kidney disease (CKD) patients die more than anything from heart disease. CKD is a risk factor for CAD, valvular heart disease, and other causes of heart disease. HTN control is critical to reduce rate of development of these cardiovascular processes. If HTN is controlled, CKD progresses more slowly.

Because the mechanism of HTN in the CKD patient is RAAS activation, ACE inhibitors and ARBs are particularly valuable agents.

PLAN FOR DISCHARGE THERAPY

The CCU patient, once discharged, must take seriously the importance of secondary prevention, for which BP control is one important component.

Lifestyle modifications that have been associated with favorable results in hypertensive patients include weight loss, increased physical activity, smoking cessation, and a low-fat, low-sodium diet. Tightly controlled dietary modification, as in the dietary approaches to stop HTN (DASH) study, for example, can reduce mean SBP by 3.0, 6.2, and 6.8 mm Hg in subjects on a low-, intermediate-, and high-sodium intake diet, respectively. Weight loss, reduced sodium intake, moderation of alcohol consumption, exercise, and an overall healthy dietary pattern are entirely appropriate for patients aiming to control HTN.

Often-times pharmacologic treatment is necessary to control BP, especially for patients discharged from the CCU. The most important question to ask when selecting initial drug treatment is which class of drug will deliver the most effective blood pressure lowering for this patient. As mentioned above, certain medications have beneficial effects for certain disease states that go beyond the medication's BP-lowering effects (β-blockers for HF). However, it must be emphasized that blood pressure lowering is in itself a driver of benefit.[23] In other words, regardless of the drug used, the goal should be to in fact lower BP. The response to different classes of drugs is similar when compared head-to-head in heterogeneous populations. However, individual responses can differ strikingly. For example, in patients older than 55 or those of black ethnic origin at any age, blood pressure lowering will generally be greatest with a thiazide-type diuretic such as chlorthalidone or CCB such as amlodipine.[24] In young people, who generally have a more active renin–angiotensin system than older individuals, BP is lowered effectively with inhibitors of the renin–angiotensin system (ACE inhibitors, ARBs).[25] For patients whose BP is already 20 mm Hg or more above their goal, guidelines recommend initial treatment with a two-drug combination because monotherapy is likely to be insufficient.[26]

REFERENCES

1. Herzog E, Frankenberger O, Aziz E, et al. A novel pathway for the management of hypertension for hospitalized patients. *Crit Pathw Cardiol.* 2007;6:150–160.
2. Fleckenstein-Grün G, Thimm F, Czirfuzs A, et al. Experimental vasoprotection by calcium antagonists against calcium-mediated arteriosclerotic alterations. *J Cardiovasc Pharmacol.* 1994;24(suppl 2):S75–S84.
3. Abernethy DR, Schwartz JF. Calcium-antagonist drugs. *N Engl J Med.* 1999;341:1447–1457.
4. Amenta F, Lanari A, Mignini F, et al. Nicardipine use in cerebrovascular disease: a review of controlled clinical studies. *J Neurol Sci.* 2009;283:219–223.
5. Aronson S, Dyke CM, Stierer KA, et al. The ECLIPSE trials: comparative studies of clevidipine to nitroglycerin, sodium nitroprusside, and nicardipine for acute hypertension treatment in cardiac surgery patients. *Anesth Analg.* 2008;107(4):1110–1121.
6. Dzau VJ. Tissue angiotensin and pathobiology of vascular disease: a unifying hypothesis. *Hypertension.* 2001;37:1047–1052.
7. Rosdendorff C. The renin-angiotensin system and vascular hypertrophy. *J Am Coll Cardiol.* 1996;28:803–812.
8. Vemmos KN, Spengos T, Tsivgoulis G, et al. Factors influencing acute blood pressure values in stroke subtypes. *J Hum Hypertens.* 2004;18:253–259.
9. Johnston KC, Mayer SA. Blood pressure reduction in ischemic stroke: a two-edged sword? *Neurology.* 2003;61:1030–1031.
10. Powers WJ. Acute hypertension after stroke: the scientific basis for treatment decisions. *Neurology.* 1993;43(pt 1):461–467.
11. Adams HP, del Zoppo G, Alberts MJ, et al. Guidelines for the early management of adults with ischemic stroke: a guideline from the American Heart Association/American Stroke

Association Stroke Council, Clinical Cardiology Council, Cardiovascular Radiology and Intervention Council, and the Atherosclerotic Peripheral Vascular Disease and Quality of Care Outcomes in Research Interdisciplinary Working Groups. Stroke. 2007;115:2761-2788.

12. Zhang Y, Reilly KH, Tong W, et al. Blood pressure and clinical outcome among patients with acute stroke in Inner Mongolia, China. *J Hypertens.* 2008:26:1446–1452.

13. Sare GM, Ali M, Shuaib A, et al. Relationship between hyperacute blood pressure and outcome after ischemic stroke: data from the VISTA collaboration. *Stroke.* 2009;54:769–774.

14. Adams HP, Zoppo G, Alberts M, et al. Guidelines for the early management of adults with ischemic stroke: a guideline from the American Heart Association/American Stroke Association Stroke Council, Clinical Cardiology Council, Cardiovascular Radiology and Intervention Council, and the Atherosclerotic Peripheral Vascular Disease and Quality of Care Outcomes in Research.

15. Potter JF, Robinson TG, Ford GA, Mistri A, James M, Chernova J, Jagger C. Controlling hypertension and hypotension immediately post-stroke (CHHIPS): a randomised, placebo-controlled, double-blind pilot trial. Lancet Neurol. 2009 Jan;8(1):48-56. Epub 2008 Dec 4.

16. Turan TN, Cotsonis G, Lynn MJ, et al. Relationship between blood pressure and stroke recurrence in patients with intracranial arterial stenosis. *Circulation.* 2007;115:2969–2975.

17. Schrader J, et al. Acute Candesartan Cilexetil Therapy in Stroke Survivors Study Group. The ACCESS study. *Stroke.* 2003;34:1699–1703.

18. Feigl EO. Coronary physiology. *Physiol Rev.* 1983;63:1.

19. Franklin SS, Gustin W IV, Wong ND, et al. Hemodynamic patterns of age-related changes in blood pressure. *Circulation.* 1997:96:308–315.

20. Oparil S, Zaman MA, Calhoun DA. Pathogenesis of hypertension. *Ann Intern Med.* 2003;139:761–776.

21. Packer, M, O'Conner, CM, Ghali, JK, et al. Effect of amlodipine on morbidity and mortality in severe chronic heart failure. *N Engl J Med.* 1996; 335:1107.

22. Shusterman NH, Elliott WJ, White WB. Fenoldopam, but not nitroprusside, improves renal function in severely hypertensive patients with impaired renal function. *Am J Med.* 1993;95:161–168.

23. Julius S, Kjeldsen SE, Weber M, et al. Outcomes in hypertensive patients at high cardiovascular risk treated with regimens based on valsartan or amlodipine: the VALUE randomized trial. *Lancet.* 2004;363:2022–2031.

24. The ALLHAT Officers and Coordinators for the ALLHAT Collaborative Research Group. Major outcomes in high-risk hypertensive patients randomized to angiotensin-converting enzyme inhibitor or calcium channel blocker vs. diuretic: the Antihypertensive and Lipid-Lowering Treatment to Prevent Heart Attack Trial (ALLHAT). *JAMA.*2002;288:2981–2987.

25. Dickerson JE, Hingorani AD, Ashby MJ et al. Optimization of antihypertensive treatment by crossover rotation of four major classes. *Lancet.* 1999;353:2008–2013.

26. Chobanian AV, et al. The seventh report of the Joint National Committee on Prevention, Detection, Evaluation and Treatment of High Blood Pressure: The JNC VII Report. *JAMA.* 2003;289:2560–2572.

PATIENT AND FAMILY INFORMATION FOR:

Hypertension

CARDIOVASCULAR SYSTEM AND HYPERTENSION

The cardiovascular system serves to propel and transport blood, which carries the elements necessary for healthy functioning of all the organs of body. Oxygen, glucose, electrolytes, immune cells, clotting, cells and a variety of other blood components must travel to every part of the body.

The cardiovascular system is sometimes compared to a water system with a pump and water pipes. It is a closed system, in that the system is self-contained; there are no openings to the outside. All the blood that starts in the heart returns to the heart (unless of course there is damage to the system, as in a tear to a vessel which results in internal or external bleeding). The pipes that leave the pump are larger as they must bear the greater volumes and pressures. The pipes let off more and more branches as they get farther from the source and therefore get smaller and thinner. The vessels that leave the heart are arteries which feed capillaries before the blood makes its way back to the heart in veins.

Blood Pressure (BP) is an index of the force per unit area inside the arteries. Factors that influence BP are the rate of blood flow through the vessel and the flexibility of the blood vessel wall. The rate of blood flow ejected from the heart through the arteries and veins per minute (cardiac output) depends on the number of heart beats per minute (heart rate) and the amount of blood ejected per beat (stroke volume). The flexibility or resistance of blood vessel walls depends on many factors including age, the nervous system, and hormones. In summary, the heart pump and its cardiac output along with the blood vessels and their resistance are what determine a person's BP. This is important because it serves as basis for understanding how such factors as age, medications, and lifestyle influence our BP.

The medical term for high BP is Hypertension (HTN). HTN is defined as a BP of 140/90 mm Hg or above. The first number represents the systolic BP; the second is the diastolic BP. As mentioned above, the heart beats to propel blood, and does so on average between 60 and 80 times per minute. When the heart ejects blood the pressure in arteries goes up because the pressure generated in the heart's largest chamber is transmitted throughout the closed cardiovascular system and there is a surge in the rate of blood flow through the arteries; this yields the systolic BP. After the heart muscle contracts, it must relax to prepare for the next contraction and in so doing allows for blood, which returns through veins, to refill the chambers of the heart. This yields the diastolic BP: the pressure in arteries during the heart muscle's relaxation phase.

CCU AND HYPERTENSION

The cardiac intensive care unit, or CCU, is where a patient goes when they are too sick to be adequately managed on a general hospital floor. The CCU patient needs more specialized care and to this end is managed by nurses and doctors with specialized training in critical care and cardiovascular medicine. The nurses are responsible for fewer patients than on a general floor, and thus are able to dedicate greater level of attention to each patient. The team of doctors assigned to the CCU remains in that unit throughout the day, rather than moving throughout the hospital.

Patients can be admitted to the CCU for a variety of conditions, such as heart attack, heart failure (HF), tears in the aorta (the major artery that leaves the heart), and very high BP. BP is an important component of every disease condition that warrants a CCU admission. In some cases, BP can be dangerously high, in others dangerously low. In some cases aberration in BP (too high or too low) is the source of the problem (hypertensive emergency causing HF), while in others it is the result of the problem (heart attack causing dangerously low BP). Regardless, BP is something the CCU doctor must manage for every CCU patient, and something the CCU patient must be educated about and take seriously, both for the short-and long-term.

DRUGS

Surely, patients and their families have heard doctors use an overwhelming number of names of drugs. Not only are there a seemingly endless number of medications, but every medication has at least two names, a generic name and a brand name (i.e., Metoprolol is also Lopressor and Toprol). It makes things simpler to think of drugs in terms of drug classes. This is how doctors think, and for good reason. Drugs that make up a drug class perform a similar function via a similar mechanism. ß-Blockers, for example, help block activity of the ß-receptor, found on the surface of many cells including those of the heart and blood vessels. ß-Blockers are very important in the treatment of and HTN (among other things). Furthermore, most drugs in a class have a similar-sounding generic name. ß-Blockers, for example, end in "lol" (i.e., metoprolol, carvedilol, atenolol). So, for example, one remembers the ß-blockers as the "-lol" drugs, which are used to treat HF. ACE inhibitors are the "-pril" drugs (i.e., lisinopril, captopril, enalapril) most commonly used to treat HTN, HF, and kidney disease. A drug class which is similar to the ACE inhibitors is the ARB family or "-artan" drugs (i.e., irbesartan, candesartan, losartan). These drugs have similar clinical indications as the ACE inhibitors, and have the benefit of a lesser likelihood of causing cough as an adverse effect. The calcium channel blockers (CCBS) can be subdivided into the dihydropyridne and nondihydropyridines. The dihydropyridine CCB's are commonly used BP medicines, and can be remembered as the "-dipine" drugs (i.e., amlodipine, nicardipine, nifedipine). The α-blocker medicines mediate their BP-reducing effects by blocking a receptor on blood vessels responsible for vessel constriction (as the vessel diameter gets smaller the pressure within the vessel increases). These "-osin" (i.e., tamsulosin, terazosin, doxazosin) medicines have a second use in relieving the symptoms of urinary frequency, hesitancy, and urgency associated with benign prostatic hyperplasia, or BPH. Thinking in terms of classes of medicines, which conveniently tend to have similar-sounding and thus easier-to-remember names, is much easier and more intuitive than remembering individual drugs.

HYPERTENSION AND IT ROLE IN THE COMMON CCU DISEASE PROCESSES

As mentioned above, patients are admitted to the CCU for a variety of conditions, most if not all of which have HTN as a significant consideration, either as cause, effect, or as important comorbidity.

HYPERTENSION AND DISEASES OF THE AORTA

The aorta is the largest artery of the body. Because it is the first vessel that blood travels through once it leaves the heart, within it travels all of the blood that leaves the heart. Whereas all other vessels are branches of a larger vessel and therefore will only receive a fraction of the cardiac output (blood leaving the heart per minute), the aorta must withstand the volume and pressure of the entire cardiac output. It is no surprise then, that the aorta is the largest, thickest-walled blood vessel in the body. One can imagine that diseases of the aorta are potentially catastrophic; for example, while a ruptured vessel in the finger will cause that vessel to spill its fraction of cardiac output, a rupture of the aorta will lead to rapid loss of a huge proportion of the body's blood. Motor vehicle accidents, for example, in which the passenger is propelled forward, then held back by a seat belt can cause the aorta to tear, leading to immediate death.

Patients admitted to the CCU for disease of the aorta often have an acute aortic syndrome, subdivided into three conditions: aortic dissection, intramural hematoma, and aortic ulcer. An aortic dissection is a tear in the innermost lining of the aorta; an intramural hematoma is a pooling of blood in the wall of the aorta without any tear in the lining of the vessel; an aortic ulcer occurs when a plaque in the

inner lining of the vessel leads to erosion of the inner part of the vessel wall and swelling of the vessel contained by the outermost lining of the wall. Patients with any of the acute aortic syndromes will usually feel sudden onset, severe, "ripping" or "tearing" pain that often feels like it goes through the chest and into the back.

Aortic dissection is a tear in the innermost lining of the aorta such that blood begins infiltrating the wall of the vessel. The problem is that this infiltrating blood pushes the inner lining into the pathway of oncoming blood, leading to obstruction to flow and an expansion of the tear. If the tear is in the first "ascending" part of the aorta, the patient needs surgery; if the tear is in the "descending" aorta the treatment is medical and not surgical. Aortic dissection may be a consideration for a patient who presents with chest pain, especially patients who smoke and/or have HTN. Aortic dissection can easily be confused with heart attack; this is important because not only are the treatments different but certain treatments for heart attack, for example, clot breaking medication, can be harmful for a patient with aortic dissection.

High BP is the major risk factor for both types of aortic dissection, and BP is also the major target of medical treatment. Whereas precipitous reductions in BP can sometimes be dangerous in other condition such as ischemic stroke, for acute aortic dissection the physician can and should be aggressive in lowering BP. BP reduction helps prevent extension of the tear, which could lead to stroke, cardiac tamponade, or other major complications. Every time the heart beats, a surge of blood exerts a force against the vessel wall, forcing blood into the tear and potentially causing the tear to enlarge and extend. ß-Blockers, the "-lol" drugs, are often used because not only do they lower BP, but they also lower heart rate. Intravenous ß-blockers such as labetalol are used for rapid BP and heart rate reduction to a target of under 120 mm Hg BP and under 60 beats per minute heart rate, or as low as tolerated by the patient (lowering heart rate or BP too much can lead to such symptoms as dizziness). The patient is sent to the CCU to continuously monitor heart rate and BP in response to intravenous medication and also to monitor electrocardiogram readings in case the dissection leads to complications. Once BP is controlled, the patient can be switched to oral medications. The patient must understand the importance of compliance with medical and lifestyle recommendations to prevent future complications of aortic dissection.

HYPERTENSION AND ACUTE NEUROLOGIC SYNDROME

Patients may often be admitted to the CCU for stroke or hypertensive encephalopathy. Stroke, or cerebrovascular accident (CVA), is caused by decreased oxygenated blood supply to the brain. Whereas a heart attack is death of heart muscle caused by decreased blood flow to the heart, stroke is death of brain cells caused by impaired blood flow to the brain. If blood flow is restored before cell death occurs, brain function may recover completely; this condition is referred to as a TIA or transient ischemic attack. Stroke can be thought of as coming in two forms: stroke caused by a blockage (ischemic stroke) versus bleeding (hemorrhagic stroke) of an artery supplying the brain. The end result, brain cell death, is similar for both. In addition, stroke may increase pressure in the skull and thus cause compression of surrounding healthy brain tissue, caused by edema or swelling in ischemic stroke and accumulation of blood in hemorrhagic stroke. In hypertensive encephalopathy, on the other hand, severe HTN causes not localized brain ischemia but rather global brain dysfunction with its associated symptoms. As a result, although stroke patients often have focal neurologic deficits (weakness in a limb, slurring of speech, and facial drooping), patients with hypertensive encephalopathy lack focal symptoms and present instead with nausea, blurry vision, he adache and/or altered consciousness.

The first step in the assessment of a patient with suspected neurologic syndrome is a head CT scan to evaluate for bleeding in the skull. CT scans are effective for detecting blood, and while not necessarily helpful in the diagnosis of hypertensive encephalopathy or early ischemic stroke, a CT scan is the first test because an intracranial bleed, if found, might require immediate neurosurgery.

HTN is a major risk factor for acute neurologic syndrome, and a major target of therapy. For hemorrhagic stroke, BP must be lowered promptly but not to such an extent that arterial pressure becomes inadequate to sufficiently overcome intracranial pressure; cerebral perfusion pressure, or the net BP gradient responsible for blood flow to healthy brain tissue, depends on adequate arterial pressure. For ischemic stroke, the data is not clear enough to make precise recommendations, but it has been commonly accepted in the medical community that aggressive lowering of BP may do more harm than good. On the other hand, high BP increases the risk for expansion of edema and/or conversion of an ischemic stroke into a hemorrhagic one. Many patients have spontaneous declines in BP during the first 24 hours after stroke onset. Largely because data was ambiguous, in 2007 an expert panel recommendation was that for acute ischemic stroke, antihypertensives should be withheld unless BP is more than 220/120 mm Hg. There is an ongoing shift in this approach. Recent data suggests this "permissive hypertension" may be dangerous and that BP in acute ischemic stroke should, in fact, be treated, although carefully, as decreasing BP too much has a detrimental effect. Target BP in the acute phases postischemic stroke remain yet to be defined.

For hypertensive encephalopathy, the baseline BP must be taken into consideration to avoid excessive BP lowering and to prevent cerebral ischemia. Lowering the mean pressure by 25% and diastolic pressure to 100 to 110 mm Hg is usually safe.

HYPERTENSION AND ACUTE CORONARY SYNDROME

An acute coronary syndrome (ACS) is a decreased blood supply to the heart (myocardial cell ischemia) that may or may not result in myocardial cell injury or death and that is caused by coronary artery disease (CAD). The three forms of ACS are unstable angina, non-STEMI, and STEMI.

These three entities are manifestations of the same disease process and are extensively discussed in Section A of this book.

The heart is thought of as the organ that supplies blood to the rest of the body; in fact, the heart supplies blood to the rest of the body *and* to itself. It does so through vessels known as coronary arteries, which come off the aorta immediately after the blood leaves the heart. There are three large coronary arteries that travel along the surface of the heart before diving deep to feed all the cells of the heart muscle. A blockage to flow in any of the coronary arteries can cut off supply enough to starve cells and lead to their death. If cells of a certain portion of the heart fail to beat adequately, the heart may not generate enough force to sustain cardiac output. A heart attack, or myocardial infarction, may cause the heart to stop beating effectively (HF), or stop beating all together (sudden cardiac death). HTN is considered a major risk factor for CAD, and thus for myocardial infarction and HF.

The key concept to understand regarding coronary blood supply is that of supply and demand. The heart is unique in that it is responsible for both its supply and demand. As the heart beats harder, it supplies more blood flow, but it also demands more blood flow. HTN affects demand: higher BP forces the heart to beat harder, thus increasing the heart's demand for blood. A 70% blockage may still allow the necessary blood supply to the normotensive patient's heart but for the hypertensive patient's more demanding heart, a 70% blockage may result in chest pain or worse, myocardial cell damage. HTN also affects supply: higher BP leads to the development of the blockages themselves. Through mechanisms, many still to be completely understood, HTN promotes atherogenesis, or the development of plaques within the inner lining of arteries such as the coronary arteries. Not only do plaques make passageways for blood flow narrower over time, but also plaques can rupture releasing contents that can immediately clot and completely block blood flow. This plaque rupture is what usually causes devastating myocardial infarctions.

Initial therapy of HTN in patients presenting to the CCU with an ACS should use medications that improve myocardial supply, lessen demand, or both. ß-Blockers, for example, not only lower BP, they also lower heart rate, and thus lessen the amount of energy the heart expends and the amount of blood flow it demands. Nitrates lower BP but they also lessen the amount of blood returning to the heart, thus lessening the volume of blood the heart must pump per beat, which also lessens demand. Nitrates and ß-blockers are often first-line BP medications in patients with ACS. One exception is in the patient whose heart is so damaged that lowering heart rate may further lessen cardiac output; in this situation, ß-blockers should not be used. ACE inhibitor and ARBs can also be used to lower BP.

Target BP is 130/80 mm Hg. Diastolic BP should not be lowered too significantly, because it is the diastolic pressure that provides the force to send blood through the coronary arteries; too low a diastolic BP may be harmful.

Upon discharge, the patient who has suffered a heart attack should be on a ß-blocker and ACE inhibitor, if possible.

These medications lower BP and help the heart preserve or even regain function.

HYPERTENSION AND HEART FAILURE

The heart as described above is a pump that allows blood to be propelled throughout the cardiovascular system of blood vessels. To effectively perform this task, the heart must fill with an adequate volume of blood, pass this blood between each of its four chambers, and have sufficient muscle strength to eject blood against a significant resistance in the aorta to the entire body.

Chambers divide the heart into a right (right atrium and right ventricle) and left (left atrium and left ventricle) side. When blood returns to the heart through veins, it passes through the right atrium and ventricle before passing through the lungs to pick up oxygen and then pass to the left atrium and ventricle where sufficient pressure is generated to propel blood to the entire body. The left ventricle is the heart's strongest and largest chamber.

HF is failure of the heart to propel blood, either because the muscle is weak or the heart does not fill adequately, such that either cardiac output is insufficient to meet the demands of the body's tissues or these demands are met at the expense of blood "backing up" in the direction of the lungs. In other words, HF can be caused by poor forward flow or adequate forward flow but with concomitant inappropriate backward flow.

HF caused by a multitude of abnormalities: ischemia such as in the form of a heart attack, damaged valves, drugs such as alcohol or certain chemotherapies, and of course, HTN are among the many possible causes of HF.

HTN forces the heart to pump harder to overcome the greater resistance to forward flow, and over time the heart muscle starts to fail; it may become stiff or weak or both, resulting in forward and/or backward flow failure.

Acute HF is one of the most common reasons for admission to the CCU. A patient may have already been diagnosed with HF, and for some reason (not taking medications, not abiding to a dietary regimen, an irregular heart rhythm, a heart attack, and uncontrolled BP) suffer an insult that disrupts the delicate balance and throws the patient into acutely symptomatic HF. It is also possible that a patient admitted to the CCU with HF never had any symptoms of HF. A previously adequately-functioning heart may go into failure because of a heart attack, or severe damage to a heart valve, or severe HTN. A heart that is accustomed to beating against a BP of 120/80 mm Hg may fail to overcome a sudden burden of 220/120 mm Hg, or a heart that is forced to beat against a pressure of 150/100 mm Hg for years and years may do well in the beginning but with time stretch and thicken and eventually decompensate. Regardless of the scenario, to treat HTN is to relieve the burden against which the failing heart is struggling to pump.

HTN is a common cause of HF; about 75% of patients admitted with HF have HTN. HTN is also a major target of therapy for HF. In fact, the medications that treat HF—ß-blockers ("-lol" meds), ACE inhibitors ("pril" meds), ARBs ("-artan" meds), and diuretics or water pills—also have effects on BP.

The initial urgent step is to stabilize the patient. A doctor will aim to reduce BP, ultimately to 130/80 mm Hg or lower, although not too quickly as to potentially starve certain tissues of adequate blood supply. Once the patient is stabilized, tight BP control becomes a fundamental component of long-term care. The HF patient can easily decompensate again if he has a drinking binge, or salty-food binge, or skips a couple days' doses of medicines. Managing HTN must be emphasized as crucial for preventing future decompensations and giving the heart the best chance of recovering over time.

HYPERTENSION AND RENAL FAILURE

The kidneys filter blood; they excrete much of what is not needed and retain much of what is needed. They also help to maintain total body water and electrolyte (sodium, potassium, calcium, etc.) concentrations within a rather narrow healthy range. When a person becomes dehydrated, the kidneys are able to retain fluid and reduce urine output dramatically; if a person were to drink excessively, the kidneys could excrete liters and liters of free water daily. The elegant and delicate mechanism that allows such regulation involves an intricate series of blood vessels and kidney tubules and electrolyte channels; this delicate structure can be disrupted when forced to withstand the forces of high BP for many years.

Renal failure can be acute or chronic; in other words, it can develop over hours to days often times with obvious symptoms, or it can develop slowly over years often times without symptoms until several years after kidney damage first begins. HTN can cause both acute and chronic kidney damage. In fact, HTN is the second leading cause of CKD, second to diabetes. Renal failure can be a reason for admission to the CCU (when because of hypertensive emergency), but more likely, it is a common complication of another disease process that warrants admission to the CCU.

Hypertensive emergency is defined as BP high enough (often diastolic BP above 120 mm Hg) to cause end-organ damage. "End-organs" most commonly affected by extremely high BP are the brain, heart, and kidneys. The high BP damages the delicate system of arteries feeding the kidney and disrupts the filtering mechanism leading to such symptoms as decreased urine output, nausea, swelling in the legs, and generalized malaise. The goal in management of acute renal failure because of severe HTN is to limit further renal damage through BP control. The choice of optimal drug therapy is controversial. Although nitroprusside is the drug with the longest track record, it does have potential cyanide and thiocyanate toxicity especially with prolonged infusions of high doses of nitroprusside. Other antihypertensive drugs that preserve renal blood flow are CCBs and adrenergic blocking agents. One sequence of add-on drugs are dihydropyridine CCB ("-pine" drugs), alfa-blocker ("-osin" drugs), loop diuretics, RAS blocker ("-pril" or "-artan" drugs), and clonidine. We recommend a goal of lowering systolic BP to below 140 mm Hg within 12 hours, doing so by reducing mean arterial pressure by 15% to 20% during the first 1 to 2 hours, and then further by 10% to 15% during the next 6 to 12 hours.

It is worth mentioning that kidney damage is not only a consequence of HTN but also a cause of HTN. Patients with CKD, especially those on dialysis, are at very high risk of having HTN.

As mentioned above, although kidney disease because of hypertensive emergency is cause for CCU admission, more commonly a patient in the CCU for some other reason (heart attack, HF) develops renal failure concomitantly because the heart attack or HF, for example, led to decreased blood supply to the kidneys. The renal failure makes more complicated the treatment of heart disease and becomes, in itself an important target of treatment. For example, diuretics, often referred to as "water pills" are critical for HF treatment. A patient in the CCU with HF is often "volume-overloaded," sometimes as much as 20 or 30 pounds heavier than usual caused by water retention. The goal is to remove this water, but (1) this fluid removal can damage the kidneys and (2) kidney damage coupled with the low output state of HF can make the fluid removal difficult. The kidney damage, at least partly brought on by the HF and/or its treatment, has made treatment of the HF more difficult. In recent years some doctors have used the term "cardiorenal syndrome" precisely to emphasize how strongly linked are kidney and heart, in that function and treatment of one very often affects function and treatment of the other.

In summary, kidney damage can be a reason for CCU admission as in the case of hypertensive emergency but more often kidney damage is related secondarily to, and complicates treatment of, the primary disease process that necessitated CCU admission. Good management of HTN can help preserve both kidney and cardiovascular health. When the patient with kidney damage recovers and leaves the hospital, BP control is of paramount importance. ACE inhibitors ("-pril") and ARBs ("-artan") not only lower BP, they delay progression of kidney disease for certain patients.

Lipid Management in the Cardiac Care Unit

Prevention can take place at many levels. Primary prevention targets people who may have asymptomatic or preclinical coronary artery disease (CAD) or have risk factors for developing CAD. Secondary prevention targets people who have clinically manifest CAD. This chapter focuses on secondary prevention, in particular lipid management after acute coronary syndrome (ACS).

The American Heart Association and American College of Cardiology issued an update to their guidelines for secondary prevention in 2006. The statement emphasizes the importance of aggressive control of dyslipidemia.[1] The principal author, Sidney Smith, comments that patients do not receive treatment for risk factors after ACS for many reasons. Hospital stays after heart procedures are short, which limits the time a patient can be educated.[2] However, hospitalization after ACS represents an ideal time to work with patients to diagnose and treat dyslipidemia.

DEFINITION OF DYSLIPIDEMIA

Lipids are a group of naturally occurring molecules to which cholesterol and triglycerides belong. Risk for CAD has been focused primarily on low-density lipoprotein cholesterol (LDL-C) as well as high-density lipoprotein cholesterol (HDL-C), and triglycerides (TG). LDL-C makes up approximately 65% of total serum cholesterol and each particle contains one apolipoprotein B-100. HDL-C makes up approximately 25% of total serum cholesterol and contains apolipoprotein A. The apolipoproteins are structural proteins that transport lipids and carry out other functions. TGs contain glycerol and three fatty acids.

Other lipid particles involved in atherosclerosis include apolipoprotein B (apoB), VLDL cholesterol, lipoprotein (a), and lipoprotein phospholipase A2. Subclasses of LDL (small, dense, large, or buoyant) and LDL particle number can also be measured. Of note, apoB levels reflect the number of atherogenic particles. One apoB particle is present on each LDL particle and is also present in other lipid particles.

Lipoprotein metabolism is complex and interrelated; a complete description is outside the scope of this chapter but more in-depth information can be found in several texts.[3–5]

In the mid-1960s, the Frederickson classification system for dyslipidemia was developed based on lipoprotein classes. Types I through V were described. This system was not particularly relevant to the clinician. There are also other classifications that include familial hypercholesterolemia (FH), familial combined hypercholesterolemia, hypertriglyceridemia, and low HDL-C." FH is common; it is an autosomal codominant

monogenic disorder primarily resulting from mutations in the LDL-receptor gene. Most people with FH are heterozygotes; homozygotes are rare at about one in one million persons and result in markedly elevated LDL starting at a young age.

The National Cholesterol Education Program Adult Treatment Program (NCEP ATP III) guidelines focus on LDL, HDL, and TG as targets for treatments. The guidelines also recommend calculating non-HDL cholesterol that closely approximates apoB levels, therefore the atherosclerotic burden. Non-HDL cholesterol is calculated as total cholesterol—HDL, that is, the difference of HDL from total cholesterol.

LDL has remained the primary target for those with either CAD or risk factors, and the NCEP guidelines stratify goals based on risk. All patients with CAD should have LDL <100 mg/dL with an optional goal of <70 mg/dL. HDL goals are ≥40 mg/dL and TGs are <150 mg/dL. Non-HDL cholesterol goal is 30 mg/dL greater than LDL goal. Of note, The revised guidelines (ATP IV) are scheduled to be published in 2012 and may have more aggressive goals.[6]

TREATMENT OF DYSLIPIDEMIA IN THE SETTING OF ACUTE CORONARY SYNDROME

During hospitalization for ACS, it is important to address risk factors prior to leaving the hospital to help in lowering the risk of having another event. Treatment of lipids is especially important as research suggests that statins have a role in the acute setting.

MEASUREMENT OF LIPIDS IN THE ACUTE SETTING

Lipid values are felt to be relatively stable in the outpatient population. TGs are influenced by the fasting or nonfasting state and therefore lipid profiles are generally obtained in the fasting state. However, LDL, HDL, and TG are considered acute phase reactants, and their levels will be altered in ACS: HDL and LDL decrease whereas TG increases.

As indicated in figure 34.1, it is important to determine the onset of ACS and obtain a fasting lipid panel within 24 hours, if possible. Research has shown that lipids levels begin to alter within 24 hours and continue to change for approximately 7 days. Levels return to baseline at about 4 weeks. Greater changes are seen with larger and more severe infarcts with peak LDL decreases up to 30% of baseline.[7–9] Pitt et al.[10] examined

507 ACS patients and found that LDL levels decreased in the first 24 hours after admission followed by an increase over the next 2 days, a change that did not appear to be clinically meaningful. Similar changes were seen with total cholesterol and HDL, although fasting TG levels did not change.

Levels may also be influenced by prior treatment with lipid medications although it is unclear how much preexisting treatment may influence degree of change in the setting of ACS.

Ideally a lipid panel should be obtained on presentation to the hospital. If the time of onset of ACS is unclear, a lipid panel will be still helpful to estimate presence and extent of dyslipidemia. Secondary causes of dyslipidemia should also be considered including hypothyroidism, nephritic syndrome, obstructive liver disease, chronic renal failure, and use of LDL-altering drugs (progestins, anabolic steroids, estrogen, corticosteroids, and protease inhibitors for the treatment of HIV disease).

Total cholesterol, HDL cholesterol, and TG should be measured. For patients with TG <400 mg/dL LDL is generally calculated using the Friedewald formula. For patients with TG >400 mg/dL most labs will automatically perform a direct measurement of LDL cholesterol. It is helpful to have liver function tests (AST, ALT) and creatinine kinase (CK) to evaluate patients who may not be able to tolerate some lipid medications. Also recommended is thyroid-stimulating hormone (TSH) to screen for thyroid disease.

BENEFIT OF LIPID TREATMENT IN ACUTE CORONARY SYNDROME

Research supports the use of lipid-lowering therapy, in particular statin use, in the setting of ACS. Less known are the benefits of other drugs such as niacin, bile acid sequestrants, intestinal absorption inhibitors, and Ω-3 fatty acids. As indicated in figure 34.1, research to date suggest giving atorvastatin 80 mg for patients with ACS if there are no contraindications.

The MIRACL Study was a randomized, double-blind trial in the late 1990s enrolling 3,086 patients with unstable angina or non-Q wave myocardial infarction (NQWMI). Patients received 80 mg a day of atorvastatin or placebo between 24 and 96 hours after hospital admission and followed for 16 weeks. There were no significant differences in death, nonfatal MI, or coronary revascularization between the two groups but the atorvastatin group had less symptomatic ischemia episodes requiring emergency hospitalization.[11]

The PROVE IT-TIMI 22 trial enrolled 4,162 patients with ACS occurring within the previous 10 days and were randomly assigned 80 mg atorvastatin daily (labeled "intensive lipid lowering") or pravastatin 40 mg daily ("moderate lipid lowering"). Patients were followed up for 2 years. The endpoints of death, reinfarction, stroke, recurrent unstable angina, and coronary revascularization were reduced from 26.3% in the pravastatin group to 22.4% in the atorvastatin group, and this difference was significant at $P = .005$.[12]

In the A to Z trial, approximately 4,500 patients with ACS were enrolled and randomized to either simvastatin 40 mg daily for 1 month followed by 80 mg a day or placebo for 4 months followed by simvastatin 20 mg a day for 4 months. Follow up was for 6 months at least and up to 24 months. Cardiovascular death occurred in 4.1% in the first group and 5.4% in the second group ($P = .05$), but there were no other differences in the other primary endpoints.[13] Factors felt to have influenced the

lack of positive findings in the A to Z trial include intensity and timing of therapy.

A more recent study, the Japan assessment of pitavastatin and atorvastatin in ACS (JAPAN-ACS) study, was a randomized, open-label parallel group study in Japan of 252 ACS patients undergoing intravascular ultrasound (IVUS)-guided percutaneous coronary intervention. Patients received either 4 mg of pitavastatin or 20 mg of atorvastatin daily. Subjects underwent repeat IVUS at 8 and 12 months to assess percentage change in nonculprit coronary plaque volume (PV). Both drug regimens achieved significant reduction in PV with neither agent demonstrating superiority.[14]

STATIN USE IN ACS PATIENTS UNDERGOING PERCUTANEOUS CORONARY INTERVENTION

Several studies have investigated whether statin use benefits ACS patients undergoing percutaneous coronary intervention (PCI). In the ARMYDA-ACS trial, 171 patients with NSTEMI going for PCI were randomized to pretreatment with atorvastatin 80 mg, 12 hours before with further 40 mg preprocedure dose or placebo. After PCI all patients were given atorvastatin 40 mg daily. Periprocedure infarct, elevation of creatine kinase-MB and troponin-I was less in the pretreated group demonstrating a short-term benefit of statins in ACS patients undergoing PCI.[15]

A substudy PROVE IT-TIMI 22 investigated patients who had ACS and underwent PCI who received either atorvastatin 80 mg or pravastatin 40 mg daily. The atorvastatin group had less all-cause mortality, myocardial infarction, unstable angina leading to hospitalization, and revascularization after 30 days.[16]

MECHANISMS BY WHICH STATINS CONFER BENEFIT IN ACS

All studies showed greater LDL lowering with statin, or in the case of PROVE IT TIMI 22, greater lowering with atorvastatin 80 mg compared with pravastatin 40 mg daily. However, benefits were seen in the short term perhaps before the lower LDL could have conferred benefits. In addition, statins have been shown to have non-LDL lowering or pleiotropic effects. Statins have also been shown to reduce inflammation (a component of ACS), be antithrombic, and improve endothelial function all of which may be beneficial for ACS patients.[17–19] In addition to LDL lowering, statins raise HDL and lower TG.

LIPID-LOWERING DRUGS

At present, the statin drugs are the only class of lipid drugs that has been clearly shown to have a benefit in ACS. Tables 34.1 and 34.2 list currently available statins and equivalent doses.

STATIN DRUGS

Statins act by competitively inhibiting HMG-CoA reductase, an enzyme in the pathway that produces cholesterol in the liver. This ultimately reduces cholesterol through several mechanisms. Cholesterol synthesis is decreased. Liver cells sense the reduced levels of liver cholesterol and seek to compensate by synthesizing LDL receptors to draw cholesterol out of the circulation. The LDL receptor then relocates to the liver cell

TABLE 34.1	Statin Drugs		
Generic/Trade Name	*Doses*	*Manufacturer*	*Generic*
Lovastatin/Mevacor	10, 20, 40, 60 mg	Merck, Whitehouse Station, NJ	Y
Pravastatin/Pravachol	10, 20, 40, 80 mg	BMS, New York, NY	Y
Simvastatin/Zocor	5, 10, 20, 40, 80 mg	Merck, Whitehouse Station, NY	Y
Fluvastatin/Lescol	20, 40, 80 mg	Novartis, Switzerland	
Atorvastatin/Lipitor	10, 20, 40, 80 mg	Pfizer, New York, NY	Y
Rosuvastatin/Crestor	5, 10, 20, 40 mg	Astrazeneca, Wilmington	
Pitavastatin/Livalo	1, 2, 4 mg	Kowa, Montgomery AL	

membrane and binds to passing LDL and VLDL particles and VLDL are drawn out of circulation into the liver where the cholesterol is reprocessed into bile salts. These are excreted, and subsequently recycled mostly by an internal bile salt circulation.

Cholesterol synthesis appears to occur mostly at night, so statins with short half-lives are usually taken at night to maximize their effect. Studies have shown greater LDL and total cholesterol reductions in the short-acting simvastatin taken at night rather than the morning, but have shown no difference in the long-acting atorvastatin.

Currently available statins, dosing, and expected treatment effects are listed in Tables 34.1 and 34.2.

Side effects and monitoring of statin drugs.

MONITORING. Liver function tests and CK should be checked at baseline and during the hospital stay. A common side effect is muscle symptoms or elevation in the muscle enzyme CK.

Patients may complain of bilateral muscle soreness generally in large muscle groups such as the thigh. Another common side effect is elevation in liver enzymes (transaminitis) with rare acute liver failure, cholestasis, and hepatitis. Less common but potentially fatal is rhabdomyolysis. Absolute contraindications are in acute or severe liver disease and pregnancy.

MYOPATHY. The NCEP guidelines recommend an initial CK measurement and evaluation of muscle symptoms. Muscle symptoms should be evaluated at each follow-up visit and a CK level obtained when there is a complaint of muscle soreness, tenderness, or pain. Patients on high doses of statins or on combinations of lipid-lowering agents may be at greater risk for myopathy and elevations of CK.[6]

The incidence of statin-related myopathy is low (0.1% to 0.2%) but mild elevations in CK (less than three times the upper limit of normal) with or without muscle soreness are more common but should not preclude the use of statins.[20]

TABLE 34.2	Statin Lowering and Equivalent Dosages[24]					
Rearrange in terms of potency						
	Statin Equivalent Dosages					
%LDL Reduction (Approximate)	*Fluvastatin*	*Lovastatin*	*Pravastin*	*Simvastatin*	*Atorvastatin*	*Rosuvastatin*
10%–20%	20 mg	10 mg	10 mg	5 mg	—	—
20%–30%	40 mg	20 mg	20 mg	10 mg	—	—
30%–40%	80 mg	40 mg	40 mg	20 mg	10 mg	5 mg
40%–45%	—	80 mg	80 mg	40 mg	20 mg	5–10 mg
46%–50%	—	—	—	80 mg	40 mg	10–20 mg
50%–55%	—	—	—	—	80 mg	20 mg
56%–60%	—	—	—	—	—	40 mg
STARTING DOSE						
Starting dose	20 mg	10–20 mg	10 mg	20 mg	10–20 mg	10 mg; 5 mg if hypothyroid, >65 y, Asian
If higher LDL reduction goal	40 mg if >25%	20 mg if >20%		40 mg if >45%	40 mg if >45%	40 mg if >190
Optimal timing	Evening	With evening meals	Anytime	Evening	Anytime	Anytime

It is important to rule out other causes of muscle soreness or elevated CK (exercise, trauma, strenuous work, hypothyroidism, inflammatory muscle weakness). If CK elevation or symptoms are mild, use of a statin with regular monitoring (every 6 to 8 weeks) is recommended. For elevations 3 to 10 times the upper limit of normal, stopping statin therapy and workup for elevated CK should be considered.[6,20]

In 2011, the FDA announced changes in labeling of simvastatin to help prevent myopathy. The recommendations advised limiting use of the 80 mg dose unless a patient has been on this dose for 12 months or more without signs and symptoms of muscle soreness or damage. Simvastatin is also contraindicated with several antifungal and antibacterial medications, protease inhibitors, gemfibrozil, and cyclosporine. (HYPERLINK "http://www.fda.gov/drugsafety/ucm/htm" \t "_blank" www.fda.gov/drugsafety/ucm/htm.)

LIVER EFFECTS. The NCEP guidelines recommend a baseline evaluation of alanine aminotransferase and aspartate aminotransferase (ALT/AST) and approximately 12 weeks after beginning statin therapy.[6]

Acute liver failure, hepatitis, and cholestasis are relatively rare. Transaminitis, the asymptomatic elevation of AST and ALT greater than three times the upper limit of normal is reported in approximately 1% of patients on statin drugs. This is usually dose related and occurs within the first 3 to 6 months and is reversible. Patients with these mild elevations should be evaluated for secondary causes of elevations. If other causes are not found, they may be kept on a statin with routine monitoring. For higher elevations, patients should have the statin dose reduced or stopped and a complete evaluation performed. Nonalcoholic fatty liver disease may be a cause of elevated liver enzymes. Once diagnosed, statins may be continued in some patients with careful monitoring.[6,21]

Comparative effectiveness of statins. No large-scale study exists that compares the relative effectiveness of the various statins. Although many benefits of statins are felt to be a class effect, there are differences in potency and metabolism of the various statin drugs.

Statins differ in their ability to reduce cholesterol levels. Doses should be individualized according to patient characteristics such as goal of therapy and response. After initiation and/or dose changes, lipid levels should be analyzed within 1 to 3 months and dosage adjusted accordingly every 6 to 12 months afterwards. More frequent monitoring is suggested for those at risk of side effects.

OTHER CONSIDERATIONS FOR LIPID TREATMENT

In most of the studies investigating statin use in ACS, statin dose was either not titrated to level of LDL or given at the highest dose. In particular, atorvastatin 80 mg is generally given to ACS patients. Guidelines do not address whether patients should be kept on this particular statin and at this highest dose. LDL levels of 40-50 mg/dL have been shown to be sate (Treating to New Targets (TNT) Study." Keep the same reference number.[22,23]

For patients who may not be able to tolerate a statin medication, NCEP guidelines should be followed in terms of getting

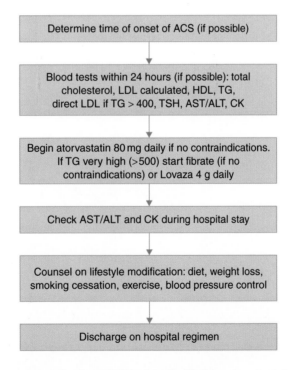

Lipids should return to baseline (non-ACS) in 4 weeks. Ideal time to recheck fasting lipid panel, AST/ALT, CK is approximately 6 weeks. If no myopathy, AST/ALT and CK within normal limits continue therapy. Goals for therapy: LDL <100 mg/dl with optional goal <70 mg/dl, HDL > 40 mg/dl, TG <150 mg/dl, non-HDL cholesterol <70 mg/dl.

Figure 34.1. Algorithm for the management of hyperlipidemia in the CCU. ACS, acute coronary syndrome; ALT, alanine aminotransferase; AST, aspartate aminotransferase; CK, creatinine kinase; LDL, low-density lipoproteins; HDL, high-density lipoproteins; TG, triglyceride.

patient to goal for LDL, HDL, and TG using one or more of nonstatin lipid medications.

DISCHARGE PLANNING

Patients should always be counseled on lifestyle modification including diet, weight loss, smoking cessation, exercise, and blood pressure control. They should be discharged on their hospital regimen and have a follow-up lipid panel. Lipids return to baseline in about 4 weeks although the ideal time frame to check for statin effects are approximately 6 weeks.

An algorithm for the management of lipids in the CCU is provided in Figure 34.1.

REFERENCES

1. Smith SC Jr, Allen J, Blair SN, et al. AHA/ACC guidelines for secondary prevention for patients with coronary and other atherosclerotic vascular disease: 2006 update. *Circulation.* 2006;113:2263–2372.
2. Mitka M. Guidelines update: aggressively target cardiovascular risk factors. *JAMA.* 2006;296:30–31.
3. Ballantyne CM, ed. *Clinical Lipidology.* Philadelphia, PA: Saunders Elsevier; 2009.
4. Davidson MH, Toth P, Maki KC, eds. *Therapeutic Lipidology.* Totawa, NJ: Humana Press; 2007.
5. Kwiterovich PO Jr. *The Johns Hopkins Textbook of Dyslipidemia.* Philadelphia, PA: Wolters Kluwer, Lippincott Williams & Wilkins; 2010.
6. Third Report of the National Cholesterol Education Program (NCEP) expert panel on detection, evaluation, and treatment of high blood cholesterol in adults (adult treatment panel III). www.nhlbi.nih.gov/guidelines/cholesterol/index.htm.
7. Rosenson RS. Myocardial injury: the acute phase response and lipoprotein metabolism. *J Am Coll Cardiol.* 1993;22:933–940.
8. Fresco C, Maggione AP, Signorini S, et al. Variations in lipoprotein levels after myocardial infarction and unstable angina: the LATIN trial. *Ital Heart J.* 2002;3:587–592.
9. Henkin Y, Crystal E, Goldberg Y, et al. Usefulness of lipoprotein changes during acute coronary syndromes for predicting post-discharge lipoprotein levels. *Am J Cardiol.* 2002;89:7–11.
10. Pitt B, Loscalzo J, Ycas J, et al. Lipid levels after acute coronary syndromes. *J Am Coll Cardiol.* 2008;51:1440–1445.
11. Schwartz GG, Olsson AG, Ezekowitz MD, et al. Effects of atorvastatin on early recurrent ischemic events in acute coronary syndromes. *JAMA.* 2001;285:1711–1718.
12. Cannon CP, Braunwald E, McCabe CH, et al. Intensive versus moderate lipid lowering with statins after acute coronary syndromes. *N Engl J Med.* 2004;350:1495–1504.
13. De Lemos JA, Blazing MA, Wiviott SD. Early invasive vs. a delayed conservative simvastatin strategy in patients with acute coronary syndromes. *JAMA.* 2004;292:1307–1316.
14. Hiro T, Kimura T, Morimoto T, et al. Effect of intensive statin therapy on regression of coronary atherosclerosis in patients with acute coronary syndromes. *J Am Coll Cardiol.* 2009;54:293–302.
15. Patti G, Pasceri V, Colonna G, et al. Atorvastatin pretreatment improves outcomes in patients with acute coronary syndromes undergoing early percutaneous coronary intervention. *J Am Coll Cardiol.* 2007;49:1272–1278.
16. Gibson CM, Pride YB, Hochberg CP. Effect of intensive statin therapy on clinical outcomes among patients undergoing percutaneous coronary intervention for acute coronary syndrome. *J Am Coll Cardiol.* 2009;54:2290–2295.
17. Ray KK, Cannon CP. The potential relevance of the multiple lipid-independent (pleiotropic) effects of statins in the management of acute coronary syndromes. *J Am Coll Cardiol.* 2005;46:1425–1433.
18. Liu P-Y, Liu Y-W, Lin L-J, et al. Evidence for statin pleiotropy in humans. *Circulation.* 2009;119:131–138.
19. Robinson JG, Smith B, Maheshwari N, et al. Pleiotropic effects of statins: benefits beyond cholesterol reduction. *J Am Coll Cardiol.* 2005;46:1855–1862.
20. Thompson PD, Clarkson PM, Rosenson RS. An assessment of statin safety by muscle experts. *Am J Cardiol.* 2006;97(suppl):69C–76C.
21. Calderon RM, Cubeddu LX, Goldberg RB, et al. Statins in the treatment of dyslipidemia in the presence of elevated liver aminotransferase levels: a therapeutic dilemma. *Mayo Clin Proc.* 2010;85:349–356.
22. LaRosa JC, Grundy SM, Waters DD, et al. Intensive lipid lowering with atorvastatin in patients with stable coronary disease. *N Engl J Med.* 2005;352:1425–1435.
23. Wiviott SD, Cannon CP, Morrow DA, et al. Can low-density lipoprotein be too low? *J Am Coll Cardiol.* 2005;46:1411–1416.
24. www.gripa.org/Documents/Pharmacy-tidbits/Aproximate-Dose-Conversions-10-06-Pharmacy.

PATIENT AND FAMILY INFORMATION FOR:
Lipid Management

Patients who have had a myocardial infarction (heart attack) or ACS often have risk factors that were either not diagnosed or not fully treated. Even if a person has had an ACS, treatment of risk factors can help reduce the chance for having another event and also improve overall cardiovascular health.

CHOLESTEROL AND LIPIDS

Cholesterol is a fat-like substance that is made by our body (in the liver) and also taken in by some of the foods (animal products) we eat. Cholesterol is a part of a class of substances called "lipids." It is an important component of our body because it is in cell membranes and is a component of some hormones and body organs. Cholesterol is carried in our blood stream. However, too much cholesterol can lead to a buildup inside blood vessels called arteries and result in atherosclerotic plaque. When the plaque becomes unstable or completely blocks off an artery an ACS can result.

SEVERAL FORMS OF CHOLESTEROL

There are several forms of cholesterol that are important.

Low-density lipoprotein cholesterol (LDL-C): This is known as the "bad" cholesterol and is the primary culprit in building up atherosclerotic plaque.

High-density lipoprotein cholesterol (HDL-C): This is known as the "good" cholesterol because it helps to take LDL-C out of the blood stream and return it to the liver from where it is passed out from the body.

Triglycerides: This is another form of fat that is made in the liver and also comes from some foods that are eaten. Having too high TG levels can also increase the risk for ACS.

Total cholesterol: A blood test report will also list a "total" number. This number is made up of the LDL, HDL, and TG. Even if the "total" number is at goal, it is important to make sure that each component is at goal.

WHAT SHOULD CHOLESTEROL NUMBERS BE?

LDL-C : In a person who has a heart attack or ACS, research studies have shown that a lower number is better. Current guidelines have <100 mg/dL as a goal with an "optional" goal of <70 mg/dL. Levels lower than this (50 to 70 mg/dL)

have also been shown to be safe and beneficial for patients with coronary artery disease.

HDL-C: Goal is >40 mg/dL. A level >60 mg/dL is considered excellent.

TG: Goal is <150 mg/dL.

WHAT TEST SHOULD A PATIENT HAVE?

A fasting blood test called a "lipid panel" with total cholesterol, LDL, HDL, and TG profile should be done. After an ACS, blood tests may not be accurate but can give doctors information about lipids. Lipid tests will again be fully accurate in about 1 month after an ACS. Many people have had this test before their ACS and the information may be available to the doctors in the hospital.

MEDICATIONS FOR LIPIDS

There are several prescription medications for high cholesterol. Often patients who have had an ACS have already been on one or more medications. Research studies investigating how to treat patients who have had an ACS have found that using a high dose of a "statin" drug is very beneficial, not only to lower LDL but also to reduce risk for further problems with coronary artery disease. There are several statin drugs and doses. Each drug has a slightly different treatment effect as well (see Tables 34.1 and 34.2) Atorvastatin (Lipitor) 80 mg daily is most often used as this has been most investigated in the setting of ACS.

If TG are very elevated (>500 mg/dL) a drug specific for lowering TG may be used, particularly a "fibrate" or a prescription of fish oil.

SIDE EFFECTS

Medications for dyslipidemia are generally considered safe but as with any medication it is important to monitor for side effects.

Common but not serious side effects when using a statin drug are muscle ache, mildly elevated liver enzymes, and mildly elevated muscle enzyme. Blood tests can check for AST, ALT, and CK.

Serious side effects are rare and include a severe condition known as rhabdomyolysis owing to muscle damage and subsequent kidney failure and death. Statin drugs can also cause severe liver damage or hepatitis.

Other medications used to treat dyslipidemia may have side effects as well. It is also important to check for interactions with other medications you may be taking.

LIFESTYLE

In addition to medication, it is very important to make lifestyle modifications. These include a heart health, low-cholesterol diet, weight loss, regular aerobic exercise, and smoking cessation.

DISCHARGE

After discharge from the hospital many patients are continued on the medications at discharge. It is important to have monitoring and review for any changes.

Diet, Nutrition, Obesity, and Weight Loss in Cardiac Care Unit Patients

A patient who presents to the cardiac care unit (CCU) with an acute myocardial infarction (AMI) or acute coronary syndrome (ACS) has by definition atherosclerotic cardiovascular disease (CVD) and requires help in mitigating morbidity and mortality from this. Appropriate nutrition will be a key element in both treatment and secondary prevention against further cardiac events.

Initially, there needs to be a focus on traditional risk factors. These include lipids and lipoproteins, blood pressure, smoking, and sedentariness. Behavioral change to healthy lifestyle practices need to be initiated, with intervention beginning immediately on entrance in the CCU, when the patient is aware of the seriousness of his/her condition, and the need to embark in an effort to restructure lifestyle habits of the past. It is important that when persons are admitted to the CCU for acute coronary events, a careful medical dietary and family history be taken as well as appropriate laboratory tests including lipid biochemistry measures.

This chapter will not deal with the cessation of smoking or with physical activity. It will address only nutrition. The discussion will focus first on lipids and lipoproteins, then on hypertension, third on metabolic syndrome (MetS) followed by discussion on diabetes and obesity, and finally on dietary patterns that may be used to reach appropriate goals.

LIPIDS AND LIPOPROTEINS

LDL CHOLESTEROL

This fraction of circulating cholesterol has been defined by numerous health care agencies and associations as the primary target of therapy for both primary and secondary prevention of coronary heart disease (CHD). It is the major cholesterol-carrying lipoprotein particle in plasma. As the level of low-density lipoprotein cholesterol (LDL-C) increases, so does the risk of CHD.[1,2] The Third Report of the National Cholesterol Education Program (NCEP) Expert Panel on Detection, Evaluation, and Treatment of High Blood Cholesterol in Adults (Adult Treatment Panel or ATP III)[3] recommended that the level of LDL-C is optimal at <100 mg per dl. In secondary prevention, lowering LDL-C reduces morbidity and mortality from CHD.[3]

Recommendations of NCEP[3] are as follows:

<100 mg per dl optimal

100 to 129 mg per dl near optimal

130 to 159 mg per dl borderline high

160 to 189 mg per dl high

>190 mg per dl very high.

For patients admitted to the CCU with evidence of ACS, we believe that the level of LDL-C should be <70 mg per dl, but this has not yet been incorporated into the official guidelines.

HDL CHOLESTEROL

This fraction of circulating cholesterol is considered the second most important fraction that needs to be assessed. It is called the "good" cholesterol because it is protective against CHD.[4,5] High-density lipoprotein cholesterol (HDL-C) is important in reverse cholesterol transport, which is the transport of cholesterol from peripheral tissues to the liver for excretion. So HDL-C protects against the development and progression of CHD. A low HDL-C is a strong independent predictor of CHD. The ATP III report defined a level of <40 mg per dl as a risk. Other organizations, such as the American College of Cardiology, have defined the risk according to gender: <40 mg per dl for men and <50 mg per dl for women.[6]

SERUM TRIGLYCERIDES

Elevated serum triglycerides are also an independent risk factor for CHD.[7,8] Levels are defined as normal if they are <150 mg per dl.[3]

HIGH BLOOD PRESSURE

Although an abnormal blood pressure has been defined as 140/90 mm Hg, recent recommendations from agencies and associations have suggested levels below 120/80 mm Hg,[9] because this lowers the risk of CHD morbidity considerably. Blood pressure is a strong risk factor for CVD (7th report). The risk of CVD increases beginning at 115/75 mm Hg. There is no threshold, rather it is a continuously increasing risk.[10] A large study by Stamler[11] showed the impressive effects of a small reduction of BP on reduction of mortality. A number of subsequent studies have confirmed the excellent impact of weight loss in lowering blood pressure in overweight individuals.[12,13]

METABOLIC SYNDROME

Matabolic Syndrome (MetS) consists of a cluster of risk factors that are predictive of the progression to type 2 diabetes and CHD. It has five components and is considered to be present if three of five components are present in an individual.[3] MetS, as defined in the United States, is shown in Table 35.1.[3] Defining the MetS has not been an attempt to declare the existence of a new disease produced by a single pathogenesis but an effort to put together risk factors that as a group have a greater ability to predict disease than is the case if they are considered separately. This cluster of lipid and nonlipid risk factors enhances the risk for CHD at any given level of LDL-C. Patients who present such a cluster are at much greater danger of morbidity and mortality from type 2 diabetes and CHD than are patients who do not.[14,15] It is therefore an alert for physicians that they should pay particular attention to these patients and address their risk factors vigorously to prevent progression to serious disease. The MetS has been described as a secondary target of therapy by ATP III.[3]

DIABETES

Macrovascular disease is the leading cause of death in diabetic persons. Many patients presenting with an AMI have either impaired glucose tolerance, impaired fasting glucose, or type 2 diabetes. Individuals with type 2 diabetes have great risk of developing CHD and eventual AMI.[16] Adults with diabetes have heart disease death rates and risks for stroke two- to fourfold higher than adults without diabetes.[17] Furthermore, the mortality rate for those diabetic individuals who have already suffered one AMI is higher than for nondiabetic persons who have suffered an AMI.[18,19] It is critical to try to improve all risk factors for AMI in these patients.

The improvement in glucose control does not in itself seem to have a great deal of effect in improving morbidity and mortality from coronary artery disease (CAD). It is likely that the pathogenesis for this accelerated CAD in diabetic patients is the dyslipidemia seen with central obesity and diabetes. This is characterized by elevated very-low-density lipoproteins (VLDL) leading to hypertriglyceridemia. There is overproduction of VLDL triglyceride and VLDL apoB, and also a defect in clearance. The composition of LDL particles is altered, with smaller and denser particles being present, which are significantly more atherogenic.[20,21] In addition, the elevated prevailing glucose can enhance the glycosylation of the LDL particles adding to their atherogenicity. Moreover, an increased susceptibility of the LDL particles to oxidation makes them more atherogenic. Finally, HDL production is decreased in obesity and diabetes, so that circulating levels are lower. These patients have elevated

triglycerides also.[22] Each of these lipid abnormalities has been shown to increase the risk for CAD in patients with type 2 diabetes.[23,24]

In type 2 diabetes, weight loss not only improves glycemic control but also ameliorates coexisting disorders such as dyslipidemia and hypertension. With dieting, the elevated triglyceride levels of obese patients with type 2 diabetes rapidly decline.[25,26] Furthermore, with weight loss, significant increases in HDL-C levels have been reported in studies that have been of sufficient duration.[27,28]

OBESITY

Approximately 65% of U.S. adults are overweight or obese.[29] Overweight and obesity are associated with an increased risk for CHD and heart failure. Obesity increases the risk of CVD. This has been well documented in the Framingham trial[30] and the Nurses Health Study.[31] In a more recent report, Wilson et al.[32] have shown increased relative and population-attributable risk for hypertension and cardiovascular sequelae in Framingham Heart Study obese participants. This is thought to be related to the increased prevalence of dyslipidemia in obesity. The dyslipidemia, as in type 2 diabetes, comprises primarily of an elevation in triglycerides and a decrease in the level of HDL-C. Levels of total cholesterol and LDL-C may be elevated but are often normal. Although LDL-C levels are not elevated, the LDL particles are, nevertheless, qualitatively different, showing a shift to smaller, denser particles that are more atherogenic.[33] These abnormalities are made worse by increased central or intra-abdominal fat.[34–36]

The evidence for the effect of weight loss as secondary prevention on reduction of adverse cardiac events is not large. Not many intervention studies have been carried out focusing on this question. Williamson et al.[37] and Gregg et al.[38] carried out retrospective analyses in women and men on the effect of intentional weight loss on mortality. They examined the life expectancy of >43,000 white U.S. women in the American Cancer Society Study. Overweight women with obesity-related health conditions had significantly higher mortality rates compared with women with no preexisting illness. Women with obesity-related conditions who intentionally lost weight showed a significant reduction in all-cause mortality compared with women whose weight remained stable. The risk of cardiovascular mortality was reduced by 14% to 24% in obese women who intentionally lost weight.[37] Gregg et al.[38] then carried out a similar study in men, using the same American Cancer Society database. They found that men with obesity-related conditions who intentionally lost weight had a reduced all-cause and cardiovascular mortality. A 4-year prospective study of >7,500 middle-aged men found an independent decrease in cardiovascular

TABLE 35.1	NCEP Adult Treatment Panel III Definition of the Metabolic Syndrome (Needs to Have at least Three of the Five Features)

Waist circumference >102 cm (40 in) in men and >88 cm (35 in) in women
Serum triglycerides >150 mg/dl (1.7 mmol/L)
HDL cholesterol <35 mg/dl (1.3 mmol/L) in men and <40 mg/dl (1.0 mmol/L) in women
Blood pressure >130/85 mm Hg
Serum glucose >100 mg/dl (5.6 mmol/L)—changed in 2004 from 110 mg/dl (6.1 mmol/L)

mortality of almost 50% in those whose weight loss brought them below a body mass index (BMI) of 28 and a reduction of 77% in those who had associated hypertension.[39] It has been suggested that CHD mortality could be reduced by 15% if everyone had a BMI between 21 and 25.

Because many obese persons also manifest hypertension and dyslipidemia, it has sometimes been difficult to assign causality for the CHD to obesity independent of these other conditions. Because obesity is associated with a number of CHD risk factors, it is not surprising that it has been related directly to greater cardiovascular risk.[40]

In both obesity and diabetes, there is an increased inflammatory environment. Obesity and fat cell size correlate with macrophage infiltration into adipose tissue.[41] Cytokines released from both adipocytes and macrophages in adipose tissue contribute to a state of chronic systemic and local vascular inflammation and enhanced coagulation.[42–44] These lead to increased insulin resistance and the progression of MetS, diabetes, and CHD.[45] This inflammation is decreased with weight loss.[45]

NUTRITIONAL BEHAVIORAL LIFESTYLE CHANGE

For the past three decades, behavior modification has been used to treat obesity. No single definition of behavior modification exists. Definitions range from the applications of operant conditioning, classical conditioning, or principles of learning theory, to more broadly based cognitive behavioral models. The primary goal is to change an individual's eating and physical activity habits; changes are gradual. Following achievement of a weight that is maintainable without excessive exercise or overly restrictive eating limitation, relapse prevention training is used to teach the individual how to cope with emotional and social situations associated with eating relapse. Unfortunately, in the few studies available, most of 3- to 5-year follow-ups show gradual return to baseline.

In the past, physicians and their patients have been overwhelmed by the magnitude and complexity of nutrition information and behavior changes they have been asked to make to achieve health benefits. However, nutrition intervention to reduce cardiovascular risk factors and cardiovascular events is achievable in primary care or cardiology practice. The focus should be initially on one to two nutrition behavior changes that are easy to implement and are supported with physician and patient educational materials. The nutrition behavior changes should result in measurable changes in endpoints over time. The physician should initiate the nutrition intervention process through nutrition messages to increase credibility and

seriousness. These messages should be reinforced and followed up by office practice members over time. The messages should focus on the key nutrient that is most problematic and where intervention will a effect the most measurable change over time (it is usually fat, but may be sugar or other carbohydrates). The nutrition behavior messages and changes should be framed positively (e.g., substitution rather than restriction). The focus should be on the total diet, rather than on individual foods. There should be a companion message to increase physical activity.

Physicians generally lack formal training in nutrition as do their office staff and have a poor understanding of how to apply nutrition intervention. They also have serious time constraints in their office. Moreover, many have experienced patient failure previously and so have lost their enthusiasm for pursuing a course of nutrition change. Furthermore, they face unrealistic patient expectations: that nutrition change needs to be only temporary, that small changes will give major weight loss, that weight loss will solve most of life's many other problems. Patients underestimate the amount of planning needed for change and many find the change inconvenient. Many are bored by the substituted food items.

Many have misconceptions about their risk often bolstered by cultural beliefs.

Many lack family or social support.

There is a need for rapport, communication, and education of the patient, and also empathy. Reasonable goals should be developed with the patient. These should be written down for the patient as a prescription. Help will be required in problem solving as a patient encounters barriers to success. Clear and explicit educational materials about nutrition are also extremely important.

LDL-C LOWERING

To lower the LDL-C, the AHA has proposed dietary goals. These AHA diet and lifestyle goals for cardiovascular risk reduction are shown in Table 35.2.[46]

The first recommendation is to "consume a healthy diet." This suggests that rather than look at one or two specific components, the whole diet be appraised so that not only macronutrients (carbohydrates, fats, and proteins) but also appropriate amounts of micronutrients (vitamins and minerals) are taken.

The NCEP guidelines for someone with already existing CHD suggest following the therapeutic lifestyle changes (TLC) diet.[3] This is shown in Table 35.3.

It is recommended that the intake of saturated fats be <7% of total energy, trans fat <1%, and cholesterol <200 mg per day. This can be best done by eating less meat, choosing lean meat

TABLE 35.2	AHA 2006 Diet and Lifestyle Goals for Cardiovascular Disease Risk Reduction

Consume an overall healthy diet.
Aim for a healthy body weight.
Aim for recommended levels of low-density lipoprotein (LDL) cholesterol, high-density lipoprotein (HDL) cholesterol, and triglycerides.
Aim for a normal blood pressure.
Aim for a normal blood glucose.
Be physically active.
Avoid use of and exposure to tobacco products.

TABLE 35.3	Nutrient Composition of the Therapeutic Lifestyle Changes Diet

Nutrient	Recommended Intake
Saturated fat[a]	Less than 7% of total calories
Polyunsaturated fat	Up to 10% of total calories
Monounsaturated fat	Up to 20% of total calories
Total fat	25%–35% of total calories
Carbohydrate[b]	50%–60% of total calories
Fiber	20–30 g/day
Protein	Approximately 15% of total calories
Cholesterol	Less than 200 mg/day
Total calories (energy)[c]	Balance energy intake and expenditure to maintain desirable body weight/prevent weight gain

[a]Trans fatty acids are another LDL-raising fat that should be kept at a low intake.
[b]Carbohydrate should be derived predominantly from foods rich in complex carbohydrates including grains, especially whole grains, fruits, and vegetables.
[c]Daily energy expenditure should include at least moderate physical activity (contributing approximately 200 kcal per day).

over more fatty meat, using fat-free or 1% fat milk, taking low-fat dairy products, and avoiding partially hydrogenated fats.

The major sources of saturated fatty acids are animal fats (meat and dairy) and the primary sources of trans fatty acids are partially hydrogenated fats used to prepare commercially fried and baked foods.

Dietary cholesterol comes from foods of animal origin such as eggs, dairy products, and meat; therefore these should be decreased. In reducing saturated fat and cholesterol, the foods that contain these are replaced with mono (MUFA) or poly-unsaturated (PUFA) fat containing foods as well as choosing lower fat versions of foods. Meats can be replaced with legumes, vegetables, and fish. Overall, it is suggested by the Institute of Medicine (IOM), NCEP,[3] and the 2005 Dietary guidelines for Americans[47] that a range of 25% to 35% fat is an appropriate level of intake. The balance of fats will be PUFA or MUFA. It has generally been suggested that PUFA be about 7% of calories whereas MUFA can vary from 7% to 20%.

Fish (particularly oily fish) is rich in very long-chain Ω-3 PUFAs, eicosapentaenoic acid (C20:5n-3) and docosahexaenoic (C22:6n-3). Eating at least two portions of fish per week is recommended. In cooking the fish, care should be taken not to add saturated or trans fats. Despite mercury contamination, two servings of fish per week are acceptable and safe.[47] Fish oil supplements are a possible route to obtain enough n-3 PUFA but to date have not been shown to improve cardiovascular prognosis.

TOTAL CALORIES (WEIGHT LOSS)

A number of randomized clinical trials have been done on the effect of weight loss on lipid levels. With sustained weight loss, there is generally a decrease in triglycerides and an increase in HDL-C.[48–50] There is also a change in the spectrum of LDL particles with a move to larger, less dense particles. In various randomized clinical trials using a hypocaloric diet, weight loss of 5% to 10% from baseline weight has been documented to decrease triglycerides from 8% to 40%, LDL-C from 1.7%

to 20%, total cholesterol from none to 19%, and to increase HDL-C from none to 38%. Results of a meta-analysis of some 70 studies, published in MEDLINE from 1966 to 1989, showed that intentional weight loss with dieting was associated with significant decrease of total cholesterol, LDL-C, VLDL-C, and total triglycerides. For every kilogram decrease in body weight, there was a 0.05 mmol per L decrease in total cholesterol, a 0.01 mmol per L decrease in LDL-C, a 0.009 mmol per L increase in HDL-C, at a stabilized body weight.[50]

In conclusion, weight loss is a powerful improver of lipid risk factors. The effect occurs in both hyperlipemic and normolipemic individuals. Weight loss also decreases inflammation, which is likely to reduce cardiovascular events.[45]

A change in nutrition is a key component of a weight-reduction effort. Obese persons consume a very large amount of calories and these must be reduced. A calorie-deficit diet can lead to significant weight loss and to improvement in an obese person with CHD. The typical American diet consists of about 15% protein, 35% fat, and 50% carbohydrates.[51] Americans eat about 30% to 35% of calories as fat and 18% as sugar. Fat should be decreased and total calories reduced. Sugar should be discouraged. High-fiber foods such as fruits and vegetables and whole grains should be encouraged. Alcohol should be eliminated or curtailed. One should aim at a deficit of about 1,000 cal per day; this would translate to about 1 kg of weight loss per week.

Many persons can benefit from a low-calorie formula diet for a period, usually 12 to 16 weeks.[52] Initially, this can be for all meals, and eventually it can be used for one or two meals a day. The advantage is that it can provide a very good mechanism of control for reducing calorie intake. The disadvantage is that it can become extremely monotonous.

The aim of weight loss is to lose fat without losing too much lean body mass. The loss of some lean body mass is inevitable, but it should be kept as low as possible. This is done by eating enough protein and making it high-quality protein (e.g., egg whites, low-fat dairy products, lean meat, fish, and poultry). The intake of protein should be at a level of 1.0 to 1.5 g per kg of ideal body weight (calculated as a BMI of 25 for each individual). The ideal body weight can be calculated using a BMI of 25 and finding the patient's appropriate weight in a BMI table. Otherwise it can be calculated as $25 \times$ height (in cm^2). A vegetarian diet can be used but protein complementation is required to ensure appropriate essential amino acid intake.[53] Total fat should not exceed 30% of calories, with saturated fat not more than 7%. This is also true of PUFA, whereas MUFA can be as high as 15% to 20%. The daily carbohydrate intake should include 20 to 30 g of fiber from fruits, vegetables, legumes, and grains. Fiber seems to help satiety at lower levels of caloric intake. It is also important that adequate amounts of vitamins and minerals are taken daily. A supplement can be helpful in this regard.

The effort to achieve a caloric deficit of between 500 and 1,500 cal per day requires a careful dietary history. This can lead to a loss of between 1 and 2 lb per week.[13] A low-calorie diet includes 800 to 1,500 cal per day. A diet of 1,200 to 1,500 cal per day for men and one of 1,000 to 1,200 cal per day for women is usually about right, but it needs to be individualized in relation to original intake and physical activity. These kinds of diets can cause a 10% weight loss in 6 months, with 75% being fat and 25% lean body mass.[54] Very-low-calorie diets of 300 to 800 cal per day have been used in the past but are not recommended. They require careful medical supervision because of potential electrolyte abnormalities, cardiac changes, and excess diuresis. Moreover, they have not been shown to produce greater weight loss long term.[55] Furthermore, there tends to be a rapid regain once the very-low-calorie diet is abandoned.[54]

In general, with such caloric deficits, weight loss continues for 4 to 6 months and then plateaus off. This plateau is due to a new equilibrium in which energy intake once again is equivalent to energy expenditure. Maintenance of the weight loss requires continuing the same lower-energy intake and a physical activity at least as great as a patient has been doing for weight loss. Therefore, there can be no liberalization of food intake or reduction of physical activity, or else weight regain will occur.

All low-calorie diets will produce weight loss in the short term, and current evidence suggests that the macronutrient composition does not play a significant role.[56] There is no optimal macronutrient composition (e.g., protein, carbohydrate, fat content) of weight loss diets. There have been long-term trials (1 year or more) of both low-fat balanced diet and the Mediterranean diet that have shown their effectiveness and their safety.[13,57,58] One long-term trial of the high-carbohydrate/low-fat diet[59] also showed its effectiveness and safety over time. A number of randomized clinical trials comparing high-fat, low-carbohydrate diets with more balanced diets have been done, showing as good or better weight loss with the former as the latter.[60–64] In a recent prospective randomized clinical trial in which several popular weight loss plans (Atkins, Ornish, Weight Watchers, Zone) were compared, all diets produced a similar amount of weight loss at the end of 1 year.[65] This finding is in agreement with results from a previous study in which a low-carbohydrate, high-protein diet was compared with a low-calorie, low-fat diet.[63] Although a low-carbohydrate, high-protein diet produced more loss of weight after 6 months; weight loss at the end of 1 year was the same regardless of dietary intervention.[63]

In its report on dietary reference intakes from macronutrients, the IOM of the NAS set the acceptable macronutrient distribution range for carbohydrate at 45% to 65%, for fat from 20% to 35% and for protein from 10% to 35%.[66]

Weight loss diets comprising single foods or food groups, severely restrict a particular macronutrient or eliminate specific foods or food groups are not recommended, as the potential for health risks (calciuria, increased saturated fat intake) and nutrient deficiencies is more likely utilizing an unbalanced approach.[67]

To be successful, dietary guidance should be individualized, allowing for patient food preferences and individual approaches to reducing caloric intake.[68] Techniques for decreasing caloric intake may include reducing portion sizes, selecting low-calorie foods, and using cooking methods that lower fat intake.[69,70]

DIETARY EFFECTS ON HIGH BLOOD PRESSURE

Dietary modifications that can improve elevated blood pressure include a reduced salt intake, reduced calorie intake leading to weight loss, increased potassium intake, and moderation of alcohol consumption.

Many clinical trials have documented that weight loss lowers blood pressure.[71–73]

Blood pressure goes up as intake of dietary salt (sodium chloride) increases.[74] Some salt intake is required for health, but the salt intake is very high in the United States. There have been some excellent dose–response trials of salt intake. Whether on a control (usual) or dietary approaches to stop hypertension (DASH) diet, lowering sodium lowers blood pressure. Although the response to lowering sodium is variable, there is a response in everyone.

Three excellent trials have tested the effect of lowered sodium intake and shown a strong effect on BP lowering.[75,76] In a recent meta-analysis,[77] a median reduction of urinary sodium (1.8 mg per day; 78 mmol per day) had a very beneficial effect lowering both systolic and diastolic BP by 2.0 and 1.0 mm Hg, respectively, in nonhypertensive patients and by 5.0 and 2.7 mm Hg, respectively, in hypertensive individuals.

The IOM set an adequate intake level at 1.5 g per day (65 mmol per day) of sodium. However lowering it to 1.5 g per day is very difficult. The AHA has suggested an upper limit of 2.3 g per day (100 mmol per day) as doable. To reduce salt intake, it is important to choose foods low in salt as well as limiting the amount of salt added to food in cooking or at the table. About 75% of consumed salt comes from processed foods,[78] therefore it is important to reduce their intake.

It is known from observational studies that a high potassium intake is associated with a reduced blood pressure. Meta-analyses have reported that there is an inverse relationship between potassium intake and blood pressure in both nonhypertensive and hypertensive persons.[79–84] The effect of a higher potassium intake is greater in Black persons.[80] A high potassium intake can be achieved through diet rather than pills. Fruits and vegetables that are high in potassium should be eaten. These also are rich in other micronutrients. A level of 4.7 g per day (120 mmol per day) has been recommended by the AHA and the IOM.

Excessive alcohol intake increases blood pressure. Whereas moderate alcohol intake can be helpful for prevention of CHD, excess leads to elevation of blood pressure. Reduction of alcohol intake reduces blood pressure.[85] According the AHA, alcohol consumption should be limited to less than two alcoholic drinks per day in most men and less than one in women and lighter weight men. One drink is defined as 12 oz of regular beer, 5 oz of wine (12% alcohol), and 1.5 oz of 80 proof distilled spirits.

DIETARY PATTERNS

It is often best to advise individual patients by seeking a dietary pattern that is acceptable to them and has enough of the required characteristics so that it is effective in lowering weight, blood pressure, and improving lipids and glucose levels. Both TLC and AHA diets are excellent diets to recommend. There are a few other patterns that are reasonable for long-term use.

MEDITERRANEAN DIET

A Mediterranean diet has been shown to significantly decrease cardiovascular and total mortality.[86] The PREDIMED trial (Prevencion con Dieta Mediterranea) is testing >9,000 high-risk persons. There is randomization to a low-fat group, to the Mediterranean diet plus 1 L of free virgin olive oil per week, or to Mediterranean diet plus 1 oz of free mixed nuts daily. In an interim analysis, those in either of the two Mediterranean diet intervention arms had lower mean glucose, lower systolic blood pressure, and a lower total cholesterol-to-HDL ratio than those randomized to the low-fat control.[87] This is a pleasant diet that appears to be cardioprotective.

DASH DIET

The DASH diet has been tested in three trials that have documented its effectiveness in lowering blood pressure. The DASH diet calls for an increased intake of fruits, vegetables, and low-fat dairy products. It includes whole grains, poultry, fish, and nuts. It reduces intake of fats, red meat, sweets, and sugar-containing vegetables.[88] The diet is rich in potassium, magnesium, calcium, and fiber and is reduced in total fat, saturated fat, and cholesterol. There is a slight increase in protein. It is very similar to a Mediterranean diet.

PREMIER DIET

The Premier diet is like the DASH diet but has been adapted to be hypocaloric so that it will be an effective diet not only for blood pressure lowering but also for weight loss.[89]

VEGETARIAN DIET

Persons eating a vegetarian diet have a lower blood pressure than nonvegetarians.[90,91] Some of the effect is clearly from the diet (no meat, high fiber) but much is related to the healthful lifestyle of many of its adherents (low weight, high exercise).

FINAL RECOMMENDATIONS

It is very important that follow-up by the physician occurs. The physician can have a very strong influence in persuading and helping a patient to change his/her lifestyle towards a healthier one.[92] If the issue is ignored at subsequent visits, there is little likelihood of success. An important component for success is to weigh and measure waist circumference at each visit, to address nutritional and physical activity issues, and to counsel a patient who is confronting barriers to pursuing a healthier lifestyle.

REFERENCES

1. Pekkanen J, Linn S, Heiss G, et al. Ten-year mortality from cardiovascular disease in relation to cholesterol level among men with and without preexisting cardiovascular disease. N Engl J Med. 1990;322:1112–1119.
2. Stamler J, Wentworth D, Neaton JD; for the MRFIT Research Group. Is relationship between serum cholesterol and risk of premature death from coronary heart disease continuous and graded? Findings in 356,222 primary screenees of the Multiple Risk Factor Intervention Trial (MRFIT). JAMA. 1986;256:2823–2828.
3. National Cholesterol Education Program. Third Report of the National Cholesterol Education Program (NCEP) Expert Panel on Detection, Evaluation, and Treatment of High Blood Cholesterol in Adults (Adult Treatment Panel III). Bethesda, MD: National Heart, Lung, and Blood Institute; National Institutes of Health; 2002. NIH publication 02-5215.
4. Wilson PWF, D'Agostino RB, Levy D, et al. Prediction of coronary heart disease using risk factor categories. Circulation. 1998;97:1837–1847.
5. Gordon DJ, Probstfield JL, Garrison RJ, et al. High-density lipoprotein cholesterol and cardiovascular disease: four prospective American studies. Circulation. 1989;79:8–15.
6. Gotto AM Jr, Brinton EA. Assessing low levels of high-density lipoprotein cholesterol as a risk factor in coronary heart disease: a working group report and update. J Am Coll Cardiol. 2001;43:717–724.
7. Austin MA, Hokanson JE, Edwards KL. Hypertriglyceridemia as a cardiovascular risk factor. Am J Cardiol. 1998;81:7B–12B.
8. Assman G, Schulte H, Funke H, et al. The emergence of triglycerides as a significant independent risk factor in coronary artery disease. Eur Heart J. 1998;19(suppl M):M8–M14.
9. Chobanian AV, Bakris GL, Black HR, et al.; Joint National Committee on Prevention, Detection, Evaluation, and Treatment of High Blood Pressure. National Heart, Lung, and Blood Institute; National High Blood Pressure Education Program Coordinating Committee. Seventh report of the Joint National Committee on Prevention, Detection, Evaluation, and Treatment of High Blood Pressure. Hypertension. 2003;42:1206–1252.
10. Lewington S, Clarke R, Qizilbash N, et al.; for the Prospective Studies Collaboration. Age-specific relevance of usual blood pressure to vascular mortality: a meta-analysis of individual data for one million adults in 61 prospective studies. Lancet. 2001;360:1903–1913.
11. Stamler R. Implications of the INTERSALT study. Hypertension. 1991;17(suppl I):I-16–I-20.
12. Whelton PK, Appel LJ, Espeland MA, et al.; TONE Collaborative Research Group. Sodium reduction and weight loss in the treatment of hypertension in older persons: a randomized controlled trial of nonpharmacologic interventions in the elderly (TONE). JAMA. 1998;279:839–846.
13. Knowler WC, Barrett-Connor E, Fowler SE, et al.; for the Diabetes Prevention Program Research Group. Reduction in the incidence of type 2 diabetes with lifestyle intervention or metformin. N Engl J Med. 2002;346:393–403.
14. Lakka HM, Laaksonen DE, Lakka TA, et al. The metabolic syndrome and total and cardiovascular disease mortality in middle-aged men. JAMA. 2002;288:2709–2716.
15. Ford ES. Risks for all-cause mortality, cardiovascular disease, and diabetes associated with the metabolic syndrome: a summary of the evidence. Diabetes Care. 2006;29:123–130.
16. Haffner SM. Diabetes, hyperlipidemia, and coronary artery disease. Am J Cardiol. 1999;83:17F–21F.
17. Haffner SM, Lehto S, Ronnema T, et al. Mortality from coronary heart disease in subjects with type 2 diabetes and in nondiabetic subjects with and without prior myocardial infarction. N Engl J Med. 1998;339:229–234.
18. Herlitz J, Karlson BW, Edrardsson N, et al. Prognosis in diabetics with chest pain or other symptoms suggestive of acute myocardial infarction. Cardiology. 1992;80:237–245.
19. Mieinen H, Lehro S, Salomaa V, et al.; for the FINMONICA Myocardial Infarction Register Study Group. Impact of diabetes on mortality after the first myocardial infarction. Diabetes Care. 1998;21:69–75.
20. Feingold KR, Grunfeld C, Png M, et al. LDL subclass phenotypes and triglyceride metabolism in non-insulin dependent diabetes. Arterioscler Thromb. 1992;12:1496–1502.
21. Anderson JW, Brinkman-Kaplan V, Hamilton CC, et al. Food-containing hypocaloric diets are as effective as liquid-supplement diets for obese individuals with NIDDM. Diabetes Care. 1994;17:602–604.
22. Stern MP, Patterson JK, Haffner SM, et al. Lack of awareness and treatment of hyperlipidemia in type II diabetes in a community survey. JAMA. 1989;262:360–364.
23. Fontbonne A, Eschwege E, Cambien F, et al. Hypertriglyceridemia as a risk factor of coronary heart disease mortality in subjects with impaired glucose tolerance in diabetes: results from the 11-year follow-up of the Paris prospective study. Diabetologia. 1989;32:300–304.
24. Nikkila EA. High-density lipoproteins in diabetes. Diabetes. 1981;30:82–87.
25. Howard WA, Savage PJ, Nagulesparan M, et al. Changes in plasma lipoproteins accompanying diet therapy in obese diabetics. Atherosclerosis. 1979;33:445–456.
26. Bauman WA, Schwartz E, Rose HG, et al. Early and long-term effects of acute caloric deprivation in obese diabetic patients. Am J Med. 1988;85:38–46.
27. Uusitupa MIJ, Laakso M, Sarlund H, et al. Effects of a very-low calorie diet on metabolic control and cardiovascular risk factors in the treatment of obese non-insulin-dependent diabetics. Am J Clin Nutr. 1990;51:768–773.
28. Wing RR, Blair E, Marcus M, et al. Year-long weight loss treatment for obese patients with type II diabetes: does including an intermittent very-low calories diet improve outcome? Am J Med. 1994;97:354–362.
29. Flegal KM, Carroll MD, Ogden CL, et al. Prevalence and trends in obesity among US adults, 1999–2008. JAMA. 2010;303:235–241.
30. Hubert HB, Feinleib M, McNamara PM, et al. Obesity as an independent risk factor for cardiovascular disease: a 26-year follow-up of participants in the Framingham Heart Study. Circulation. 1983;67:968–977.
31. Manson JE, Willett WC, Stampfer MJ, et al. Body weight and mortality among women. N Engl J Med. 1995;333:677–685.

32. Wilson PW, D'Agostino RB, Sullivan L, et al. Overweight and obesity as determinants of cardiovascular risk: the Framingham experience. *Arch Intern Med.* 2002;162:1867–1872.

33. Austin MA, Breslow JL, Hennekens CH, et al. Low-density lipoprotein subclass patterns and risk of myocardial infarction. *JAMA.* 1988;2000:1917–1921.

34. Despres JP, Moorjani S, Lupien PJ, et al. Regional distribution of body fat, plasma lipoproteins, and cardiovascular disease. *Arteriosclerosis.* 1990;10:497–511.

35. Pouliot MC, Despres JP, Nadeau A, et al. Visceral obesity in men: associations with glucose tolerance, plasma insulin, and lipoprotein levels. *Diabetes.* 1992;41:826–834.

36. Matsuzawa Y, Shimomura I, Nakamura T, et al. Pathophysiology and pathogenesis of visceral fat obesity. *Diabetes Res Clin Pract.* 1994;24:S111–S116.

37. Williamson DF, Pamuk E, Thun M, et al. Prospective study of intentional weight loss and mortality in never-smoking overweight US white women aged 40–65 years. *Am J Epidemiol.* 1995;141:1128–1141.

38. Gregg EW, Gerzoff RB, Thompson TJ, et al. Intentional weight loss and death in overweight and obese US adults 35 years of age and older. *Ann Intern Med.* 2003;138:383–389.

39. Wannamethee SG, Shaper AG, Lennon L, et al. Metabolic syndrome vs Framingham Risk Score for prediction of coronary heart disease, stroke, and type 2 diabetes mellitus. *Arch Intern Med.* 2005;165:2644–2650.

40. Calle EE, Thun MJ, Petrelli JM, et al. Body-mass index and mortality in a prospective cohort of US adults. *N Engl J Med.* 1999;341:1097–1105.

41. Weisberg SP, McCann D, Desai M, et al. Obesity is associated with macrophage accumulation in adipose tissue. *J Clin Invest.* 2003;112:1796–1808.

42. Trayhurn P, Wood IS. Adipokines: inflammation and the pleiotropic role of white adipose tissue. *Br J Nutr.* 2004;92:347–355.

43. Fantuzzi G. Adipose tissue, adipokines, and inflammation. *J Allergy Clin Immunol.* 2005;115:911–919.

44. Lyon CJ, Law RE, Hsueh WA. Minireview: adiposity, inflammation, and atherogenesis. *Endocrinology.* 2003;144:2195–2200.

45. Pi-Sunyer FX. The relation of adipose tissue to cardiometabolic risk. *Clin Cornerstone.* 2006;8:S14–S23.

46. Lichtenstein AH, Appel LJ, Brands M, et al. Diet and lifestyle recommendations revision 2006: a scientific statement from the American Heart Association Nutrition Committee. *Circulation.* 2006;114:82–96.

47. *Report of the Dietary Guidelines Advisory Committee on the Dietary Guidelines for Americans, 2005.* Washington, DC: Agricultural Research Service, US Department of Agriculture; 2005.

48. Goldstein DJ. Beneficial effects of modest weight loss. *Int J Obes.* 1992;16:397–415.

49. Pi-Sunyer FX. Review of long-term studies evaluating the efficacy of weight loss in ameliorating disorders associated with obesity. *Clin Ther.* 1996;18:1006–1035.

50. Dattilo AM, Kris-Etherton PM. Effects of weight reduction on blood lipids and lipoproteins: a meta-analysis. *Am J Clin Nutr.* 1992;56:320–328.

51. Centers for Disease Control and Prevention. *Dietary Intake of Macronutrients, Micronutrients, and Other Dietary Constituents, USA 1988–1994.* Hyattsville, MD: National Center for Health Statistics; 2002. Series 11, No. 245.

52. Flechner-Mors M, Ditschuneit HH, Johnson TD, et al. Metabolic and weight loss effects of long-term dietary intervention in obese patients: four year results. *Obes Res.* 2000;8:399–402.

53. Johnston PK. Vegetarian nutrition: proceedings of a symposium held in Arlington, VA. *Am J Clin Nutr.* 1994;59:1099S–1262S.

54. Yang MU, Van Itallie TB. Reducing primary risk factors by therapeutic weight loss. In: Wadden TA, Van Itallie TB, eds. *Treatment of the Seriously Obese Patient.* New York, NY: Guilford Press; 1992:83–106.

55. Wadden TA, Foster GD, Letizia KA. One year behavioral treatment of obesity: comparison of moderate and severe caloric restriction and the effects of weight maintenance therapy. *N Engl J Med.* 1994;62:165–171.

56. NIH and NHLBI, NIDDK. *Clinical Guidelines on the Identification, Evaluation, and Treatment of Overweight and Obesity in Adults.* Bethesda, MD: NIH; 1998.

57. Tuomilehto J, Lindstrom J, Eriksson JG, et al. Prevention of type 2 diabetes mellitus by changes in lifestyle among subjects with impaired glucose tolerance. *N Engl J Med.* 2001;344:1343–1350.

58. De Lorgeril M, Salen P, Martin JL, et al. Mediterranean diet, traditional risk factors, and the rate of cardiovascular complications after myocardial infarction: final report of the Lyon Diet Heart Study. *Circulation.* 1999;99:779–785.

59. Ornish D, Brown SE, Scherwitz LW, et al. Can lifestyle changes reverse coronary heart disease? The Lifestyle Heart Trial. *Lancet.* 1990;336:129–133.

60. Skov AR, Toubro S, Ronn B, et al. Randomized trial on protein vs carbohydrate in ad libitum fat reduced diet for the treatment of obesity. *Int J Obes Relat Metab Disord.* 1999;23:528–536.

61. Brehm BJ, Seeley RJ, Daniels SR, et al. A randomized trial comparing a very low carbohydrate diet and a calorie-restricted low fat diet on body weight and cardiovascular risk factors in healthy women. *J Clin Endocrinol Metab.* 2003;88:1617–1623.

62. Samaha FF, Iqbal N, Seshadri P, et al. A low-carbohydrate as compared with a low-fat diet in severe obesity. *N Engl J Med.* 2003;348:2074–2081.

63. Foster GD, Wyatt HR, Hill JO, et al. A randomized trial of a low-carbohydrate diet for obesity. *N Engl J Med.* 2003;348:2082–2090.

64. Stern J, Iqbal N, Seshadri P, et al. The effects of a low-carbohydrate versus conventional weight loss diets in severely obese adults: one-year follow-up of a randomized trial. *Ann Intern Med.* 2004;140:778–785.

65. Dansinger ML, Gleason JA, Griffith JL, et al. Comparison of the Atkins, Ornish, Weight Watchers, and Zone diets for weight loss and heart disease reduction. *JAMA.* 2005;293:43–53.

66. Institute of Medicine of the National Academies. *Dietary Reference Intakes for Energy, Carbohydrate, Fiber, Fat, Fatty Acids, cholesterol, protein, and amino Acids (Macronutrients).* Washington, DC: National Academy Press; 2002.

67. Bonow RO, Eckel RH. Diet, obesity, and cardiovascular risk. *N Engl J Med.* 2003;348:2057–2058.

68. NIH, NHLNI, NHLBI Obesity Education Initiative, and North American Association for the Study of Obesity. *The Practical Guide. Identification, Evaluation, and Treatment of Overweight and Obesity in Adults.* Bethesda, MD: NIH; 2000.

69. Serdula MK, Khan LK, Dietz WH. Weight loss counseling revisited. *JAMA.* 2003;289:1747–1750.

70. Wing RR, Hill JO. Successful weight loss maintenance. *Annu Rev Nutr.* 2001;21:323–341.

71. Neter JE, Stam BE, Kok FJ, et al. Influence of weight reduction on blood pressure: a meta-analysis of randomized controlled trials. *Hypertension.* 2003;42:878–884.

72. Stevens VJ, Corrigan SA, Obarzanek E, et al. Weight loss intervention in phase 1 of the Trials of Hypertension Prevention: the TOHP Collaborative Research Group. *Arch Intern Med.* 1993;153:849–858.

73. Stevens VJ, Obarzanek E, Cook NR, et al.; for the Trials for the Hypertension Prevention Research Group. Long-term weight loss and changes in blood pressure: results of the Trials of Hypertension Prevention, phase II. *Ann Intern Med.* 1998;128:81–88.

74. Johnson AG, Nguyen TV, Davis D. Blood pressure is linked to salt intake and modulated by the angiotensinogen gene in normotensive and hypertensive elderly subjects. *J Hypertens.* 2001;19:1053–1060.

75. MacGregor GA, Makandu ND, Sagnella GA, et al. Double-blind study of three sodium intakes and long-term effects of sodium restriction in essential hypertension. *Lancet.* 1989;2:1244–1247.

76. Sacks FM, Svetkey LP, Vollmer WM, et al.; for the DASH–Sodium Collaborative Research Group. Effects on blood pressure of reduced dietary sodium and the Dietary Approaches to Stop Hypertension (DASH) diet: DASH–Sodium Collaborative Research Group. *N Engl J Med.* 2001;344:3–10.

77. He FJ, MacGregor GA. Effect of modest salt reduction on blood pressure: a meta-analysis of randomized trials: implications for public health. *J Hum Hypertens.* 2002;16:761–770.

78. Mattes RD, Donnely D. Relative contributions of dietary sodium sources. *J Am Coll Nutr.* 1991;10:383–393.

79. Cappuccio FP, MacGregor GA. Does potassium supplementation lower blood pressure? A meta-analysis of published trials. *J Hypertens.* 1991;9:465–473.

80. Whelton PK, He J, Cutler JA, et al. Effects of oral potassium on blood pressure; meta-analysis of randomized controlled clinical trials. *JAMA.* 1997;277:1624–1632.

81. Geleijnse JM, Kok FJ, Grobee DE. Blood pressure response to changes in sodium and potassium intake: a metaregression analysis of randomized trials. *J Hum Hypertens.* 2003;17:471–480.

82. Brancati FL, Appel LJ, Seidler AJ, et al. Effect of potassium supplementation on blood pressure in African Americans on a low-potassium diet: a randomized, double-blind, placebo-controlled trial. *Arch Intern Med.* 1996;156:61–67.

83. Naismith DJ, Braschi A. The effect of low-dose potassium supplementation on blood pressure in apparently healthy volunteers. *Br J Nutr.* 2003;90:53–60.

84. Obel AO. Placebo-controlled trial of potassium supplements in black patients with mild essential hypertension. *J Cardiovasc Pharmacol.* 1989;14:294–296.

85. Xin X, He J, Frontini MG, et al. Effects of alcohol reduction on blood pressure: a meta-analysis of randomized controlled trials. *Hypertension.* 2001;38:1112–1117.

86. Martinez-Gonzalez MA, Bes-Rastrollo M, Serra-Majem L, et al. Mediterranean food pattern and the primary prevention of chronic disease: recent developments. *Nutr Rev.* 2009;67(suppl 1):S111–S116.

87. Salas-Salvado J, Bullo M, Babio N, et al.; for the PREDIMED Study. Reduction in the incidence of type 2-diabetes with the Mediterranean diet: results of the PREDIMED-Reus nutrition intervention randomized trial. *Diabetes Care.* 2011;34:14–19.

88. Karanja NM, Obarzanek E, Lin PH, et al. Descriptive characteristics of the dietary patterns used in the Dietary Approaches to Stop Hypertension Trial: DASH Collaborative Research Group. *J Am Diet Assoc.* 1999;99:S19–S27.

89. Maruthur NM, Wang NY, Appel LJ. Lifestyle interventions reduce coronary heart disease risk: results from the PREMIER Trial. *Circulation.* 2009;119:2026–2031.

90. Sacks FM, Rosner B, Kass EH. Blood pressure in vegetarians. *Am J Epidemiol.* 1974;100:390–398.

91. Armstrong B, Von Merwyk AJ, Coates H. Blood pressure in Seventh-day Adventist vegetarians. *Am J Epidemiol.* 1977;105:444–449.

92. Krauss RM, Eckel RH, Howard B, et al. AHA Dietary Guidelines: revision 2000: a statement for healthcare professionals from the Nutrition Committee of the American Heart Association. *Circulation.* 2000;102:2284–2299.

PATIENT AND FAMILY INFORMATION FOR:

Diet, Nutrition, Obesity, and Weight Loss

A patient admitted to the CCU with an AMI or ACS has by definition atherosclerotic CVD and requires help in slowing down further progression of disease. Dietary changes will be necessary to prevent further cardiac events.

Traditional risk factors for heart disease need to be checked. These include blood lipids, blood pressure, smoking, and sedentariness. Changes to healthier lifestyle practices need to be initiated right away.

This chapter does not deal with the cessation of smoking or with physical activity. It only addresses nutrition. It will focus first on lipids and lipoproteins, then on hypertension, followed by MetS, diabetes and obesity, and finally dietary patterns that may be used to reach healthy goals.

LIPIDS AND LIPOPROTEINS

LDL CHOLESTEROL

This fraction of blood cholesterol is the primary target of therapy for prevention of progression of CHD. As the level of LDL-C increases, so does the risk of CHD. The level of LDL-C is optimal at <100 mg per dl. Lowering LDL reduces progressive disease and mortality from CHD.

HDL CHOLESTEROL

This fraction of circulating cholesterol is considered the second most important one. It is called the "good" cholesterol. HDL-C is important in getting rid of cholesterol from the body. In this way it protects against the development and progression of CHD. A low HDL-C level is a strong independent predictor of CHD. A plasma level of <40 mg per dl for men and <50 mg per dl for women is considered a risk for heart disease.

SERUM TRIGLYCERIDES

Elevated serum triglycerides are also an independent risk factor for CHD. Levels are defined as normal if they are <150 mg per dl.

HIGH BLOOD PRESSURE

Blood pressure is a strong risk factor for CHD. An abnormal blood pressure has been defined as 140/90 mm Hg, and levels below 120/80 mm Hg are recommended because this lowers the risk of CHD morbidity. The risk increases continuously beginning at 115/75 mm Hg. A number of studies have confirmed that weight loss lowers blood pressure in overweight individuals.

METABOLIC SYNDROME

Metabolic Syndrome (MetS) consists of a cluster of risk factors that are predictive of the progression to type 2 diabetes and CHD. It has five components and is considered to be present if three of five components are present in an individual. MetS, as defined in the United States, is shown in Table 35.1. This cluster increases the risk for CHD at any given level of LDL-C. Patients with the MetS should pay particular attention to improving their risk factors to prevent progression of heart disease.

DIABETES

Disease of large arteries (atherosclerosis) is the leading cause of death in diabetic persons. Many patients who present with an AMI have either impaired glucose tolerance, impaired fasting glucose, or type 2 diabetes. Diabetic persons have heart disease death rates and risks for stroke two- to fourfolds higher than adults without diabetes. It is critical to try to improve all risk factors for AMI in these patients.

The improvement in glucose control does not in itself seem to have a great deal of effect in improving morbidity and mortality from CAD. It is likely that the causes of accelerated CHD in diabetic patients are the abnormal lipids that are present: high LDL-C, low HDL-C, and high triglycerides. In type 2 diabetes, weight loss not only improves glucose levels but also ameliorates coexisting disorders such as dyslipidemia and hypertension.

OBESITY

Approximately 65% of U.S. adults are overweight or obese. Overweight and obesity are associated with an increased risk for CHD. This is probably related to the abnormal blood lipids in obesity. As in type 2 diabetes, this consists primarily of an elevation in triglycerides and a decrease in HDL-C. Levels of total cholesterol and LDL-C may be elevated but are often normal.

Because many obese persons also manifest hypertension and dyslipidemia, it has sometimes been difficult to assign causality to obesity independent of these other conditions.

In both obesity and diabetes, there is an increased chronic vascular inflammation and enhanced coagulation. These lead to increased insulin resistance and the progression of MetS, diabetes, and CHD. This inflammatory state decreases with weight loss.

NUTRITIONAL BEHAVIORAL LIFESTYLE CHANGE

For the past three decades, behavior modification has been used to treat obesity. The primary goal is to change an individual's eating and physical activity habits. Changes are gradual. Following achievement of a weight that is maintainable without excessive exercise or overly restrictive eating, relapse prevention training is used to teach the individual how to cope with emotional and social situations associated with relapse.

The focus should be initially on one to two nutrition behavior changes that are easy to implement and are supported with educational materials. The physician should initiate the nutrition intervention through nutrition messages to increase credibility and seriousness. The nutrition messages should be reinforced and followed up by office practice members over time. The nutrition messages should focus on the key nutrient that is most problematic and where intervention a will effect the most measurable change over time (it is usually fat, but may be sugar or other carbohydrates). The nutrition behavior messages and changes should be framed positively (e.g., substitution rather than restriction). The focus should be on the total diet rather than on individual foods. The nutrition message should have a companion message to increase physical activity.

Unrealistic patient expectations are common: that nutrition change only needs to be temporary, small changes will give major weight loss, and weight loss will solve most of life's many other problems. Patients underestimate the amount of planning needed for change and many find the change inconvenient. Many are bored by the substituted food items. Many have misconceptions about their risk often bolstered by cultural beliefs. Many lack family or social support.

Reasonable goals should be developed by the doctor and the patient. These should be written down for the patient as a prescription. Help will be required in problem solving as a patient encounters barriers to success. Clear and explicit educational materials about nutrition are also extremely important.

LDL LOWERING

To lower the LDL, the AHA has proposed dietary goals. These AHA diet and lifestyle goals for cardiovascular risk reduction are shown in Table 35.2.

The first recommendation is to "consume a healthy diet." This suggests that rather than look at one or two specific components, the whole diet be appraised so that not only macronutrients (carbohydrates, fats, and proteins) but also appropriate amounts of micronutrients (vitamins and minerals) be taken.

The NCEP guidelines for someone with already existing CHD suggest following the TLC diet. This is shown in Table 35.3.

It is recommended that the intake of saturated fats be <7% of total energy, trans fat be <1%, and total cholesterol be <200 mg per day. This can be done best by eating less meat, choosing lean meat over more fatty meat, using fat-free or 1% fat milk, taking low-fat dairy products, and avoiding partially hydrogenated fats.

The major sources of saturated fatty acids are animal fats (meat and dairy), and the primary sources of trans fatty acids are partially hydrogenated fats used to prepare commercially fried and baked foods.

Dietary cholesterol comes from foods of animal origin such as eggs, dairy products, meat, and these should be decreased. In reducing saturated fat and cholesterol, the foods that contain these are replaced with mono (MUFA) or polyunsaturated (PUFA) fat containing foods as well as choosing lower fat versions of foods. It has generally been suggested that PUFA be about 7% of calories whereas MUFA can vary from 7% to 20%. Overall, a range of 20% to 30% fat is an appropriate level of intake. Meats can be replaced with legumes, vegetables, and fish.

Fish (particularly oily fish) is rich in very-long-chain Ω-3 PUFAs. Eating at least two portions of fish per week is recommended. In cooking the fish, care should be taken not to add saturated or trans fats. Despite mercury contamination, two servings of fish per week are acceptable and safe. Fish oil supplements are a possible route to obtain enough n-3 PUFA but to date have not been shown to improve cardiovascular prognosis.

TOTAL CALORIES (WEIGHT LOSS)

A number of randomized clinical trials have been done on the effect of weight loss on lipid levels. With sustained weight loss, there is generally an improvement in blood lipids. Weight loss also decreases inflammation, which is likely to reduce cardiovascular events.

Obese persons consume a very large amount of calories and these must be reduced. A calorie-deficit diet can lead to significant weight loss and to improvement in an obese person with CHD. The typical American diet consists of about 15% protein, 35% fat, and 50% carbohydrates. Americans eat approximately 30% to 35% of calories as fat and 18% as sugar. Fat should be decreased and total calories reduced. Sugar should be discouraged. High-fiber foods such as fruits and vegetables and whole grains should be encouraged. One should aim at a deficit of about 1,000 kcal per day; this would translate to about 1 kg of weight loss per week.

Many persons can benefit from a low-calorie formula diet for a period, usually 12 to 16 weeks. Initially, this can be for all meals, and eventually it can be used for one or two meals a day. This is a very good way to reduce calorie intake.

The aim of weight loss is to lose fat without losing too much lean body mass. The loss of some lean body mass is inevitable, but it should be kept as low as possible. This is done by eating enough high quality-protein (e.g., egg whites, low-fat dairy products, lean meat, fish, and poultry). The intake of protein should be at a level of 1.0 to 1.5 g per kg of ideal body weight. A vegetarian diet can be used but protein complementation is required to ensure appropriate essential amino acid intake. Total fat should not exceed 30% of calories, with saturated fat not more than 7%. This is also true of PUFA, whereas MUFA can be as high as 15% to 20%. The daily carbohydrate intake should include 20 to 30 g of fiber from fruits, vegetables, legumes, and grains. Fiber seems to help satiety at lower levels of caloric intake. It is also important that adequate amounts of vitamins and minerals are taken daily. A supplement can be helpful in this regard.

The effort to achieve a caloric deficit of between 500 and 1,500 cal per day requires a careful dietary history. This can lead to a loss of between 1 and 2 lb per week. A low-calorie diet includes 800 to 1,500 cal per day. A diet of 1,200 to 1,500 cal per day for men and one of 1,000 to 1,200 cal per day for women is usually about right, but it needs to be individualized in relation to original intake and physical activity. These kinds of diets can lead to a safe 10% weight loss in 6 months, with 75% being fat and 25% lean body mass. Very-low-calorie diets of 300 to 800 cal per day have been used in the past but are not recommended. They require careful medical supervision because of potential adverse effects. They also do not produce greater weight loss long term. Moreover, there tends to be a rapid regain once the very-low-calorie diet is abandoned.

In general, with such caloric deficits, weight loss continues for 4 to 6 months and then plateaus off. This plateau is due to a new equilibrium in which energy intake is once again equivalent to energy expenditure. Maintenance of the weight loss requires continuing the same lower-energy intake and a physical activity at least as great as a patient has been doing for weight loss. Therefore, there can be no liberalization of food intake or reduction of physical activity, or else weight regain will occur.

All low-calorie diets will produce weight loss in the short term and current evidence suggests that the macronutrient composition does not play a significant role. There is no optimal macronutrient composition (e.g., protein, carbohydrate, fat content) of weight loss diets. In a recent prospective randomized clinical trial in which several popular weight loss plans (Atkins, Ornish, Weight Watchers, Zone) were compared, and all of the diets produced a similar amount of weight loss at the end of 1 year. This finding is in agreement with results from a previous study in which a low-carbohydrate, high-protein diet was compared with a low-calorie, low-fat diet. Although a low-carbohydrate, high-protein diet produced more loss of weight after 6 months, weight loss at the end of 1 year was the same regardless of dietary intervention.

To be successful, dietary guidance should be individualized, allowing for patient food preferences and individual approaches to reducing caloric intake. Techniques for decreasing caloric intake may include reducing portion sizes, selecting low-calorie foods, and using cooking methods that lower fat intake.

HIGH BLOOD PRESSURE

Dietary modifications that can improve elevated blood pressure include a reduced salt intake, reduced calorie intake leading to weight loss, increased potassium intake, and moderation of alcohol consumption.

Many clinical trials have documented that weight loss lowers blood pressure.

Blood pressure goes up as intake of dietary salt (sodium chloride) increases. Some salt intake is required for health, but the salt intake is very high in the United States. There have been some excellent dose–response trials of salt intake showing that lowering sodium lowers blood pressure. The AHA has suggested an upper limit of 2.3 g per day as doable. To reduce salt intake, it is important to choose foods low in salt as well as limiting the amount of salt added to food in cooking or at the table. Because approximately 75% of consumed salt comes from processed foods, it is important to reduce their intake.

It is known from observational studies that a high potassium intake is associated with a reduced blood pressure. There is an inverse relationship between potassium intake and blood pressure in both nonhypertensive and hypertensive persons. The effect of a higher potassium intake is greater in Black persons. A high potassium intake can be achieved through diet rather than pills. Fruits and vegetables that are high in potassium should be eaten. These also are rich in other micronutrients. A level of 4.7 g per day has been recommended.

Excessive alcohol intake increases blood pressure, whereas reduction of alcohol intake reduces it. Alcohol consumption should be limited to less than two alcoholic drinks per day in most men and less than one in women and lighter weight men. One drink is defined as 12 oz of regular beer, 5 oz of wine (12% alcohol) and 1.5 oz of 80 proof distilled spirits.

DIETARY PATTERNS

Individual patients may seek a dietary pattern that is particularly acceptable to them and has enough of the required characteristics so that it is effective in lowering weight, blood pressure, and improving lipids and glucose levels. Both the TLC and the AHA diets are excellent diets to recommend. There are a few other patterns that are reasonable for long-term use.

MEDITERRANEAN DIET

A Mediterranean diet has been shown to significantly decrease cardiovascular and total mortality. The PREDIMED trial is testing >9,000 high-risk persons in Spain. In an interim analysis, those in either of the two Mediterranean diet intervention arms (one olive oil, one nuts) had lower mean glucose, lower systolic blood pressure, and a lower total cholesterol-to-HDL ratio than those randomized to the low-fat control. This is a pleasant diet that appears to be cardioprotective.

DASH DIET

The DASH diet has been tested in three trials that have documented its effectiveness in lowering blood pressure. The DASH diet calls for an increased intake of fruits, vegetables, and low-fat dairy products. It includes whole grains, poultry, fish, and nuts. It reduces intake of fats, red meat, sweets, and sugar-containing vegetables. The diet is rich in potassium, magnesium, calcium, and fiber and is reduced in total fat, saturated fat, and cholesterol. There is a slight increase in protein. It is very similar to a Mediterranean diet.

PREMIER DIET

The Premier diet is like the DASH diet but has been adapted to be hypocaloric so that it will be an effective diet for not only blood pressure lowering also for weight loss.

VEGETARIAN DIET

Persons eating a vegetarian diet have a lower blood pressure than nonvegetarians. Some of the effect is clearly from the diet (no meat, high fiber) but much is related to the healthful lifestyle of many of its adherents (low weight, high exercise).

FINAL RECOMMENDATIONS

It is very important that follow-up between patient and physician occurs. If this issue is ignored, there is little likelihood of success. An important component for success is to weigh and measure waist circumference at each visit, to address nutritional and physical activity issues, and to counsel a patient who is confronting barriers to pursuing a healthier lifestyle.

36

Barry A. Franklin

Exercise and Physical Activity

Exercise training appears to play an important role in the medical management and rehabilitation of patients with coronary heart disease (CHD). The salutary effects of chronic exercise training, increased lifestyle physical activity, or both are well documented. Numerous studies also suggest that cardiorespiratory fitness, expressed as metabolic equivalents (METs; 1 MET = 3.5 mL O_2/kg/minute), is one of the strongest prognostic markers in persons with and without CHD.[1] Accordingly, sedentary patients should be counseled to engage in regular walking at moderate exercise intensities so they can move out of the least fit, least active, "high-risk" cohort (bottom 20%).[2]

There are, however, limitations to the benefits that exercise training offers relative to the prevention of initial and recurrent cardiovascular events. Contrary to the speculation of a few overzealous enthusiasts, regular exercise training, regardless of the intensity, duration, or frequency, does not confer "immunity" to CHD.[3] Furthermore, exertion-related cardiovascular events have been reported in the medical literature[4] and the lay press,[5] suggesting that strenuous physical activity may actually trigger cardiac arrest or acute myocardial infarction (AMI) in selected individuals.

This chapter reviews the physiologic basis and rationale for exercise therapy in patients with CHD, with specific reference to the liberalization of physical activity in the treatment of patients with AMI, cardiorespiratory adaptations to exercise training, fitness and mortality, cardioprotective effects of exercise, exercise prescription, exercise-related cardiovascular events, and strategies to increase patient compliance to exercise regimens.

EARLY CONVALESCENCE AFTER ACUTE MYOCARDIAL INFARCTION

Although in his classic cardiology text, Friedberg[6] still recommended 2 to 3 weeks in bed and an additional period of 3 to 4 weeks in hospital for patients with AMI, prolonged bed rest is no longer recommended in the care of patients with acute cardiovascular events because of an abbreviated hospital stay. Moreover, extended bed rest has been shown to result in physiologic deconditioning and significant decreases in peak or maximal oxygen consumption (VO$_2$ max), stroke volume, and cardiac output.[7] Other adverse sequelae include increased muscle fatigue associated with reduced muscle blood flow, red cell volume, capillary growth, and oxidative enzymes; loss of muscle mass and bone density; constipation; urinary retention; thrombophlebitis; pulmonary embolism; hypostatic pneumonia; orthostatic intolerance; and depression.[8]

A seminal report by Levine and Lown,[9] involving 81 patients with AMI who were subjected to "armchair treatment," further prompted liberalization of activity restriction soon after an acute coronary event. Most patients were out of bed and sitting in a chair for up to 2 hours on their first day of hospitalization. Their time in the chair was progressively increased during hospital convalescence and most were encouraged to feed themselves and use the bedside commode or bathroom. Nearly all were discharged after 4 weeks. There were no complications attributed to the intervention, and the mortality rate of patients treated with chair rest, was lower than that of a control group who had received conventional therapy (e.g., bed rest). These findings have now been supported by numerous controlled clinical trials, providing convincing evidence that early mobilization and hospital discharge of patients with uncomplicated myocardial infarction is a safe practice that is associated with numerous physiologic, psychological, and economic benefits. Today, many uncomplicated postmyocardial infarction patients are being discharged from the hospital within 3 to 4 days.

Numerous studies now suggest that the lack of orthostatic stress is more important than physical inactivity in producing many of the deleterious effects of bed rest; consequently, interventions to simulate gravitational stress are widely used in preventing or attenuating these consequences. Convertino et al.[10] studied changes in VO$_2$ max before and after 14 days of bed rest using daily treatments with a reverse gradient garment that simulated the effects of standing. Aerobic capacity decreased only 6% in subjects who received venous pooling treatments, compared with a 15% decrease in nontreated (control) subjects (Table 36.1). These data have important practical implications for inpatient cardiac rehabilitation and early home convalescence.[11] The loss of exposure to gravitational stress during the hospital stay contributes to the decrease in VO$_2$ max after AMI, independent of related clinical variables (e.g., ejection fraction). Thus, it appears that the deterioration in VO$_2$ max with bed rest may be lessened simply by regular exposure to orthostatic stress, such as intermittent sitting or standing. Structured, formalized in-hospital exercise programs after AMI appear to offer little additional physiologic or behavioral benefits over routine medical care.[12]

TABLE 36.1	Mean Changes in Maximal Oxygen Uptake (VO$_2$ max) Before and After Bed Rest		
Remedial Treatment Mode	*Bed Rest (Days)*	*VO$_2$ max (L/min)*	
		%Δ	*Before*	*After*
None	14	−15	3.9	3.3
Venous pooling	14	−6	3.3	3.1

Adapted from COnvertino VA, Sandler H, Webb P, et al. Induced venous pooling and cardiorespiratory responses to exercise after bed rest. *J Appl Physiol.* 1982;52:1343–1348.

CARDIORESPIRATORY ADAPTATIONS TO EXERCISE TRAINING

Regular endurance exercise training increases physical work (functional) capacity and provides relief of angina pectoris in many patients with CHD. These are particularly beneficial outcomes because many cardiac patients have a reduced functional or aerobic capacity (50% to 70% age, sex predicted), whereas others are limited by anginal chest pain at relatively low levels of effort. The postconditioning improvement in aerobic capacity appears to be mediated by increased central and/or peripheral oxygen transport and utilization, whereas relief of angina pectoris may result from a decreased rate–pressure product at rest and during any given level of submaximal exercise, increased oxygen delivery, or both.

Studies of physical conditioning in patients with CHD have generally demonstrated a 10% to 40% increase in preconditioning values of VO_2 max; the wide variation in improvement is attributed to numerous factors affecting exercise trainability, including the patient's age, clinical status, initial fitness, time from the acute cardiac event, the exercise prescription, and compliance to the conditioning program. Because a given submaximal task requires a relatively constant rate of oxygen uptake, expressed as METs, the cardiac patient finds that after an exercise training program, he/she is working at a lower percentage of his/her aerobic capacity, with a greater functional reserve (Figure 36.1).[13]

CARDIORESPIRATORY FITNESS AS A PREDICTOR OF MORTALITY

To examine the relationship between aerobic fitness and mortality in patients with documented cardiovascular disease (CVD), Vanhees et al.[14] studied 527 men who were referred to an outpatient cardiac rehabilitation program. Peak oxygen uptake on a cycle ergometer was directly measured 12.9 ± 2.7 weeks after AMI (n = 312) or coronary artery bypass surgery

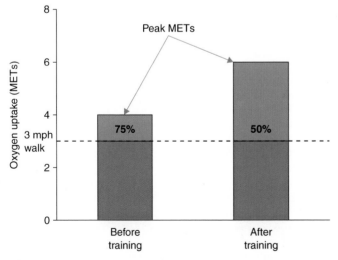

Figure 36.1. The effect of physical conditioning on peak oxygen uptake (METs) and relative oxygen cost (activity METs/peak METs) of walking at 3 miles per hour (mph) on a level grade is shown. Following a physical conditioning program, peak oxygen uptake increased from 4 to 6 METs, decreasing the relative oxygen cost of a 3 mph walk from 75% to 50%.

(n = 215). During the average follow-up duration of 6.1 years, 33 and 20 patients died of cardiovascular and noncardiovascular causes, respectively. Those with the highest cardiovascular and all-cause mortality averaged ≤4.4 METs. In contrast, there were no deaths among patients who averaged ≥9.2 METs.

In a cohort of men (n = 6,213) reported by Myers et al.,[15] 3,679 with an abnormal exercise-test result and/or known CVD were referred for treadmill exercise testing. The average follow-up was 6.2 ± 3.7 years. Those with an exercise capacity of ≤4.9 METs had the highest relative risk of death, whereas those with a fitness level ≥10.7 METs had the lowest relative risk of death (4.1 and 1.0, respectively). For the total group, every 1-MET increase in exercise capacity conferred a 12% improvement in survival. Similarly, long-term findings from the National Exercise and Heart Disease Project among postmyocardial infarction patients demonstrated that every 1-MET increase in exercise capacity after a training period was associated with a reduction in mortality from any cause that ranged from 8% to 14% over the course of 19 years follow-up.[16]

Kavanagh et al.[17,18] evaluated the predictive value of cardiopulmonary exercise testing in 12,169 men (55.0 ± 9.6 years) and 2,380 women (59.7 ± 9.5 years) with known CHD who were referred for exercise-based cardiac rehabilitation. The men and women were followed for an average of 7.9 and 6.1 years, respectively. Directly measured peak oxygen uptake on a cycle ergometer at program entry proved to be a powerful predictor of cardiovascular and all-cause mortality. The cutoff point, above which there was a marked benefit in prognosis, was 13 mL/kg/minute (3.7 METs) in women and 15 mL/kg/minute (4.3 METs) in men. For each 1 mL/kg/minute increase in exercise capacity, there was a 10% reduction of cardiac mortality in women versus 9% in men.

More recently, Dutcher et al.,[19] using the well-described primary angioplasty in AMI (PAMI-2) database, reported that exercise capacity more accurately predicts 2- and 5-year mortality than does left ventricular ejection fraction in patients with ST-elevation myocardial infarction who were emergently treated with percutaneous coronary intervention. Those who had an exercise capacity ≥4 METs had better long-term survival; in contrast, those with an exercise capacity <4 METs were at a substantially increased risk of mortality, which was worsened in the presence of left ventricular dysfunction (ejection fraction <40%). The investigators concluded that exercise capacity was a better predictor of mortality than was left ventricular ejection fraction in this escalating patient subset. Accordingly, these data have important implications for the medical management and triaging of postmyocardial infarction patients who may benefit the most from an exercise-based cardiac rehabilitation program.

CARDIOPROTECTIVE EFFECTS OF EXERCISE

Two meta-analyses[20,21] have now shown that regular exercise participation can decrease the overall risk of cardiovascular events by up to 50%, presumably from multiple mechanisms, including antiatherosclerotic, anti-ischemic, antiarrhythmic, antithrombotic, and psychological effects (Figure 36.2). Regular aerobic exercise can result in moderate losses in body weight, moderate-to-large losses in body fat, and small-to-moderate increases in lean body weight. Endurance exercise can promote decreases in blood pressure (particularly in hypertensives), total blood cholesterol, serum triglycerides, and low-density lipoprotein

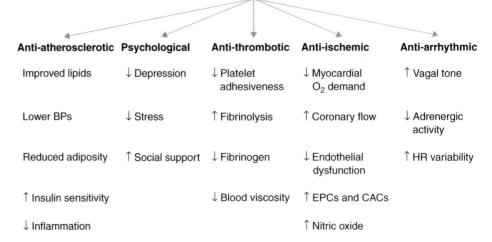

Potential cardioprotective effects of regular physical activity

Anti-atherosclerotic	Psychological	Anti-thrombotic	Anti-ischemic	Anti-arrhythmic
Improved lipids	↓ Depression	↓ Platelet adhesiveness	↓ Myocardial O₂ demand	↑ Vagal tone
Lower BPs	↓ Stress	↑ Fibrinolysis	↑ Coronary flow	↓ Adrenergic activity
Reduced adiposity	↑ Social support	↓ Fibrinogen	↓ Endothelial dysfunction	↑ HR variability
↑ Insulin sensitivity		↓ Blood viscosity	↑ EPCs and CACs	
↓ Inflammation			↑ Nitric oxide	

Figure 36.2. A structured endurance exercise program sufficient to maintain and enhance cardiorespiratory fitness may provide multiple mechanisms to reduce nonfatal and fatal cardiovascular events. BP, blood pressure; CACs, cultured angiogenic cells; EPCs, endothelial progenitor cells; HR, heart rate; ↑, increased; ↓, decreased; O₂, oxygen.

cholesterol, and increases in the "antiatherogenic" high-density lipoprotein cholesterol subfraction. Moreover, exercise has favorable effects on glucose and insulin homeostasis, inflammatory markers (e.g., C-reactive protein), coagulability, fibrinolysis, and coronary endothelial function.[22]

Because >40% of the risk reduction associated with exercise cannot be explained by changes in conventional risk factors, Green et al.[23] proposed a cardioprotective "vascular conditioning" effect, including enhanced nitric oxide vasodilator function, improved vascular reactivity, altered vascular structure, or combinations thereof. Decreased vulnerability to arrhythmias and increased resistance to ventricular fibrillation have also been postulated to reflect exercise-related adaptations in autonomic control. As a consequence of endurance training, sympathetic drive at rest is reduced and vagal tone is increased. Moreover, ischemic preconditioning before coronary occlusion, at least in animal models, can reduce subsequent infarct size and/or the potential for malignant ventricular arrhythmias.[24,25]

EXERCISE PRESCRIPTION

COMPONENTS

Structured exercise training sessions should include a preliminary aerobic warm-up (approximately 10 minutes), a continuous or accumulated conditioning phase (≥30 minutes or multiple 10 to 15 minutes exercise bouts), and a cool-down (5 to 10 minutes) followed by stretching activities. The warm-up facilitates the transition from rest to the conditioning phase, reducing the potential for ventricular ectopy and ischemic electrocardiographic (ECG) responses, which can occur with sudden strenuous exertion.[26] A walking cool-down enhances venous return during recovery, decreasing the possibility of hypotension and related sequelae, and ameliorates the potential, deleterious effects of the postexercise rise in plasma catecholamines.[27]

MODALITIES/INTENSITIES

The most effective exercises for the conditioning phase include walking, jogging, stationary or outdoor cycling, swimming, rowing, stair climbing, and combined arm–leg ergometry. To improve cardiorespiratory fitness in the coronary patient,

the threshold intensity for training should approximate 45% of the oxygen uptake reserve, which corresponds approximately to 69% of the highest heart rate achieved during peak or symptom-limited exercise testing.[28] For ≥90% of the men and women participating in early outpatient cardiac rehabilitation programs, this intensity can be achieved by walking on a level surface at speeds of 2.9 to 3.3 miles per hour.[29] Over time, the exercise intensity should be increased to 50% and up to 75% of the oxygen uptake reserve (or maximal heart rate reserve) to further increase aerobic fitness.

THE MET CONCEPT

The metabolic costs of many household, recreational/training (Table 36.2), and occupational activities have been defined in terms of oxygen uptake. Consequently, activity prescription can also be made in terms of METs.[30] This involves recommendation of activities that are sufficiently below the maximal MET level (estimated or directly measured) achieved during progressive exercise testing to volitional fatigue. Average healthy young to middle-aged adults generally have an exercise capacity of 8 to 12 METs. In other words, at maximal exercise, they can consume 8 to 12 times the amount of oxygen used at rest (1 MET). Heart failure patients and those who are elderly or morbidly obese could be as low as 2 to 4 METs. On the other hand, elite endurance athletes are often in the range of 20 to 25 METs.

For example, consider the woman who achieves 1 minute of stage III of the Bruce treadmill protocol (3.4 mph, 14%), which corresponds to approximately 8 METs. At this workload, the patient experienced moderately severe shortness of breath and rated the effort as "very hard." Her recommended training intensities at average expenditure and peak expenditure during the training session are approximately 4.5 and 6.2 METs, respectively. Table 36.2 provides a wide choice of activities for these aerobic requirements: walking (3.5 to 4.0 mph), doubles tennis, badminton, and so on.[30] However, activities requiring an expenditure ≥7 to 8 METs (e.g., jogging [5 mph], basketball, competitive handball) would appear contraindicated, as they would presumably require near-maximal, maximal, or supramaximal efforts. The concept is attractive, easy to understand, and is frequently adopted as a training and activity prescription guide.

Unfortunately, there are several inherent limitations in using estimated METs in activity prescription. One limitation is

TABLE 36.2	Approximate Metabolic Cost of Various Recreational and Training Activities
Activity	*Aerobic Requirement (METs)*
Walking (1 mph)	1.5–2.0
Walking (2 mph), bicycling (5 mph), billiards, bowling, golf (power cart)	2.0–3.0
Walking (3 mph), bicycling (6 mph), volleyball, golf (pulling bag cart), archery, badminton (social doubles)	3.0–4.0
Walking (3.5 mph), bicycling (8 mph), table tennis, golf (carrying clubs), badminton (singles), tennis (doubles), many calisthenics	4.0–5.0
Walking (4 mph), bicycling (10 mph), ice skating, roller skating	5.0–6.0
Walking (5 mph), bicycling (11 mph), badminton (competitive), tennis (singles), square dancing, light downhill skiing, water skiing	6.0–7.0
Jogging (5 mph), bicycling (12 mph), vigorous downhill skiing, basketball, ice hockey, touch football, paddleball	7.0–8.0
Running (5.5 mph), bicycling (13 mph), squash (social), handball (social), fencing, basketball (vigorous)	8.0–9.0
Running (6.0 mph), handball (competitive), squash (competitive)	10.0 plus

MET, metabolic equivalents. Data derived from Fox SM, Naughton JP, Gorman PA. Physical activity and cardiovascular health. III. The exercise prescription; frequency and type of activity. *Mod Concepts Cardiovasc Dis.* 1972;41:21–24.

that the MET values of selected physical activities represent average energy expenditure levels, and these may vary considerably among individuals. The manner in which individuals participate in activity varies widely in terms of energy expenditure, ranging from the lackadaisical to the frenetic. Aerobic demands are also highly dependent on speed and efficiency (skill). Moreover, it cannot be assumed that occupational and recreational activities demanding oxygen consumption equal to that registered during leg exercise testing produce similar cardiac demands. Additional factors at work include the stresses of emotions, excitement, cognition, and environment (temperature and humidity) as well as the activation of muscle groups not used during the exercise tests. Finally, the oxygen costs listed for many common occupational and domestic activities were derived from continuous steady-state work (≥3 minutes), whereas activities of daily life are predominantly intermittent. For example, a patient with a 5-MET capacity would be counseled to refrain from digging in the garden (a requirement of 5 to 7 METs), as it presumably represents maximal or supramaximal effort. However, if the activity is performed intermittently (i.e., 2 minutes work, 1 minute rest), the task can easily be accomplished at oxygen consumption levels well below those estimated for the task. Thus, using the MET method for prescribing activity may considerably underestimate the patient's capacity for physical work.

In summary, the MET concept has limited applicability in the recommendation of activities for coronary patients. Heart rate response and rating of perceived exertion (Table 36.3)[31] immediately after physical effort usually provide a better assessment of cardiac and somatic demands than metabolic equivalent tables.

UPPER-BODY TRAINING

The lack of transfer of training benefits from the legs to the arms, and vice versa, seems to discredit the practice of prescribing exercise for the lower extremities alone (e.g., walking, jogging, cycle ergometry).[32] Consequently, patients with and without CHD who rely on their upper extremities for occupational or leisure-time activities should be advised to train the legs as well as the arms, with the goal of developing muscle-specific adaptations to both types of effort.[33,34] Although upper-extremity exercise for cardiac patients was traditionally proscribed, numerous studies have now demonstrated the safety and effectiveness of arm exercise training in patients with CHD.[35] Guidelines for dynamic arm exercise training are shown in Table 36.4.

RESISTANCE TRAINING

Many cardiac patients lack the physical strength and/or self-confidence to perform common activities of daily living. Mild-to-moderate resistance training can provide an effective

TABLE 36.3	Rating of Perceived Exertion (RPE)
6	
7	Very, very light
8	
9	Very light
10	
11	Fairly light
12	
13	Somewhat hard
14	
15	Hard
16	
17	Very hard
18	
19	Very, very hard
20	

From Borg GAV. Psychophysical bases of perceived exertion. *Med Sci Sports Exerc.* 1982;14:377–381, with permission.

TABLE 36.4	Guidelines for Dynamic Arm Exercise Training
Variable	Comment
Target heart rate	-10–15 beats/min lower than for leg training
Work rate	-50% ± 10% of the power output (kgm/min) used for leg training
Equipment	Arm ergometer, combined arm–leg ergometer, rowing machine, wall pulleys, simulated cross-country skiing devices

~=approximately

method for improving muscular strength and endurance, preventing and managing a variety of chronic medical conditions, modifying coronary risk factors, and enhancing psychosocial well-being.[36,37] Weight training has also been shown to attenuate the rate–pressure product when any given load is lifted.[38] Thus, resistance training can decrease myocardial demands during daily activities such as carrying groceries or lifting moderate-to-heavy objects. Moreover, recent studies have shown that muscular strength is inversely associated with all-cause mortality and the presence of metabolic syndrome, independent of cardiorespiratory fitness levels.[39,40]

Although the traditional weight-training prescription has involved performing each exercise three times (e.g., three sets of 10 to 15 repetitions per set), it appears that one set provides similar improvements in muscular strength and endurance.[41] Consequently, single-set programs performed at least two times a week are recommended rather than multiset programs, especially among novice exercisers, because they are highly effective, less time-consuming, and less likely to cause musculoskeletal injury or soreness. Such regimens should include 8 to 10 different exercises at a load that permits 8 to 15 repetitions per set. Heavy resistance exercise, which may increase the hemodynamic response to and risk of strength training, offers little additional benefit in strength gains, at least in cardiac patients.[37]

LIFESTYLE PHYSICAL ACTIVITY

Despite contemporary exercise guidelines[42] and the much-heralded Surgeon General's report,[43] structured exercise programs have been only marginally effective for getting people to be more physically active. Randomized clinical trials have now shown that a lifestyle approach to physical activity among previously sedentary people has similar effects on cardiorespiratory fitness, body composition, and coronary risk factors as a structured exercise program.[44,45] These findings have important implications for public health, suggesting an alternative approach to sedentary people who are not ready to comply with a formal exercise program. Accordingly, physicians and allied health professionals should counsel patients to integrate multiple short bouts of physical activity into their daily lives.[46] Pedometers can be helpful in this regard, as can programs that use them (e.g., America on the Move) to enhance awareness of physical activity by progressively increasing daily step totals. According to one systematic review, pedometer users significantly increased their physical activity by an average of 2,491 steps per day more than their control counterparts.[47] The activity pyramid (Figure 36.3) presents a tiered set of weekly goals, building on a base that emphasizes the importance of accumulating 30 minutes or more of moderate-intensity activity on at least 5 days per week.[48]

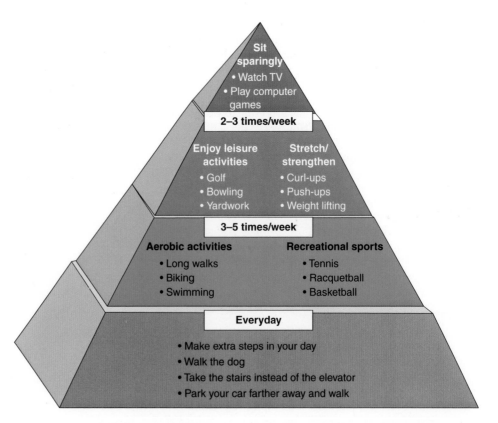

Figure 36.3. The activity pyramid has been suggested as a model to facilitate public and patient education for adoption of a progressively more active lifestyle. (Reprinted with permission from 1996 Park Nicollet Healthsource Institute for Research and Education.)

EXERCISE-RELATED CARDIOVASCULAR EVENTS

Pathophysiologic evidence suggests that vigorous physical exertion may precipitate AMI or cardiac arrest in selected persons with known or occult CVD. Several hypotheses have been suggested as triggering mechanisms for plaque rupture and acute coronary thrombosis (Table 36.5).[49] By increasing myocardial oxygen consumption and simultaneously shortening diastole and coronary perfusion time, exercise may evoke a transient oxygen deficiency at the subendocardial level, which is exacerbated by abrupt cessation of activity. Ischemia can alter depolarization, repolarization, and conduction velocity, triggering threatening ventricular arrhythmias (Figure 36.4) that, in extreme cases, may be harbingers of ventricular tachycardia or fibrillation. In addition, symptomatic or silent myocardial ischemia, sodium–potassium imbalance, increased catecholamine excretion, and circulating free fatty acids may all be arrhythmogenic.[49]

To a large extent, the cause of exertion-related cardiovascular complications depends on the exerciser's age. Coronary atherosclerosis is the most frequent autopsy finding in individuals over the age of 40 who die suddenly. However, inherited structural cardiovascular abnormalities are the major cause of sudden cardiac death (SCD) during exercise in younger athletes.[50] One of the commonest congenital abnormalities leading to SCD in young athletes is hypertrophic cardiomyopathy, which affects approximately 1 in 500 and is found in about one-third to one-half of the fatalities among young athletes. Thus, it is the combination of vigorous physical exertion and a diseased or susceptible heart, rather than the exercise itself, that seems to be the major cause of SCD.

The incidence of cardiovascular events during very light-to-moderate intensity activities is similar to that expected by chance alone. However, strenuous physical exertion (Table 36.6), especially when it is sudden, unaccustomed, or involving high levels of anaerobic metabolism, appears to transiently increase the risk of AMI and SCD in susceptible individuals.[50] The aerobic and

TABLE 36.5	Physiologic and Clinical Mechanisms That May Be Responsible for Exertion-Related Plaque Rupture and Acute Myocardial Infarction

Induces plaque rupture via
  Increased heart rate, blood pressure, and shear forces
  Altered coronary artery dimensions
  Exercise-induced spasm in diseased artery segments

Renders a fissured plaque more thrombogenic by
  Deepening the fissure
  Increasing thrombogenicity

Induces thrombogenesis directly via
  Catecholamine-induced platelet aggregation

cardiac demands of these activities are influenced by a host of extraneous variables, including team members, opponent expertise, and superimposed environmental stressors (e.g., cold, heat, and humidity). Moreover, the excitement of competition may increase sympathetic activity and catecholamine levels and lower the threshold to ventricular fibrillation. Recreational and domestic activities that are associated with an increased incidence of cardiovascular events include competitive running events, deer hunting,[51] and snow removal.[52] Indeed, during the 2009 *Detroit Free Press* Marathon, three deaths occurred within five blocks and 15 minutes of each other![53]

Although the relative risk of AMI and SCD appears to increase transiently during strenuous physical exertion compared with the risk at other times, the absolute risk is small. Exercise-related cardiovascular events are more likely to occur among susceptible persons, that is, habitually sedentary individuals with known or occult CVD who were performing unaccustomed vigorous physical activity.[49] On the other hand, the net effect of regular physical activity and/or increased cardiorespiratory fitness is a

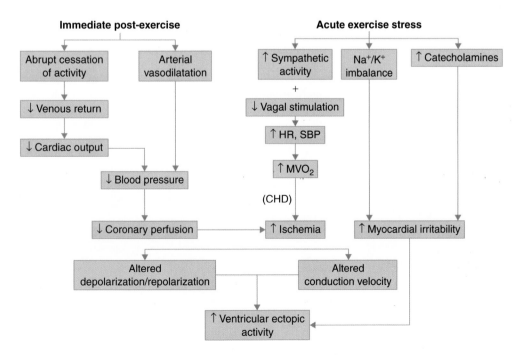

Figure 36.4. Physiologic alterations accompanying acute exercise and recovery and their possible sequelae. HR, indicates heart rate; SBP, systolic blood pressure; MVO$_2$, myocardial oxygen consumption; CHD, coronary heart disease.

| TABLE 36.6 | Common Activities Classified as "Strenuous Physical Exertion" (≥6 METs) |

Self-Care or Home	Occupational	Recreational	Exercise Training
Digging in garden	Carpentry[a]	Tennis (singles)	Race walking (≥4.5 mph)
Lawn mowing	Shoveling dirt[a]	Water skiing[a]	Swimming (breast stroke)
Climbing stairs	Pneumatic tools[a]	Basketball	Jogging (≥5 mph)
Carrying objects (≥30 lb)[a]	Digging ditches[a]	Mountain climbing[a]	Rowing
Sawing wood[a]	Lumberjack[a]	Paddleball	Heavy calisthenics[a]
Heavy shoveling[a]	Heavy laborer[a]	Handball	Rope jumping
Snow shoveling[a]		Competitive running events	
		Deer hunting[a]	

[a]May produce excessive myocardial demands because of arm work or isometric exercise.

lower overall risk of mortality from CVD.[50] Recommendations to potentially reduce the risk of cardiovascular events during exercise include the following: encourage sedentary individuals to engage in regular walking so as to move them out of the least fit, least active, "high-risk" cohort; counsel inactive individuals to avoid unaccustomed, vigorous physical activity (e.g., racquet sports, squash, snow shoveling); advocate appropriate warm-up and cool-down procedures; promote education of warning signs/symptoms (e.g., chest pain or pressure, light-headedness, heart palpitations/arrhythmias); emphasize strict adherence to prescribed training pulse rates; use continuous or instantaneous ECG monitoring in selected coronary patients[54]; minimize competition and modify recreational games to decrease the energy cost and heart rate response to play; and adapt the exercise to the environment.[50] Because symptomatic or silent myocardial ischemia may be highly arrhythmogenic, the target heart rate for endurance exercise should be set safely below (≥10 beats per minute) the ischemic ECG or anginal threshold.[55]

STRATEGIES TO ENHANCE EXERCISE COMPLIANCE

Although many patients can be encouraged to initiate an exercise program, motivating them to continue can be challenging. Unfortunately, negative variables often outweigh the positive variables contributing to sustained interest and enthusiasm, including

| TABLE 36.7 | Strategies to Enhance Exercise Compliance |

- Assess exercise habits and counsel patients to be physically active
- Evaluate the patient's "Readiness to Change," and target interventions accordingly
- Establish short-term, attainable goals
- Minimize injury with a moderate (initial) exercise prescription
- Advocate exercising with others (i.e., social support)
- Avoid overemphasis of regimented calisthenics
- Consider gender differences in activity programming
- Provide positive reinforcement through periodic testing
- Recruit spouse support of the exercise program
- Use progress charts to record exercise achievements
- Encourage patients to use certified, enthusiastic exercise leaders and to engage in activities that are enjoyable

inadequate supervision/coaching, time inconvenience, musculoskeletal problems, exercise boredom, cost issues, accessibility, lack of progress awareness, and work or family-related conflicts. Collectively, these deterrents often lead to a decline in adherence, and therefore program effectiveness diminishes. According to one study, the single most important factor determining coronary patients' participation in exercise was a strong recommendation from their cardiologist or primary care physician.[56] Several research-based counseling and motivational strategies may enhance patient interest and facilitate initiation of and compliance with a structured exercise program, increased lifestyle activity, or both (Table 36.7).[22]

CONCLUSIONS

There are multiple mechanisms by which moderate-to-vigorous physical activity and increased cardiorespiratory fitness may decrease morbidity and mortality rates associated with CVD and improve psychosocial well-being and quality of life. The challenge for physicians and other health care providers is to bring this accessible, cost-effective intervention to fruition by referring increasing numbers of patients, with and without CVD, to home, club, or medically based exercise programs so that many more individuals may realize the cardioprotective and general health benefits that regular physical activity can provide.

We must conclude as William C. Robert's, M.D., Editor-in-Chief, *American Journal of Cardiology*, summarized it in 1984: "Exercise training? An agent with lipid-lowering, anti-hypertensive, positive inotropic, negative chronotropic, vasodilating, diuretic, anorexigenic, weight-reducing, cathartic, hypoglycemic, tranquilizing, hypnotic and anti-depressive qualities."

Like all statements of wisdom, this observation is both elegant and unadorned, so clearly evident and acceptable today that we feel we should have known it all along.

REFERENCES

1. Franklin BA. Fitness: the ultimate marker for risk stratification and health outcomes? *Prev Cardiol.* 2007;10:42–45.
2. Franklin BA, McCullough PA. Cardiorespiratory fitness: an independent and additive marker of risk stratification and health outcomes. *Mayo Clinic Proc.* 2009;84:776–779.
3. Bassler TJ. Marathon running and immunity to heart disease. *Phys Sportsmed.* 1975;3:77–80.
4. Cantwell JD, Fletcher GF. Cardiac complications while jogging. *JAMA.* 1969;210:130–131.
5. Kidder K. Doctors urged Byron to give up jogging. *The Baltimore Sun.* October 16, 1978:1C–2C.
6. Friedberg CK. *Diseases of the Heart.* 3rd ed. Philadelphia, PA: WB Saunders Company; 1966.

7. Convertino VA, Bloomfield SA, Greenleaf JE. An overview of the issues: physiological effects of bed rest and restricted physical activity. *Med Sci Sports Exerc.* 1997;29:187–190.

8. Winslow EH. Cardiovascular consequences of bed rest. *Heart Lung.* 1985;14:236–246.

9. Levine SA, Lown B. Armchair treatment of acute coronary thrombosis. *JAMA.* 1952;148:1365–1369.

10. Convertino VA, Sandler H, Webb P, et al. Induced venous pooling and cardiorespiratory responses to exercise after bed rest. *J Appl Physiol.* 1982;52:1343–1348.

11. Convertino VA. Effect of orthostatic stress on exercise performance after bed rest: relation to inhospital rehabilitation. *J Card Rehabil.* 1983;3:660–663.

12. Sivarajan ES, Bruce RA, Almes MJ, et al. In-hospital exercise after myocardial infarction does not improve treadmill performance. *N Engl J Med.* 1981;305:357–362.

13. Franklin BA, Rubenfire M. Exercise training in coronary heart disease: mechanisms of improvement. *Pract Cardiol.* 1980;6:84–99.

14. Vanhees L, Fagard R, Thijs L, et al. Prognostic significance of peak exercise capacity in patients with coronary artery disease. *J Am Coll Cardiol.* 1994;23:358–363.

15. Myers J, Prakash M, Froelicher V, et al. Exercise capacity and mortality among men referred for exercise testing. *N Engl J Med.* 2002;346:793–801.

16. Dorn J, Naughton J, Imanmura D, et al. Results of a multicenter randomized clinical trial of exercise and long-term survival in myocardial infarction patients: the National Exercise and Heart Disease Project (NEHDP). *Circulation.* 1999;100:1764–1769.

17. Kavanagh T, Mertens DJ, Hamm LF, et al. Prediction of long-term prognosis in 12 169 men referred for cardiac rehabilitation. *Circulation.* 2002;106:666–671.

18. Kavanagh T, Mertens DJ, Hamm LF, et al. Peak oxygen intake and cardiac mortality in women referred for cardiac rehabilitation. *J Am Coll Cardiol.* 2003;42:2139–2143.

19. Dutcher JR, Kahn J, Grines C, et al. Comparison of left ventricular ejection fraction and exercise capacity as predictors of 2- and 5-year mortality following acute myocardial infarction. *Am J Cardiol.* 2007;99:436–441.

20. Powell KE, Thompson PD, Caspersen CJ, et al. Physical activity and the incidence of coronary heart disease. *Annu Rev Public Health.* 1987;8:253–287.

21. Berlin JA, Colditz GA. A meta-analysis of physical activity in the prevention of coronary heart disease. *Am J Epidemiol.* 1990;132:612–628.

22. Franklin BA, Gordon NF. *Contemporary Diagnosis and Management in Cardiovascular Exercise.* Newtown, PA: Handbooks in Health Care Company; 2009:74–88.

23. Green DJ, O'Driscoll G, Joyner MJ, et al. Exercise and cardiovascular risk reduction: time to update the rationale for exercise? *J Appl Physiol.* 2008;105:766–768. Epub 2008 Jan 3.

24. Billman GE, Schwartz PJ, Stone HL, et al. The effects of daily exercise on susceptibility to sudden cardiac death. *Circulation.* 1984;69:1182–1189.

25. Hull SS, Vanoli E, Adamson PB, et al. Exercise training confers anticipatory protection from sudden death during acute myocardial ischemia. *Circulation.* 1994;89:548–552.

26. Barnard RJ, MacAlpin R, Kattus AA, et al. Ischemic response to sudden strenuous exercise in healthy men. *Circulation.* 1973;48:936–942.

27. Dimsdale JE, Hartley LH, Guiney T, et al. Postexercise peril. Plasma catecholamines and exercise. *JAMA.* 1984;251:630–632.

28. Swain DP, Franklin BA. Is there a threshold intensity for aerobic training in cardiac patients? *Med Sci Sports Exerc.* 2002;34:1071–1075.

29. Quell KJ, Porcari JP, Franklin BA, et al. Is brisk walking an adequate aerobic training stimulus for cardiac patients? *Chest.* 2002;122:1852–1856.

30. Fox SM, Naughton JP, Gorman PA. Physical activity and cardiovascular health. III. The exercise prescription; frequency and type of activity. *Mod Concepts Cardiovasc Dis.* 1972;41:21–24.

31. Borg GAV. Psychophysical bases of perceived exertion. *Med Sci Sports Exerc.* 1982;14:377–381.

32. Clausen JP, Klausen K, Rasmussen B, et al. Central and peripheral circulatory changes after training of the arms or legs. *Am J Physiol.* 1973;225:675–682.

33. Fardy PS, Webb D, Hellerstein HK. Benefits of arm exercise in cardiac rehabilitation. *Phys Sportsmed.* 1977;5:30–41.

34. Franklin BA. Aerobic exercise training programs for the upper body. *Med Sci Sports Exerc.* 1989;21(suppl 5):S141–S148.

35. Franklin BA, Vander L, Wrisley D, et al. Trainability of arms versus legs in men with previous myocardial infarction. *Chest.* 1994;105:262–264.

36. Braith RW, Stewart KJ. Resistance exercise training: its role in the prevention of cardiovascular disease. *Circulation.* 2006;113:2642–2650.

37. Williams MA, Haskell WL, Ades PA, et al. Resistance exercise in individuals with and without cardiovascular disease: 2007 update: a scientific statement from the American Heart Association Council on Clinical Cardiology and Council on Nutrition, Physical Activity, and Metabolism. *Circulation.* 2007;116:572–584.

38. McCartney N, McKelvie RS, Martin J, et al. Weight-training-induced attenuation of the circulatory response of older males to weight lifting. *J Appl Physiol.* 1993;74:1056–1060.

39. FitzGerald SJ, Barlow CE, Kampert JB, et al. Muscular fitness and all-cause mortality: prospective observations. *J Phys Act Health.* 2004;1:7.

40. Jurca R, Lamonte MJ, Barlow CE, et al. Association of muscular strength with incidence of metabolic syndrome in men. *Med Sci Sports Exerc.* 2005;37:1849–1855.

41. Feigenbaum MS, Pollock ML. Strength training: rationale for current guidelines for adult fitness programs. *Phys Sportsmed.* 1997;25:44–64.

42. Haskell WL, Lee IM, Pate RR, et al. Physical activity and public health: updated recommendation for adults from the American College of Sports Medicine and the American Heart Association. *Circulation.* 2007;116:1081–1093.

43. United States Department of Health and Human Services. *Physical Activity and Health: A Report of the Surgeon General.* Atlanta, GA: U.S. Department of Health and Human Services, Centers for Disease Control and Prevention, National Center for Chronic Disease Prevention and Health Promotion; 1996.

44. Dunn AL, Marcus BH, Kampert JB, et al. Comparison of lifestyle and structured interventions to increase physical activity and cardiorespiratory fitness: a randomized trial. *JAMA.* 1999;281:327–334.

45. Andersen RE, Wadden TA, Bartlett SJ, et al. Effects of lifestyle activity vs structured aerobic exercise in obese women: a randomized trial. *JAMA.* 1999;281:335–340.

46. Gordon NF, Kohl HW III, Blair SN. Life style exercise: a new strategy to promote physical activity for adults. *J Cardiopulm Rehabil.* 1993;13:161–163.

47. Bravata DM, Smith-Spangler C, Sundaram V, et al. Using pedometers to increase physical activity and improve health: a systematic review. *JAMA.* 2007;298:2296–2304.

48. Leon AS, Norstrom J. Evidence of the role of physical activity and cardiorespiratory fitness in the prevention of coronary heart disease. *Quest.* 1995;47:311–319.

49. Thompson PD, Franklin BA, Balady GJ, et al. Exercise and acute cardiovascular events: placing the risks into perspective. A Scientific Statement from the American Heart Association Council on Nutrition, Physical Activity, and Metabolism and the Council on Clinical Cardiology. *Circulation.* 2007;115:2358–2368.

50. Franklin BA. Cardiovascular events associated with exercise. The risk-protection paradox. *J Cardiopulm Rehab.* 2005;25:189–195.

51. Haapaniemi S, Franklin BA, Wegner JH, et al. Electrocardiographic responses to deer hunting activities in men with and without coronary artery disease. *Am J Cardiol.* 2007;100:175–179.

52. Chowdhury PS, Franklin BA, Boura JA, et al. Sudden cardiac death after manual or automated snow removal. *Am J Cardiol.* 2003;92:833–835.

53. Wilkins K. Triumph and tragedy: record field but 3 deaths in annual race. *Detroit Free Press.* October 19, 2009:1A.

54. Franklin BA, Reed PS, Gordon S, et al. Instantaneous electrocardiography: a simple screening technique for cardiac exercise programs. *Chest.* 1989;96:174–177.

55. American College of Sports Medicine. *Guidelines for Exercise Testing and Prescription.* 7th ed. Baltimore, MD: Lippincott Williams & Wilkins; 2005.

56. Ades PA, Waldmann ML, McCann JW, et al. Predictors of cardiac rehabilitation participation in older coronary patients. *Arch Intern Med.* 1992;152:1033–1035.

PATIENT AND FAMILY INFORMATION FOR:
Exercise and Physical Activity

It's easy to double your risk of developing a chronic health problem. Just remain physically inactive. Approximately 70% of American adults do not meet current daily physical activity recommendations—that is, they have sedentary jobs (or sit most of the day); do not have a regular regimen of physical activity; don't do much work around their homes and yards. Yet gradually increasing your level of physical activity is especially important after a heart attack, angioplasty procedure, or bypass surgery.

GETTING STARTED? EXERCISE AFTER A CARDIAC EVENT

Although doctors traditionally recommended 2 to 3 weeks in bed and an additional period of 3 to 4 weeks in the hospital for patients who experienced a heart attack, prolonged bed rest has adverse effects and is no longer advised in the care of heart patients. Extended bed rest has been shown to result in numerous deleterious effects, including deconditioning, reduced heart–lung fitness, increased muscle fatigue, loss of muscle mass and bone density, blood clots, pneumonia, and depression. A classic report showed that heart attack patients who were counseled to engage in self-care activities and sit in a chair on their first day of hospitalization actually had better outcomes than their counterparts who received conventional therapy (e.g., bed rest). More recent studies have shown that the deterioration in fitness with bed rest may be lessened simply by intermittent sitting or standing.

During the first few weeks after you have been discharged from the hospital, your exercise should consist of progressive walking at a comfortable pace. Start by walking for about 10 minutes and increase it to 30 minutes or more as your physical condition improves. After that, you can gradually increase the exercise intensity (e.g., walking speed), duration, frequency, or combinations thereof. Ask your doctor for a referral to a medically supervised, exercise-based cardiac rehabilitation program.

EXERCISE FOR HEART PATIENTS: BENEFITS AND LIMITATIONS

Regular physical activity plays an important role in promoting cardiovascular health. However, new studies indicate that having a high aerobic fitness (or capacity) reduces ones risk of heart disease, and the reduction is greater than that obtained merely by being physically active. According to a recent landmark study, a low level of fitness more accurately predicts early mortality than does obesity, cigarette smoking, elevated blood cholesterol, or diabetes. Aerobic fitness, not merely physical activity, greatly reduces the risk of stroke and heart attack. A measure of aerobic fitness, called METs (metabolic equivalents), appears to be one of the most powerful predictors of cardiovascular health and longevity.

UNDERSTANDING METS

Aerobic fitness is measured in METs, which can be determined during a progressive treadmill test to peak effort. In general, the longer you last on the treadmill, the higher your MET capacity. If you undergo a treadmill stress test, ask your test supervisor (or your physician) to tell you your MET capacity, along with such standard measures as heart rhythm and blood pressure responses.

One MET equals the amount of oxygen your body uses when resting. A comfortable walking pace expends about 3 METs. Singles tennis requires 6 to 7 METs, whereas jogging requires 8 to 10 or more METs, depending on the speed. The average healthy adult has an aerobic capacity of 8 to 12 METs. Someone who is sedentary has about 5 to 8 METs. Persons with <5 METs are generally considered unfit and have the highest mortality rate. However, middle-aged and older adults with an aerobic capacity >8 METs are considered moderate-to-high fit, and have the best health outcomes. Regular exercise raises your MET capacity. For each MET you gain, you reduce your chances of dying from a heart attack by 10% to 15%.

DECREASED HEART RATE AND BLOOD PRESSURE

When you perform aerobic exercise regularly, your body becomes physically conditioned. This decreases the heart rate and blood pressure when you are at rest and at any level of exercise. Consequently, the heart does not need to work as hard to achieve a given amount of work. The reduced workload on the heart also raises the level of activity that can be tolerated without experiencing anginal chest pain and/or abnormal electrocardiographic changes.

WHY IMPROVE AEROBIC CAPACITY?

When the body's ability to transport and deliver oxygen improves, people have added energy and less fatigue. Any task requires a certain amount of oxygen, expressed as METs. People who aren't aerobically fit may use their entire aerobic capacity to, say, work in the garden. People who are aerobically fit may use the same amount of oxygen to do gardening, but because they have a higher aerobic capacity, they have more "energy reserve."

IMPROVED RISK FACTORS FOR HEART DISEASE

Exercise improves many of the risk factors associated with the development and progression of heart disease. These include the following:

- Lowers blood pressure, especially in patients with hypertension.
- May reduce triglyceride and total cholesterol levels, increase HDL-C levels (the good cholesterol), and lower LDL-C levels (the bad cholesterol).
- Helps control body weight and reduce body fat stores.
- Relieves stress, anxiety, and depression.
- Helps regulate blood sugar levels in patients with diabetes.

LIMITATIONS OF EXERCISE

There is limited scientific evidence that exercise alone increases the diameter of the coronary arteries, or the number of tiny interconnecting blood vessels called "collaterals" that feed the heart muscle. Moreover, exercise training has little or no effect on improving the pumping effectiveness of a damaged heart or reducing heart rhythm irregularities. Furthermore, exercise alone has little or no effect on halting or reversing atherosclerotic plaques. This is why patients benefit more from a comprehensive rehabilitation program, that includes healthy dietary modifications, weight loss, and smoking cessation (if appropriate), and selected cardioprotective medications such as aspirin, ß-blockers, and cholesterol-lowering statins.

YOUR EXERCISE PROGRAM

To protect your cardiovascular system (including the heart and blood vessels), you should perform regular aerobic activity. The most effective exercises for the conditioning phase include horizontal or graded walking, jogging, swimming, cycling, or working out on a stair-climber, elliptical machine, exercise bike, or rowing machine. Training sessions should include a preliminary aerobic warm-up (approximately 10 minutes), a continuous or accumulated conditioning phase (at least 30 minutes in duration or multiple 10 to 15 minutes exercise bouts), and a cool-down (5 to 10 minutes) followed by stretching activities. The warm-up and cool-down are vital to maximize safety and reduce the likelihood of complications. However, the key to effectiveness is to exercise at a sufficient intensity level.

For improvements in heart–lung fitness, you need to exercise at approximately 40% to 60% of your maximum MET capacity (as determined from a treadmill test). If your maximum exercise capacity is only 5 METs, then your exercise intensity should be in the 2 to 3 MET range. For most patients, this intensity approximates 70% of the highest heart rate achieved during peak or symptom-limited exercise testing. Alternatively, if you stay in the 11 to 13 range on the perceived exertion scale during your workouts, corresponding to "fairly light" to "somewhat hard" exertion, you'll be exercising at an intensity that is sufficient to improve cardiovascular health. The aerobic activity should be complemented by upper body exercises, light-to-moderate resistance (weight) training, and increased lifestyle activity. Quality pedometers (e.g., Yamax Digiwalker, Omron Pocket Pedometer) can be helpful in this regard, by recording daily step totals. Ideally, your goal should be 8,000 to 10,000 steps daily.

RISK OF CARDIOVASCULAR COMPLICATIONS

People who have heart disease or have experienced a heart attack may be afraid to perform strenuous exertion. In fact, some are afraid to undertake everyday leisure-time and occupational activities, feeling they may precipitate further heart problems. The risk of having a heart attack during exercise, however, is very small. Probably the most important question we can ask is: Do the benefits of exercise outweigh the risks?

Numerous studies have shown that the risk of cardiovascular events increases transiently during vigorous exercise. This seems to be especially true in people with known or occult heart disease who perform unaccustomed vigorous physical exertion and in those who have recently experienced a worsening in their symptoms, such as increasing shortness of breath or chest pain during exercise. However, the overall risk of heart problems appears to be reduced in people who are regular exercisers. For most heart patients, the benefits of moderate-to-vigorous intensity exercise far outweigh the risks.

HIGH RISK ACTIVITIES

Highly strenuous activities that involve sudden starts and stops are not as beneficial as exercise in which the workload is more constant and regular. Such activities are more likely to place undue stress on the heart, increasing the risk of cardiovascular complications. Recreational and domestic activities that are associated with an increased incidence of heart attack and sudden cardiac death include competitive running events, deep sea diving, racquet sports, water skiing, cross-country skiing, deer hunting, and automated or manual snow removal.

SAFETY TIPS

Recommendations to potentially reduce the risk of cardiovascular events during exercise include the following: undergo exercise testing periodically to assess your progress and screen for abnormal signs and symptoms; start gradually; warm up before and cool down after exercise; exercise regularly (e.g., don't try to cram all your exercise into 1 day per week); avoid unaccustomed high-intensity physical exertion; don't exercise outdoors on extremely hot or cold days, or when the humidity is high or it is very windy; and, if warning signs or symptoms transiently occur (e.g., chest pain/pressure, unusual shortness of breath, heart rhythm irregularities, dizziness or lightheadedness, sudden weight gain, and/or swelling of the ankles), stop exercising and consult with your physician.

BEHAVIORAL STRATEGIES TO INCREASE EXERCISE COMPLIANCE

There are several things you can do, beyond relying on mere willpower, to maintain your interest in and enthusiasm for exercise. These include the following:

- List your exercise goals in writing and look at them frequently throughout the day.

- Use visualization. Keep your ideal body image of yourself in mind.

- Make structured exercise a priority. Set aside a regular exercise time and do not let anything interfere.

- Decrease the likelihood of injury with a moderate exercise prescription—at least initially.

- Keep a record of your daily exercise achievements.

- Exercise with others. Social reinforcement strengthens your commitment.

- Participate in activities you enjoy. It is easier to stay motivated when exercise is fun.

- Obtain periodic evaluations (e.g., body fatness, cholesterol level, treadmill test performance [peak METs]) to measure your progress.

- Disguise your exercise. Incorporating more physical activity into everyday life is just as important as setting up a formal exercise routine.

A CALL TO ACTION: START EXERCISING GRADUALLY—BUT START!

If you are doing no exercise at the present time, start by exercising for 10 to 15 minutes at a time, three to four times per week. That may not sound like much—but if you go from doing nothing to doing this amount of exercise, you will improve your health more than a person who goes from running 30 miles per week to running 35 miles a week.

How could this be? Recent pioneering research has shown that people who do not exercise at all (we refer to them as the least active, least fit cohort—or the bottom 20%) have the greatest risk of developing cardiovascular problems. If you get out of this "high-risk" category by doing even a modest amount of cardioprotective exercise each week, you will substantially decrease your risk for a heart attack or stroke.

In conclusion, people follow the physics principle of inertia: A body at rest tends to remain at rest and a body in motion tends to remain in motion. By simply starting, you overcome inertia and build momentum! You may be surprised at how soon you will begin to exercise longer than you ever thought was possible.

Smoking Cessation in the Cardiac Patient

For patients with cardiac heart disease, quitting smoking is associated with a 36% reduction in all-cause mortality.[1] For patients with left ventricular (LV) dysfunction after myocardial infarction (MI), smoking cessation is associated with a 40% lower hazard of all-cause mortality over a median follow-up of 42 months.[2] Current smoking is a powerful independent risk factor for sudden cardiac death among patients with a previous MI or stable angina. Those who quit have the same risk of sudden death as those who have never smoked.[3] The impact of smoking cessation in this population is therefore of at least the same magnitude as that of angiotensin-converting enzyme (ACE) inhibitors (19% relative risk decrease), β-blockers (23% relative risk decrease), and aldosterone antagonists (15% relative risk decrease).[4–6]

The effects of smoking on heart rate, blood pressure, cardiovascular blood flow, myocardial oxygen demand, and thrombosis are largely reversible. Because the benefit is of immediate onset, and as there are effective tools available, smoking cessation for the cardiac patient is an essential component of care.[7] In this chapter we will review how cigarettes induce cardiac disease, the role of nicotine in this process, the pharmacologic tools available, their safety profile in the cardiac patient, and the basics of behavioral modification for the smoking addiction. Helping patients to quit smoking is certainly more challenging than simply ordering a medication. Understanding the biology involved assists us in helping our patients break this notoriously severe addiction.

HOW DOES SMOKING CAUSE HEART DISEASE?

Although the entry portal for cigarette smoke is the lung, where the chemicals present in the smoke are quickly and easily absorbed, the resulting inflammatory cascade has a profound effect well beyond the confines of the lung. The systemic effects of cigarette smoking include a variety of complicated processes that induce, in the genetically susceptible individual, vascular and hematologic abnormalities that can result in accelerated atherosclerosis as well as the acute events of MI and sudden death. The chemicals that are inhaled induce oxidative stress, systemic inflammation with activation and release of both inflammatory cells and inflammatory mediators, endothelial dysfunction, and abnormalities of coagulation and hemostasis[8]:

1. *Oxidative stress.* The particulate (tar) phase of cigarette smoke contains $>10^{17}$ free radicals per gram, and the gas phase contains $>10^{15}$ free radicals per puff. Many of the damaging effects of smoking are induced by these molecules. The sustained release of reactive free radicals from the tar and gas phases of smoke imposes an oxidant stress, inducing a variety of chemical injuries including the promotion of lipid peroxidation. Also, the inhaled oxidant molecules significantly deplete the body's antioxidant defense system.[8,9]

2. *Systemic inflammation.* Long-term cigarette smoking increases total WBC counts. There is an increased early bone marrow release of polymorphonuclear leukocytes (PMNs) and platelets into the circulation. These activated inflammatory cells then produce a variety of inflammatory mediators, acute phase proteins, and cytokines, among them C-reactive protein (CRP), fibrinogen, IL-6, and tumor necrosis factor. Some of the inflammatory mediators and hematologic effects of smoking decline rapidly after smoking cessation. However, CRP can remain elevated for 10 to 19 years.[10] These mediators may not be just markers of disease but may be actively involved in the proinflammatory and proatherogenic effects of chronic smoke exposure.

3. *Endothelial dysfunction.* Smoking-induced endothelial dysfunction is mainly caused by decreased production or availability of nitric oxide (NO) resulting in impaired vasodilatory function at the macrovascular level (e.g., coronary arteries) as well as at the microvascular level.[11,12] NO is also affected by cigarette smoke through the changes induced on low-density lipoprotein (LDL). In cigarette smokers, LDL gets oxidatively modified by the inhaled oxidant molecules. The modified LDL then interferes with the protective effect of NO on the arterial wall. The result is increased inflammatory cell entry into the arterial wall. The oxidatively modified LDL is taken up by the macrophages that enter the arterial wall; cholesterol esters are deposited and foam cells form.

4. *Abnormalities of coagulation and hemostasis.* Smoking cigarettes induces a hypercoaguable state that is the predominant cause of *acute* cardiovascular events induced by smoking. Viscosity is increased, with increased levels of fibrinogen, lipoproteins, and hematocrit. Antithrombotic, prothrombotic factors, and platelet function are affected. There is impaired release of the t-PA, the main fibrinolytic activator resulting in impaired fibrinolysis. Hypercoaguability is responsible for 25% to 50% of the link between smoking and coronary artery disease (CAD)[3] and is especially involved in acute cardiac events. This is borne out in multiple clinical situations:

   • Smoking increases the risk of MI and sudden death much more than it increases the risk of angina, reflecting the importance of acute thrombus formation.[13]

- Similarly, the prognosis after thrombolysis is better in smokers than in nonsmokers. This reflects the greater part that clot plays in the disease process.[14]
- Sudden cardiac death is correlated with the presence of acute thrombosis and not the level of plaque burden.[13]
- Smokers who continue to smoke after thrombolysis or angioplasty have a substantially increased risk of reinfarction or reocclusion.[15,16]
- At least a part of the thrombotic effects of smoking are induced by even passive smoke.[17,18] The remarkable sensitivity of the coagulation system to the effect of cigarette smoke[19] mandates that the cardiac patient must cease all smoking, not just cut down their habit, to achieve reversal of these effects. Patients should be taught the seriousness of this issue.

Although some of the effects of smoking on inflammatory markers may persist for years, a great portion of these effects are reversible by stopping smoking.

WHAT IS THE ROLE OF CARBON MONOXIDE IN THIS PROCESS?

CO acutely poisons the oxygen delivery system, placing the patient at risk for arrhythmia and MI.[13]

HOW DOES NICOTINE PARTICIPATE IN THIS PROCESS?

Although much of the toxic effects of cigarette smoke are due to the other chemicals present, nicotine is the chemical that is responsible for the addiction. It is inhaled in cigarette smoke and rapidly reaches the nicotinic cholinergic receptors, found both in the peripheral and central nervous system, resulting in the release of a variety of neurotransmitters including dopamine, glutamate, γ-aminobutyric acid, norepinephrine, acetylcholine, serotonin, and endorphins, which are important in the development of addiction in the susceptible individual. The pleasure derived from the dopamine release contributes to the addictive process.

Nicotine dependence is highly heritable. It is determined by a number of genes that are receptors for the drug, and they determine its rate of metabolism, its pleasurable effects as well as its withdrawal syndrome. One of the primary genes involved is the CYP2A gene that is a controller of the rate of metabolism of nicotine, the vulnerability to tobacco dependence, the response to smoking treatment, and is involved with lung cancer risk. The α3β4 nicotinic acetyl choline receptor is believed to mediate the cardiovascular effects of nicotine.[20]

With repeated exposure, nicotine tolerance develops through a desensitization of the receptors to the effect of nicotine and an increase in the number of nicotine receptors. Nicotine withdrawal is a complex process—not unlike that of withdrawal from alcohol, cocaine, opiates, and cannabinoids—that results in a state of anxiety, stress, generalized discomfort, inability to concentrate, and depressed mood.[20]

Thus smokers learn to use the cigarette's nicotine as a modulator of anxiety, concentration, depressive symptoms, and pleasure; a major tool for handling life's stresses. At the same time, those who are genetically susceptible to the addiction, after a relatively short period of use, become trapped by an inability

to function without the satisfaction of the increased number of less-responsive nicotine receptors. By smoking, not only does the intense discomfort of withdrawal get relieved within 10 seconds, but the relief is accompanied by significant pleasure.

With time the smoker associates certain situations with smoking: after a meal, drinks with friends, coffee, stress, and so on. This association is learned and contributes significantly to the activity of the nicotine receptors and the expectation of immediate relief. These conditioned responses play a significant role in maintaining the addiction and become a significant impediment to the process of quitting. Understanding the biology makes clear the importance of the behavioral component of smoking cessation.[20] As we will see from the studies on smoking cessation in the cardiac patient, the behavioral component of therapy is as important as the pharmacologic component. The permanence of the receptors and the persistence of the learned behavior make the incidence of relapse very high; thus the importance of "learning" new sources of pleasure, stress management, concentration, and mood regulation.

WHAT IS THE ROLE OF NICOTINE IN THE DEVELOPMENT OF CARDIOVASCULAR DISEASE?

Sympathetic overactivity is a significant factor by which smoking, and at least in part nicotine, induces cardiovascular disease.[13] Nicotine releases catecholamines, increases heart rate and cardiac contractility, constricts cutaneous and coronary blood vessels, and transiently increases blood pressure.[21] There is an increase of myocardial work and oxygen consumption through an increase of blood pressure, heart rate, and myocardial contractility.[22] Nicotine also reduces sensitivity to insulin and may contribute to endothelial dysfunction.[23,24] How much of the sympathetic overactivity induced by smoking results from the effect of nicotine in the cigarette is unclear, but this is of obvious concern when we are considering using nicotine replacement therapy (NRT) in the cardiac patient.

IS THE USE OF NICOTINE REPLACEMENT THERAPY SAFE?

In a 2010 meta-analysis of adverse events associated with the use of NRT among 177,390 participants, Mills et al.[25] found that NRT is associated with increased risk of GI complaints and insomnia. There was an observed risk of skin irritation and, with orally administered NRT, oropharyngeal complaints. Although NRT was associated with an increased risk of heart palpitations and chest pain, there was no increased incidence of heart attack or death. Their conclusion was that NRT is associated with adverse effects that may be discomforting for the patient but are not life-threatening. In a study of electrocardiographic effects of NRT, improvements were seen with reduced heart rate and heart rate corrected QT during a cold-turkey smoking quit attempt as well as during NRT pharmacotherapy.[26]

In a clinical trial of nicotine patches in smokers with cardiovascular disease, Joseph et al.[27] showed no increased risk of cardiovascular events compared with placebo. The dose–response curve for the cardiovascular effects, such as heart rate acceleration or the release of catecholamines is flat, such that adding nicotine medication to smoking produces no further effect.[13]

Even high-dose transdermal patches did not result in changes of blood pressure or heart rate.[28] Increased cardiovascular risk owing to nicotine medication does not appear to be a problem.[20]

IS THE USE OF NICOTINE REPLACEMENT THERAPY IN THE CARDIAC PATIENT SAFE?

Early case reports suggested cardiovascular risk associated with use of NRT, especially if the patient smoked while using nicotine replacement. Data are now available[13,27,29–33] from randomized controlled trials, efficacy studies, observational data, and physiologic studies supporting the safety of NRT used in the stable cardiac patient. There was no increased risk of angina, MI, stroke, arrhythmia, or death. These studies looked at patients with stable cardiovascular disease who had no cardiac event requiring an intervention in the prior 2 weeks.

There is only one study[34] that looks at use of NRT among patients who were admitted for acute coronary syndromes and who received transdermal NRT during hospitalization. In this retrospective propensity analysis from Duke University, patients who had undergone a cardiac catheterization for an acute coronary syndrome and received NRT were retrospectively compared with comparable patients from their database. After propensity matched analysis, they found no difference in short- or long-term mortality in patients who did or did not receive the patch. There was no significant difference between the groups in the need for undergoing coronary artery bypass graft (CABG) surgery or percutaneous transluminal angioplasty. Nonetheless, nicotine does have hemodynamic effects that could contribute to acute cardiovascular events.

There are two troubling retrospective reports regarding the use of nicotine replacement in critically ill patients. One is among medical intensive care unit patients[35] and the other among patients undergoing CABG.[36] In each study, the use of NRT was associated with an increased mortality. In the intensive care unit (ICU) study, it was postulated that the increased myocardial oxygen consumption induced by nicotine in the face of reduced oxygen delivery may have been a contributing mechanism. Although they controlled for chronic obstructive pulmonary disease (COPD), they could not exclude the fact that the patients who received NRT may have had more severe nicotine dependence and associated comorbidities than controls. In the study of the CABG patients, the patients in the NRT group had an increased pack year history and an increased incidence of COPD which, as the authors discuss, may have predisposed that group to a higher mortality risk. The retrospective nature of these studies and their small size, along with not being able to control for the severity of the patients nicotine dependence, limits the weight we can place on them. However, they most definitely indicate the need for prospective work and raise a need for caution.

The hemodynamic effects of NRT appear to be very mild, and its use in the stable cardiac patient appears to be quite safe. Its use in the cardiac care unit (CCU) remains an issue needing study.

BUPROPION FOR SMOKERS WITH CARDIOVASCULAR DISEASE

Bupropion, an atypical antidepressant with a structure related to amphetamine, has, like nicotine replacement and has been shown to be an effective smoking cessation tool.

After approximately 10 days of treatment, the desire to smoke diminishes significantly. In addition, the depression that not uncommonly surfaces in patients stopping smoking is prevented. The contraindications include a seizure history, alcoholism, bipolar disorder, bulimia, and panic attacks. The side effects include dry mouth, headache, agitation, and insomnia. Hypertension has been described, especially in patients taking both bupropion and the nicotine replacement. The treatment is usually begun at bupropion 150 mg SR and subsequently increased to 150 mg SR twice a day. The side effects are dose-dependent and some patients may obtain an adequate therapeutic benefit with the 150 mg daily dose. The drug is metabolized in the liver, so dose adjustment is advised with significant liver disease. The drug inhibits the activity of CYP2D6 isoenzyme, which metabolizes β-blockers, anti-arrhythmics, certain antidepressants, selective serotonin reuptake inhibitors (SSRIs), and antipsychotics. There have been a number of case reports of death and severe adverse cardiovascular reactions occurring in patients taking bupropion. The contribution of bupropion SR to these deaths is not known, because as retrospective case reports, they could not control for other significant risk factors and therefore contribute little to safety assessment.[37]

More recently, in a five hospital, double-blind placebo controlled trial, patients who were admitted with acute cardiovascular disease were randomized to receive either bupropion SR 150 mg twice a day and intensive counseling versus placebo and intensive counseling for 3 months. The bupropion and placebo groups did not differ in cardiovascular mortality at 1 year, in blood pressure at follow-up, or in cardiovascular events at end-of-treatment or 1 year. The bupropion group did have improved short-term quit rates (37.1% vs. 26.8%) but not improved long-term quit rates (25% vs. 21.3%) over intensive counseling, but bupropion did appear to be safe for smokers hospitalized with acute cardiovascular disease. When controlled for cigarettes per day, depression symptoms, prior bupropion use, hypertension, and length of stay the smoke-free adjusted odds ratio was 1.51 (95% CI, 0.81 to 2.8) at 1 year. After 30 days off the drug, there was a borderline significant increase in cardiac events; 75% of the subjects were smoking before the event. Although this study was only powered to identify a doubling of cardiac events, it did within those limits support its safety in hospitalized patients with acute cardiac events. The patients enrolled in the study were significantly addicted, and 40% of them had been smoking with known CAD prior to admission, a highly challenging group. In addition to supporting the safety of the use of bupropion in the CCU patient, this study raises several additional points: the significant benefit of intensive ongoing counseling in this population, and the possible indication for longer-term therapy with bupropion to help maintain the abstinence advantage seen at 3 months.[38]

There is one randomized trial for smoking cessation comparing bupropion SR 150 mg twice a day with placebo in outpatients with stable cardiovascular disease.[39] At 1 year, the quit rates were 27% for the bupropion arm versus 11% for the placebo arm. There were no clinically significant changes in blood pressure and heart rate throughout the treatment phase.

In studies of bupropion SR being used as an antidepressant in patients with cardiac disease, few cardiac adverse effects were seen. There was occasional hypertension but no effect on cardiac conduction or ejection fraction.

Despite the concern raised by case reports, current evidence suggests that bupropion SR may be a safe and possibly efficacious treatment for smoking cessation for patients with cardiovascular disease. Full evaluation of bupropion SR in patients with cardiac disease is needed. Bupropion may be used in combination with nicotine replacement. The success rate of this combination has not been shown to be statistically superior[40,41] and has not been evaluated in the cardiac patient. It is suggested that while on combined therapy, blood pressure should be monitored.

WHAT IS THE ROLE OF VARENICLINE FOR THE CARDIAC PATIENT?

Varenicline is a highly effective smoking cessation medication that is both a partial nicotine agonist and an antagonist. After the first week taking this drug, the patient experiences little to no cravings and if they do smoke they derive no pleasure. It is used alone, not in combination with nicotine replacement or bupropion. Although this drug has had the highest quit rates among healthy individuals, postmarketing data raised serious concerns regarding the risk of depression, aggressive behavior, suicidal ideation, and suicide. It is well known that depression may surface in patients attempting to quit smoking. Many patients use the nicotine in cigarettes, to treat a full-blown or borderline depression, and when they stop smoking depression may be uncovered. Whether the psychiatric effects of varenicline are above and beyond the usual rate of depression that is seen with stopping smoking is an area of ongoing research, and caution is advised.

For the cardiac patient considering use of varenicline, two questions arise. First, is there any excess cardiovascular risk? Second, what is the risk of depression? This is of special concern in this often depressed population.[42]

Theoretically, varenicline should have little to no cardiovascular effects. The sympathomimetic cardiovascular effects of nicotine are mediated primarily by binding to $\alpha 3\beta 4$ nicotinic acetylcholine receptors. Varenicline binds to a different nicotinic receptor, $\alpha 4\beta 2$, and was therefore theorized not to have cardiovascular effects. In 2010, Rigotti et al.[43] published a multicenter randomized, double-blind placebo-controlled trial comparing the efficacy of 12 weeks of varenicline with counseling versus counseling alone in 714 smokers with stable cardiovascular disease. At the end of a year, the quit rate was 19.2% for the varenicline group versus 7.2% for placebo. Although the trial was small, there was no increase of cardiovascular events or mortality. For this study, patients had to be otherwise well, including no psychiatric history. Mood was not systematically assessed, but there was no difference in spontaneously reported psychiatric symptoms in the varenicline versus placebo group.

Varenicline is our most effective pharmacotherapy for smoking cessation to date. The psychiatric risks remain a major concern, and it is advised to use the drug only in patients who do not have a psychiatric history and who have family who can watch the patient for signs of developing change of mood.

Further work is needed to further clarify the psychiatric risk and to ensure the cardiac safety profile. No data are available for the use of this agent in the acute cardiac setting. These data however do provide a strong evidence base to support the use of varenicline for outpatient smokers with stable cardiovascular disease.

BEHAVIORAL MODIFICATION

Although 30% to 45% of smokers who suffer an initial cardiac event stop smoking,[44] 60% to 70% of those relapse within a year. No matter which pharmacologic therapy one uses to stop smoking, there is a 50% relapse rate. The problem is that nicotine addiction is permanent. The patient who smokes immediately on waking, or who is uncomfortable in places where they cannot smoke for any length of time, is very addicted. The faster and stronger the craving, the more addicted the patient. Other patients are able to wait for hours before their first cigarette. They are less affected by the decreased nicotine level that occurs over a night without smoking. They have fewer or no cravings. They have a larger behavioral component to their habit and are less in need of medication to quit.

Patients who are highly addicted need more than medication to have a sustained success. They need to learn behavioral techniques to allow them to remain smoke free through a lifetime. We know that smoking cessation programs that do not include postdischarge counseling and that do not provide follow-up for more than a month are ineffective.[45–48] Follow-up of at least 3 months is indicated.[49] Cardiologists should attend to these simple techniques and the importance of lifestyle modification on an ongoing basis.[50,51]

WHAT ARE THE PRINCIPLES INVOLVED?

- Convince the patient that he or she can succeed. You will provide the medication and behavioral techniques required for success.

- Ask the patient what do they use the cigarette for: depression, boredom, anxiety, or stress; pleasure, concentration, relief from cravings, or all of the above? Together consider alternative approaches to those problems, which may require antidepressants,[42] stress and anger management techniques, exercise, keeping oneself busy at all times, finding alternate pleasures, and avoiding the situations that lead to the urge to smoke.

- Have the patient make a concrete plan for what he or she will do to cope with cravings (e.g., gum, water, or deep breathing).

- Identify and plan for avoidance of triggers such as coffee, alcohol, or friends who smoke.

- Identify substitutes that the patient likes and can look forward to, for example, movies, museums, friends who do not smoke, or magazines.

- Encourage the patient to be busy as much as possible, especially immediately after meals.

- Most important, discuss with the patient the permanence of the addiction and the need to be on guard even years later, especially in situations of stress. Unfortunately, the thought of picking up another cigarette recurs for a very long time and one puff can lead to full relapse.

- Patients should never allow others to smoke around them or endanger their sobriety. As their cardiologist, you are giving them the license to inconvenience others, within limits, because it is so important that they succeed that nothing should be allowed to endanger their success.

Smoking cessation in the cardiac patient covers a spectrum of therapy from simple behavioral modification to complex decisions involving pharmacotherapeutic options. We have ample data indicating that the approach must be a combination of techniques, with months of ongoing support. However, the relapse rate remains unacceptably high. As we have reviewed, the risks of ongoing smoking are high as are the benefits from quitting. Clearly, we need more physician participation in this process and those who could be more effective in guiding the patient to success than their own cardiologist.

REFERENCES

1. Critchley J, Capewell S. Smoking cessation for the secondary prevention of coronary heart disease. *Cochrane Database Syst Rev.* 2004;(4):CD003041.
2. Shah AM, Pfeffer MA, Hartley LH, et al. Risk of all-cause mortality, recurrent myocardial infarction, and heart failure hospitalization associated with smoking status following myocardial infarction with left ventricular dysfunction. *Am J Cardiol.* 2010;106:911–916.
3. Goldenberg I, Jonas M, Tenenbaum A, et al.; Bezafibrate Infarction Prevention Study Group. Current smoking, smoking cessation, and the risk of sudden cardiac death in patients with coronary artery disease. *Arch Intern Med.* 2003;163:2301–2305.
4. Pfeffer MA, Braunwald E, Moyé LA, et al. Effect of captopril on mortality and morbidity in patients with left ventricular dysfunction after myocardial infarction: results of the Survival and Ventricular Enlargement trial. *N Engl J Med.* 1992;327:669–677.
5. Yusuf S, Hawken S, Ounpuu S, et al.; INTERHEART Study Investigators. Effect of potentially modifiable risk factors associated with myocardial infarction in 52 countries (the INTERHEART study): case-control study. *Lancet.* 2004;364:937–953.
6. Conroy RM, Pyorala K, Fitzgerald AP, et al.; SCORE Project Group. Estimation of ten-year risk of fatal cardiovascular disease in Europe: the SCORE project. *Eur Heart J.* 2003;24:987–1003.
7. Thomson CC, Rigotti NA. Hospital- and clinic-based smoking cessation interventions for smokers with cardiovascular disease. *Prog Cardiovasc Dis.* 2003;45(6):459–479.
8. Yanbaeva D, Dentener M, Creutzberg EC, et al. Systemic effects of smoking. *Chest.* 2007;131:1557–1566.
9. Pasupathi P, Bakthavathsalam G, Saravanan G, et al. Effect of cigarette smoking on lipids and oxidative stress biomarkers in patients with acute myocardial infarction. *Res J Med Med Sci.* 2009;4(2):151–159.
10. Wannamethee SG, Lowe GD, Shaper AG, et al. Associations between cigarette smoking, pipe/cigar smoking, and smoking cessation, and haemostatic and inflammatory markers for cardiovascular disease. *Eur Heart J.* 2005;26:1765–1773.
11. Pryor WA, Stone K. Oxidants in cigarette smoke radicals, hydrogen peroxides, peroxynitrate and peroxynitrite. *Ann N Y Acad Sci.* 1993;686(1):12–27.
12. Ludwig PW, Hoidal JR. Alterations in leukocyte oxidative metabolism in cigarette smokers. *Am Rev Respir Dis.* 1982;126:977–980.
13. Benowitz NL, Gourlay SG. Cardiovascular toxicity of nicotine: implications for nicotine replacement therapy. *J Am Coll Cardiol.* 1997;29:1422–1431.
14. Barbash GI, Reiner J, White HD, et al. Evaluation of paradoxic beneficial effects of smoking in patients receiving thrombolytic therapy for acute myocardial infarction: mechanism of the "smoker's paradox" from the GUSTO-I trial, with angiographic insights. Global Utilization of Streptokinase and Tissue-Plasminogen Activator for Occluded Coronary Arteries. *J Am Coll Cardiol.* 1995;26(5):1222–1229.
15. Rivers JT, White HD, Cross DB, et al. Reinfarction after thrombolytic therapy for acute myocardial infarction followed by conservative management: incidence and effect of smoking. *J Am Coll Cardiol.* 1990;16:340.
16. Galan KM, Deligonul U, Kern MJ, et al. Increased frequency of restenosis in patients continuing to smoke cigarettes after percutaneous transluminal coronary angioplasty. *Am J Cardiol.* 1988;61:260.
17. Glantz SA, Parmley WW. Passive smoking and heart disease: mechanisms and risk. *JAMA.* 1995;273:1047–1053.
18. Barnoya J, Glantz SA. Cardiovascular effects of secondhand smoke: nearly as large as smoking. *Circulation.* 2005;111(20):2684–2698.
19. Ambrose JA, Barua RS. The pathophysiology of cigarette smoking and cardiovascular disease: an update. *J Am Coll Cardiol.* 2004;43:1731–1737.
20. Benowitz NL. Pharmacology of nicotine: addiction, smoking-induced disease, and therapeutics. *Annu Rev Pharmacol Toxicol.* 2009;49:57–71.
21. Benowitz NL. Cigarette smoking and cardiovascular disease: pathophysiology and implications for treatment. *Prog Cardiovasc Dis.* 2003;46:91–111.
22. Najem B, Houssiere A, Pathak A, et al. Acute cardiovascular and sympathetic effects of nicotine replacement therapy. *Hypertension.* 2006;47:1162–1167.
23. Eliasson B. Cigarette smoking and diabetes. *Prog Cardiovasc Dis.* 2003;45:405–413.
24. Puranik R, Celermajer DS. Smoking and endothelial function. *Prog Cardiovasc Dis.* 2003;45:443–458.
25. Mills EJ, Wu P, Lockhart I, et al. Adverse events associated with nicotine replacement therapy (NRT) for smoking cessation. A systematic review and meta-analysis of one hundred and twenty studies involving 177,390 individuals. *Tob Induc Dis.* 2010;8:8.
26. Lewis MJ, Balaji G, Dixon H, et al. Influence of smoking abstinence and nicotine replacement therapy on heart rate and QT time-series. *Clin Physiol Funct Imaging.* 2010;30(1):43–50.
27. Joseph AM, Norman SM, Ferry LH, et al. The safety of transdermal nicotine as an aid to smoking cessation in patients with cardiac disease. *N Engl J Med.* 1996;335:1792–1798.
28. Hatsukami D, Mooney M, Murphy S, et al. Effects of high dose transdermal nicotine replacement in cigarette smokers. *Pharmacol Biochem Behav.* 2007;86(1):132–139.
29. Ludvig J, Miner B, Eisenberg MJ. Smoking cessation in patients with coronary artery disease. *Am Heart J.* 2005;149:565–572.
30. Ford CL, Zlabek JA. Nicotine replacement therapy and cardiovascular disease. *Mayo Clin Proc.* 2005;80:652–656.
31. Hubbard R, Lewis S, Smith C, et al. Use of nicotine replacement therapy and the risk of acute myocardial infarction, stroke, and death. *Tob Control.* 2005;14:416–421.
32. Fishbein L, O'Brien P, Hutson A, et al. Pharmacokinetics and pharmacodynamic effects of nicotine nasal spray devices on cardiovascular and pulmonary function. *J Investig Med.* 2000;48:435–440.
33. Tzivoni D, Keren A, Meyler S, et al. Cardiovascular safety of transdermal nicotine patches in patients with coronary artery disease who try to quit smoking. *Cardiovasc Drugs Ther.* 1998;12:239–244.
34. Meine TJ, Patel MR, Washam JB, et al. Safety and effectiveness of transdermal nicotine patch in smokers admitted with acute coronary syndromes. *Am J Cardiol.* 2005;95:976–978.
35. Lee A, Alessa B. The association of nicotine replacement therapy with mortality in a medical intensive care unit. *Crit Care Med.* 2007;35:1517–1521.
36. Paciullo C, Short M, Steinke DT, et al. Impact of nicotine replacement therapy on postoperative mortality following coronary artery bypass graft surgery. *Ann Pharmacother.* 2009;43:1197–1202.
37. Joseph A, Fu S. Safety issues in pharmacotherapy for smoking in patients with cardiovascular disease. *Prog Cardiovasc Dis.* 2003;45(6):429–441.
38. Rigotti NA, Thorndike A, Regan S, et al. Bupropion for smokers hospitalized with acute cardiovascular disease. *Am J Med.* 2006;119:1080–1087.
39. Tonstad S, Farsang C, Klaene G, et al. Bupropion SR for smoking cessation in smokers with cardiovascular disease: a multicentre, randomized study. *Eur Heart J.* 2003;24:946–955.
40. Jorenby D, Leischow S, Nides M, et al. A controlled trial of sustained-release bupropion, a nicotine patch, or both for smoking cessation. *N Engl J Med.* 1999;340:685–691.
41. Simon J, Duncan C, Carmody T, et al. Bupropion for smoking cessation. *Arch Intern Med.* 2004;164:1797–1803.
42. Thorndike AN, Rigotti NA. A tragic triad: coronary artery disease, nicotine addiction and depression. *Curr Opin Cardiol.* 2009;24:447–453.
43. Rigotti NA, Pipe AL, Benowitz NL, et al. Efficacy and safety of varenicline for smoking cessation in patients with cardiovascular disease. *Circulation.* 2010;121:221–229.
44. Rigotti NA, Singer DE, Mulley AG Jr, et al. Smoking cessation following admission to a coronary care unit. *J Gen Intern Med.* 1991;6:305–311.
45. Aziz O, Skapinakis P, Rahman S, et al. Behavioural interventions for smoking cessation in patients hospitalised for a major cardiovascular event. *Int J Cardiol.* 2008;137:171–174.
46. Quist-Paulsen P, Gallefoss F. Randomised controlled trial of smoking cessation intervention after admission for coronary heart disease. *BMJ.* 2003;327:1254–1257.
47. Rigotti NA, Munafo MR, Stead LF. Smoking cessation interventions for hospitalized smokers. *Arch Intern Med.* 2008;168(18):1950–1960.
48. Smith P, Burgess E. Smoking cessation initiated during hospital stay for patients with coronary artery disease: a randomized controlled trial. *CMAJ.* 2009;180(13):1297–1303.
49. Mohiuddin SM, Mooss AN, Hunter CB, et al. Intensive smoking cessation intervention reduces mortality in high-risk smokers with cardiovascular disease. *Chest.* 2007;131:446–452.
50. Chow CK, Jolly S, Rao-Melacini P, et al. Association of diet, exercise, and smoking modification with risk of early cardiovascular events after acute coronary syndromes. *Circulation.* 2010;121:750–758.
51. Bullen C. Impact of tobacco smoking and smoking cessation on cardiovascular risk and disease. *Expert Rev Cardiovasc Ther.* 2008;6(6):883–895.

PATIENT AND FAMILY INFORMATION FOR:
Smoking Cessation

As a cardiac patient who smokes, you have an urgent need to understand not only how much cigarettes endanger your survival but also how rapidly and thoroughly stopping smoking will improve your health and outcome. For patients with coronary heart disease, quitting smoking produces a 36% reduction in death from any cause. As you well know, cigarette addiction can be very intense for many people. However, despite the intensity of this addiction, with your determination and a little help from medication and behavioral techniques, you will really succeed.

HOW DOES IT BEGIN?

You most likely began smoking as a teenager, when you were very vulnerable to the addictive properties of nicotine. You tried a cigarette and found that it gave you a certain degree of confidence and pleasure. That feeling came from a substance called dopamine, which the nicotine in cigarette smoke causes to be released in the brain. Quickly, as you developed tolerance to nicotine, you found that to get the same effect you needed two cigarettes. Eventually, you found that you needed a cigarette to get going in the morning. Nowadays, it is hard to function without that morning cigarette and maybe a cup of coffee. The discomfort before that first cigarette in the morning is called withdrawal and when you first felt it you were hooked.

WHY CAN SOME PEOPLE STOP "COLD TURKEY" AND I CAN'T?

The level of addiction varies from person to person. It is determined genetically, by how your body handles nicotine, the addicting substance in the cigarette. Some people can be "social" smokers and just have an occasional cigarette. They experience the harmful effects of the cigarette, but they are not addicted. Their bodies handle nicotine differently. They do not have the genetic makeup that causes them to be susceptible to the addictive properties of nicotine. Why is this important to understand? Accepting that your smoking is an addiction is a heavy burden, but it is important for you and your loved ones to understand it, accept it, and look forward to getting you the help you need to quit.

HOW DO YOU KNOW IF YOU ARE ADDICTED?

The easiest way to know if you are addicted to cigarettes is to ask yourself how soon after you wake up you have your first cigarette. If it is within minutes, you are very addicted and quitting may be tough for you. We therefore suggest that for you, quitting will be most successful if you combine medication with behavioral changes. Participating in a program with ongoing support such as a smoking cessation clinic is likely to be a major help.

WHAT IS NICOTINE WITHDRAWAL?

Nicotine withdrawal is a real physical brain dysfunction. You cannot do your day's work. You get irritable, unable to concentrate. What makes cigarettes so addicting is that within 10 seconds of smoking, not only is that uncomfortable feeling gone, but you experience real pleasure.

IS IT TOO LATE TO QUIT?

Absolutely not! Much of the effect of smoking on the heart and circulation is reversible and, within 3 years of quitting, the risk for recurrent coronary events becomes that of someone who never smoked. The benefits begin immediately. Within hours of quitting smoking, the CO that poisons your oxygen delivery system and the chemically induced tightening of your blood vessels dissipates.

An important part of what happens when a person has a heart attack is caused by the development of clot in the coronary arteries. That is why your doctor is giving you medicines such as aspirin and other anticoagulants to thin your blood. Smoking, however, causes your blood to clot and that effect is not blocked by aspirin. The clotting system is so sensitive to the effect of smoking that even one cigarette can disrupt it. It is therefore very important to understand that it is not enough to cut down on your smoking. You must quit entirely. Even one cigarette endangers your survival. The good news is that your clotting system renews itself very well and fairly rapidly such that the benefits of quitting begin almost immediately.

Smoking also contributes to vascular damage over the years; damage not just to your coronary arteries but to all the vessels in your body. If you are also diabetic, this effect is further enhanced with an increased risk of blindness, kidney damage, stroke, and loss of limb.

HOW DO I STOP?

There are two parts of this process: medication for the physical withdrawal and behavioral change for the habit.

You may be disturbed by the idea of taking another medication and believe that you can do this without pharmacologic support. The truth is, if you are addicted, you double your chance of success with treatment, and stopping smoking is as important for your cardiac health as taking some of your cardiac medications, ACE inhibitors, or ß-blockers.

MEDICATION

Your doctor will speak with you about using medication to help with nicotine withdrawal. It may be a nicotine patch or gum or even an inhaler, a medication called bupropion that can be used with or without nicotine replacement or varenicline that is used alone.

If you have been a heavy smoker and are using Nicotine Replacement Therapy (NRT), you will need higher doses of nicotine replacement or possibly a combination of medications such as the patch and gum. If you used nicotine replacement before and felt that it did not help, be aware that the dose must be just right for you. Also, it may seem strange to take nicotine to quit smoking when it is nicotine that you are trying to get away from. The reason this works is that the patch satisfies your need for nicotine without giving you any pleasure. It also breaks the ritual of the smoking habit, doubling your chance of success. As you become comfortable not smoking, the dose of nicotine is gradually reduced and finally stopped.

Your doctor may prescribe a medicine called bupropion that helps with the desire to smoke, cravings as well as with depression. If you have been depressed, it is important to let your doctor know because bupropion may be very helpful.

There is also a newer, highly effective medicine for stopping smoking called varenicline. It may cause nausea and strange dreams, but after taking it for 7 days you will not feel like smoking. You continue to take varenicline for several months. Unfortunately, some people can become very depressed and even suicidal while taking varenicline. Your doctor may ask a family member to be aware of this and monitor you for any change of mood. If you do experience any change of mood, you need to stop varenicline immediately and speak to your doctor. Although warnings of mood change and depression are concerning, the effectiveness of this drug is very real. You and your doctor need to discuss this option in light of previous quit attempts, level of addiction, and the vulnerability of your cardiac status.

No matter which pharmacotherapy you use, a year later the relapse rate is the same. Something more is needed to remain smoke free and this is called behavioral therapy—learning new life skills to cope with the issues that made you want to smoke is the first place.

WHAT IS THE BEHAVIORAL PART OF MY TREATMENT?

In addition to dealing with the nicotine withdrawal, you must have a plan for handling the behavioral part of your addiction. Do you use cigarettes for stress, boredom, anger, pleasure, socializing? It is important to look at the reasons for your smoking to plan a lifetime change, not just while you are taking medication but a whole new approach to handling those situations that make you want to smoke.

Develop a clear plan for limiting your stress and avoiding situations that upset you. Exercise regularly, giving yourself real rewards. Put relaxation into your day. Develop hobbies that you can substitute for the pleasure that you derived from cigarettes: music, reading, meditation, yoga, sketching, deep breathing, or whatever gives you pleasure. Bring a magazine to work for what used to be your smoking break. Have a game on your cell phone to play when you are waiting for the bus.

Some tips to avoid smoking are as follows:

- Develop a list of activities that you can use to keep yourself busy happy and relaxed.
- Don't let anyone interfere with or endanger your success. No one can smoke around you!
- Avoid alcohol; it is the strongest trigger.
- For some coffee is a trigger. Get a substitute, tea or juice or chocolate at least for the first day, to change your routine and make it easier to quit.
- Purchase healthy snacks and keep them on hand to relieve the cravings and avoid weight gain.

Pick a quit day and have all your tools ready to go. Choose a busy, nonstressful day, have no cigarettes in the house, throw out all your ashtrays. Keep very busy and go to bed early.

Cigarette addiction can be overcome, but it never goes completely away, even as your body becomes much healthier. If you do have a relapse, get back to your plan immediately. Relapse is very common, but it is best to think of it as a learning opportunity—how you could handle that situation differently in the future. It is all part of the process of becoming smoke free.

An Integrative Behavioral Approach for Adopting a Healthy Lifestyle After the Diagnosis of Heart Disease

John is a 53-year-old lawyer and father of two teenage girls. Recently, John has experienced arm pain on a number of occasions while driving his car. His father had died of a heart attack at the age of 57. Concerned that his symptoms may represent heart disease, John makes an appointment to see a cardiologist. On physical examination, John is found to have normal findings except for mild elevation in his blood pressure and excess weight. He is 5 feet 8 inches and weighs 190 pounds. His resting electrocardiogram is normal. Because of the concern for heart disease, his physician orders blood work and a coronary artery calcium scan. The latter is ordered to assess if there is direct evidence of any atherosclerotic build-up in John's coronary arteries. John's blood work reveals an elevated cholesterol level and a borderline elevation in his blood sugar level. His coronary calcium score is substantial elevated (score of 620), thus indicating the presence of extensive underlying atherosclerosis in John's coronary arteries. A stress test is subsequently ordered. The test reveals that John is quite deconditioned but as the test is normal, John's physician informs him that consideration of a coronary stent placement or bypass surgery is currently not necessary. However, he advises John that it is important that he now work to control his risk factors for heart disease. Motivated by his newly discovered risk, John tells his physician he wants to do "whatever it takes." John is placed on blood pressure and cholesterol-lowering medication and is told to go on a heart-healthy weight loss diet and to start exercising. In the past, however, John has not been successful in initiating a better diet and exercise and even sometimes forgets to take prescribed medications. Now that John is at risk, how can he be assisted in doing "whatever it takes"?

Heart disease is the most common chronic disease and the leading cause of death in the United States and other industrialized countries. Each year, >800,000 people die from heart disease in the United States and >1.2 million have either a new or recurrent heart attack. Since the 1960s, major risk factors for heart disease have been identified. The ones most commonly assessed and targeted for treatment include high blood pressure, high cholesterol, diabetes, smoking, obesity, and lack of exercise. The treatment of cardiac risk factors can slow the progression of heart disease and decrease the possibility of heart attack or fatal cardiac events.

It is often hard for people to fully adopt the lifestyles that can help prevent the progression of heart disease. Some patients become highly motivated to change their diet and start exercising after a heart attack, but then wane in their enthusiasm for maintaining their new health habits over time. Many other patients succeed in taking medications to control risk factors for heart disease but do not succeed in initiating behaviors that require a frank change in lifestyle. A surprising number of patients even find it difficult to just take the medications that have been ordered by their physicians.[1]

Generally people need guidance and help in adopting healthier lifestyles after the diagnosis of heart disease. Accordingly, this chapter will serve as a primer for physicians and patients alike regarding the full context of behavioral changes that can be adopted to promote a healthier lifestyle.

RISK FACTORS FOR HEART DISEASE

Besides the traditional behavior risk factors for heart disease (poor diet, lack of exercise, and smoking), over time a wide variety of other behaviors and psychosocial factors have been linked to the development of heart disease. These factors are listed in Table 38.1 and discussed below.

LACK OF ADEQUATE REST AND RELAXATION

The importance of rest and relaxation is being increasingly studied by physicians. A large category in this domain is sleep problems, which can be divided into three principal forms: (1) sleep apnea and other forms of sleep disordered breathing problems; (2) chronic insomnia; and (3) a voluntary restriction of sleep time. Both sleep apnea and insomnia can adversely affect health but the medical effects of undue voluntary sleep loss have only been recently delineated. Experimental work indicates that when volunteers are asked to curtail their sleep by 2 hours per night, a stress response is elicited in the body, consisting of diminished insulin sensitivity, increase in evening cortisol levels, and production of inflammatory proteins.[2,3] In addition, short sleep has been linked to increase in appetite and weight. In part, this effect is due to a reduction in the secretion of an appetite suppressing hormone called leptin and an increase in an appetite stimulating hormone called ghrelin as people get less sleep.[4] Recent epidemiologic data now also link short sleep to adverse clinical events.[5,6] These results are of increasing interest because our society as a whole obtains less sleep than yesteryear. In 1960, the mean sleep time for Americans averaged around 8 hours per night but currently only averages approximately 6.5 hours per night.

TABLE 38.1	Spectrum of Behavioral Risk Factors for Heart Disease

"Traditional" behavioral factors

1. Overeating and poor nutritional habits
2. Lack of physical activity
3. Smoking

Non traditional risk factors

1. Rest and relaxation
   Poor sleep or voluntary sleep loss
   Lack of unwinding
2. Chronic stress
   Work stress
   Marital stress and dissatisfaction
   Caregiver strain
   Effects of trauma and abuse
   Pool socioeconomic status
3. Chronic negative thought and emotional patterns
   Depressive syndromes
   Anxiety syndromes and worry
   Hostility and anger
   Worry
   Rumination
   Pessimism
   Perfectionism
4. Unmet psychological needs
   Need for purpose
   Need for social connectedness

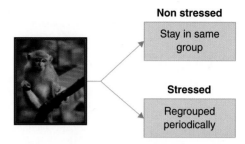

Figure 38.1. Use of cynomolgus monkeys to study the effects of chronic stress. Cynomolgus monkeys develop atherosclerosis in a manner pathologically similar to humans. When grouped together, male monkeys fight with each other until a clear pecking order is established. If the monkeys are regrouped every few months, fighting continually ensues.

Difficulty in unwinding is also an increasingly studied area that has become more relevant as modern technology makes it possible and often routine for individuals to continue work after hours. Although more study is needed, a series of studies have now demonstrated an increase in clinical events among individuals who report difficulty in unwinding after work.[7,8] Difficulty in unwinding after work may be physical or psychological in nature. Physically impaired unwinding is most commonly because of continued involvement in work on nights and weekends or demanding domestic duties after work. Psychologically impaired unwinding may be due to physiological arousal resulting from undue worry or rumination about work or other matters after leaving one's job.

CHRONIC STRESS

Modern medical science has identified the presence of a strong link between chronic stress and heart disease. Chronic stress

is unique among psychosocial stresses because it can be easily produced and well quantified in animals. An important animal species in this regard is cynomolgus monkeys. This is because these animals develop atherosclerosis in a manner that is similar to humans. The experimental production of stress in such monkeys is based on their social tendencies.[9] Specifically, when male monkeys are placed into a new group, they fight with each other until a pecking order from most dominant to submissive monkeys has been established. A stable order then ensues. However, if male monkeys are regrouped into new groups every few months, a situation of chronic stress is established (Figure 38.1). Male dominant monkeys who live under such stress are found upon necropsy to have substantially more atherosclerosis than their submissive counterparts or males that live in stable social groups[9] (Figure 38.2).

Over time, the mechanisms that account for the increased risk for atherosclerosis under conditions of chronic stress has been identified (Figure 38.3). Chronic stress is associated with a continuously elevated stimulation of two central brain systems: the hypothalamic–pituitary–adrenocortical (HPA) axis and the sympathetic nervous system (SNS) system.[10] This stimulation results in elevated secretion of two "stress hormones": cortisol and norepinephrine. Such chronic hormonal elevations are highly detrimental to health, resulting in metabolic abnormalities that favor the development of hypertension,[11] insulin resistance (a precursor to diabetes),[12] increased storage of fat in the abdomen,[13] elevation in inflammatory proteins within the body,[14,15] a tendency to increased coagulabilty of the blood,[16] and a pathologic state of the inner lining of blood vessels (the "endothelium") that prevents these blood vessels from properly vasodilating during periods of stress (a condition termed

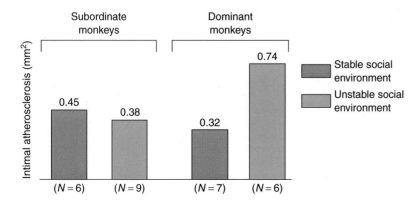

Figure 38.2. The comparison of the measured amount of atherosclerosis (plotted on the vertical axis) when the cynomolgus monkeys came to necropsy. Despite each monkey having been fed exactly the same controlled diet, the dominant male monkeys who had been living in the unstable social environment condition developed substantially more atherosclerosis than the other monkey groups.

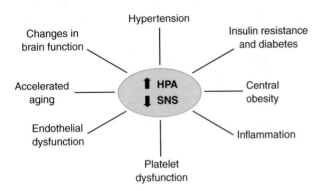

Figure 38.3. The chronic activation of the hypothalamic–pituitary–adrenocortical (HPA) axis and the sympathetic nervous system (SNS) that is associated with chronic stress sets the stage for health damaging sequelae. The principal mechanisms by which chronic stress is health damaging is shown here.

"endothelial dysfunction").[17] Chronic stress can also promote ovarian dysfunction.[18]

Among other effects, people under chronic stress are more likely to become physiologic "hyperreactors," meaning that there is a tendency for heart rate and blood pressure responses to rise higher and recover more slowly following acute stimulations compared with people who are not under stress.[19] More recently, Epel et al.[20] have demonstrated that people under chronic stress are more likely to suffer from DNA evidence of accelerated aging, and McEwen[21] demonstrated that chronic stress can cause adverse remodeling of the brain: an increase in size of the amygdala (the brain's fear center), and reduction in the size of the hippocampus (involved in regulating long-term memory and other functions) and the prefrontal cortical regions of the brain (regulating "executive functions") (Figure 38.4).

Many forms of chronic stress have been documented to cause heart disease and/or reduce longevity, including work stress, marital strain, and caregiver stress. However, in understanding stress, it is important to distinguish between stress that is "good" and "bad." As depicted in Figure 38.5, whether a given life challenge is viewed as "good" or "bad" may depend on a number of factors, including the intensity of the stress, how manageable or controllable it is, how meaningful the stress experience is relative to one's value systems and the chronicity of stress. For

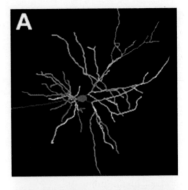

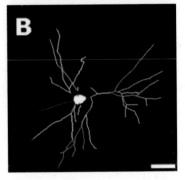

Figure 38.4. Illustration of the amount of dendrites in neurons of the hippocampus present at baseline (**A**) and after the experimental induction of chronic stress (**B**). Similar functional atrophy occurs within the prefrontal cortex during chronic stress. By contrast, chronic stress causes growth and expansion of dendrites in the neurons of the brain's fear center, the amygdala. (Figure provided by McEwen BS).

example, two people having the same amount of challenge in providing caregiving for an incapacitated elderly person may experience the challenge quite differently according to whether they find the experience to be personally meaningful or not. The more worthwhile the caregiving is viewed, the less likely there is to be early burnout.

When stress is well handled, it builds people's coping skills, sense of self-mastery, and self-esteem. By contrast, as stress becomes more uncontrollable and prolonged, there is increasing likelihood that the chronic stress response that is outlined in Figure 38.3 will ensue.

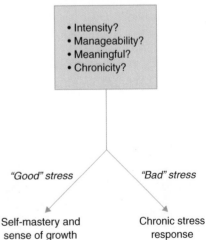

Figure 38.5. Important determinants of how challenging stresses are perceived and their consequential effects include the intensity of the stress, whether it is manageable or feels uncontrollable, how meaningful the stress is, and the chronicity of the stress. Stress that is favorably handled and is viewed as fitting into a meaningful purpose tends to build individual's personal resources (e.g., sense of self-mastery and desire for growth) and thus has the connotation of being "good stress." In contrast, unrelenting or uncontrollable stress that is not viewed as meaningful is viewed as "bad stress" and has the capacity to evoke a chronic stress response.

CHRONICALLY NEGATIVE THOUGHT PATTERNS AND EMOTIONS

The presence of chronic negative emotions—chronic depression and chronic anxiety in particular and chronic negative thought patterns such as worry, hostility, and pessimism are health-damaging. Depression has been the most studied of the common negative emotional states. Depressive orders can vary from mild to severe. Major depression—characterized by a severely depressed mood, loss of interest, or pleasure in most activities, and somatic symptoms such as fatigue and insomnia—is a particularly disabling disorder that at any one time is present in approximately 5% of Americans. By contrast, major depression is consistently noted in approximately 15% of cardiac patient populations and another 15% have lesser but still concerning depressive symptoms.[10] Thus, nearly one-third of cardiac patients have some level of depressive symptoms. This association is due to a bidirectional relationship between depression and heart disease: depression is a direct causative risk factor for heart disease but chronic illnesses such as heart disease can also help precipitate or worsen depressive symptoms in some patients. Study indicates a gradient relationship between the magnitude of depressive symptoms and the risk for adverse clinical outcomes (Figure 38.6).[22]

The mechanisms by which chronic depression causes heart disease is not dissimilar to mechanism by which chronic stress causes disease, but some difference in mechanisms is present. Like chronic stress, chronic depression is associated with high cortisol and norepinephrine secretion, resulting in insulin resistance and a threefold increased risk for diabetes, the development of abdominal obesity, elevation in inflammatory proteins, the development of platelet dysfunction, and presence of endothelial dysfunction.[23–29] These changes combine to accelerate the development and progression of atherosclerosis. In addition, female patients experiencing chronic depression are at increased risk for developing osteoporosis[30,31] (Figure 38.7). Thus, it is not surprising that epidemiologic study indicates that chronic depression is as potent as hypertension, diabetes, smoking, and other CAD risk factors in promoting heart disease.[19]

Anxiety syndromes that have now been strongly linked to heart disease include general anxiety disorder,[32] phobic anxiety,[33] panic disorder,[34] and posttraumatic stress disorder.[35] Another commonly studied negative thought–emotion complex that has been linked to heart disease has been chronic anger and/or hostility.[36] More recently, there has been consistent study demonstrating the negative health effects of pessimism.[37–40] In addition, pending further study, chronic worry,[41] rumination,[42] and even perfectionism[43,44] are additional factors that have been preliminary linked to either a heightened frequency of clinical disease or to disturbances in the normal functioning of human physiology.

SATISFACTION OF PSYCHOLOGICAL NEEDS

Humans have unique basic psychological needs.[45–48] The satisfaction of these needs produces a sense of vitality—an energetic sense that is pleasing to people (Figure 38.8). By contrast, the failure to meet basic psychological needs produces a sense of dissatisfaction or tension. The feeling of dissatisfaction or tension resulting from failure to meet one's basic psychological needs may be hard to identify because these feelings may be vague and muted and easily attributable to other factors. Nevertheless, increasing medical data indicate that the failure to satisfy basic psychological needs can be health-damaging.

Theorists vary on what constitutes the gamut of basic psychological needs.[45–48] However, there is unanimity that one of these needs is the need for social connectedness. The earliest large-scale epidemiologic study to this issue was the Alameda Country study, published in 1979.[49] That study, which followed healthy residents over a period of years, found that longevity during follow-up was inversely related to the number of social connections that people had: those with the least number of social connections had the shortest longevity, and those with the highest number of social connections had the longest longevity in this study. Many subsequent epidemiologic studies have established that quality of one's social life is a strong long-term predictor of health.

An increasingly studied basic psychological need is the need for a sense of purpose. This need was first popularized by Victor Frankl,[46] a psychiatrist who survived the Holocaust. In his seminal book on his experiences, he noted that those who had a sense of meaning while trying to survive within Nazi concentration camps had a greater chance of doing so. A number of

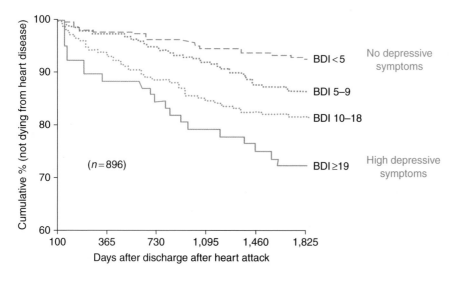

Figure 38.6. After sustaining a heart attack, 896 patients were assessed for the presence of depressive symptoms and then followed up for 5 years (1,825 days). Depression was measured by a questionnaire, the Beck Depression Inventory (BDI), with low scores (<5) indicating that no depressive symptoms were present. Progressively higher BDI scores are indicative of increasing depression. The vertical axis indicates the percent of patients who did *not* die from heart disease during the next 5 years. Survival was highest in those without depressive symptoms. As depressive symptoms increased, so too did the percentage of patients who died from heart disease in the next 5 years following their heart attack. (Reproduced from Lesperance F, Frasure-Smith N, Talajiv M, et al. Five-year risk of cardiac mortality in relation to initial severity and one-year changes in depression symptoms after myocardial infarction. *Circulation.* 2002;105:1049–1053, with permission.)

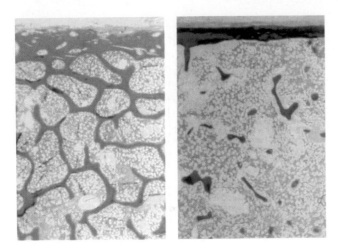

Figure 38.7. Case examples of two matched 40-year women, one with depression and one without depression, who had bone biopsies of the anterior iliac crest. The biopsy from the woman without depression is on the left and that from the women with depression is on the right. (Reproduced by permission from Macmillan Publishers Ltd: Gold PW, Chrousos GP. Organization of the stress system and its dysregulation in melancholic and atypical depression: high *vs* low CRH/NE states. *Mol Psychiatry.* 2002;7:254–275.)

recent epidemiologic studies have now linked the presence or absence of a sense of life purpose to health outcomes (Figure 38.9).[50–52] Various other basic psychological needs are operative in individuals, such as a need for autonomy and a need to feel self-competent, but prospective epidemiologic study is needed to assess the potential impact of these needs on human health.

POSITIVE FACTORS

Since the advent of modern epidemiologic study, medical studies focused on the health damaging effects of negative psychosocial factors. In recent years, however, there has been an increasing focus on the health-promoting effects of positive psychosocial factors. This research has found that positive psychosocial factors are health buffering, improving human physiologic functioning, and improving longevity as indicated in a recent summary of 70 studies.[53] Thus, many psychological factors are more properly measured along a continuum from negative to positive. For example, just like pessimists have a reduced lifespan, those who are optimists have an increased

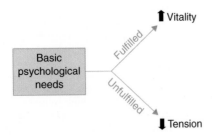

Figure 38.8. People have universal basic psychological needs such as the need to have a sense of purpose in life and the need to feel socially connected to others. When these needs are fulfilled, they produce a sense of energizing vitality. If these needs are not met, they produce a vague sense of dissatisfaction and tension.

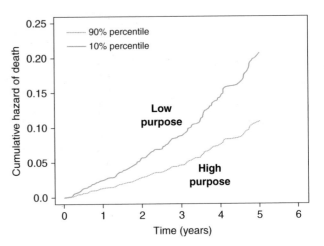

Figure 38.9. An example of a study that evaluated the health effects of having or not having a sense of purpose is shown in this figure. Shown on the vertical axis is the cumulative hazard of death during 5 years of follow-up among 1,238 elderly individuals who were divided according to their reported sense of life purpose at baseline (high vs. low). Among those with a high sense of life purpose, the hazard ratio for mortality was approximately 57% lower than those with a low sense of purpose. (Reproduced from Boyle PA, Barnes LL, Buchman AS, et al. Purpose in life is associated with mortality among community-dwelling older persons. *Psychosom Med.* 2009;71:575–579, with permission.)

lifespan compared with those individuals who are intermediate between optimism and pessimism.[37–40]

HELPING JOHN

John's physician is attuned to screening for psychosocial factors that can affect patients' health. He is aware that considering and counseling patients in accordance with psychosocial influences and principles that can affect health behaviors improves his ability to help his patients. After discussing John's exercise and diet habits, his physician also asks John about the quality of his sleep and his ability to unwind after work and on weekends, how energetic John generally feels, whether he feels under pressure at work or at home, whether he has someone to turn to for support, how his general mood has been, and his overall sense of life balance. He also asks John how confident he feels about making the recommended changes in his diet and physical activity.

John responds by explaining that he has always been a hard-driving and successful lawyer, but over the last 2 years his firm has been downsizing and is feeling increasing competitive pressures. As a result, he has been working longer hours. John has gotten into the habit of checking his e-mails, working using the Web, and surfing the Web for pleasure at night. As a consequence, he always gets to bed at least 1 hour later than he would like. John tends to feel less energetic and sometimes even light-headed in the late afternoon. He has made several attempts to get going with an exercise program, but it always peters out. His last real vacation was more than 2 years ago. It is clear from John's description that he is experiencing substantial work stress and a sense of chronic time pressure.

With this added knowledge, an integrated health plan can be devised for John, which takes cognizance not only of the specific health behaviors that he has to initiate, such as starting an exercise program, but also of the larger psychosocial factors that need to be addressed for John to become successful in improving his health and reducing his risk for developing a future heart attack.

UNDERSTANDING THE DETERMINANTS OF BEHAVIORAL CHANGE

The ability to change our behaviors does not occur in a vacuum. Examples of factors that can influence our ability to change our behaviors include the "mood" we are in, our level of energy, and how stressed or time pressed we feel. A basic approach to changing any behavior can be organized around three basic questions that you should ask yourself (Figure 38.10): (1) How motivated are you to initiate your new behavioral goal? (2) Do you have the right plan and principles in place for "executing" your new goal? and (3) What can you do to maintain your new health behavior over the long term? Examples of approaches to help you address each of these questions are discussed below.

AM I MOTIVATED?

It takes motivation to initiate new health practices. As a first step, you have to decide whether what you are planning to take on is something that you truly want to do, or whether you are doing it only because your doctor or a significant other wants you to do so. It is human nature to be more enrolled when a given choice is made of your own volition. The concept of choosing a goal based on your own volition rather than being told by someone else what to do is termed autonomy by behavioral scientists.

Important research has indicated that when a patient leaves the doctor's office with a sense of autonomy regarding a suggested health goal, greater adherence to the health goal occurs over time.[54,55] For instance, let us say your physician wants you to lose weight, provides you with good reasons to do so, and prescribes a certain diet approach. If the doctor is attuned to the concept of autonomy, the doctor may then pause and ask you, "*Based on what I have just told you, do you see a reason why you might personally want to lose weight?*" If you identify a reason, your physician may then further ask, "*Are you okay with the plan I am suggesting for losing your weight or do you have another idea that might work for you?*"

If your physician does not bring up such questions, it is still helpful to raise these questions to yourself and even discuss your thoughts with your physician if the situation is conducive for such a conversation. The more you embrace a suggested health goal and the plan for its execution based on your own volition rather than outside influences, the more you are likely to be successful.

Another foundational principle in spurring motivation is aligning your goal with your belief that you can accomplish the goal. Health professionals refer to this belief as self-efficacy. Study indicates that the more someone believes that a certain goal can be accomplished (i.e., the greater their sense of self-efficacy), the more that person is willing to try to succeed.[56]

Practically, this means that you should modulate your health goals towards "small wins" that you know that you can achieve. For example, let us say your physician tells you that you need to lose 30 pounds. If you do not believe you can lose this amount of weight, you should be frank about this and modulate your goal according to whatever minimal weight loss you think is a reasonable goal for yourself. There should be, however, some "stretch" beyond your comfort zone in trying to achieve new health goals—just not too much.

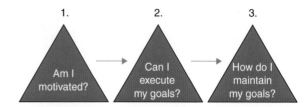

Figure 38.10. Three key questions to address in developing a plan for successful behavioral change.

Modulating health goals to meet one's sense of self-efficacy works, in part, because behavioral change is frequently nonlinear. That is, small changes in health behaviors at the outset can lead to progressively larger changes later. However, if one does not get "on the playing field," success is not possible. Based on the recommendations of medical societies,[57] patients may read or hear from their physicians that they should obtain a minimum of 30 minutes of moderate intensity (endurance) exercise 5 days per week.

However, if this aerobic goal is too difficult for you, beginning with a goal that is as minimal as 5 minutes of dedicated physical activity per day may be all that it takes to get you "on the playing field" towards progressive growth in exercise activity.

DO I HAVE A GOOD PLAN FOR EXECUTING MY HEALTH GOAL?

There is an old saying that "the road to hell is paved with good intentions." This saying reflects the fact that motivation itself is generally not sufficient to accomplish a given goal. Although being motivated is a foundational step, behavioral science indicates that lack of success in achieving an intended goal is more often the result of lack of adequate execution in the pursuit of that desired goal. This lack of execution can be due to many factors.

One of the common causes for poor success in this regard is difficulty in balancing multiple life priorities and thus feeling time-pressed. Time pressure can plan an important role in distorting how competing life goals are valued. This distortion is because of a universal human tendency to *overvalue* goals that are *present-centered* and *undervalue* goals that are *future-oriented* (Figure 38.11). This phenomenon is termed temporal discounting by behavioral scientists.

Temporal discounting is particularly relevant with respect to the execution of health goals. When physicians discuss health goals with patients, these discussions are frequently held in the abstract, without consideration of patients' other real-life priorities. That is, after patients leave the confines of their doctors' offices, upon return to their daily routine, health goals face competition with patients' other goals and responsibilities. Health goals are commonly not perceived as pressing as other daily life obligations such as work deadlines or important family obligations.

To illustrate this essential point, let us say your physician has advised you to lose weight on discovering that you are borderline hypertensive and have a mildly elevated blood sugar level, as is the case with John. While you are in the doctor's office, you sincerely embrace your physician's advice and leave the office convinced, along with your physician, that you will start a

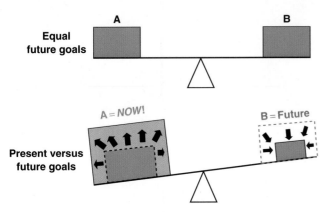

Figure 38.11. Schematic representation of the impact of temporal discounting on goal pursuit. Suppose two goals "A" and "B" are deemed of equal weight when considered in the abstract, without any consideration of any temporal issues. However, if goal "A" is a present-centered goal (e.g., a work deadline that is due now) and goal "B" is not, goal "A" will tend to be overvalued in its importance, and goal "B" will tend to become undervalued in its importance relative to when these goals were considered in the abstract. This type of temporal influence is commonplace, can be strong in influence, and may exert its effects nonconsciously.

new diet plan that your physician has suggested. However, at work the day after your doctor's visit, pressing job deadlines may loom large and thus assume greater value for *that day* while losing weight on that day is downplayed, under the rationalization: *"My weight will lead to serious health problems over time but it will not make much difference if I start tomorrow instead of today."*

Quite often, that same scenario is replayed the next day and the next and that "tomorrow" never comes.

When the phenomenon of temporal discounting is recognized and dealt with, a more realistic and successful program to initiate behavioral change can be accomplished. Of note, the technological advances of modern life, such as e-mail and text messaging, cell phone use, Internet use and the like, have the propensity to inadvertently increase the degree to which people temporally discount, owing to their tendency to make routine daily matters appear or become more important and urgent.

Implementation intentions. One of the approaches to dealing with temporal discounting is to rely on the use of "implementation intentions." Implementation intentions are conditional statements that were developed and tested in research that was devised by Peter Gollwitzer and colleagues.[58] They take the following formation: *"When it is X, I will do Y"* (Figure 38.12). "X" in this formulation is an external cue, such as a given time of day or a given situation, such as the completion of work.

To illustrate the use of implementation intentions, consider a woman who has been advised to periodically perform breast self-examination because of a family history of breast cancer. This woman may declare an implementation intention such as, *"When I take my shower on Sunday nights, then I will perform my breast self-examination."* Research indicates that women who are asked to form an implementation intention concerning breast self-examination at the time of being counseled about this health practice comply more frequently compared with women who are similarly counseled but are not asked to form an implantation intention[59] (Figure 38.13). Extensive other research

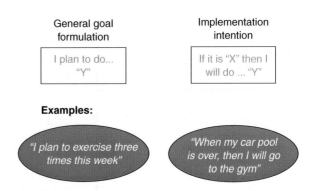

Figure 38.12. Comparison of a generally formulated goal versus that designed as an implementation intention. Implementation intentions lead to specific goal plans based on a preagreed external cue for the desired goal behavior. The cue, for example, can be a specific time, place, or designated situation.

has demonstrated the utility of implementation for improving the execution of many other health and/or other life goals.[60]

Implementation intentions were devised, in part, as a technique to deal with the recognition that new behaviors are essentially "practices" that are generally vulnerable to such factors as time pressure, stress, feelings of fatigue or boredom with a new practice. This is in contradistinction to our habits, which are ingrained and automatic. Implementation intentions make new practices function similar to habits in that they force us to rely on preagreed external cues instead of continually negotiating our competing agendas in our head such as, *"Do I have enough time?"* or *"Am I too tired for this?"* However, for implementation intentions to work, there first has to be a reasonably high level of motivation in place.

Self-monitoring. Another approach to improving execution of a health goal is to commit to self-monitoring actions that can be

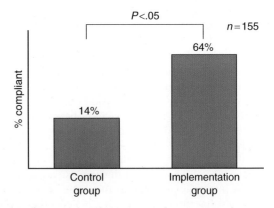

Figure 38.13. Example of the results of a study that assessed the value of implementation: 155 women were randomized into two groups that received a lecture on the importance of breast self-examination. One-half of these subjects were in addition asked to form an implementation intention regarding breast self-examination before they left the lecture (implementation group) and the other half were not (control group). A survey 1 month later reveals substantially greater compliance with the behavioral injunction to perform breast self-examination within the implementation group compared with the control group. (Adapted from Orbeil S, Hodgldns S, Sheeran P. Implementation intentions and the theory of planned behavior. *Pers Soc Psychol Bull.* 1997;23:945.)

performed on a daily basis. Such actions serve to anchor health goals by providing specific measurable results that can be followed by patients. Self-monitoring can also provide a measure of daily self-awareness that helps to counter the tendency to forget about one's health goals because they are generally not as immediately pressing as work or other life goals.

An obvious method of self-monitoring is using a scale to weigh oneself daily. Studies indicate that overweight individuals who weigh themselves daily are more successful in maintaining weight loss compared to individuals who do not.[61,62] More recently, the use of pedometers as a means of self-monitoring one's physical activity has become increasingly promulgated. Pedometers are portable motion sensor devices that can accurately measure the number of physical steps taken per day by detecting motion at individuals' hips. In recent years, a goal of 10,000 steps per day has gained popularity as a recommended health goal, and a scale of low-to-high daily physical activity has been proposed based on pedometer steps[63] (Table 38.2). In a recent study that summarized the results of 26 medical studies, the use of pedometers was associated with a 27% increase in physical activity compared with physical activity before initiating pedometer use. Pedometer use was also associated with reduction in weight and in blood pressure levels.[64]

However, the goal of 10,000 steps per day should be applied with caution as this goal may not be practical for older adults, those with chronic illnesses, or those who are significantly deconditioned. Rather, for such individuals, an incremental approach towards increased physical activity is best applied. That is, individuals should first wear a pedometer for a number of days without any increase in physical activity, to ascertain one's baseline physical activity level. Then, subjects can be asked to increase their physical activity by a mere 100 to 200 steps per day, with progressive increases according to individuals' sense of what constitutes a reasonable progression of steps for themselves.

HOW CAN I MAINTAIN MY NEW BEHAVIOR OVER THE LONG TERM?

It is quite common for people to initially succeed in losing weight, starting exercise, or other health goals, only to relapse into old behavioral patterns over time. Maintaining a new health goal over the long term can be challenging for a variety of reasons. For instance, as people succeed in an initial goal, they may take their success for granted or lose enthusiasm as the novelty of the new health activity wears off, resulting in sentiments like the following: "W*hen my doctor told me I had developed mild hypertension, I joined the gym and went consistently for 3 months. However, it then became increasingly boring for me. I came to view it as a big grind.*" Other common barriers to long-term maintenance include the development of intervening illness, increasing work stress, new family demands, unexpected life events, and the like. Because breakdowns in initially successful behavioral change are so commonplace, it behooves individuals to develop contingency plans for supporting the long-term maintenance of new health goals. Discussed below are basic support mechanisms that can be put into place.

Creating a "floor" for your health goal. A key aspect of guarding your health goal is to identify a minimum "floor" of activity to maintain your health goal. For instance, let us say you are accustomed to working out at your local gym for 30 to 60 minutes

TABLE 38.2	Preliminary Indices for Classifying Pedometer Use According to Tudor-Locke and Basset[63]
Daily Step Count	*Activity Range*
<5,000 steps	Sedentary
5,000–7,499 steps	Low active
7,500–9,999 steps	Somewhat active
10,000–12,500 steps	Active
>12,500 steps	Highly active

most days of the week. Now owing to various work and travel obligations, your ability to get to the gym has been impaired. However, you previously identified a contingency that at times such as this; you will at least take two 10-minute brisk walks during the course of your daily activities. Keeping to this floor of physical activity ensures that you will remain "on the playing field," making it easier to resume your original health plans after a period of personal difficulty has passed.

Social support. Adequate social support is often an important mediator in the long-term maintenance of new health habits. Medical studies reveal that when social support is lacking, patients experience more difficulty in adhering to their physician's suggested recommendations.[65]

Building appropriate social support is a highly individualist matter that is dependent on many factors, such as one's personal need for social support, time availability, the degree of social opportunities in one's community, and one's recognition as to the value of social support. Some forms of social support may occur naturally such as in the formation of gym friendships. Other forms of social support require effort and initiative such as in finding an appropriate exercise buddy or finding the "right" community or hospital group program for weight loss. Important as it is, the value of social support is one of the arenas that tends to be temporally discounted when people are under substantial work stress or time pressure.

Energy management. Our innate level of vitality is an important determinant of our ability to do hard things. An important phenomenon in this regard was elucidated by Robert Thayer and colleagues[66] some years ago. They asked volunteer subjects to record their energy levels, their level of tension, their moods, and what activities they were doing at different times over a course of days. The results of their research indicated that one's perceived energy level is an important determinant of our moods and various subconscious behaviors (Figure 38.14). Specifically, they found that when people are both tense and tired, the presence of negative moods were more commonplace than at other times and "quick fix" behaviors to reduce tension and/or increase energy such as reaching for a candy bar or a cigarette, or turning towards distracting activities, such as watching television. However, if people were tense but energetic, predominantly positive moods predominated and "quick fix" behaviors were less common.

In other words, when both high-tension and high-energy are both present, our energy level tends to "trump" our stress level relative to our moods and tendency towards quick fix behaviors.

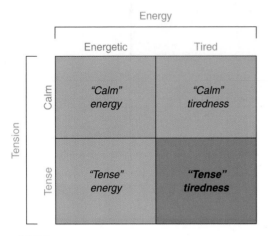

Figure 38.14. Thayer and colleagues proposed a model for linking moods to energy and tension levels based on their experimental study. They found that when people were relatively calm and had either high energy ("calm energy") or felt unenergetic ("calm tiredness"), positive moods prevailed. Under conditions of high tension, relatively positive moods prevailed when individuals still felt energetic ("tense energy"). However, if people had low energy and also felt tense ("tense tiredness"), there was a substantial increase in negative moods and "quick fix" coping behaviors.

However, people are not generally accustomed to consciously monitoring and guarding their energy level. Prophylactically learning how to protect your energy level can be very useful in this regard. Potential prophylaxis can be quite varied, ranging from getting to bed earlier, taking naps, introducing planned diversions that can serve to break up the "grind" of daily work life, learning to downsize the size of one's "to-do" list, and many other potential approaches. A good litmus is to ask yourself on a scale of 1 (lowest) to 10 (highest) how energetic you now feel compared with an extended period when you were younger? If your answer is in the 5 to 7 range or below, you have some work to do. In John's case, his answer had been a "5," indicating that he needed to work on his energy management.

Stress management. The presence of chronic stress poses an important barrier towards successful maintenance of recommended behavioral changes. Besides its direct detrimental effects on health, as discussed earlier in this chapter, chronic stress impairs overall quality-of life by making people more prone to "tense-tiredness" and low-mood states. For instance, data indicate that the frequency of depression is increased threefold among individuals experiencing chronic work stress.[67] Because of its complexity, a full discussion of stress management techniques is beyond the scope of this chapter, but certain principles can be applied generically for its management:

1. *Managing energy first.* As mentioned earlier, increasing your energy can trump reducing your tension as a means for dealing with the tense tiredness that is associated with chronic stress. It is useful in this regard to learn to identify and anticipate your low mood and/or energy points during the day. For example, if you find yourself sagging from work pressure in the late afternoon, a common low point for many people, rather than pushing ahead with your work agenda, you may benefit from taking a 10 to 15 minutes physical or mental breather that is restorative of energy.

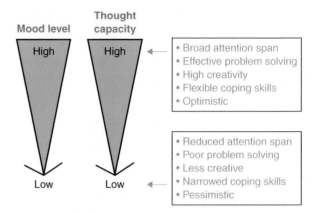

Figure 38.15. As mood levels drop and become negative or depressive, there is a corresponding decrease in the quality of one's overall thinking capacity. Experimental study indicates that high mood tends to be associated with more expansive thinking, characterized by a broader attention span, and other parameters of thinking shown in this figure, and low moods are characterized by thinking that is the opposite.

Learning to catch your progression towards fatigue, however, can be difficult to do when you are caught up in the momentum of your daily work. Rather people tend to commonly rely on quick fix methods to raise energy while working and commonly do so completely subconsciously. Easy methods for boosting energy include the reliance on caffeine or calorie-dense foods, such as candy bars. However, the reliance on such quick fixes is not necessarily inconsequential. For example, in experimental work that compared the effects of ingesting a candy bar with that of a short burst of 5 to 10 minutes of exercise, both produced a short-term increase in energy, but ingestion of the candy bar led to increase in perceived tension 1 to 2 hours later, whereas exercising reduced subsequent tension levels.[68]

2. *Managing the tension associated with chronic stress.* Chronic stress causes a build of tension. The break-up of continuous tension can be physiologically and psychologically beneficial. Of note in this regard, the presence of tension can be reduced without trying to actively manage the *source* of your tension.

Examples of tension reducers include simple breathing and meditation exercises, turning towards entertainment or mental interests that are relaxing, or engaging in social diversions. In addition, individuals may turn to specific forms of stress-reducing physical activities such as yoga and tai-chi.[69–71]

3. *Learning to turn your focus away from stress.* The low mood associated with chronic stress can have secondary negative effects on one's level of thinking, thus causing a negative vicious cycle relative to stress management. In important work, Barbara Fredrickson[72] and associates have demonstrated that when in positive mood states, individuals manifest a broader span of attention, better problem solving, more creativity, higher optimism, greater friendliness, and more flexible thinking patterns. As mood lowers, our thought capacity becomes increasingly restrictive and present-centered (Figure 38.15). Thus, we do not have our best "wits" about us when we are in a low mood.

Paradoxically, however, problems often appear to assume more importance and feel more urgent when we are in a low mood. It is then when people often become intolerant of problems that did not bother them as much when they were in a high mood. This is a very ineffective way of dealing with stress that may serve to make people feel even more tense-tired and stressed. Thus, a useful step in managing stress is learning not to take your thinking so seriously during times of low moods or high stress. Learning to do so requires that you learn how to become an observer of your thinking, so that you can "catch" yourself getting caught up in your negative thinking. However, it is important to emphasize this is a high-level skill that usually requires outside assistance for its development if you are not naturally inclined in this area. Some practitioners in the field of positive psychology can be helpful in this regard.

4. *Stress management counseling.* When stress feels intractable or unmanageable, seeking the advice of trained mental health professionals may be quite helpful. If significant depression and/or anxiety have developed, patients require professional psychotherapeutic counseling and may also be candidates for the use of pharmacologic agents such as selective serotonin reuptake inhibitors, a first-line medication for treating either significant depression or significant anxiety. Notably, just as the field of preventive cardiology emphasizes the early recognition and treatment of traditional risk factors for heart disease such as high blood pressure or physical inactivity, so too, can *early* intervention for problems such as marital or work stress or poor time management be considered as intervention for warding off subsequently greater psychosocial dysfunction and attendant health consequences. Both for physical risk factors and those of a psychosocial nature, *"An ounce of prevention is worth a pound of cure."*

JOHN'S COURSE

After his physician's questioning, the two agreed upon a health strategy. John bought a pedometer and then wore it for a week to establish his baseline steps per day. He averaged only 4,800 steps per day, a clear indication that he was too sedentary. John followed his physician's instruction to start increasing his steps by at least 100 to 200 steps per week. After a few months, John joined a gym and found that he could add more than 2,500 aerobic steps to his daily average by exercising on a treadmill. Within 6 months, John was averaging close to 10,000 steps per day and going to the gym on a regular basis. By 1 year, he was close to 12,000 steps per day.

John's physician helped him to establish a modest weight loss goal: to lose 5 pounds over 6 months. John met with a dietician who helped him understand that he needed to eat more whole grains, fruits, and vegetables, make more use of polyunsaturated fats, and limit his exposure to saturated fats and refined sugars. He applied her tips about controlling his food portions. Of note, John was a habitual "nosher," particularly when tired or when feeling time pressed by his work deadlines. His dietician advised him to not restrain from this eating pattern but to substitute healthier "nosh" foods. Thus, John got his daughter to make him a daily container of carrot sticks and a bag of unsalted and unbuttered air-popped popcorn, and he brought a can of almond butter to work, which he applied sparingly to whole grain crackers as part of his new snack repertoire. John succeeded in losing 7 lb over 6 months on his new diet regimen.

John also realized it would behoove him to do something about his lack of adequate sleep and lack of rest and relaxation. He realized that this would also require him to improve his time management skills. To that end, John bought a book on time management recommended by a friend and also took a 1-day time management seminar. Among the steps deriving from this experience was John's creation of a "not-to-do"

list and increased attention to better delegating some of his activities to his secretarial staff. John found a back room in his office where he could lie down for 10 to 15 minutes in the late afternoon and he used this period to listen to his favorite music on his Ipod. John also took a 10-day vacation with his family and another 6-day vacation with his wife alone. Initially, John found it hard to break his habit of going to sleep too late, but he decided to schedule a late morning start for Wednesdays so that he could sleep in for an extra hour that morning of each week. Eventually, with prodding from his wife, John did succeed in going to sleep half-an-hour earlier on weekday evenings.

Upon his physician visit 1 year later, John was now found to have normal blood pressure and he had lost five additional pounds. His blood sugar level was now also normal, as was his cholesterol level, aided by the use of cholesterol-lowering medication. When asked to re-rate his energy level on a scale of 1 to 10, John now responded a "10." Although John would have preferred not to have heart disease, he also recognized the blessing that had come out of his diagnosis. Although John was now 54, he felt like he was 20 again!

REFERENCES

1. Newby LK, LaPointe NMA, Chen AY, et al. Long-term adherence to evidence-based secondary prevention therapies in coronary artery disease. *Circulation.* 2006;113:203–212.
2. Knuston KL, Speigel K, Penev P, et al. The metabolic consequences of sleep deprivation. *Sleep Med Rev.* 2007;11:163–178.
3. Irwin MR, Wang M, Compomayor CO, et al. Sleep deprivation and activation of morning levels of cellular and genomic markers of inflammation. *Arch Intern Med.* 2006;166:1756–1762.
4. Speigel K, Talasi E, Penev P, et al. Sleep curtailment in healthy young men is associated with decreased leptin levels, elevated ghrelin levels and increased hunger and appetite. *Ann Intern Med.* 2004;141:846–850.
5. Gallicchio L, Kalesan B. Sleep duration and mortality: a systematic review and meta-analysis. *J Sleep Res.* 2009;18(2):145–158.
6. Cappuccio FP, D'Elia L, Strazzullo P, et al. Sleep duration and all-cause mortality: a systematic review and meta-analysis of prospective studies. *Sleep.* 2010;33(5):585–592.
7. Van Amselvoort LGPM, Bultmann IJK, Swaen GMH, et al. Need for recovery after work and the subsequent risk of cardiovascular disease in a working population. *Occup Environ Med.* 2003;60:183–187.
8. Kivimaki M, Leino-Arjas P, Kaila-Kangas L, et al. Is incomplete recovery from work a risk marker of cardiovascular death? Prospective evidence from industrial employees. *Psychosom Med.* 2006;68:402–407.
9. Kaplan JR, Manuck SB, Clarkson TB, et al. Social status, environment and atherosclerosis in cynomolgus monkeys. *Arteriosclerosis.* 1982;2:359–368.
10. Rozanski A, Blumenthal JA, Kaplan J. Impact of psychological factors on the pathogenesis of cardiovascular disease and implications for therapy. *Circulation.* 1999;99:2192–2217.
11. Schnall PL, Schwartz JE, Landsbergis PA, et al. A longitudinal study of job strain and ambulatory blood pressure: results from a three-year follow-up. *Psychosom Med.* 1998;60:697–706.
12. Brunner EJ, Hemmingway H, Walker BR. Adrenocortical, autonomic, and inflammatory causes of the metabolic syndrome: nested case-control study. *Circulation.* 2002;106:2659–2665.
13. Brunner EJ, Chandola T, Marmot MG. Prospective effect of job strain on general and central obesity in the Whitehall II Study. *Am J Epidemiol.* 2007;165:828–837.
14. Kiecolt-Glaser JK, Preacher KJ, MacCallum RC, et al. Chronic stress and age-related increases in the proinflammatory cytokine IL-6. *Proc Natl Acad Sci U S A.* 2003;100:9090–9095.
15. Jain S, Mills PH, Kanel RV. Effects of perceived stress and uplifts on inflammation and coagulability. *Psychophysiology.* 2007;44:154–160.
16. Brydon L, Magid K, Steptoe A, et al. Platelets, coronary heart disease, and stress. *Brain Behav Immun.* 2006;20(2):113–119.
17. Mausbach BT, Roepke SK, Ziegler MG, et al. Association between chronic caregiving stress and impaired endothelial function in the elderly. *J Am Coll Cardiol.* 2010;55:2599–2606.
18. Kaplan JR, Manuck SB. Ovarian dysfunction, stress, and disease: a primate continuum. *ILAR J.* 2004;45:89–115.
19. Rozanski A, Blumenthal JA, Davidson KW, et al. The epidemiology, pathophysiology, and management of psychosocial risk factors in cardiac practice: the emerging field of behavioral cardiology. *J Am Coll Cardiol.* 2005;45:637–651.
20. Epel ES, Blackburn EH, Lin J, et al. Accelerated telomere shortening in response to life stress. *Proc Natl Acad Sci U S A.* 2004;101:17312–17315.
21. McEwen BS. Physiology and neurobiology of stress and adaptation: central role of the brain. *Physiol Rev.* 2007;87:873–904.
22. Lesperance F, Frasure-Smith N, Talajiv M, et al. Five-year risk of cardiac mortality in relation to initial severity and one-year changes in depression symptoms after myocardial infarction. *Circulation.* 2002;105:1049–1053.
23. Koschke M, Boettger MK, Schulz S, et al. Autonomy of autonomic dysfunction in major depression. *Psychosom Med.* 2009;71:852–860.

24. Timonen M, Salmenkaita I, Jokelainen J, et al. Insulin resistance and depressive symptoms in young adult males: findings from Finnish Military Conscripts. *Psychosom Med.* 2007;69:723–728.

25. De Groot M, Anderson R, Freedland KE, et al. Association of depression and diabetes complications: a meta-analysis. *Psychosom Med.* 2001;63:619–630.

26. Vaccarino V, McClure C, Johnson D, et al. Depression, the metabolic syndrome and cardiovascular risk. *Psychosom Med.* 2008;70:40–48.

27. Everson-Rose SA, Lewis TT, Karavolus K, et al. Depressive symptoms and increased visceral fat in middle-aged women. *Psychosom Med.* 2009;71:410–416.

28. Howren MB, Lamkin DM, Suls J. Associations of depression with C-reactive protein, IL-1, and IL-6: a meta-analysis. *Psychosom Med.* 2009;71:171–186.

29. Broadley AJM, Jones CJH, Frenneaux MP. Arterial endothelial function is impaired in treated depression. *Heart.* 2002;88:521–524.

30. Michelson D, Stratakis C, Hill L, et al. Bone mineral density in women with depression. *N Engl J Med.* 1996;335:1176–1181.

31. Gold PW, Chrousos GP. Organization of the stress system and its dysregulation in melancholic and atypical depression: high *vs* low CRH/NE states. *Mol Psychiatry.* 2002;7:254–275.

32. Frasure-Smith N, Lesperance F. Depression and anxiety as predictors of 2-year cardiac events in patients with stable coronary artery disease. *Arch Gen Psychiatry.* 2008;65:62–71.

33. Kawachi I, Colditz GA, Ascherio A, et al. Prospective study of phobic anxiety and risk of coronary heart disease in men. *Circulation.* 1994;89:1992–1997.

34. Smoller JW, Pollack MG, Wassertheil-Smoller S, et al. Panic attacks and risk of incident cardiovascular events among postmenopausal women in the Women's Health Initiative Observational Study. *Arch Gen Psychiatry.* 2007;64:1153–1160.

35. Kubzansky LD, Koenen KC, Spiro A, et al. Prospective study of posttraumatic stress disorder symptoms and coronary heart disease in the normative aging study. *Arch Gen Psychiatry.* 2007;64:109–116.

36. Chida Y, Steptoe A. The association of anger and hostility with future coronary heart disease. *J Am Coll Cardiol.* 2009;59:936–946.

37. Kubzansky LD, Sparrow D, Vokonas P, et al. Is the glass half empty or half full? A prospective study of optimism and coronary heart disease in the normative aging study. *Psychosom Med.* 2001;63:910–916.

38. Giltay EJ, Kamphuis MH, Kalmijn S, et al. Dispositional optimism and the risk of cardiovascular death. *Arch Intern Med.* 2006;166:431–436.

39. Grodbardt BR, Bower JH, Geda YE, et al. Pessimistic, anxious, and depressive personality traits predict all-cause mortality: The Mayo Clinic Cohort Study of Personality and Aging. *Psychosom Med.* 2009;71:491–500.

40. Tindle HA, Chang YF, Kuller LH, et al. Optimism, cynical hostility, and incident coronary heart disease and mortality in the women's health initiative. *Circulation.* 2009;120:656–662.

41. Kubzansky LD, Kawachi I, Spiro A III, et al. Is worrying bad for your heart? A prospective study of worry and coronary heart disease in the Normative Aging Study. *Circulation.* 1997;95:818–824.

42. Glynn LM, Christenfeld N, Gerin W. The role of rumination in recovery from reactivity: cardiovascular consequences of emotional states. *Psychosom Med.* 2002;64:714–726.

43. Wirtz PH, Elsenbruch S, Emini L, et al. Perfectionism and the cortisol response to psychosocial stress in men. *Psychosom Med.* 2007;69:249–255.

44. Fry PS, Debats DL. Perfectionism and the five-factor personality traits as predictors of mortality in older adults. *J Health Psychol.* 2009;14:513–524.

45. Maslow A. *Motivation and Personality.* New York, NY: Harper; 1954.

46. Frankl VE. *Man's Search for Meaning: An Introduction to Logotherapy.* New York, NY: Simon & Schuster; 1959.

47. Ryff CD, Singer B. The contours of positive human health. *Psychol Inq.* 1998;9:1–28.

48. Ryan RM, Deci EL. Self-determination theory and the development, and well-being. *Am Psychol.* 2000;55:68–78.

49. Berkman LF, Syme SL. Social networks, host resistance, and mortality: a nine-year follow-up study of Alameda county residents. *Am J Epidemiol.* 1979;109:186–204.

50. Okamoto K, Tanaka Y. Subjective usefulness and 6-year mortality risks among elderly persons in Japan. *Psychol Sci.* 2004;59B:P246–P249.

51. Boyle PA, Barnes LL, Buchman AS, et al. Purpose in life is associated with mortality among community-dwelling older persons. *Psychosom Med.* 2009;71:575–579.

52. Gruenewald TL, Karlamangla AS, Greendale GA, et al. Feelings of usefulness to others, disability, and mortality in older adults: The MacArthur Study of Successful Aging. *J Gerontol.* 2007;62B:P28–P37.

53. Chida Y, Steptoe A. Positive psychological well-being and mortality: a quantitative review of prospective observational studies. *Psychosom Med.* 2008;70:741–756.

54. Williams G, Cox E, Kouides R. Presenting the facts about smoking to adolescents. *Arch Pediatr Adolesc Med.* 1999;153:959–964.

55. Williams GC, Grow VM, Freeman ZR, et al. Motivational predictors of weight loss and weight-loss maintenance. *J Pers Soc Psychol.* 1996;70:115–126.

56. Bandura A. *Social Learning Theory.* Englewood Cliffs, NJ: Prentice Hall; 1977.

57. Haskell W, Lee IM, Pate R, et al. Physical activity and public health: updated recommendation for adults from the American College of Sports Medicine and the American Heart Association. *Circulation.* 2007;116:1081–1093.

58. Gollwitzer PM. Implementation intentions: strong effects of simple plans. *Am Psychol.* 1999;54:493–503.

59. Orbeil S, Hodgldns S, Sheeran P. Implementation intentions and the theory of planned behavior. *Pers Soc Psychol Bull.* 1997;23:945.

60. Gollwitzer PM, Sheeran P. Implementation intentions and goal achievement: a meta-analysis of effects of processes. *Adv Exp Soc Psychol.* 2006;38:69–119.

61. O'Neil PM, Brown JD. Weighing the evidence: benefits of regular weight monitoring for weight control. *J Nutr Educ Behav.* 2005;37:319–322.

62. Linde JA, Jeffrey RW, French S, et al. Self-weighing in Weight Gain Prevention and Weight Loss Trials. *Ann Behav Med.* 2005;30(3):210–216.

63. Tudor-Locke C, Bassett DR Jr. How many steps/day are enough? Preliminary pedometer indicies for public health. *Sports Med.* 2004;34(1):1–8.

64. Bravata DM, Smith-Spangler C, Sundaram V, et al. Using pedometers to increase physical activity and improve health. *JAMA.* 2007;298(19):2296–2304.

65. DiMatteo MR. Social support and patient adherence to medical treatment: a meta-analysis. *Health Psychol.* 2004;23:207–218.

66. Thayer RE, Newman R, McClain TM. Self regulation of mood: strategies for changing a bad mood, raising energy and reducing tension. *J Pers Soc Psychol.* 1994;67:910–925.

67. Mausner-Dorsch H, Easton WW. Psychosocial work environment and depression: epidemiologic assessment of the demand-control mode. *Am J Public Health.* 2000;90:1765–1770.

68. Thayer RE. Energy, tiredness, and tension effects of a sugar snack vs moderate exercise. *J Pers Soc Psychol.* 1987;52:119–125.

69. Kiecolt-Glaser JK, Christian L, Preston H, et al. Stress, inflammation, and yoga practice. *Psychosom Med.* 2010;72:113–121.

70. Motivala SJ, Sollers J, Thayer J, et al. Tai chi acutely decreases sympathetic nervous system activity in older adults. *J Gerontol.* 2006;11:1177–1180.

71. Pace TWW, Negi LT, Adame DD, et al. Effect of compassion meditation on neuroendocrine, innate immune and behavioral responses to psychosocial stress. *Psychoneuroendocrinology.* 2009;34:87–98.

72. Fredrickson BL. The role of positive emotions in positive psychology: the broaden-and-build theory of positive emotions. *Am Psychol.* 2001;56:218–226.

Index

Note: Page numbers followed by '*f*' and '*t*' refer to figures and tables respectively.